midwifery
Preparation for Practice 5e

midwifery
Preparation for Practice 5e

Sally Pairman, Sally K Tracy, Hannah G Dahlen, Lesley Dixon

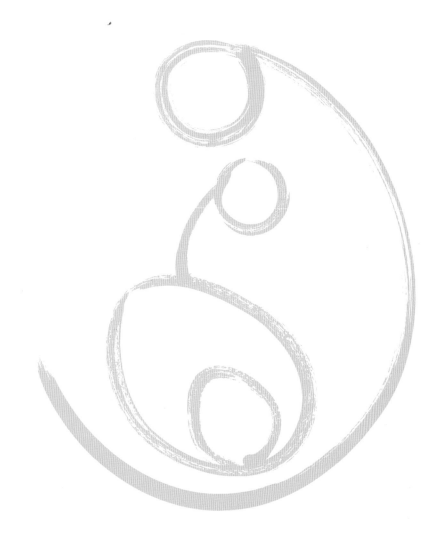

ELSEVIER

ELSEVIER

Elsevier Australia. ACN 001 002 357
(a division of Reed International Books Australia Pty Ltd)
Tower 1, 475 Victoria Avenue, Chatswood, NSW 2067

ISBN (Two-Book set): 978-0-7295-4381-1
ISBN (Book 1): 978-0-7295-4382-8

Notice

National Library of Australia Cataloguing-in-Publication Data

A catalogue record for this book is available from the National Library of Australia

---

Content Strategist: Libby Houston
Content Project Manager: Shruti Raj
Edited by Laura Davies
Proofread by Melissa Faulkner
Copyrights Coordinator: Saravanan Murugan
Cover and internal design by Georgette Hall
Index by Innodata Indexing

Typeset by GW Tech

Printed in Inidia by Multivista Global Pvt. Ltd, Chennai.

Contents

Contents

Detailed contents

Book 1:   Contextual implications for midwifery practice

Preface

This midwifery textbook is the first to reflect Australasian historical and sociopolitical contexts for midwifery practice and the first to frame content within the philosophy and standards of the New Zealand and Australian Colleges of Midwives. It is endorsed by the New Zealand College of Midwives and the Australian College of Midwives. Now in its fifth edition, this text provides an up-to-date evidence- and practice-based resource for midwives who work in partnership with women in woman-centred models of midwife-led care.

As such, this text is designed for midwifery students and practising midwives in New Zealand and Australia, and will also be relevant to midwives in other parts of the world where midwifery autonomy is acknowledged and emerging, such as Canada, Europe, Scandinavia, Japan and the United Kingdom.

We acknowledge that not all contexts in Australia and elsewhere currently support midwifery autonomy as we have described it. However, the primary purpose of this text is to equip midwives to practise autonomously and in partnership with women once contextual constraints to midwifery autonomy have been removed through political action and an enabling environment for midwife-led care is in place. This text provides a model of midwifery to which midwives can aspire and for which they can be prepared. We hope that this knowledge will strengthen midwives' determination to find ways to work with women and with each other that will enhance midwifery autonomy and woman-centred midwifery practice.

Philosophical Framework

The philosophical framework of this text is shaped by our vision for maternity services: that each woman should have access to a midwife of her choice and that each midwife should be able to work within the full scope of midwifery practice. The context within which midwives practise may either support or limit the individual midwife's ability to practise in a way that is congruent with this philosophy. A primary purpose of this textbook is to articulate and exemplify the way in which midwifery partnership is, or can be, actualised in practice.

We believe that midwifery is both an art and a science. It occurs within historical, social, cultural, political and legal contexts. Midwifery knowledge is derived from the wisdom of women and experienced midwives, and from scientific research. The individual midwife's knowledge develops by scholarship and praxis.

A midwife forms a partnership with a woman as she experiences the life process of childbearing and early parenting. Midwifery care is woman centred; however, care of the woman includes those she considers to be her family. The midwife shares knowledge, experience and wisdom reciprocally with the woman and her family. The midwife protects and promotes the rights and dignity of each woman and accepts her culture, beliefs, values, expectations and previous experiences. The midwife and the woman make decisions together through a process of negotiation.

Midwives are autonomous health professionals who, like other healthcare practitioners, have a social mandate to practise within legally defined professional boundaries. The scope of midwifery practice involves care of the woman and her family pre-pregnancy and during all phases of childbearing and early parenting up until 6 weeks after the birth. The midwife works on her own responsibility, but in partnership with the woman, as long as the woman and her baby remain well and healthy.

When there is an indication that the woman or the baby requires the service of another healthcare provider, the midwife works collaboratively with the other healthcare provider. The midwife maintains her relationship with the woman and her family even if referral to another healthcare provider is needed, and in most cases continues to provide care in collaboration with the other provider.

Structure of the Textbook

Aim

The overall aim of this textbook is to support the development of competent and confident midwifery practitioners who are able to make professional judgments, in partnership with women, on their own responsibility. These practitioners will:

- have a woman-centred approach
- work in partnership with women as autonomous practitioners in all settings
- have a sound knowledge base
- be critical thinkers
- be reflective practitioners
- be ethical decision makers
- critically appraise the literature and provide evidence-based midwifery care
- be accountable and responsible for their practice
- contribute to the development of midwifery knowledge and the profession.

Structuring concepts

The text is broadly structured around the following concepts derived from its philosophical framework:
1. *Context*—a reflection of the history of colonisation and the impact on the indigenous peoples of Australia and

New Zealand, our current bicultural and multicultural societies, our laws and legal systems, our political structures and processes, our healthcare systems, the organisation of maternity services and the payment of maternity care providers. Childbirth and midwifery practice have been constructed within these different contexts. All individuals involved in childbearing are affected by the context from which they have emerged and bring with them their individual life histories and culturally moulded attitudes, values and beliefs.

2. *Woman*—includes the self of each woman and encompasses the baby that each woman carries within her body and to which she gives birth. This concept also includes each woman's partner, family / whānau, and cultural and subcultural group, and incorporates each woman's experience(s) of childbearing.

3. *Midwife*—includes the self of each midwife, her knowledge, attitudes and beliefs, her partner and / or family / whānau, her cultural or subcultural group and her professional role as midwife. A midwife cares for and supports a woman as she grows and nurtures her baby, and strengthens the woman in her role as a mother.

4. *Partnership*—implies a relationship of trust, reciprocity and equity through which both partners are strengthened. Each midwife strives to ensure that she does not impose her professional and personal power onto women; rather, through negotiation a midwife seeks to establish relationships in which each woman is the primary decision maker. (*Note*: because most midwives are women we have chosen to use the feminine pronoun throughout this text.)

5. *Autonomous practice*—occurs when a midwife provides care to a woman and her baby on her own responsibility. As autonomous practitioners, midwives have the knowledge and skills to provide care independently without a requirement to refer to another healthcare professional. This does not mean that midwives practise alone; rather, midwives work in partnership with midwifery colleague(s). Nor are midwives independent of women, because all midwifery professional judgments emerge from midwife–woman relationships.

6. *Collaborative practice*—means working with other healthcare professionals/providers when the health of a woman or baby is outside the scope of midwifery practice. The relationship and responsibilities of each woman, each midwife and other health professionals need to be negotiated.

Sections of the textbook

These structuring concepts are reflected in the ordering of the chapters. As in the fourth edition, the text is provided in two books. Book One focuses on the background for midwifery practice with sections on context, on each of the two partners within a midwifery partnership—the woman and the midwife—and on how partnership is practised. Book Two focuses on midwifery practice. Section One explores autonomous midwifery practice and Section Two explores collaborative midwifery practice.

Several chapters have been refocused to avoid repetition, to consolidate content and to reflect emerging midwifery and childbirth issues and contemporary discourses. Some chapters have been significantly updated and new content has been added.

We acknowledge that a number of disciplines contribute to the knowledge, attitudes and skills that a midwife needs, but the focus of this book is on midwifery-specific knowledge and the application of knowledge from other disciplines where it directly relates to the scope of midwifery practice. Where additional depth is required, readers are referred to more specific texts from other disciplines.

Each chapter provides:
- learning outcomes
- midwifery practice scenarios where relevant
- reflective and critical thinking exercises, and sometimes research exercises
- questions for review
- a list of online resources.

This text provides a new approach to midwifery education. In focusing on the midwife as an autonomous practitioner with a specific scope of practice, we have endeavoured to show how professional judgments and practice decisions rely on strong assessment skills, knowledge and understanding of physiology, application of evidence-based practice knowledge and integration of attitudes and philosophy within a professional framework for practice. Midwives who approach practice in this way will be able to provide individualised and woman-centred care. They will be able to identify when they have reached their level of expertise and when it is necessary to consult and collaborate with others to ensure that the needs of women and their babies are met. It is this awareness and midwifery 'thinking' that ensures midwives are competent and safe practitioners.

We hope you enjoy using this textbook.

Sally Pairman
Sally K Tracy
Hannah G Dahlen
Lesley Dixon

About the editors

Sally Pairman BA, MA, MNZM, DMid, RM, RGON is Chief Executive of the International Confederation of Midwives (ICM) and is based in The Hague, The Netherlands. Sally took up this role in January 2017 after more than 30 years employed at Otago Polytechnic, Dunedin, New Zealand in various positions, including Professor of Midwifery, Director of Learning and Teaching and Head of Midwifery. Sally has been actively involved in the New Zealand College of Midwives in various roles, including President, since its inception in 1989. She was made an honorary member in 1997. She was appointed to the Midwifery Council of New Zealand on its establishment and served as the inaugural Chair of the Council (2003–11) throughout her term in office. In 2008, Sally was appointed as co-chair of the International Confederation of Midwives Regulation Standing Committee, a role she held until 2017 when she joined the ICM as Chief Executive. Sally was at the forefront of establishing midwifery autonomy and degree-level direct-entry midwifery education in New Zealand, and throughout her career has actively worked to strengthen midwifery regulation and education at national, regional and global levels. In 2008, Sally was made a Member of the Order of New Zealand for her services to midwifery and women's health.

Sally is co-author with Karen Guilliland of *The Midwifery Partnership: A Model for Practice*, a monograph describing a theoretical model of midwifery as a partnership between a woman and a midwife. Sally's Master's research resulted in refinement of the model. First published in 2005, with a second edition in 2010, the midwifery partnership model is foundational to New Zealand midwifery practice and has been widely adopted by midwives around the world as a model for practice. Sally's professional Doctorate in midwifery further analysed midwifery partnership in relation to midwifery leadership, midwifery education and midwifery regulation in her exploration of New Zealand midwifery's professionalising strategies from 1986 to 2005. Sally has published and presented extensively on these and other related topics including *Women's Business: The Story of the New Zealand College of Midwives 1986–2010*, co-authored with Karen Guilliland and published in 2010. Sally, along with Sally Tracy, was one of the inaugural authors and editors of *Midwifery: Preparation for Practice*.

Sally is married to Michael Lucas and they have two sons, Oscar and Felix.

Sally K Tracy BNurs, AdvDipN, MA, DMid, RM, RGON is Professor Emerita, Midwifery, at the University of Sydney, and conjoint Professor of Midwifery at the Molly Wardaguga Research Centre at Charles Darwin University. She previously held the Chair in Midwifery at the University of Sydney, based at the Midwifery and Women's Health Research Unit at the Royal Hospital for Women in Sydney. She was one of a progressive group of midwives and obstetricians who oversaw the introduction of midwifery group practice care as a mainstream option for all women. Sally was the lead researcher on three large National Health and Medical Research Council of Australia project grants. The first was a randomised controlled trial of caseload midwifery care for women regardless of identified risk factors—the M@NGO trial; the second, a prospective cohort study of freestanding primary-level maternity units in Australia and New Zealand (EMU), and the third was the Amniotic Fluid Lactate Study, which aimed to ascertain the role of amniotic fluid lactate in the diagnosis of labour dystocia. All these studies contributed valuable research data to maternity policy regarding the efficacy of midwifery group practice care and safety of the place of birth. She is currently a lead researcher on an NHMRC partnership grant to promote Birth on Country.

Sally was educated as a midwife in New Zealand and the United Kingdom, and has extensive community and hospital midwifery experience in New Zealand and Australia.

Sally was awarded the world's first professional Doctorate in midwifery at the University of Technology Sydney in 2003, and has published widely on the epidemiology of obstetric intervention in labour and birth, pre-term birth and birth centres using large population data sets, and more recently on the outcomes of caseload midwifery and the safety of stand-alone maternity units.

Sally was one of the inaugural authors and editors of *Midwifery: Preparation for Practice*, along with Sally Pairman.

She is married to Mark and has four children, Gabriel, Raphael, Amy and Imogen, and three grandchildren, Charlie, Max and Atem.

Hannah G Dahlen BN (Hons 1st), Grad Cert (Mid-Pharm), MCommN, PhD, RN, RM, FACM is Professor of Midwifery, Associate Dean Research and Higher Degree Research and Midwifery Discipline Lead in the School of Nursing and Midwifery at Western Sydney University. She is a leading midwifery researcher in Australia, with an international reputation as an outstanding midwifery scholar. This is demonstrated through publication of over 250 papers and book chapters, presentation at over 100 conferences, more than half being invited keynotes and strong national and international collaborations. Hannah has been cited in numerous key documents guiding healthcare, including the World Health Organization. In 2019 Hannah was awarded a Member (AM) of the Order of Australia (General Division) in the Queen's Birthday Honours list for her significant services to midwifery, nursing and medical education and research. In November 2012, Hannah was named in the *Sydney Morning Herald*'s list of 100 'people who change our city for the better' as one of the leading 'science and knowledge thinkers' owing to her research and public profile. Hannah regularly appears in the media on issues to do with midwifery and childbearing women. She has appeared in five documentaries to do with birth: *Hannah's Story* (2005), *Face of Birth* (2012), *Microbirth* (2014), *Untying Breastfeeding* (2018) and *Birth Time* (2021).

Hannah has been a midwife for more than 30 years. She is one of the first midwives in Australia to gain Eligibility and access to a Medicare provider number following government reforms in 2010. Prior to working in the university sector, Hannah had a mainly clinical role working as clinical midwife specialist, clinical midwifery educator and a midwifery consultant. Hannah worked more recently as a privately practising midwife in a group practice in Sydney. Hannah is married to Malcolm and has two girls, Lydia and Bronte, and she also gave birth to two boys who both died (Luke and Ethan) and their stories feature in Chapter 43 of this textbook.

Lesley Dixon BA (Hons), MA (Midwifery), PhD, RM, RGON is a midwifery advisor with the New Zealand College of Midwives. In this role she provides midwifery practice advice, reviews evidence, and the impact on midwifery practice, and leads, coordinates and supports research projects. She is the co-editor of the *New Zealand College of Midwives Journal*. Her Doctoral research investigated the woman's perspective of labour progress and she has subsequently been the lead investigator and co-author for a number of international and New Zealand midwifery research collaborations. Her current research focus has two aspects: the first explores continuity of care and the effects on women's experiences of maternity care; the second explores how midwives work, their emotional health and the challenges, barriers and enablers of care provision. Both of these issues are important to the sustainability of the profession and the New Zealand model of continuity of maternity care.

Lesley has over 30 years' experience as a practising midwife, gaining her midwifery qualification in England and moving to New Zealand in 1999, where she has worked in both community and hospital settings. She provides midwifery expertise on several national clinical maternity guideline review groups and has had positions on the Maternal Mortality Review Working Group, the Maternal Morbidity Working Group and the Maternity Clinical Indicators Expert Working Group. She was appointed the co-chair of the International Confederation of Midwives (ICM) Research Standing Committee from 2017 to 2019. Lesley is married to David, and has one daughter, Rachel, and three grandchildren, Ava, Theo and Hope.

Foreword by Lesley Page

It is an absolute delight to write this foreword.

Over a long and varied career in midwifery, I have become increasingly aware of the importance of the time around birth as a critical point in human life and society: critical not only for the individual baby, woman becoming mother, other parent and family, but also for communities and society. The birth of a baby is a time of promise and potential for us all.

The question is, how might we realise the promise of childbirth, the potential of new life, and make safe, humanised childbirth a sustainable reality, for every childbearing woman and her baby, every parent, every family, no matter what their circumstances and where they live? It is clear that midwifery and midwives play a vital role in fulfilling this promise and potential.

The wide sweep, the sheer depth, the science base and clarity, even amongst the complexity, of this fifth edition, make this vital importance clear, and show clearly how this vital contribution may be made.

I was struck by the wide sweep of understanding of history, society, healthcare systems, politics and legal aspects, as well as the depth of understanding of the science base, and the art and science of midwifery practice.

This is a book that will advance midwifery, and help midwives work to their full scope of practice. Philosophy of midwifery and a clear model of practice are woven together. This philosophy and model centres midwifery and midwives on the women we serve, and supports and protects midwives. It will help midwives understand the wide world around them, including the position of women in society, particularly in Australia and Aotearoa New Zealand, amid the impact and long shadow of colonisation, thinking about, working with and understanding indigenous populations and cultures. A new chapter explores sustainability, from a global perspective, but also the meaning of sustainability for midwives and midwifery.

I was struck by the importance of midwifery preparation for practice, to preparation for leadership. Human rights, ethics as they apply to childbirth, considerations of risk and understanding of healthcare systems are essential to aspiring midwives and leaders, and will help every midwife, no matter what their role, advance midwifery and healthcare.

Substantial chapters on midwifery practice are interwoven with the art. Beautiful writing takes us into the nuanced language of working in partnership, working with the woman, reciprocity and relational care, the psychological impact of complex care and life-threatening emergencies. This is humanising care at its best.

Midwifery: Preparation for Practice is born from midwifery in Aotearoa New Zealand and Australia. This is fundamental to the approaches expressed and is of great importance. While geographically close, the two countries have grown midwifery in different ways. The differences are clearly set out. These differences reflect different cultures, governments and health services. But we should be in no doubt: Aotearoa New Zealand and Australia have been world leaders in political change, making real-world change in policy and practice, developing knowledge and philosophy, and putting a human rights framework into practice. They have been world leaders in making midwifery woman-centred and responsive to present-day needs. We all have much to learn from their leadership.

This is a book that is an essential resource for any part of the world. It would form the basis of autonomous, effective, compassionate midwifery, establishing appropriate healthcare systems, and work in influencing health service change, anywhere.

The success of *Midwifery: Preparation for Practice* comes in great part from the editors: Sally Pairman, Sally Tracy, Hannah Dahlen and Lesley Dixon. The editors are active leaders internationally as well as nationally in advancing midwifery, through policy, research and science, activism, practice development and regulation. Their experience and strong knowledge base are clear in the structure, content and approach.

It is no mean feat to prepare a textbook composed, as this is, of so many different strands of knowledge and understanding, of art and science. This fifth edition shows just how far we have come and helps us see just how far we have to go. Sally Pairman talks of strengthening midwives' determination to work with women and each other. Reading *Midwifery: Preparation for Practice* has certainly strengthened my determination to advance midwifery, and given me a valuable resource for helping to do it.

**Professor Lesley Page CBE, BA, MSc, PhD, Honorary DSc, Honorary PhD midwifery, RM, HFRCM
Visiting Professor, Florence Nightingale Faculty of Nursing, Midwifery and Palliative Care, King's College London
Adjunct Professor, University of Technology Sydney**

Foreword by Joanne Gray and Alison Eddy

The New Zealand and Australian Colleges of Midwives welcome and endorse the fifth edition of *Midwifery: Preparation for Practice*. This edition builds on its success by further refining and expanding the profession's growing knowledge base.

Skilfully written by midwives and other contributors with longstanding involvement in both midwifery practice and education, and the wider disciplines that inform the profession, the chapters have been updated and revised to ensure the content is up to date and the present-day context of midwifery practice in both Aotearoa New Zealand and Australia is acknowledged throughout.

Due to the high calibre of the authors and their inspiring evidence-based contributions, this book is a 'must have' for every student of midwifery. We would also strongly recommend it for all registered midwives, for another reason: this book makes a unique contribution to midwifery knowledge and practice, through its focus on the universal principles that underpin midwifery philosophy. These are partnership with women/wāhine, midwifery autonomy in practice and continuity of care. The midwifery partnership in which a woman and midwife work together to achieve the best outcome for that woman/wahine and baby/pēpi differentiates it from other models of care, where the healthcare professional assumes expertise within the relationship. Continuity of care is a strong enabler for this partnership, with care provided through a relational model over the course of pregnancy, labour and birth and the postpartum. This book draws on these universal principles and approaches midwifery care from the perspective of the midwife as a primary healthcare practitioner, based in the community, who interfaces with hospitals and specialists as necessary to meet the needs of individual women. It explores both autonomous practice and collaborative practice, and it was the first textbook to discuss midwifery practice in the context of community and primary health rather than hospital-based maternity services.

This updated version reorganises previous chapters on the historical development of midwifery and maternity services in Australia and New Zealand, and contemporary midwifery and maternity services into a single chapter, and includes two new chapters on sustainability and environmental healthcare, and ethical frameworks for practice. For Aotearoa New Zealand, the importance of Te Tiriti o Waitangi as a foundational document is described in the updated chapter of this edition with Māori

recognised as Tangata Whenua along with our evolving understanding of the importance of cultural competence, and its essential place alongside clinical competence in midwifery care.

These contributions further strengthen the content which recognises the broader social, cultural, ethical, political and historical context that shapes the practice of midwifery in any given time and place.

Just as childbirth is far more than a physiological process, the art and science of midwifery is more than a study of the female human body and its reproductive powers. It is therefore essential that all midwives have a sound understanding of not only the physiological processes of pregnancy, birth and the postpartum, but also the broader context in which they work, and an awareness of how it may influence their own practice in providing care to women. This includes the increasing influence of risk and fear paradigms impacting clinical practice. The discussions on risk underpin many of the issues facing midwifery today and are essential reading for those trying to understand what drives practitioners' behaviour and women's choices and preferences.

Although there may be structural and systems differences between Australia and New Zealand, our model of maternity care is slowly converging with an increasing number of women in Australia now receiving midwifery-led continuity of maternity care, the model which has been predominant in New Zealand for over two decades now.

In Australia, over 70% of midwives are employed within the public healthcare system, providing professional care to women within a fragmented system, yet pleasingly the number of midwives engaged in midwifery continuity of care models is increasing. However, times are changing in Australia and this edition documents the expansion of access to a known midwife in the country's public maternity services, including the provision of public homebirth services. These reforms mark a new era in Australian midwifery practice.

Midwives in New Zealand have been free to practise in either hospitals or the community since 1990. All midwives have access to public funding for their professional services, have prescribing rights, and work in partnership with women and with each other if they choose to. This edition tracks the successful midwifery workforce redesign and the continued progress in improved outcomes for women and babies. However, the New Zealand health system is undergoing major structural reform. It is essential that, whatever structures and arrangements develop, midwifery remains enabled to work in a manner which maintains women as central to the birthing process, and at the centre of care, through ensuring midwifery professional and clinical autonomy is preserved.

In focusing on midwifery autonomy and midwifery partnership, this textbook reinforces, for all midwives, the achievements of women and midwives in giving childbirth back to women/wāhine and their families/whanau. It reminds us of how important it is to keep women central to the birthing process. Each chapter provides valuable knowledge and guidance to both experienced and new midwives that will help to ensure that they have the knowledge and confidence to keep women and their babies' needs at the centre of practice decisions.

Despite the differences in culture, politics, health systems and maternity services between our two countries, this textbook confirms that midwifery remains universally constant, and guided by the same theoretical and practice knowledge and skills that combine to make midwifery such a vital profession for women and babies. The commonalities far outweigh the differences, and this edition further enriches with up-to-date and relevant information aimed at supporting all midwives to practise autonomously and ever with an eye on the needs of the women for whom they care.

Joanne Gray
President, Australian College of Midwives
Alison Eddy
Chief Executive, New Zealand College of Midwives

Contributors

Jacqui Anderson RM, RGON, MMid
Midwifery Advisor, New Zealand College of Midwives |
Te Kāreti o ngā Kaiwhakawhānau ki Aotearoa,
Christchurch,
Aotearoa New Zealand

Sally Baddock PhD, Dip Tchng, BSc
Professor, School of Midwifery and Research and
Postgraduate Studies,
Te Kura Matatini ki Otago | Otago Polytechnic;
Te Pūkenga | NZ Institute of Skills and Technology,
Hamilton,
Aotearoa New Zealand

Carol Bartle MNZM, RN, RM, MHealSc (Otago), PGDip
ChAd (Otago)
Policy Analyst, New Zealand College of Midwives | Te
Kāreti o ngā Kaiwhakawhānau ki Aotearoa,
Christchurch,
Aotearoa New Zealand

Rebecca Bear PhD, PGDipSci, BSc, BVSc
Policy Director, Mental Health Lived Experience Peak
Queensland,
Brisbane, QLD,
Australia

Elaine Burns RM, RN, BN, MCN, PhD
Associate Professor of Midwifery,
Western Sydney University,
Sydney, NSW,
Australia

Shea Caplice RN, RM, Post Grad Dip Ind. Practice, MMid
Clinical Midwifery Consultant, Royal Hospital for
Women,
Sydney, NSW,
Australia

Megan Cooper BMidwif, BHlthSc(Hons),
GradDipEdStud(DigitLrn), MBA(HlthServMgt), CHIA,
PhD, FACM
Senior Lecturer and Course Coordinator—Midwifery
Programs, College of Nursing and Health Sciences,
Flinders University,
Adelaide, SA,
Australia

Hannah G Dahlen AM (RN, RM, BN(Hons), MCommN,
PhD, FACM)
Professor of Midwifery, Associate Dean Research and
HDR, Midwifery Discipline Lead,
School of Nursing and Midwifery,
Western Sydney University,
Sydney, NSW,
Australia

Lorna Davies RM, BSc, MA, PGCEA, PhD
Principal Lecturer/ Midwifery Consultant, Te Kura
Matatini ki Otago | Otago Polytechnic,
Aotearoa New Zealand

Deborah Davis RM, BN, MNS, PhD
Professor/Clinical Chair, Midwifery, University of
Canberra; ACT Health,
Canberra, ACT,
Australia

Jennifer Dawson RN, PhD
Nurse Researcher, The Royal Women's Hospital,
Sydney, NSW,
Australia

Lesley Dixon RM, PhD
Midwifery Advisor: Kaiwhakawhānau Tohutohu,
New Zealand College of Midwives | Te Kāreti o ngā
Kaiwhakawhānau ki Aotearoa,
Christchurch,
Aotearoa New Zealand

Catherine Donaldson RM, RN, ADM, MSc
Lecturer Midwifery, Bachelor of Midwifery,
Griffith University,
Brisbane,
Australia

Natasha Donnolley BSc(HIM), PhD
Research Project Manager, National Perinatal
Epidemiology and Statistics Unit, Centre for Big Data
Research in Health, University of New South Wales,
Sydney, NSW,
Australia

Alison Eddy RN, RM MPH
Chief Executive, New Zealand College of Midwives | Te
Kāreti o ngā Kaiwhakawhānau ki Aotearoa,
Christchurch,
Aotearoa New Zealand

Terri Foran MB BS (Syd), M Clin Ed (UNSW), FAChSHM
Sexual Health Physician; Conjoint Senior Lecturer,
University of New South Wales,
Sydney, NSW,
Australia

Andrea Gilkison RM, MEd, PhD
Associate Professor, Midwifery, Auckland University of
Technology,
Auckland,
Aotearoa New Zealand

Elaine Gray MM(Hons), DipALT, RM
Midwifery Advisor: Kaiwhakawhānau Tohutohu, New
Zealand College of Midwives | Te Kāreti o ngā
Kaiwhakawhānau ki Aotearoa,
Christchurch,
Aotearoa New Zealand

Michelle Gray PhD, Mast Prof Learning, BSc (Hons) Mid,
PGDE, SFHEA, RM, RN
Associate Professor in Midwifery, Course Coordinator
I80 Master of Midwifery Practice
Course Coordinator L90 Graduate Certificate in
Midwifery Diagnostics and Prescribing

Celia Grigg BA(Educ), BMid, MMid(Distinc), PhD
Midwife, Te Whatu Ora Waitaha Canterbury; Honorary
Academic, Liggins Institute, University of Auckland;
Independent Midwifery Researcher,
Aotearoa New Zealand

Donna Hartz RN, RM, MMID Studies, PhD, FACM
Associate Professor, School of Nursing and Midwifery,
College of Health Medicine and Wellbeing, the
University of Newcastle,
Newcastle, NSW,
Australia

Leonie Hewitt RM, MMid, MRes, PhD candidate
Western Sydney University,
Sydney, NSW,
Australia

Caroline SE Homer RM, MN, MScMed(ClinEpi), PhD,
FAAHMS
Professor, Maternal, Child and Adolescent Health,
Burnet Institute and University of Technology Sydney,
Sydney, NSW,
Australia

Carla Humphrey LLB
Legal Advisor, Barrister and Solicitor, New Zealand
College of Midwives | Te Kāreti o ngā Kaiwhakawhānau
ki Aotearoa;
Carla Humphrey Law Firm,
Christchurch,
Aotearoa New Zealand

Marion Hunter RGON, RM, ADN, BA, MA (Hons 1st
class), DHSc
Consultant Midwifery Education
Auckland,
Aotearoa New Zealand

Bashi Kumar-Hazard B Eco (Soc Sci), LLB (Hons I) USyd,
PhD (USyd);
Solicitor (High Court of Australia); Chair, Human Rights
in Childbirth,
Sydney, NSW
Australia

Kaniwa Kupenga-Tamarama RM, BHSC (Midwifery),
PGDip (Midwifery), Dip Life Coaching, Masters of Health
Practice Student at AUT University; Director of Kia Kaha
Mama; Nāti Pēpi Midwifery Project Manager; Ngāti
Porou Hauora,
Gisborne,
Aotearoa New Zealand

Nicky Leap RM, MSc, DMid
Adjunct Professor of Midwifery, Centre for Midwifery,
Child and Family Health, University of Technology
Sydney; The Molly Wardaguga Research Centre, Charles
Darwin University,
Sydney, NSW,
Australia

Nigel Lee RM BHlthSc, MMid, PhD, FHEA
Midwifery Research Fellow, School of Nursing,
Midwifery and Social Work,
University of Queensland,
Brisbane, QLD,
Australia

Emma Le Lievre RM, PHDip ClnRes, BMid, BApSc
Lecturer, Te Kura Matatini ki Otago | Otago Polytechnic,
Dunedin,
Aotearoa New Zealand

Claire MacDonald RM, MPH
Midwifery Advisor, New Zealand College of Midwives |
Te Kāreti o ngā Kaiwhakawhānau ki Aotearoa,
Christchurch,
Aotearoa New Zealand

Suzanne Miller PhD, MMid, RM, GCTLT
Associate Professor, Te Kura Atawhai ka Kaiākapono te
Hākuitaka | School of Midwifery, Te Kura Matatini ki
Otago | Otago Polytechnic,
Wellington,
Aotearoa New Zealand

Jane Morrow RM, RN, BHlthSci, MHlthAdmin, PhD
Sessional Academic, Midwife, Australian Catholic
University and Epworth Freemasons,
Melbourne, VIC,
Australia

Sally Pairman MNZM, DMid, MM, RM, RGON
Chief Executive, International Confederation of
Midwives,
The Hague,
The Netherlands

Holly Priddis BM, BN(Hons), PhD, GC(Autism Studies)
Adjunct Fellow, Western Sydney University,
Sydney, NSW,
Australia

Virginia Schmied RM, RN, BA, MA(Hons), PhD
Professor of Midwifery, Western Sydney University,
Sydney, NSW,
Australia

Juanita Sherwood
Professor of First Nations Health and Education
Research and Policy,
Jumbunna, University of Technology Sydney,
Sydney, NSW,
Australia

Megan Tahere RM, BHSc Midwifery, GradCert HSc—Te
Ara Hauora Māori, PGDip Midwifery, PhD Candidate
Public Health
Tāhuhu Rangapū—Chief Māori Health and Equity
Officer, Midwife, Principal Advisor Kahu Taurima—
Maternity and Early Years, Te Whatu Ora—Health New
Zealand Taranaki, Te Aka Whai Ora—Māori Health
Authority,
Aotearoa New Zealand

Tricia Thompson RM, MPhil, GCTLT
Senior Lecturer, School of Midwifery, Te Kura Matatini ki
Otago | Otago Polytechnic,
Aotearoa New Zealand

Juliet Thorpe RCompN, NZRM, MMid
Employed Midwife at Oromairaki Birthing Unit,
Christchurch,
Aotearoa New Zealand

Sally K Tracy DMid, MA, BNurs, GradDip(Mid), RGON,
RM
Professor Emerita, Midwifery, Faculty of Medicine and
Health, University of Sydney,
Sydney, NSW
Australia

Emma Tumilty PhD (Bioethics), GCHELT,
PGDipHealthSci (Bioethics), BA (Philosophy)
Assistant Professor, Bioethics and Health Humanities,
University of Texas Medical Branch Galveston,
Galveston, Texas,
United States

Hope Tupara PhD, RM
Māori Health Research and Development Consultant,
Hamilton,
Aotearoa New Zealand

Karen Walker RGN, RSCN, BAppSc, MN, PhD
Clinical Professor, Clinical Nurse Consultant, University
of Sydney and Royal Prince Alfred Hospital,
Sydney, NSW,
Australia

Jill White RN, RM, BEd, MEd, MHPol, PhD, FACN, FAAN
Professor Emerita, University of Sydney and University
of Technology Sydney,
Sydney, NSW,
Australia

Jade Wratten BM, RM, MM, GCTLT
Principal Midwifery Lecturer, Te Kura Matatini ki Otago |
Otago Polytechnic,
Dunedin,
Aotearoa New Zealand

Reviewers

Janice Butt RN, RM, ADM, PGCEA, MA(Ed) (UK)
Coordinator Midwifery and Nursing Staff Development,
Women and Newborn Health Service, King Edward
Memorial Hospital,
Perth, WA,
Australia

Kym Davey RN, RM, BN, Master of Advanced Nursing (in
progress)
Level B Lecturer, Monash University,
Melbourne, VIC,
Australia

Deborah Fox B Mid, RM, M Sc, PhD
Senior Lecturer in Midwifery, University of Technology
Sydney,
Sydney, NSW,
Australia

Elaine Jefford PhD, MSc, BSc(Hons) Midwifery,
BSc(Hons) Nursing
Associate Professor Midwifery, University of
South Australia,
Adelaide, SA,
Australia

Hazel Keedle PhD, Masters (Hons) Nursing, Grad Dip
Midwifery, Grad Cert Midwifery, RM, RN
Lecturer of Midwifery, Western Sydney University,
Sydney, NSW,
Australia

Suzanne Miller PhD, MMid, RM, GCTLT
Associate Professor, Te Kura Atawhai ka Kaiākapono te
Hākuitaka | School of Midwifery, Te Kura Matatini ki
Otago | Otago Polytechnic,
Wellington,
Aotearoa New Zealand

Annabel Sheehy BMid(Hons), PhD, BHSc
Lecturer in Midwifery, University of Technology Sydney,
Sydney, NSW,
Australia

Rachel Taylor BA, CertNatTherapies, BMid/Registered
Midwife (RM), PGCertComplexCare, PGCertTERTL,
Master of Professional Practice (Midwifery)
Senior Lecturer and Year Two Program Coordinator,
School of Midwifery, Centre for Health and Social
Practice, Waikato Institute of Technology (Wintec),
Hamilton,
Aotearoa New Zealand

Acknowledgements

This revised edition has taken many months to prepare and would not have been completed without the support of many people. We give heartfelt thanks to the following:

- all the authors who worked so hard to complete their chapters on time despite their very busy lives and personal challenges
- the manuscript reviewers, in conjunction with Elsevier Australia, for their insightful comments
- David Vernon for use of a birth story from the book titled *Having a Good Birth in Australia*
- David Hancock for the photographs in Chapter 27
- Hinke van Belzen-Slappendel (Midwife) for the photographs in Chapter 36
- the New Zealand College of Midwives, Archives New Zealand and the Alexander Turnbull Library (NZ) for the photographs in Chapters 7 and 23
- our professional organisations—the New Zealand College of Midwives and the Australian College of Midwives—for their support of our vision for this book
- our hard-working team from Elsevier Australia—Libby Houston and Shruti Raj—and freelancers—Laura Davies (editor), Melissa Faulkner (proofreader), Georgette Hall (designer), Alan Laver (illustrator) and Saravanan Murugan (permissions editor)—for their diligence, perseverance and endless patience
- and, finally, our families and friends, who supported us in so many ways over the long months of writing and reviewing, and who encouraged us when the end seemed nowhere in sight.

**Sally Pairman, Sally K Tracy,
Hannah G Dahlen, Lesley Dixon**

Contextual implications for midwifery practice

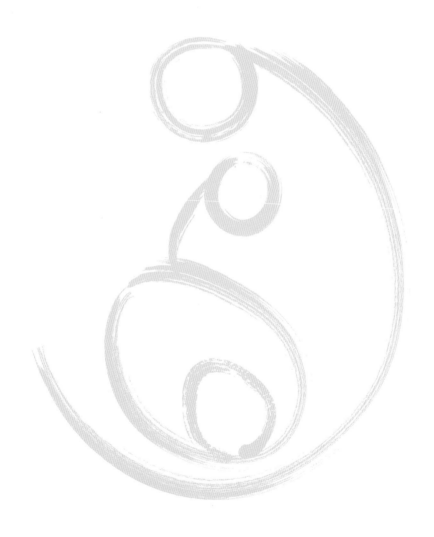

Context

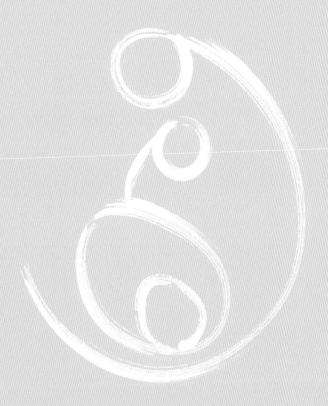

CHAPTER 1

The Australian and New Zealand context

Jill White

LEARNING OUTCOMES

Learning outcomes for this chapter are:

1. To describe the cardinal elements of the histories of Australia and New Zealand
2. To analyse the effects of European colonisation on the indigenous peoples of both countries
3. To discuss the importance of the Treaty of Waitangi to Māori and Pākehā in contemporary New Zealand society
4. To discuss the importance of the 2008 Apology to Aboriginal and Torres Strait Islands people
5. To discuss the place of women in contemporary New Zealand and Australian societies, and the influence of history on this positioning
6. To explain the key social and cultural similarities and differences between Australia and New Zealand.

CHAPTER OVERVIEW

Other chapters of this book introduce the philosophical contexts of midwifery and maternity services generally, and the specific contexts of women in the world. This chapter seeks to situate this understanding of women, mothers and their babies, and maternity services within the social, historical and cultural contexts of Australia and Aotearoa New Zealand.

Having lived as woman, mother, midwife and nurse in both countries, I am approaching this chapter as I lived in these countries. My approach was to accept that, despite their geographic closeness, they are as different as France and Germany, or the United States and Mexico. It is, I believe, important to try to understand their separateness and then to be surprised by the similarities rather than, as many do, think of them as the same and only gradually, after episodes that can only be seen as culturally insensitive, come to understand the differences. Appreciating such difference, this chapter will look at each country in turn.

In exploring the social, historical and cultural contexts of any country, looking first at the history provides an explanatory backdrop for the current relationships and attitudes as played out socially and culturally. The brief histories presented here are by no means historians' histories. The social and cultural comments are those of neither sociologist nor anthropologist. They are practitioner histories, and social and cultural commentaries, stories that highlight some salient social and historical events that give colour to a picture of a past that inevitably influences the present and the people with whom we work as midwives, and the values the women and their families express in our interactions with them in practice.

KEY TERMS

Anglo-Celtic
Australian Aboriginal
indigenous
mana

Māori
Stolen Generations
tapu
terra nullius

Treaty of Waitangi
utu

INTRODUCTION

Australia and New Zealand are closely integrated regionally, economically and politically. They share the same part of the world and their urban settlements were created by the British during the last three centuries. The two countries have enjoyed unbroken friendly diplomatic relations over the entire period of their coexistence from the early 19th century up to the present. Notwithstanding these commonalities, both countries have been subjected to differing historical and environmental influences that have resulted in significant cultural differences. Their different histories are most clearly reflected in their separate **indigenous** histories. The **Australian Aboriginal** people are descended directly from the earliest modern explorers—who migrated into Asia before finally reaching Australia about 70,000 years ago—whereas New Zealand was settled by peoples from islands in the tropical Pacific around 1250–1300AD.

AUSTRALIA

Early Australia

Australia has been home to its Aboriginal population for more than 50,000 years, and to Europeans for a mere 230 years. For Aboriginal and Torres Strait Islander people this represents 2000 generations of living, hunting and gathering in this often-harsh environment. There are estimated to have been about 300,000 Aboriginal people living in Australia in 1788 when Europeans arrived. This population was spread across over 500 tribes, each with its own dialect, history, culture and territory. While all tribes were seminomadic hunters and gatherers moving across their specific territory with seasonal purpose, the size of their tribal grounds varied from 500 square kilometres in generous coastal areas to 100,000 square kilometres in desert areas (Broome, 2010). Land connection was and is fundamental to Aboriginal being and features in their stories, songs and paintings. In particular, the lives of the Aboriginal people 'are shaped by their Dreamtime stories which were both an explanation of how the world came to be, and how people must conduct their behaviour and social relations' (Broome, *Aboriginal Australians*. 4th ed. Sydney: Allen & Unwin; 2010, p. 19; reproduced with permission of Allen & Unwin Pty Ltd).

From the time the Dutch navigated to what is now known as Indonesia in the 16th century, there had been tales of rich southern lands, and ships from many countries sought these lands. A Spaniard, de Torres, navigated the straits between northern Australia and New Guinea in 1606. In 1616 the Dutch commander Hartog found the western Australian coast. There followed many more ships from Holland, finding and naming land along the southern Australian coast. Tasman found what was to become Tasmania and named it van Diemen's Land after the Governor of the East Indies in Java, then a Dutch colony. Then, rather than travelling north along the Australian coast, Tasman sailed further east and found the coast of New Zealand. But, as these ships were in search of gold and spices, their discoveries of land that appeared undeveloped and lacking in riches was not valued by their home countries.

At the end of the 17th century an Englishman, Dampier, voyaged to western Australia but again reported he had found little of value, little water and little available food. Some signs of European life were found on the edges of the continent but were the flotsam and jetsam of wrecked ships and sailors who had perished.

So Australia became known to the European world piece by piece in multiple voyages from many different countries, but was coveted mainly by the British. When the British government sent Captain Cook to the South Seas, ostensibly to study an eclipse from the oceans near Tahiti in order to help problems of navigation, the opportunity presented itself to search for the southern land and take possession of it for Britain. International law at the time required a 'new' country to be taken only after permission was sought from the 'natives'—that is, unless the land was either uninhabited or inhabited by a people who did not appear to use the land. In 1770 James Cook 'discovered' Australia's eastern coast and he and his party landed in what has become known as Botany Bay. The ship's name and date were carved on a tree and the British flag planted in the soil. After many reported attempts to engage peacefully with the 'natives' Cook recorded in his diary, 'All they seem'd to want was for us to be gone' (Clark et al., 2000, p. 20). He recorded the lack of interest of the Aboriginal people in the trinkets, ribbons and cloth that he had left for them, and their lack of clothing, organised housing or land usage—thus attempting to justify, according to the law of the time, his taking of the land, as it had no organised system of government with which to negotiate. Cook arrived back in England in 1771; the government, far from being uninterested in his 'discovery', began to make plans to use this new land as a penal colony as England's gaols were overcrowded and they could no longer sell their prisoners to America, as had been their most recent solution to their social problem (Clark et al., 2000).

Here we have the first of many of the significant differences in the development of Australia and New Zealand as neighbouring but distinctly different countries. The organised system of Māori living, recognised by the Europeans as familiar, led to the development and signing of a treaty, rather than just a taking of 'empty' lands.

In January 1788 the 11 ships of the First Fleet entered the harbour in Botany Bay carrying 759 convicts and 200 marine guards, the chaplain and the captain who was to govern them, Captain Arthur Phillip. This was the place Cook had detailed in his week-long visit in a wet autumn 18 years earlier. But, as any antipodean knows, Sydney in January is quite a different picture to the cool of autumn, and the harsh reality of what they had before them in setting up a colony must have been a terrifying thought. They quickly realised the place they had landed would not support them and moved just north to Sydney Cove with its fresh-water source and more-fertile plains. But accidents of history are amazing. Within days of the English landing, a French ship under Captain La Perouse landed. What would have happened had storms or winds delayed the First Fleet and La Perouse attempted to claim the land for France, we will never know. How different might the outcome for the indigenous population have been? Again we cannot know, but given the similar patterns of constructing European communities one can imagine a contest would still have occurred for the best and most productive lands and for sources of fresh water.

Accounts of the early days of the settlement are of Aboriginal people being frightened off their lands by musket-discharging soldiers, and convicts and soldiers being frightened by spear-throwing 'natives'. Two groups of people were thrust together in a harsh environment, with no understanding of the way of life of the other, no common language and each with a determination and need to survive. The novel (now also a play and film) *Secret River* (Grenville, 2005) provides a graphic fictional account of early encounters in the Sydney basin. The early 1800s saw the senior members of the European colony discussing the 'native problem' and seeing 'civilising' the natives as the only solution. But these discussions concerned a fairly small colony around the area of Sydney. The rest of Australia remained relatively untouched by European settlement—that is, until the stroke of a pen on the other side of the world resulted in the slashing of duty for Australian wool compared with that of European wool producers. By 1850, some 200,000 migrants had moved from the United Kingdom to fell trees, clear land and graze sheep. By 1860, about 4000 Europeans with 20 million sheep occupied the prime river-fed land from southern Queensland to South Australia (Broome, 2010). An itinerant male workforce working in rough country with a male to female ratio of 40 men to every woman framed the beginnings of the nation that 'grew on the sheep's back', as it was colloquially described. It was a nation of burly men, of mateship and of women being seen as 'damned whores and God's police', a situation so colourfully captured by Anne Summers (1994) in the title of her book chronicling women's lives in early Australia. The small number of women compared with that of men throughout the early days of European settlement had predictable consequences for the Aboriginal people, as the Aboriginal women became 'useful' to white men as domestic servants and at times in sexual relationships, both consensual and non-consensual.

As white men moved further away from the coast, they increasingly disrupted the tribal grounds of individual Aboriginal groupings and forced them onto the traditional grounds of others. This progressively disrupted the seasonal movements across the lands and brought Aboriginal tribal groups into conflict with each other as well as with the white 'settlers'. Also, far more devastatingly, it disturbed a way of life that had existed for thousands of years, with rules of kinship and community and spirituality that were difficult to sustain away from the more nomadic lifestyle. Nutrition and infection control in the

form of sanitation were adversely affected by a static form of living and resulted in poor diet, ear, eye and chest infections and diarrhoea. Also negatively affected was the sense of purpose in what were the daily rituals associated with hunting and gathering. European infections of smallpox, influenza, measles and even the common cold also damaged the Aboriginal communities, who had no resistance to these new and foreign organisms. Fighting was particularly intense on the frontiers, with many deaths on both sides, but the balance of musket and spear was irrevocably disturbed by the introduction of the repeating rifle in 1870.

Aboriginal people were forced to live either on distant government-controlled reserves, in church-run 'missions' or close to but on the edges of white settlements in order to provide their families with safety, food and shelter. It is estimated that by the early 1900s the Aboriginal population was only a quarter of that of 1788.

Variations on the New South Wales experience were repeated throughout the country. In 1829 Captain Fremantle annexed 7000 kilometres of the western Australian coast for Britain and settlement began. By 1830, over 1500 British immigrants had landed in the Swan River region of Western Australia. However, unlike the beginnings in New South Wales, the Western Australian experience was of young people and families coming to start new lives, not of convicts and soldiers and a virtually all-male environment. In 1836 a further colony was begun, this time in South Australia at a site close to the mouth of the River Murray. This too was a settlement of 'free settlers'. Settlement by families had the potential to create very different societies to those dominated by men and may hold some explanation of the more 'cultured' reputation of Adelaide.

Other settlements that were to become state capitals grew at around the same time. They all experienced similar hardships and conflicts with those Aboriginal tribes, who also valued the land where rivers meet the sea and which are the most fertile. But there are stories of settlements with better race relations than others. Captain George Grey, for example, had developed a genuine respect for and understanding of the Aboriginal people after having experienced an accident in the north of Western Australia. He had been sheltered and fed by the 'natives' there and had come to hold them in higher esteem than did his predecessor British colonial officers. Captain George Grey's 'success' with the natives resulted in several of his subsequent government postings, first to Adelaide as Governor and then to New Zealand, as the Māori wars were causing British nervousness about the stability of that newly encountered country. We will meet up with Governor Grey later, in New Zealand, as he was very nearly to play an interesting role in Māori health and wellbeing post colonisation.

Darwin's 1859 *On the Origin of Species* and his notion of 'survival of the fittest' was well known in Australia by the late 1800s and provided what was at the time an acceptable, 'logical' and 'scientific' explanation for the racism that had come to dominate Australian attitudes to its indigenous people by the latter part of the 1800s and early 1900s.

Broome (2010, pp. 17–18) paints this picture of misunderstanding:

Cultural encounters are marked by misunderstandings. Language barriers obscure meaning. Even gestures can be misinterpreted, as winks and handshakes in one group are mere twitches or touches by the other. Governor Phillip observed cuts on Eora women's temples—marks of mourning—but to him they were signs of Aboriginal men's brutality to their women. The Eora noted Phillip's missing front tooth and mistook it for a sign of men's initiation, which to them it was. Natural misunderstandings arising from cultural difference were exaggerated as the two peoples held radically different orientations. The Eora lived a life largely without possessions, looked to the past, the community and a religiously based Great Tradition for inspiration, while the British valued material items, eyed the future and lauded the individual, science and the Enlightenment.

(Broome R. *Aboriginal Australians*. 4th ed. Sydney: Allen & Unwin; 2010; reproduced with permission of Allen & Unwin Pty Ltd)

The paternalistic attitude and overt racism that such preconceptions brought forth were a feature of Australian society until the 1970s, and many would say they are still present.

REFLECTIVE THINKING EXERCISE

- Imagine yourself a convict woman arriving on one of the early ships to settle in Port Jackson. What would be your hopes and fears?
- Imagine yourself as an Aboriginal woman and mother in the early 1800s in south-eastern Australia. What would be your hopes and fears?

Federation of the colonies into a nation: a commonwealth of Australia

On 1 January 1901 the six colonies that had developed around the coastline of Australia became a federated nation: the Commonwealth of Australia. Its population was recorded at the time as 3.75 million. Aboriginal people were not counted as part of this census; nor, when the parliament was set up, were they permitted to vote. Indeed it was not until 1962 that Aboriginal people were entitled to vote.

The perception of many Australians is of politics having been male dominated from its inception, but a study of the political history of Australia tells a different story. From the beginning of Federation, women were nominated for parliament, with three women being nominated for the senate as early as 1903, although it was 41 years before a woman was elected to federal parliament (Sawer & Simms, 1993). Clearly, women were anxious for the role but not elected into it. Thus parliament may have been male dominated but politics was not—women used the elections as opportunities to voice their concerns and lobby for change.

The new Australia was seen as full of promise and potential wealth and, as the dominant view was that the Aboriginal people would soon die out, it was seen to be a country for and of white people. Two of the first pieces of legislation passed in the new federal parliament were those restricting immigration to white people (the language used at the time to describe what is now referred to as **Anglo-Celtic** or European). Unofficially this legislation became known as the 'White Australia Policy'. This was not the first legislation to keep out or restrict the rights of those who were not white. In the mid 1800s, gold had been found in New South Wales and the gold rush began, doubling the population in less than 10 years. With wool and gold, Australia looked like the land of opportunity. People began to come not only from Europe—Chinese people flooded in, in their tens of thousands, for gold. Consequently, legislation was passed to limit Chinese immigration; those who were already here were not permitted to be naturalised and were to be regarded for generations as 'foreigners'. This dismissal of the Chinese as legitimate citizens occurred in spite of the fact that in the Northern Territory by 1879 there were only 400 Europeans but 3500 Chinese.

Federation was seen as a mechanism for integrating the whole of Australia under a British parliamentary structure and hence ensuring its 'white' future. This situation is perplexing when one looks at the already existing ethnic mix. Clark et al. (2000, p. 127) quote the following demographics at the time of Federation:

Three-quarters had been born in Australia, the greatest majority were of English, Irish or Scottish descent. But there were also 30,000 people born in China, 4,000 in Japan, 7,600 in India, 38,400 in Germany, 10,000 in Sweden, 5,600 in Italy, 6,300 in Denmark, 7,500 in the United States and 5,200 born at sea.

The First World War

The First World War was important in the formation of a sense of a national Australian identity and an identity separate from Britain. By 1914, more than 20,000 men had joined the armed forces and had landed in Egypt for training. The Australians landed at the same time as the troops from New Zealand, and collectively they became known as the ANZACs (the Australian and New Zealand Army Corps). Together they met some of the most ferocious fighting, particularly at Gallipoli, in Turkey. The way in which these men dealt with their dire and tragic situation led to the development of what became known as the 'ANZAC spirit'; more than 26,000 Australians and over 7500 New Zealanders died at Gallipoli, but the stories of the determination, mateship and bravery during that time are now legend. Following the debacle of Gallipoli, many of the survivors were taken to Europe to fight at the Western Front against the German army in different but equally atrocious conditions. The conditions faced on the Western Front are graphically represented by Sebastian Faulks (1993) in his book *Birdsong: A Novel of Love and War,* a harrowing but accessible account of the kinds of hardships the Australians and New Zealanders would have faced.

Many Australian women joined the war effort as nurses, but women were not allowed to be part of the war in any other formal capacity. They were left to undertake all the everyday jobs that had previously been the province of men, particularly in the country, including fencing, shearing and heavy farm work.

REFLECTIVE THINKING EXERCISE

What complex and conflicting emotions might you have felt at the end of the war with the men in your life returning, and (a) you having to relinquish a job you had enjoyed? and (b) where you found your loved ones unrecognisably changed by their experiences?

Wars waged between Aboriginal peoples and the colonial invaders

As explained above, the ANZAC legend and its associated myths have had a profound effect on Australian identity. Indeed, many authors contend that 'The legend of the Australian fighting man … blossomed into full flower on the bloody razorback ridges of Gallipoli during 1915', in the words of Firkins in *Australians in Nine Wars* (1973, p. 210).

Interestingly, the nine wars described by this author do not include the battles waged between Australia's first citizens and their country's invaders. The bloody and prolonged battles that accompanied colonial invasion of Australia, and claimed at least 20,000 Aboriginal lives, rate barely a mention on Canberra's Australian War Memorial, built to honour Australian deaths in battle. There are similar war memorials throughout the country in almost every community. Unlike New Zealand, where the wars that accompanied colonisation are widely recognised, in Australia there are only a handful of reminders of the many brutal events that occurred on Australian soil. Indeed, a monument to 28 Aboriginal people, mainly women and children, who were massacred in 1838 at Myall Creek in New South Wales was erected only in 2003. The Australian frontier wars are not part of the ANZAC legend, with its emphasis on mateship, service and sacrifice. Peter Stanley, who was the Australian War Memorial's chief historian, called them 'guerrilla wars … sordid and secret'. The book *Murder at Myall Creek* gives detailed insights into the atrocities and the circumstances that enabled many of them to go unpunished (Tedeschi, 2016).

Authors such as Raymond Evans and Henry Reynolds (whose works on colonial violence and Aboriginal resistance started appearing in the 1970s), Anna Haebich and Robert Manne (who have published extensively on the issue of stolen/removed children), and Russell McGregor and Tim Rowse, have brought the 'dirty wars' to the public's attention. The seven-part documentary *First Australians* (SBS, 2008) chronicles the birth of contemporary Australia as never told before—from the perspective of its first people. *First Australians* explores what unfolded when the oldest living culture in the world was overrun by the British Empire. Chronicling the experiences of Aboriginal Australians, from the first contact with whites in Botany Bay in 1788 to Eddie Koiki Mabo's 1993 legal challenge to the British **terra nullius** declaration, *First Australians* is the most exhaustive account of Aboriginal history so far broadcast on Australian television, and makes a compelling case for the argument that the invaders and, later, the Australian government introduced a number of genocidal policies that aimed to eradicate Aboriginal communities. From the Tasmanian Black War, in which Aboriginals were systematically shot, raped and eventually exiled to Flinders Island, to the policies of assimilation, under which 'half-caste' children were stolen from their families and imprisoned in Christian missions, every conceivable strategy has been employed to 'delete' Aboriginal people and their cultures and traditions from history.

The documentary series also describes the personal and political options available to Aboriginal people fighting against policies leading to colonial dominance, dispossession, relocation and threatened extinction. It refutes the argument that Aboriginal Australians accepted the theft of their land; rather, they actively resisted the white settlers' land grab. For example, Windradyne from Bathurst and Jandamarra from the Kimberley led fierce guerrilla wars against the colonists. The Coniston Massacre of 1928 was the last recorded 'official' massacre of Aboriginal people by white Australians. In Alice Springs, JC Cawood sent Constable WG Murray to Coniston Station to arrest the murderers of settler Fred Brooks and any Aboriginal Australians who had been spearing the cattle of the European settlers. The official death toll was 31, including women and children; however, Aboriginal oral tradition records almost 90 dead. It is generally agreed that the police killed up to 100 Aboriginal Australians across six sites. Although none of the perpetrators of the crime were brought to justice, public outrage ensured that the deliberate and officially sanctioned slaughter of innocent people was never repeated. The impact of the killings on the Warlpiri, Anmatyerre and Kaytetye peoples resulted in major cultural dislocation: the killings destabilised land tenure and religious groups through disruptions to ceremonial life, exchange networks and religious ceremonies.

To this day, Aboriginal Australians still fight for the return of their land, evidenced for example by the Cummeragunja Walk-off in 1989, the Freedom Rides of the 1960s and the ongoing struggle for land rights, closing

9

the health gap, reclaiming of language, and recognition in the Australian Constitution.

Australian identity

The Australian identity has long been a contradictory one. Described by Ward in *The Australian Legend* over 50 years ago as 'the rough, honest, easy-going bushman, laconic, resourceful, loyal to his mates, uncomfortable with parsons and women, facing adversity with a stoical joke' (Ward, 1958, summarised in Hudson & Bolton, 1997, p. 1), to which could be added 'Anglo-Celtic bloke', this view still permeates society despite the multicultural nature of the Australian population and the fact that more than three-quarters of the population live an urban life in coastal cities.

Hudson & Bolton (1997) exhort us to look to Australia's multiple personalities rather than find attachment in a single, perhaps only briefly existing, 'rural ideal' and to be cognisant of the amazing diversity that is the essence of the different regions within Australia. What it is to be Australian and live in Australia is very different if one is in inner-city Sydney or in Bourke or Broken Hill, and different again if one is in Perth or Broome. Even within the large cities there are now suburbs with such ethnic homogeneity that the shop signs are in Vietnamese, Arabic or Greek, and the norms of behaviour and identity vary in each.

The single Australian story may have been male, with the female either absent or as the shadow behind the man, but the women's history is a varied one too. Early attempts to tell a women's story, such as Miriam Dixon's *The Real Matilda* (1999, first published in 1976), paint a picture of an oppressed group. The introduction to Dixon's book begins, 'In this exploratory book I propose that Australian women, women in the land of mateship, "the Ocker", keg-culture, come pretty close to top rating as the "Doormats of the Western World"' (Dixon, 1999, p. 11). However, the women's story is populated also by gutsy feminists at the turn of the 20th century standing for parliament, and fighting for peace and for pensions for the aged and invalided. These women broke down the barriers to women's entry to medicine (1897), law (1903) and architecture (1889), but had to wait until after the Second World War to enter the other male bastions of the Church, the armed forces and engineering. In 1902 Vida Goldstein went to Washington to the founding conference of what was to become the International Women's Suffrage Alliance, and served as its secretary. Women were also internationally published authors, for example Miles Franklin (1965), who gives us a glimpse into a gutsy heroine in Sybylla Melvyn in *My Brilliant Career* (published 1901). Jessie Street in 1946 was the Australian delegate to the United Nations. These women were part of the first wave of feminism; the second wave was to come in the 1970s.

If there was one constant in the interruption to the development of women and their voices in Australian history, it was war. War created the ANZAC legend, reinforcing the mateship ethic as central to being 'dinky-di' Australian. It gave women the unsung role of keeping the urban and rural productivity going while the men were overseas, though they were expected to relinquish these positions when the men returned and to adjust to living with a generation of men brutalised by their experiences of the inhumanity of war. Following the Second World War, women again left the jobs they had been doing—but this time they not only were childbearing but also were expected to join the workforce without the advantage of the same educational, occupational and economic opportunities as men.

The need for the country to have a single common image to relate to is seen by White (1981, 1997) to be a construction of a market that had products to sell. He writes of the relationship between the market and a sense of being a nation, citing as examples the Heidelberg school of painting's need to be iconic, as they had to be saleable to galleries rather than private collectors; the *Bulletin*'s need for a single popular market; and latterly, in the 1980s and 1990s, the advertising agencies' need to sell beer, collectively contributing to over a hundred years of image reinforcement. Women did not control the spending power and were thus rendered invisible in all but domestic commercials and image portrayals.

Thus, the quintessential Australian became a construction that was male, of mateship, of exhibiting a laconic sense of humour and, while predominantly white, of 'tolerance' to others.

The Anglo-Celtic Australian notion of multicultural tolerance is questioned by Curthoys (1997, p. 35). 'Tolerance' suggests two elements: the tolerators and the tolerated:

> Tolerance may be better than intolerance but it does not guarantee equality. Anglo-Celtic Australians, in their enthusiasm for multiculturalism and thereby the new inclusive Australian identity, are, then, still expressing power relations, still speaking from a self-confident centre, the Australian nation. They are doing the including, not being included. The politics of inclusion, based on notions of community and identity absorbs difference within a pre-given and predefined space.

Taking the argument a step further, Curthoys says: 'Everyone in Australia who is non-Indigenous, the "tolerators" and the "tolerated" alike, still share in and are advantaged by a history of colonialism.'

In speaking also of tolerance and diversity, Don Watson, in his now famous speech, 'A Toast to the Postmodern Republic', said:

> I'm only just game enough to say it: it might be the first postmodern republic, and I mean that in the nicest possible way. I mean a republic that exalts the nation less than the way of life. Whose principal value is tolerance rather than conformity, difference rather than uniformity.
>
> (quoted in Wark, 1997, p. 152)

Watson's 1997 speech predated the move to the Right and the resurgence of sexism and racism in Australian society that occurred under the Liberal Howard government up to late 2007, and has resurfaced with the Abbott/Turnbull/Morrison government since 2013 when the conservatives again came to power.

A very interesting and easily readable book that traverses Australia from the 1950s to the beginning of the 21st century is the autobiography of Wendy McCarthy (2000), *Don't Fence Me In*.

Anne Summers (2003) again became the conscience of Australia with her powerful book *The End of Equality: Work, Babies and Women's Choices in 21st Century Australia*.

> In her introduction she maintains the promise of equality is far from met amongst Australian women. In fact, sometimes it seems we are going backwards. This is despite the rhetoric and the promises of equal pay and work conditions. In Australia, more women work part time, mainly because childcare and other support conditions are not available. On the whole the conditions for women's equal work and pay have not changed over the past thirty years, and we remain behind many other industrialised countries in our dependence on welfare … "As a result of all these factors, there are more women living at the economic margin, or actual poverty than ever before".
>
> (Summers 2003 pp. 2–3).

In contradiction to a self-image of tolerance, the plight of refugees and asylum seekers in Australia has shocked many in the Australian community. The Howard government's agreement to assist the United States in a 'war against terrorism' in Iraq again divided the nation. Any notion of being a nation with a single voice was seriously challenged. Australia's stance on both these issues was in stark contrast to that of New Zealand, again reinforcing the separation of the two countries. These challenges to the Australian people about international relations, the treatment of the Aboriginal people and the failure of the Howard government to say 'sorry' appeared to play a significant role in the change of government in November 2007. 'Sorry' was an election promise of the then opposition leader Kevin Rudd, and this came to pass on 13 February 2008. The nation as a whole took part in this special day, with hundreds of thousands travelling to Canberra to bear witness. Prime Minister Kevin Rudd began the long awaited 'sorry' speech thus:

> I move:
> That today we honour the Indigenous peoples of this land, the oldest continuing cultures in human history.
> We reflect on their past mistreatment.
> We reflect in particular on the mistreatment of those who were Stolen Generations—this blemished chapter in our nation's history.
> The time has now come for the nation to turn a new page in Australia's history by righting the wrongs of the past and so moving forward with confidence to the future.
> We apologise for the laws and policies of successive parliaments and governments that have inflicted profound grief, suffering and loss on these our fellow Australians.

> We apologise especially for the removal of Aboriginal and Torres Strait Islander children from their families, their communities and their country.
> For the pain, suffering and hurt of these Stolen Generations, their descendants and for their families left behind, we say sorry.
> To the mothers and the fathers, the brothers and the sisters, for the breaking up of families and communities, we say sorry.
> And for the indignity and degradation thus inflicted on a proud people and a proud culture, we say sorry.
> We the Parliament of Australia respectfully request that this apology be received in the spirit in which it is offered as part of the healing of the nation.
> For the future we take heart; resolving that this new page in the history of our great continent can now be written.
> We today take this first step by acknowledging the past and laying claim to a future that embraces all Australians.
> A future where this Parliament resolves that the injustices of the past must never, never happen again.
> A future where we harness the determination of all Australians, Indigenous and non-Indigenous, to close the gap that lies between us in life expectancy, educational achievement and economic opportunity.
> A future where we embrace the possibility of new solutions to enduring problems where old approaches have failed.
> A future based on mutual respect, mutual resolve and mutual responsibility.
> A future where all Australians, whatever their origins, are truly equal partners, with equal opportunities and with an equal stake in shaping the next chapter in the history of this great country, Australia.
>
> (Rudd, 2008)

Under the Labor government of Rudd and Gillard there were numerous changes that moved the Australian position closer to that of New Zealand under Helen Clark and her former Labour government. Australia fleetingly had a better representation of women in government, including a woman Prime Minister, a woman Governor-General and a woman State Premier of Queensland—the state known to generations as the misogynous heartland of Australia. Typical of the see-saw between the two countries, however, Australia returned to a conservative government headed by a male Prime Minister in 2013, where it has remained, while New Zealand elected a Labour government with a female Prime Minister, Jacinda Ardern, in 2017.

CRITICAL THINKING EXERCISE

- Where were you when Kevin Rudd read the Apology to the Australian people, and what impact did it have on you?
- What are the issues that affect you as a woman in contemporary Australian society, and in what way have these issues been influenced by the history of this country?

Modern Aboriginal society

I position myself in writing this section as a middle-class Anglo-Celtic, fifth-generation Australian woman and do not presume to be able to tell authentically an Aboriginal and Torres Strait Islander story. I will therefore distil some of what other writers have seen as the cardinal events in Aboriginal society for you here so that you can form a schema from which to do your own further reading.

No version of modern Australian Aboriginal society can make sense without an understanding of the effects of European colonisation. We were briefly introduced to this earlier in the chapter. What we did not focus on at that time is the collision of paternalistic intentions to try to 'save a dying race' and the removal of children from their parents and families, which became known in Australian history as the '**Stolen Generations**'.

In 1906 Bishop Frodsman was reported to have said:

> The Aborigines are disappearing. In the course of a generation or two, at the most, the last Australian blackfellow will have turned his face to warm mother earth … Missionary work then may be only smoothing the pillow of a dying race, but I think if the Lord Jesus came to Australia he would be moved with great compassion for these poor outcasts, living by the wayside, robbed of their land, wounded by the lust and passion of a stronger race, and dying.
>
> (Broome, *Aboriginal Australians*. 4th ed. Sydney: Allen & Unwin; 2010, p. 149; reproduced with permission of Allen & Unwin Pty Ltd)

Thinking of the adults as 'lost causes', the missionaries and the government determined to 'save the children'. The main strategy used was to separate the children from their parents. Some parents agreed to this separation because they saw it as a means to enhance and protect their children's health and wellbeing, despite the grief of separation; other children were forcibly removed from their parents. The children were removed to either government reserves or church missions.

Mission or reserve schooling and life left the children between two worlds, belonging to neither. Restricting the children and young adults to life on the missions or reserves not only introduced them to European foods and language but also disturbed their learning of bush ways and independence in being able to hunt and gather their own foods, increasing their dependency and depriving them of traditional rituals such as initiations, which were often banned. Most missions introduced the notion of matrimonial monogamy and marriage without respect for traditional Aboriginal relationship rules that had stood for generations. In 1953 the Australian government financed the provision of medical and educational facilities on the missions, further entrenching their function in the assimilation of Aboriginal children into the lifestyle of white Australia.

But such a loss can remain submerged for only so long. The stories of the lives dislodged began to be recorded and the cry for self-determination for Aboriginal people became louder through the 1960s and 1970s, with several government inquiries into the treatment received on the missions and reserves, which had at times included severe physical punishment as well as family dislocation. To generalise on the experience of all missions and reserves is to do an injustice to some who valued and upheld the traditional language and customs, but they do appear to have been in the minority.

The mission story and experience dominated the northern Aboriginal settlements, but the story of south-eastern Aboriginals was of fringe settlement around the edges of the towns and cities or on government reserves, of which there were 49 in 1960 (Broome, 2010). The people on the reserves were rigidly controlled under the *Aboriginal Protection Act* of 1909 and its later amendments. In 1936, amendments to the Act gave the Aboriginal Protection Board powers to carry out compulsory medical checks and remove people to government settlements. Aboriginal children were not permitted in state schools until 1949.

REFLECTIVE THINKING EXERCISE

- If you were an Aboriginal woman whose child had been taken to a mission, how might you have consoled yourself and what effect might this have had on your life?

- If you were a young Aboriginal woman brought up on a mission with little contact with your family, how might this have affected your life physically, socially, culturally and spiritually? What are the positives, what are the negatives, and how do you heal and move forward?

- How would you feel/behave if the government kidnapped *your* daughter?

Read the *Bringing Them Home* report (HREOC, 1997) and Doris Pilkington's 1996 book *Follow the Rabbit-proof Fence*. You might like to view the episode 'The rabbit-proof fence' of the documentary series *First Australians* (SBS, 2008) as you reflect on these questions.

Discrimination and racism caused poverty and lack of political power, which reinforced the cycle of poverty and discrimination. The flow-on effects of poverty, being of course poorer health and education status, led to further cycles of alienation and despair, confusion and loss of purpose though with growing defiance for some. Alcohol became an increasing problem for some old enough to obtain it and, for some younger Aboriginal people, so did glue and petrol sniffing. Although local group identity was strong, there was no history of a broader sense of national Aboriginal solidarity. Sport and art were two of the few areas in which Aboriginal young people had had opportunities to excel, as they did in boxing, football, tennis, dance and painting.

Movements for Aboriginal rights had existed sporadically since the 1920s. One of the most public and decisive movements came from William Cooper, who in 1937 led a campaign for the 150th anniversary of the landing of the First Fleet to be proclaimed a day of mourning, commemorating instead the 150th anniversary of misery and degradation of the original inhabitants by white invaders (Broome, 2010). This was to resurface 50 years later, when the Bicentennial created a focus for national Aboriginal cohesion and a questioning of Australia Day as a cause for celebration as opposed to its recognition as a day of mourning for the Aboriginal people of Australia.

In 1961 the Federal Council for the Advancement of Aborigines was formed, changing its name in 1964 to include Torres Strait Islanders. In 1967, 89% of voters voted for Aboriginal citizenship, and the federal government, rather than the states, was given power to legislate on Aboriginal affairs; the Department of Aboriginal Affairs was created. In 1972 the first Aboriginal tent embassy was set up on the lawns of Parliament House and was a symbol of a new Aboriginal determination. In 1973 a federal inquiry into Aboriginal land rights was established. Aboriginal stories began to be recorded and in the 1980s there was an explosion of oral history recording.

But it was not until 1992 that the fiction of the empty land, *terra nullius*, was overturned by the Mabo High Court decision after more than 200 years of European colonisation. Native title was enshrined in the *Native Title Act 1993* and required proof of continuous relationship to the land. The national focus of the 1990s and into the early 2000s was on Aboriginal and Torres Strait Islander health—physical, mental and spiritual.

The Human Rights and Equal Opportunity Commission in 1995 explored, among other matters, the removal of children from their parents and families. The inquiry heard that, since 1911 in Queensland alone, over 6000 children had been removed; some thought this to be a gross underestimation. The Stolen Generations and their sequelae are now an acknowledged part of Australian history, and their impact on current social and cultural life is recognised. The Commission's report, *Bringing Them Home*, estimated that 40,000 Aboriginal children had been removed from their families in the 1900s (Human Rights and Equal Opportunity Commission (HREOC), 1997). In the decade from 1919, up to one-third of children were taken in the southern states.

The complex and troublesome issue for a generation of European Australians in attempting to come to terms with the consequences of the actions of their forebears has been explored in a highly readable book, *Being Whitefella*, edited by Duncan Graham (1994). This book is a compilation of 16 well-known and respected 'whitefellas' exploring their relationship with Aboriginal Australia.

In 1996 the then Premier of New South Wales, Bob Carr, formally apologised in parliament, saying:

I affirm in this place, formally and solemnly as Premier, on behalf of the government and people of New South Wales, our apology to Aboriginal people.

The Howard federal government consistently refused to say 'sorry', the word called for by Aboriginal Australians. It did, however, commit to the 'process of reconciliation with Aboriginal and Torres Strait Islander people, in the context of redressing their profound social and economic disadvantage'. Australia was seen to be beginning to take the necessary steps to atone for its past injustices. However, the 1996 federal election saw the election of Queensland Senator Pauline Hanson. Her maiden speech in parliament was a blatant attack on Aboriginal people and it reignited racism in Australia.

Poor health, in the form of diabetes, renal disease, mental health problems, violence, alcoholism and domestic violence, are difficulties still facing many Aboriginal families, for whom poverty is still the fundamental issue of discrimination. Indigenous people are much more likely to die before they are old than people in the rest of the Australian population (2008 research). The most recent estimates from the Australian Institute for Health and Welfare (AIHW, 2018) indicate that an Aboriginal male born in the period 2010–12 could be expected to live to 69.1 years, 10.6 years less than a non-Aboriginal male of that time (who could expect to live 79.7 years). In the same period, an Aboriginal female could be expected to live to 73.7 years, which is 9.5 years less than her non-Aboriginal counterpart (83.1 years). The Aboriginal health statistics still show an unacceptable discrepancy in life expectancy and in maternal and perinatal mortality. This will be addressed in detail later in this text (see Chs 10 and 11). In 2007 the report *Little Children Are Sacred: Report of the Northern Territory Board of Inquiry Into the Protection of Aboriginal Children From Sexual Abuse* (Northern Territory (NT) Government, 2007) was released. It prompted a most extraordinary and controversial response from the federal government in the form of the 'Northern Territory Intervention', which introduced health checks for all Aboriginal children in the Northern Territory—and included using the army to assist. The Intervention also disrupted many of the governance arrangements in place in Northern Territory communities. At issue was not a denial of the need for help for the health of these communities, but the swift, patriarchal manner in which it was instituted (Brown & Brown, 2007).

Professor Mick Dodson, the 2009 Australian of the Year, crystallises much of the debate as follows:

We must ask how the considered and sensitive discussion in 'Little Children are Sacred' of the long-term problem of handling sexual abuse, and the culturally meaningful interventions required to address this crisis, have been translated into the storm-trooper tent diplomacy of health providers dressed in battle fatigues. Have the policy playground bullies won the day?
(Dodson, 2007, p. 95)

On coming to office in late 2007, the Rudd government committed to six targets to 'close the gap' between Aboriginal and non-Aboriginal Australians in life expectancy, under-five mortality rates, access to early childhood education, literacy rates, Year 12 (end of high school) attainment and employment outcomes. The Sorry Day national apology of Prime Minister Rudd, referred to earlier, has been critical in laying the groundwork for the formation of

13

partnerships between the government and Aboriginal leaders and communities that are needed to meet these targets. However, by 2017 the 9th *Closing the Gap* report indicated that only one of the seven targets was expected to be met in that year and that, although there had been improvements in mortality statistics, in non-smoking and in chronic diseases, cancer rates were increasing. All Australians will be watching and/or working towards the closing of these gaps, particularly those who have an interest in healthcare and in improving its outcomes for all people.

This section would not, however, be complete without acknowledgement of the extraordinary accomplishment of many Aboriginal and Torres Strait Islander people, in business, parliament, sport, art, academia and indeed all aspects of life in Australia, in spite of 200 years of colonisation.

CRITICAL THINKING EXERCISE

Activist Mick Dodson stated that the Apology to indigenous Australians is not about dwelling on the past, it's about building a future. Jot down your vision of a 'new' Australia and what impact this this will have on all Australians.

NEW ZEALAND

Early New Zealand

New Zealand too is an ancient land, separating as its own land mass 80 million years ago. Yet, even in their geological and ecological foundations, Australia and New Zealand are profoundly different. The New Zealand land mass is turbulent and shaky, with large earthquakes a constant possibility and small tremors part of everyday life. The vegetation looks different, to an Australian eye, and vice versa—different green, different scrub or bush—and, as flat and solid as Australia is, New Zealand is mountainous and forever shifting its footing.

By the time of British settlement in New Zealand, **Māori** had been living in New Zealand for at least a thousand years, having come from Polynesia in canoes (waka). Belich (2001, p. 18) suggests that three cardinal features of Māori society that are still prized today were strongly present even at this time: **mana**, **utu** and **tapu**.

Mana was a kind of spiritual capital, often translated as prestige or authority, inherited, acquired and lost by both individuals and groups. Utu was not simply revenge, but reciprocity, obliging one to return gifts as well as a blow. It was particularly important in relations between groups: the exchange of gifts and hospitality were positive utu. Tapu, a system of sanctity, social constraint and sacred laws, was complemented by its opposite—noa, which can be translated as normal, ordinary or unrestricted.

Māori were and are a tribal people with specific land affiliation. They cultivated their lands for root crops, supplementing their diet through fishing and hunting. Belich (2007) describes the first Māori–European interaction thus: 'The first Māori reaction to contact with Europeans was, unambiguously enough, to kill and eat them.' Tasman, the Dutch explorer spoken of earlier, visited the New Zealand coast in 1642, and his boats were attacked and several of his crew killed. When Cook visited in 1769, similarly violent incidents occurred. However, there is evidence of trade with Pākehā (non-Māori New Zealanders, a name already in use by 1814), particularly in whaling, sealing and as missionaries (King, 2012). And there is evidence of significant movement between Port Jackson, the New South Wales colony, and the Māori world, particularly in trade for timber and flax (King, 2012). The return trade was in metals and tools and, devastatingly, muskets. Belich (2007, p. 19) summarised the interactions in the following way:

If Europeans mistreated Māori(s), they would be killed. If Māori(s) mistreated Europeans, trade would stop.

King puts a slightly different complexion on these interactions:

Where Europeans took the trouble to try to understand Maori codes of behaviour and to identify Maori expectations Maori–Pakeha relations in the nineteenth century were generally harmonious … Where they did not, there were severe disappointments on the European side, accusations of Maori unreliability and treachery, and bloodshed.

(King, 1988, p. 205)

The key to successful interaction clearly was the effort or ability to understand the importance and place of mana, utu and tapu.

As indicated above, from the early 1800s there had been small numbers of Europeans in New Zealand as missionaries, whalers and traders. Missionaries began to teach the writing of Māori languages, which until that time had been exclusively oral, as well as, of course, trying to convert the 'natives' to their God. Prior to 1840, the time of the establishment of the Treaty of Waitangi, there were only about 2000 non-Māori living in New Zealand.

Tribal warfare was part of New Zealand history, with the North Island in internal warfare from 1818 to 1833. This intertribal warfare was made worse by the phenomenon of the musket brought to them by Europeans, giving rise to the naming of these as the Musket Wars.

The interactions of Māori with the British colonies in eastern Australia brought them into increasing contact with Europeans and eventually to the attention of London. In 1832 a formal link was established, with James Busby being sent to New Zealand as a representative of the British Crown. This appointment was to protect the interests of New Zealand trade with the Australian colonies. According to King (2012), Busby's instruction from London, via the New South Wales Governor, 'was to protect "well disposed" settlers and traders, guard against the exploitation of Māori by Europeans and outrages committed against them, and recapture escaped convicts' (King, 2012, p. 153).

The British, keen to prevent expansion of the French in the southern oceans and to control the sale of land to Europeans, planned to annex and then colonise parts of New Zealand. Given that the country was clearly 'owned, governed and used' by its indigenous people, unlike the British view of Australia, some form of negotiated settlement was required by international law. Relationships with Māori chiefs had been cultivated through about 50 years of contact with New South Wales and Busby had moved these further since coming to live in New Zealand. In 1839 William Hobson was sent from London to take the constitutional steps necessary to establish a British colony. This was to be in the form of a treaty.

The original plan was to annex small portions of land only. However, the behaviour of the New Zealand Company, a British company set up to establish trading colonies, together with the threat of the French, who had set up a colony on the South Island at Akaroa and were planning further colonisation of the rich pastoral lands of the Canterbury Plains, and Baron de Thierry's attempts to establish himself at Hokianga, caused Hobson to proclaim sovereignty over the whole country in the Treaty of Waitangi, discussed more fully later.

In everyday life, British annexation had relatively little obvious effect outside the towns of Auckland, Wellington, Wanganui, New Plymouth and Nelson. Although Māori dominated the country areas, the way in which Māori tribes interacted with each other had been irrevocably disturbed by European contact and resulted in what are known as the New Zealand Wars of 1845 to 1872 (until the 1980s these were referred to as the Māori Wars). These were wars of Māori tribes against each other and the British, and resulted in an enormous influx of British military. (These wars are well documented in the book *The New Zealand Wars* by James Belich (2015), if you are interested in further reading, or Chapter 15 of King's (2012) *The Penguin History of New Zealand*.)

Governor George Grey was sent to New Zealand as Governor in 1845 at a time of great unrest between Māori and Māori, and between Māori and Pākehā. He had had contact with Australian Aboriginal people and was seen as 'good with natives'. He was particularly influential in New Zealand, attempting to ensure that the Treaty conditions were observed and Māori land rights respected. Governor Grey learned the Māori language and assisted on having Māori legends and traditions written down. His papers eventually became one of the most important repositories of Māori language in the country. Governor Grey was also concerned with Māori health and built several hospitals, and also wrote to Florence Nightingale asking how to improve the deteriorating health of the Māori people. Unfortunately, Florence Nightingale's response was not received until shortly before Grey left for South Africa and was never to be influential in New Zealand. The document that influenced health and education policy at the time was a book by Dr AS Thompson, who advocated separation of Māori into English housing and compulsory attendance at European schools. The advice was completely contrary to that suggested by Nightingale, whose letter was eventually found decades later in Grey's South African papers. Nightingale warned against too quickly seeking to educate Māori, to increase the separations between beds in marae (Māori meeting houses) and not to remove the people to individual English-style houses. The advice was not dissimilar to public health advice that may be given today, and if attended to at the time might have changed the course of Māori health history (Keith, 1988). Grey also left a legacy of a draft of the constitution that was to become the foundation for governance for 150 years. Under this constitution, Māori men were given the vote in 1867 and all women were given the vote in 1893.

The 1860s were dominated by further flare-ups of the New Zealand Wars and by the gold rush, with discoveries on both Islands—in the north in the Coromandel Peninsula and in the south in Nelson and Otago. By 1860, the European population had surpassed that of Māori.

In the towns, European development continued as if a subset of England or, in the south, Scotland. In 1848 Dunedin was established as a Scottish Free Church settlement and Christchurch in 1850 as a Canterbury Association (Church of England) settlement, both based on New Zealand Company settlement models. Dunedin and Christchurch today display visible signs of their respective Scottish and English heritages. In 1874 Dunedin had a population of 29,832, Auckland 27,840, Wellington 15,941 and Christchurch 14,270 (King, 2012, p. 209). But the landscape of the South Island was dominated not by people but by sheep, of which there were 13 million by 1878.

Again, unlike the experience in Australia, the coexistence of the two dominant cultures moved in a virtually parallel existence until after the Second World War, when the numbers of Māori seeking to live an urban lifestyle grew exponentially.

The Treaty of Waitangi and British 'annexation' in 1840

The **Treaty of Waitangi** is a foundational document for all New Zealanders and is the basis for the claim that New Zealand is a bicultural country. It is a statement of intent by two very different groups to live equitably and harmoniously together. It was, however, drawn up hastily and by non-lawyers, and translated into Māori by people other than the original authors. On 5 February 1840, copies of the Treaty in both languages were put before a gathering of Northern Chiefs at Busby's house near Waitangi.

There were three articles to the Treaty. The first declared that the chiefs would 'cede to her Majesty the Queen of England absolutely and without reservation all rights and powers of Sovereignty … over their respective Territories' (as quoted in King, 2012, p. 159).

The second article in English held a guarantee from the Queen to the chiefs and tribes and their families of 'full exclusive and undisturbed possession of their lands and Estates Forests Fisheries and other properties … So long as it is their wish and desire to retain the same in their possession' (as quoted in King, 2012, p. 159). In return, the chiefs would give exclusive right of any sale to the Crown.

The third article extends to the 'Natives of New Zealand Her royal protection and imparts to them all the Rights and Privileges of British Subjects' (as quoted in King, 2012, p. 153).

How one explained to different groups of people with different languages and cultural background the subtle meaning of these words, especially a word such as 'sovereignty', leaves significant questions of informed consent, which have been played out in courts over the past three decades. These misunderstandings were further complicated by the translation into Māori, where the word 'sovereignty' was translated as 'kāwanatanga', which to Māori means 'governorship'—vastly different from sovereignty. This misunderstanding was to be reinforced in the wording of article two, which assured the retention of 'the unqualified exercise of their chieftainship over their lands, villages and all their treasures' (King, 2012, p. 160). These discrepancies were, however, not obvious to anyone at the signing of the Treaty. As part of the Treaty negotiations there was a commitment also that all land transactions that had taken place prior to 1840 were to be investigated by a Land Claims Commissioner.

The Treaty of Waitangi was signed on 6 February 1840 by Hobson and by many, but not all, of the Māori chiefs. Hobson then travelled the country, acquiring the signatures of most of the remaining chiefs, and the document was completed on 3 September that year. Five hundred chiefs signed the Treaty, although a number of important chiefs would not, including Te Wherowhero of Waikato, Tāraia of Thames, Tupaea of Tauranga, the Te Arawa of Rotorua and the Ngāti Tūwharetoa of Taupo. Land purchases began, with land in the South Island becoming readily available as Te Rauparaha and his warring tribe had seriously depleted the number of Māori in the south. This included the purchase by the New Zealand Company of the Canterbury Plains, the most fertile pastoral land in New Zealand. The gold rush also led to European settlement of the South Island, with gold found in Nelson and large finds in Otago leading to a doubling of the Otago population in 6 months in the 1860s.

From 1840 to 1914, 90% of those migrating to New Zealand were from Britain or Ireland, most on assisted passage to the five New Zealand Company settlements, by assisted passage to the South Island to settle Canterbury or Otago, or as military persons brought in in their thousands to protect the colony.

Despite the existence of the Treaty, the mechanisms for purchasing land were by no means straightforward, as often several different chiefs were involved and negotiation with one did not mean permission of others. These complicated land contestations led to what have become known as the New Zealand Land Wars. Following these wars there was significant confiscation of lands in the North Island, and even though this was deemed unjust by a Royal Commission 60 years later the return of the lands was by then impossible. Māori retreated to their rural communities and Pākehā lived predominantly in the towns, and this segregation continued until the Second World War, when rural economic difficulties and growing job availability in the cities lured young Māori to the towns.

War and beyond

The New Zealand and Australian experiences were often shared experiences in the First World War, and this has already been explored. A major part of New Zealand's Second World War campaign took place in Greece and in Crete. As noted by King (2012, p. 398), 'Of all the New Zealand battles in World War II, none engraved itself more deeply on the national consciousness than that for Crete. It was the Gallipoli of its era.' The other major theatre of war was North Africa and included the well-known battle of El Alamein in 1942. The New Zealand armed forces also moved to Italy to continue the fight against the Germans. With the fall of Singapore to the Japanese in 1942, New Zealand also dispatched troops to the Pacific. As with the Australian experience, war appeared to unify the nation. But the postwar time was the catalyst for a disruption of the seemingly cohesive nation of parallel lives of Māori and Pākehā. The movement of Māori from the rural areas to the cities grew from a 'trickle to a torrent' (King, 2012, p. 417).

In the 1920s, New Zealand's Pākehā population was 95% 'British'. Those not British but European fitted quickly into the dominant culture. Those who did not, like the Chinese who had migrated with the gold rush, suffered similar discrimination as they had in Australia, were relegated to market gardening and were never really seen as part of the identity of the nation. It took until the 1990s for an apology to be offered by Helen Clark to the New Zealand Chinese for the discrimination shown towards them for over a century.

For women, both Māori and Pākehā, freedom was much more limited than for men. Having moved on abruptly from its anachronistic British civilisation of the period up until the 1980s, when shops had shut early and never opened on weekends and the cars looked like they belonged in the 1950s and 1960s, New Zealand in the 1980s caught up three decades in a very short period once international travel became faster and more affordable, and when tariffs and industrial relations policies changed to bring New Zealand business into closer alignment with other OECD countries. New Zealand's small size as a country had ensured a history of intellectuals, artists and writers going overseas to further their talents and creativity. From the 1970s it became possible to remain in New Zealand and still participate actively in the international community. Painters such as Colin McCahon, Toss Woollaston and Ralph Hotere stayed in New Zealand to work.

Contemporary New Zealand society

The beginnings of change to the steady and time-warped New Zealand Britishness began in the latter part of the 1960s, with the coming together of television, the Vietnam War, to which New Zealand had committed troops, and the collapse of wool prices with its flow-on effect on the economy. The late 1960s and 1970s saw protests related to land, women's issues, Māori issues and issues of sexuality. These immediately became national issues because they could be played out on television. Perhaps the most insightful and accessible writing on the change in the life of Pākehā growing up in the 1940s and 1950s in New Zealand and living through the turbulence of the 1970s and 1980s is the book by Michael King (1985), *Being Pakeha*.

New Zealand women began organising themselves through the early 1970s, having had their consciousness raised by the US women's movement and the growing movements in Australia, of which Germaine Greer's book *The Female Eunuch* (1970) was influential. One advantage of the smallness of New Zealand is that change can happen quickly and critical mass is relatively easily reached. New Zealand had a group of articulate, well-educated women who, when they began to speak and write, tilled the soil for New Zealand to become a world force in Women's Studies. Sandra Coney, Phillida Bunkle and Marilyn Waring became household names for several decades. In some ways this is not surprising, as New Zealand European settlement was by families, and New Zealand women appear to have been more-equal participants in public life than their eastern-coast Australian sisters. They have a history of working with and beside, rather than in service to, the men since colonisation.

Between 1984 and 1990 the Labour government of the time was sympathetic to women's issues and in 1984 it established the Ministry of Women's Affairs. It passed legislation important to raising women's status, including the *Parental Leave and Employment Protection Act 1987*, the *State Sector Act 1988*, which required equal employment opportunities, and the *Employment Equity Act 1990*. Under Helen Clark, the then Minister for Health, the *Nurse Amendment Act 1990* was passed with the full support in parliament of all women of both parties. This Act separated midwifery from nursing and hence from direct control by doctors. It enabled midwives to practise as independent practitioners and changed the face of childbirth in New Zealand.

Much of the political awareness of women's issues had been raised through the Cartwright Inquiry of 1987–9. The inquiry exposed the mistreatment of women's cervical cancer in Auckland for 20 years from 1966. The experience was captured in the book by Sandra Coney (1988) *The Unfortunate Experiment*. The inquiry resulted in a strong and vocal consumer movement in New Zealand, a disillusionment with the medical profession and a call for cultural sensitivity in healthcare (Guilliland & Pairman, 1995).

The late 1980s to the mid 1990s saw an economic revolution in New Zealand that disturbed the whole country. It was economic rationalism on a scale not witnessed anywhere in the world. All understandings of New Zealand's caring, socialist society were shed and a user-pays, individualistic, contractually based, privatised society dominated. Introduced by the Labour government but taken to an increased pitch by the Nationals, the country's assets were restructured and many jobs were lost. Many would contend that this revolution was necessary for New Zealand's economic survival; others would say there was no need for the haste or brutality of what occurred. This tumultuous time has since subsided and a new era of collaboration, cooperation and consultation has taken over as the New Zealand way of 'doing business'.

The progress of women in New Zealand is demonstrated in an unparalleled way with, at the beginning of the 21st century, a woman Governor-General, a woman Prime Minister and a woman Minister for Health, Attorney-General and Chief Justice.

Michael King (2012, pp. 519–20) ends *The Penguin History of New Zealand* with the following words:

> The Maori culture of the twenty-first century is not Maori culture frozen at 1769, nor at 1840. Nor should it be. It changed and grew dynamically according to changing needs and circumstances prior to the eighteenth century, and it continues to do so in the twenty-first century.
>
> Similarly, Pakeha culture continues to borrow and to learn from Maori. That was one of the features that made it different from its European cultures of origin. It took words and concepts (mana, tapu, whanau, taonga, haka, turangawaewae), attitudes (the traditional hospitality which, in the early nineteenth century, was so much more visible from the Maori side of the frontier than the Pakeha), ways of doing business (an increasing willingness to talk issues through to consensus in preference to dividing groups 'for' and 'against' a given motion), and rites of passage (loosening up of formerly formal and highly structured funeral services) ...
>
> And most New Zealanders, whatever their cultural backgrounds, are good-hearted, practical, commonsensical and tolerant. Those qualities are part of the national cultural capital that has in the past saved the country from the worst excesses of chauvinism and racism seen in other parts of the world. They are as sound a basis as any for optimism about the country's future.

REFLECTIVE THINKING EXERCISE

What are the issues that affect you as a woman in contemporary New Zealand society, and in what ways have these issues been influenced by the history of this country?

Modern Māori society

The caveat with which I introduced the section on modern Aboriginal society holds even more deeply for this section. I had the privilege of living in New Zealand for 4 years in the 1990s and travel frequently to that country, but I do not presume to do more here than highlight some respected texts and again attempt to assist in the development of a conceptual framework from which to further develop your personal understanding.

Unlike the circumstance of the Australian Aboriginal and Torres Strait Islander people, New Zealand Māori had, as we have seen, the benefit of having had a system of living recognisable to the European colonisers, leading to the existence of a founding document of living together, the Treaty of Waitangi, and until after the Second World War there was a prevailing sense of racial harmony, mainly related to the separation of Māori, predominantly to rural areas of the North Island. Postwar industrial development brought young Māori to the cities. In little over a generation, Māori had become a predominantly urban people.

> For the first time since the nineteenth century, the country's two major cultural traditions collided and generated the white water of confusion and hostility. Nobody was prepared for this outcome. Maori experienced discrimination in accommodation, employment and hotel bars. They were confronted with a world that was aggressively European in orientation at the very time that they had severed bonds with many sources of their own culture—traditional marae, hapu and extended families. Many of them became marginal people, weakened both by what they had relinquished and what confronted them. They were soon disproportionately represented in the ranks of convicted criminals, problem drinkers and the unemployed.
>
> (King, 1988, p. 12)

In 1936, 11.2% of Māori were urban; in 1945 it was 25.7% and in 1996 over 81% (King, 2012, p. 473). Distress and dislocation of urban Māori grew, Māori protest groups formed, and with the assistance of media attention their claims that the Treaty had not been honoured were heard. Māori were insisting on and gaining major changes in government departmental operations, and language nests—kōhanga reo—were set up to teach preschoolers Māori language. A Māori renaissance was being witnessed. The difficulties emerging from the dislocation of people and culture were graphically depicted in Alan Duff's 1990 novel *Once Were Warriors*, later made into a harrowing but illuminative film. This brought the issues of alcohol abuse and domestic violence into the open to be addressed by Māori themselves. Perhaps the most momentous of all the changes was the establishment of the Waitangi Tribunal in 1975, which over the next decade explored breaches of the Treaty retrospectively to 1840.

The 1980s resurgence of Māori pride and power has resulted in New Zealand being, and being seen to be, a bicultural country. Māori language infuses the national public communication. The 2002 film *Whale Rider* provides a compelling view of New Zealand Māori and their challenges.

REFLECTIVE THINKING EXERCISE

Your mother/grandmother believed that the best upbringing she could give you was to leave behind as much Māori culture as she could, in order for you to 'fit in' more easily. Imagine a conversation with your mother/grandmother in which you try to balance your respect for her decision with your position as a proud young Māori person for whom language and culture are paramount.

Pacific Islands people in New Zealand

No snapshot of New Zealand would be complete without acknowledgement of the dramatic increase in the number of Pacific Islands people who have made their home in New Zealand since the 1960s and 1970s. Sitting somewhere outside the bicultural notions of either Māori or Pākehā, the Pacific Islands people have become an integral part of New Zealand identity, art, music and culture. By the 2013 census there were 295,941 Pacific Islands people in New Zealand, representing 7.4% of the population, two-thirds of whom are New Zealand born. They have predominantly settled in south Auckland and north-west Wellington and, while they have made a significant contribution to rugby, they are disproportionately represented in manual labouring jobs. They experience significant health problems related to obesity and its sequelae. The six major cultural groups represented are Samoan, Cook Islander, Tongan, Niuean, Tokalauan and Fijian. Again, film can give access to contemporary issues and *Sione's Wedding* (2006) gives us a glimpse into the life of an Auckland-based Samoan family.

REFLECTIVE THINKING EXERCISE

You are a Pacific Islands woman living in south Auckland. You are asked by your teenage child how you see yourself in relation to New Zealand and your Pacific Island country of origin. How would you respond?

Conclusion: in celebration of similarity and difference

As we have seen, there are similarities between Australia and New Zealand in that their non-indigenous antecedents were predominantly British. This inevitably brings some commonality of culture. These bonds provide a facade of sameness in the countries but, as we have seen, the differences are significant.

The difference, for me, is symbolised in the flatness and solidity of one compared with the mountainous and unstable nature of the other, where green in one country is a very different colour to the green in the other. These differences are paralleled in the differing histories. New Zealand is a bicultural country with a recent history of immigration bringing it very much into the Pacific. This compares with Australia's recent history of immigration and trade, which positions it clearly as part of Asia.

The relationship between the indigenous and non-indigenous people is also a strong contrast, and the modern impacts of the indigenous cultures have been played out in very different ways. Australia describes itself as multicultural, New Zealand as bicultural. New Zealand everyday language is infused with Māori words; the Australian vernacular is barely touched by Aboriginal languages.

Perhaps the two countries are, in these early stages of the new millennium, at a point further away from each other than at any time since European colonisation. This may be symbolised by their differing natural disasters. Australia has recently been ravaged by drought, floods and fire, whilst New Zealand has been again rattled by earthquakes. Australia faces Asia, New Zealand faces the Pacific; metaphorically they stand with their backs to each other. Australia took an international position aligned with the United States, New Zealand an independent stance. The temptation of Australians to view New Zealand as a ninth state or territory of Australia could never be more deceptive. The richness of the multiple cultures in both countries is a cause for celebration and exploration, and for practitioners is essential if cultural inappropriateness is to be avoided and culturally appropriate and safe practice is to be achieved.

I hope this chapter has helped your understanding of these two countries, their similarities and differences.

Review questions

1. Summarise the impact that history and culture have on health in general and maternity services in particular.
2. Identify strategies that will improve the health and wellbeing of either Australian Aboriginal or Māori women and their babies.
3. Why is the health of Australian Aboriginals and Māori generally poorer than that of non-indigenous peoples? What can you, as a midwife, do about this situation?
4. What impact does history have on the conduct of midwifery in New Zealand and Australia?
5. In what ways has the Treaty of Waitangi affected policy development and midwifery in New Zealand?
6. How can midwives work in partnership with indigenous women to develop strategies for health gain and *appropriate* health and maternity services?
7. Compared with women from European backgrounds, Māori and Australian Aboriginal women do not have the same levels of participation in decision making, planning, development and delivery of health and maternity services. How can midwives work in partnership with indigenous women to remedy these inequities?
8. Do midwives have a responsibility to work with women to help safeguard their nations' heritage, cultural concepts, values and practices? If so, how should they go about this and why is it important?
9. From the 1800s to 1969, part-Australian Aboriginal babies and children were taken from their mothers and families and placed into government-run institutions or fostered or adopted by white families. Should all midwifery education programs include compulsory units of study aimed at increasing midwives' understanding of the effects of the Stolen Generations on Aboriginal culture, history and health? If so, why?

Online resources

Australian Government Department of Health: http://www.health.gov.au.

Australian Government Department of Health Aboriginal and Torres Strait Islander Health: http://www.health.gov.au/Indigenous.

Australian Government—History: http://www.australia.gov.au/information-and-services/culture-and-arts/history.

Australian Indigenous Health InfoNet: http://www.healthinfonet.ecu.edu.au/.

Australian National Library Aboriginal culture: https://www.creativespirits.info/.

New Zealand Māori Health, Ministry of Health: https://www.health.govt.nz/our-work/populations/maori-health.

New Zealand Ministry for Pacific Peoples: http://www.mpp.govt.nz/.

New Zealand Ministry for Women: http://women.govt.nz/.

New Zealand Ministry of Culture and Heritage—History: http://www.nzhistory.net.nz.

References

Unlike in most other chapters in this book, many of these references are more than 5 years old. This relates to the timelines by which history books are written. The editions stand for longer periods of time than do most other texts.

Australian Institute for Health and Welfare (AIHW). *Life expectancy & deaths.* 2018. Online: http://www.aihw.gov.au/deaths/life-expectancy/.

Belich J. *Paradise Reforged: A History of New Zealanders From the 1880s to the Year 2000.* Auckland: Penguin; 2001.

Belich J. *Making Peoples: A History of New Zealanders.* Auckland: Penguin; 2007.

Belich J. *The New Zealand Wars and the Victorian Interpretation of Racial Conflict.* Auckland: Penguin; 2015.

Broome R. *Aboriginal Australians.* 4th ed. Sydney: Allen & Unwin; 2010.

Brown A, Brown N. The Northern Territory Intervention: voices from the centre of the fringe. *Med J Aust.* 2007;187:621–623.

Clark M, Hooper M, Ferrier S. *History of Australia.* Sydney: Scholastic Books; 2000.

Coney S. *The Unfortunate Experiment.* Auckland: Penguin; 1988.

Curthoys A. History and identity. In: Hudson W, Bolton G, eds. *Creating Australia.* Sydney: Allen & Unwin; 1997:23–36.

Dixon M. *The Real Matilda.* 4th ed. Melbourne: Penguin; 1999.

Dodson M. Bully in the playground: a new stolen generation. In: Altman J, Hinkson M, eds. *Coercive Reconciliation.* Melbourne: Arena Publications; 2007:85–97.

Duff A. *Once Were Warriors.* Auckland: Tandem Press; 1990.

Faulks S. *Birdsong: A Novel of Love and War.* London: Random House; 1993.

Firkins P. *Australians in Nine Wars.* London: Pan Books; 1973.

Franklin M. *My Brilliant Career.* Sydney: Angus and Robertson; 1965.

Graham D, ed. *Being Whitefella.* Fremantle: Fremantle Arts Centre Press; 1994.

Greer G. *The Female Eunuch.* London: MacGibbon & Kee; 1970.

Grenville K. *The Secret River.* Melbourne: Text Publishing; 2005.

Guilliland K, Pairman S. *The Midwifery Partnership.* Wellington: Department of Nursing and Midwifery, Victoria University of Wellington; 1995.

Hudson W, Bolton G, eds. *Creating Australia.* Sydney: Allen & Unwin; 1997.

Human Rights and Equal Opportunity Commission (HREOC). *Bringing Them Home—A Guide to the Findings and Recommendations of the National Inquiry Into the Separation of Aboriginal and Torres Strait Islander Children From Their Families.* Sydney: HREOC; 1997.

Keith J. Florence Nightingale: statistician and consultant epidemiologist. *Int Nurs Rev.* 1988;35(5):147–150.

King M. *Being Pakeha.* Auckland: Hodder & Stoughton; 1985.

King M. *After the War: New Zealand Since 1945.* Auckland: Hodder & Stoughton; 1988.

King M. *The Penguin History of New Zealand.* 2nd ed. Auckland: Penguin; 2012.

McCarthy W. *Don't Fence Me In.* Sydney: Random House; 2000.

Northern Territory Government. *Little Children are Sacred: Report of the Northern Territory Board of Inquiry Into the Protection of Aboriginal Children From Sexual Abuse.* Darwin: NT Government; 2007.

Pilkington D (Nugi Garimara). *Follow the Rabbit-proof Fence.* Brisbane: University of Queensland Press; 1996.

Rudd K. Sorry speech. Apology to Australia's Indigenous peoples by Prime Minister Kevin Rudd, MP on Wednesday, 13 February 2008, at the Parliament of Australia, House of Representatives; 2008.

Sawer M, Simms M. *A Woman's Place: Women and Politics in Australia.* 2nd ed. Sydney: Allen & Unwin; 1993.

Summers A. *Damned Whores and God's Police.* Rev. ed. Melbourne: Penguin; 1994.

Summers A. *The End of Equality: Work, Babies and Women's Choices in 21st Century Australia.* Sydney: Random House; 2003.

Tedeschi M. *Myall Creek Massacre.* Sydney: Simon & Schuster; 2016.

Ward R. *The Australian Legend.* Melbourne: Oxford University Press; 1958.

Wark M. *The Virtual Republic: Australia's Cultural Wars of the 1990s.* Sydney: Allen & Unwin; 1997.

White R. *Inventing Australia: Images and Identity 1688–1980.* Sydney: Allen & Unwin; 1981.

White R. Inventing Australia, revisited. In: Hudson W, Bolton G, eds. *Creating Australia.* Sydney: Allen & Unwin; 1997:171.

Further reading

Altman J, Hinkson M, eds. *Coercive Reconciliation.* Melbourne: Arena Publications; 2007.

Belich J. *The New Zealand Wars and the Victorian Interpretation of Racial Conflict.* Auckland: Penguin; 2015.

Crotty M, Roberts DA, eds. *Turning Points in Australian History.* Sydney: University of New South Wales; 2009.

James B, Saville-Smith K. *Critical Issues in New Zealand Society: Gender, Culture and Power.* 2nd ed. Auckland: Oxford University Press; 1999.

Jones P. *Ochre and Rust: Artefacts and Encounters on Australian Frontiers.* Adelaide: Wakefield Press; 2007.

Kawharu I, ed. *Waitangi—Māori and Pakeha Perspectives of the Treaty of Waitangi.* Auckland: Oxford University Press; 1989.

King M. *The Penguin History of New Zealand.* Auckland: Penguin; 2012.

Pilkington D (Nugi Garimara). *Follow the Rabbit-proof Fence.* Brisbane: University of Queensland Press; 1996.

Reynolds H. *An Indelible Stain?* Melbourne: Viking; 2001.

Novels

Catton E. *The Luminaries.* Wellington NZ: Victoria University Press; 2013.

Chatwin B. *The Songlines.* New York: Viking; 1987.

Gee M. *Blindsight.* Auckland: Penguin; 2006.

Grace P. *Baby No-eyes.* Auckland: Penguin; 1998.

Grenville K. *The Lieutenant.* Melbourne: Text Publishing; 2008.

Hulme K. *The Bone People.* London: Picador; 1984.

Morgan S. *My Place.* Fremantle: Fremantle Arts Centre Press; 1988.

Olsson L. *Sonata for Miriam.* Auckland: Penguin; 2008.

Pilkington D. *Follow the Rabbit-proof Fence.* Brisbane: University of Queensland Press; 1996.

Scott K. *The Deadman Dance.* Sydney: Picador; 2010.

Winton T. *Dirt Music.* Sydney: Picador; 2001.

Winton T. *Breath.* Sydney: Picador; 2008.

Wright A. *The Swan Book.* Sydney: Giramondo; 2013.

Poets

Gilmore DM—Australian nationalism, the spirit of pioneering, motherhood, women's rights, history, Aboriginal welfare, treatment of prisoners, health and pensions.

Hunt S—contemporary New Zealand life.

Manhire B—contemporary New Zealand life.

Murray L—contemporary Australian life.

Noonucca O (Kathleen Walker)—Stolen Generation, reconciliation, recognition of Aboriginal vote.

Owen W—First World War.

Paterson B—early Australian life.

Films and television

Australia. Dir. Luhrmann B Northern Australia life at the time of WWII. 2008.

Caddie. Dir. Crombie D A woman's life in Australia in the depression. 1976.

First Australians. SBS, Sydney. 2008. Online: http://www.sbs.com.au/firstaustralians/.

Hunt for the Wilderpeople, Dir. Waititi T 2016.

Muriel's Wedding, Dir. Hogan PJ A humorous look at contemporary Australia. 1994.

Once Were Warriors, Dir. Tamahori L Māori poverty and domestic violence in Auckland in the 1980s. 1994.

Rabbit-proof Fence, Dir. Noyce P Children of the Stolen Generation finding their way back home. 2002.

Red Dog, Dir. Stenders K 2011.

Romulus, my Father, Dir. Roxburgh R Australian immigrant's son's story of his father. 2007.

Samson and Delilah, Dir. Thornton W Love story dealing with life in a remote Aboriginal community and the ways in which one young couple manage to escape from a mundane existence. 2008.

Sione's Wedding (or Samoan Wedding), Dir. Graham C Auckland-based Samoan family wedding. 2006.

Sunday Too Far Away, Dir. Hannam K Australian rural life in the early 1970s. 1976.

The Castle, Dir. Sitch R Urban Australian life. 1997.

The Dressmaker, Dir. Moorhouse J 2015.

The Piano, Dir. Campion J Early New Zealand settlement by Europeans. 1993.

They're a Weird Mob, Dir. Powell M Australia in the 1950s with Mediterranean migration. 1966.

Whale Rider, Dir. Caro N Intergenerational cultural clashes and resolution, a gentler and more hopeful Once Were Warriors. 2002.

CHAPTER 2

Contemporary Australian and New Zealand midwifery and maternity services

Alison Eddy and Sally K Tracy

LEARNING OUTCOMES

Learning outcomes for this chapter are:

1. To discuss the role of midwives within the New Zealand and Australian maternity services
2. To describe the structure and funding of New Zealand's maternity services
3. To describe the structure and funding of Australia's maternity services
4. To explain how funding models affect the provision of services
5. To discuss the outcomes of care for women and babies in both countries.

CHAPTER OVERVIEW

This chapter provides an overview of the development and current structure of the New Zealand and Australian maternity systems. It briefly discusses the role of midwives and identifies how the maternity service structure in each country supports, or does not support, the provision of midwife-led maternity care.

KEY TERMS

annualised salary agreements
District Health Boards
government financing

health systems
lead maternity carer (LMC)
National Maternity Collection

Medicare
midwifery models

INTRODUCTION

Both Aotearoa New Zealand (NZ) and Australia provide universal healthcare coverage within public **health systems** that combine taxation-based **government financing** with service provision by state-owned healthcare providers. Both countries also have private sector health service providers with a mixture of public and private (insurance-based and self-pay) financing.

Australia spends about 25% more on healthcare per capita (at purchasing power parity) than does New Zealand (OECD, 2021). Both countries have similar regulatory frameworks for the use of pharmaceuticals and medical devices and are working to establish common processes for their regulation (Streat & Munn, 2012).

All Australian and New Zealand women have access to 'free' maternity care. However, in Australia differences in the quality and quantity of these services, especially with regard to community-based midwifery, home birth and caseload midwifery care, mean that many must pay extra for services that are better able to meet their needs. For example, until very recently Western Australia was the only state to offer a publicly funded midwife-led home-birth service. In other states, some women who prefer this model of care may have access to publicly funded services if they 'conform' to rigid risk criteria. Most women, however, opt to pay for the services of a private midwife. Similarly, some women may have access to caseload midwifery through the public hospital system; however, these models very often exclude women who have complex pregnancies that require additional medical expertise. More recently, a Health Legislation Amendment (Midwives and Nurse Practitioners) Bill (2009) established a model of private (fee for service) midwifery care where women may access an eligible midwife to provide the continuum of care (see Chs 13 and 14). All these systems will be discussed in detail within this chapter.

The picture is very different in New Zealand, where all maternity care is funded publicly. All women expect to have their own **lead maternity carer** (LMC) and the majority (94.8%) are able to have a midwife LMC (Ministry of Health (MOH), 2021). Women can choose where they give birth, with primary unit and home birth supported and fully funded. Women who choose midwives or general practitioners (GPs) as their LMC are also able to freely access specialist care should the need arise. Women who do not require referral to specialist care can still choose a private obstetrician to be their LMC instead of the public obstetric service, although the private obstetrician is likely to charge a fee and be accessible only in some main cities.

CONTEMPORARY MATERNITY SERVICES IN NEW ZEALAND

The New Zealand health system

It is important to understand how the maternity system fits into the overall health services. Prior to 2021, the government and the Minister of Health (served by the Ministry of Health) set strategy and made policy and funding decisions. These were then implemented by the 20 **District Health Boards** (DHBs) spread throughout New Zealand (Fig. 2.1). With each DHB funded on a population basis, funding reflected the numbers and make-up of its community of people, and each board was responsible for ensuring that the population received the best possible range, mix and types of services its funding allows.

Primary care

General practice services were under the umbrella of Primary Health Organisations (PHOs) which were contracted by the DHBs. The PHOs provided primary care and coordinated appropriate referrals to the hospital services. People enrolled with a PHO in their area. Most PHOs were centred on GP and practice nurse services despite the original vision of a more integrated multidisciplinary organisation (see Ch 6).

Community (primary) maternity and Well Child services remained outside the management of the regional DHBs and the PHOs, and were funded nationally by the Ministry of Health.

Health service reforms (2021 onwards)

The system described above has been complex and somewhat fragmented. In April 2021, the Minister of Health announced major structural changes to the New Zealand health service. Reasons for the reforms were:

- *inequitable outcomes for Māori, Pacific communities and disabled people*
- *insufficient investment in primary and community care*
- *limited national planning*
- *resulting in a postcode lottery, meaning that the health care an individual receives depends on the place they lived.*

(Beehive.govt.nz, 2021)

The reforms are expected to simplify the health service, improve equity, enable more consistency, and coordinate healthcare with changes ongoing from 2021 (Fig. 2.2). The Ministry of Health will be focused on stewardship, strategy and policy. Commissioning and funding of services will be undertaken by a new entity titled Health NZ (at the time of writing) which will be responsible for the day to day running of the whole health system. There will be four regional divisions and a range of district offices (three in the North Island and one in the South Island) who will ensure that decisions reflect the population needs.

A new Māori Health Authority will support the Ministry in shaping system policy and strategy to ensure performance for Māori and will commission and fund healthcare to ensure the needs and expectations of Māori communities are central to the provision of care.

A Public Health Agency will provide national leadership on public health policy, strategy and intelligence. All public health units will be brought into the Health NZ entity to form a national public health service.

Primary and community care will come under locality networks of healthcare providers. These will include GPs,

Our health system is relatively complex; it involves many organisations, each with their own roles and relationships. But at the highest level, our health system broadly works like this:

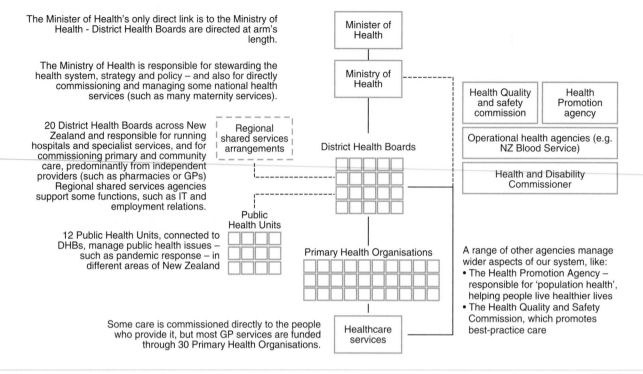

The Minister of Health's only direct link is to the Ministry of Health - District Health Boards are directed at arm's length.

The Ministry of Health is responsible for stewarding the health system, strategy and policy – and also for directly commissioning and managing some national health services (such as many maternity services).

20 District Health Boards across New Zealand and responsible for running hospitals and specialist services, and for commissioning primary and community care, predominantly from independent providers (such as pharmacies or GPs) Regional shared services agencies support some functions, such as IT and employment relations.

12 Public Health Units, connected to DHBs, manage public health issues – such as pandemic response – in different areas of New Zealand

Some care is commissioned directly to the people who provide it, but most GP services are funded through 30 Primary Health Organisations.

A range of other agencies manage wider aspects of our system, like:
• The Health Promotion Agency – responsible for 'population health', helping people live healthier lives
• The Health Quality and Safety Commission, which promotes best-practice care

FIGURE 2.1 MOH diagram of New Zealand health service prior to reforms
(Source: Department of the Prime Minister and Cabinet (DPMC): https://dpmc.govt.nz/sites/default/files/2021-04/heallth-reform-white-paper-summary-apr21.pdf)

Instead of that complex system, the health system of the future will look more like:

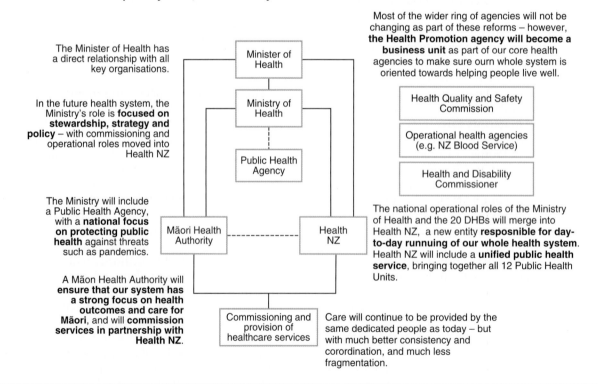

The Minister of Health has a direct relationship with all key organisations.

In the future health system, the Ministry's role is **focused on stewardship, strategy and policy** – with commissioning and operational roles moved into Health NZ

The Ministry will include a Public Health Agency, with a **national focus on protecting public health** against threats such as pandemics.

A Mãon Health Authority will **ensure that our system has a strong focus on health outcomes and care for Mãori**, and will **commission services in partnership with Health NZ.**

Most of the wider ring of agencies will not be changing as part of these reforms – however, **the Health Promotion agency will become a business unit** as part of our core health agencies to make sure ourn whole system is oriented towards helping people live well.

The national operational roles of the Ministry of Health and the 20 DHBs will merge into Health NZ, a new entity **resposnible for day-to-day runnuing of our whole health system.** Health NZ will include a **unified public health service**, bringing together all 12 Public Health Units.

Care will continue to be provided by the same dedicated people as today – but with much better consistency and coordination, and much less fragmentation.

FIGURE 2.2 Move to new configuration of health service provision in New Zealand from 2022
(Source: Department of the Prime Minister and Cabinet (DPMC): https://dpmc.govt.nz/sites/default/files/2021-04/heallth-reform-white-paper-summary-apr21.pdf)

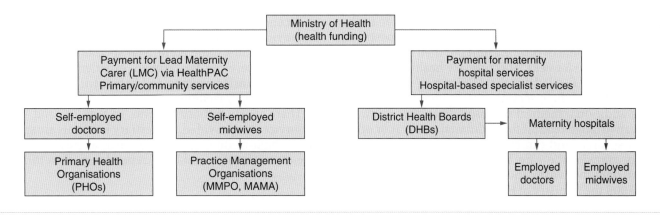

FIGURE 2.3 Funding mechanisms for New Zealand's maternity services. MAMA = Mothers and Midwives Association; MMPO = Midwifery and Maternity Providers Organisation

district nurses, allied health, maternity care and Well Child providers. The aim is that care will be seamless and accessible with digital health records and care pathways that support care closer to home. The next few years will see these changes implemented.

The maternity service

The maternity service in New Zealand takes an integrated and women-centred partnership approach. The service is placed within the primary health arena in recognition that birth is a physiological, normal life event and that women and their families should direct the care (Pairman, 2005, 2010). The service specifications are explicit and within a set budget per woman. Standardised referral guidelines give the framework for consultation and transfer of care to hospital specialists if necessary (MOH, 2017). Fig. 2.3 sets out the current funding mechanisms of New Zealand's maternity services, however this may change in July 2022, when Health NZ and the Māori health authority are formally established.

Vision for the maternity service

The 1990 Nurses Amendment Act, the maternity consumer movement and various health sector changes through the 1990s provided a context that was favourable to the establishment of New Zealand's current maternity service. The New Zealand College of Midwives has provided consensus guidance to midwives from 1993 on a collective philosophy, code of ethics and standards of practice (*Midwives Handbook for Practice*, NZCOM, 2018).

The government's initial vision for the maternity service was set out under Section 88 of the *Public Health and Disability Act 2000*:

Each woman, and her whanau, will have every opportunity to have a fulfilling outcome to her pregnancy and childbirth, through the provision of services that are safe and based on partnership, information and choice. Pregnancy and childbirth are a normal life-stage for most women, with appropriate additional care available to those women who require it. A

Lead Maternity Carer chosen by the woman with responsibility for assessment of her needs, planning her care with her and the care of her baby and being responsible for ensuring provision of Maternity Services, is the cornerstone of maternity care in New Zealand.

(MOH, 2000, p. 11)

Although the review of Section 88 in 2005 rearranged the wording to suit the contracting style favoured at the time, the vision above has remained intact.

The influence of New Zealand's pioneering women and midwives is obvious in this vision (Mein Smith, 1986; Parkes, 1991). The health system, including maternity, is overseen by a strong code of patient's rights and a culture of informed consent. In 2021, New Zealand has a free maternity service with equity of access for women to all the levels of care required. These levels of care cover primary care in the community and hospital-based specialist or secondary and tertiary care.

Equitable access can be challenging for rural women, women who identify as Māori and Pasifika and women from low sociodemographic deciles. Māori as the Tangata Whenua are the indigenous people of Aotearoa New Zealand, with Te Tiriti o Waitangi the founding document which sets out an agreement between the Crown and Māori. Principles within te Tiriti include partnership, participation and protection but indigenous determinants of health have resulted in significant issues for Māori who lag behind in key health status indicators (see Ch. 10). The health reforms signal the importance of ensuring that Hauora Māori will lead the system and make real change for Māori.

When a woman becomes pregnant she chooses an LMC (a midwife, a GP or an obstetrician) to provide and coordinate her maternity care, develop a care plan with her and attend her labour, birth and postpartum period of up to 6 weeks. The New Zealand College of Midwives has set up a website to help women identify a midwife LMC in their area (https://www.findyourmidwife.co.nz/). The LMC service is a primary health one and therefore is provided mainly in the community. Most antenatal care is in women's homes or in midwives' community clinics.

If not giving birth at home, the majority of women in the first 12 to 48 hours following birth have their postnatal care in the hospital or birthing unit but then receive visits at home for 4 to 6 weeks. This primary health service has been centrally funded by the Ministry of Health, and LMCs claim for their service fees. When a woman requires additional medical or hospital care her midwife-LMC can arrange referral for additional medical or other specialist carers and can continue to provide midwifery care, or transfer the care to a hospital team including obstetricians, midwives and paediatricians.

In 2009 the Ministry of Health consulted on a national maternity strategy as a result of disquiet in the sector over the variances between DHBs and inequity of service provision as a result of workforce shortages. The consultation reaffirmed the original maternity services vision of a woman-centred LMC model of care that is based on childbirth as usually a physiological life event and this vision later underpinned the Maternity Quality Initiative (MOH, 2011). As part of this initiative a set of maternity standards was published in 2011 and standard two states that 'maternity services ensure a woman-centred approach that acknowledges pregnancy and childbirth as a normal life stage' (MOH, 2011, p. 6).

Place of birth

(See also Ch. 7.)

New Zealand women have a variety of options as to where they can give birth. Although there are no universal booking criteria for place of birth, the national consultation and referral guidelines provide a screening tool to assist women to make appropriate choices. The maternity facilities or hospitals and their associated services are funded separately from the primary LMC budget.

Birth at home is a mainstream government-supported and funded option. The LMC is almost always a midwife. While consumer-led home-birth associations support many women, the majority of women today who choose home birth do so as a natural matter of course and no longer view it as a 'fringe' option. Between 3% and 4% of all New Zealand women have their babies at home although there is a wide range between regions of 1%–8.3% (MOH, 2021). The rates of home birth are similar in both high- and low-decile areas.

There are 54 primary birthing or maternity units throughout New Zealand, most located in rural or provincial towns, although women in most big cities also have access to a primary birthing unit either via a DHB or at a privately owned but publicly funded enterprise. A primary unit provides in-house midwifery services for labour, birth and immediate postpartum care. Women have no access to onsite obstetric and medical specialists. Approximately 10.6 % of births in 2019 were in primary units (MOH, 2021). There is an ethnic difference in usage of primary, secondary and tertiary facilities, with Māori women more likely to birth in primary facilities, whereas Pacific, Indian and Asian women are more likely to utilise tertiary hospitals (Hunter et al., 2011; MOH, 2021).

Secondary facilities or hospitals are generally found in provincial towns or the smaller cities. The secondary service provides some additional specialist obstetric and midwifery services for women experiencing complications, but transfers women and babies with intensive care needs to tertiary facilities.

There are six tertiary facilities in New Zealand. While all services are provided, the tertiary hospitals are specialists in high-technology services such as neonatal intensive care, infertility and high-dependency obstetric care.

Section 88, Public Health and Disability Act 2000

Section 88 of the *New Zealand Public Health and Disability Act 2000* is the legislative framework that outlines the model of care and gives notice of the terms and conditions for the provision of primary maternity services. The Ministry of Health originally set these terms, conditions and fees with the New Zealand College of Midwives (the College) and the New Zealand Medical Association. However, in 2007 the right to negotiate was removed and as a consequence the funding levels have not kept pace. Funding levels remained static for several years, and during this time there were increased public health screening requirements. These along with the impact of DHB midwifery workforce shortages and the changing demographics of pregnant women have all added to the workload of midwives without additional funding sources to support this work.

The Primary Maternity Services Notice, or Section 88 as it is generally referred to, provides a nationally consistent set of service specifications for midwives, GPs, obstetricians and radiologists (Box 2.1). It covers issues such as arrangements for antenatal, labour and birth, and postnatal care but does not describe specific aspects of practice; rather it provides a generic blueprint for service delivery. The College provides a detailed framework for midwifery practice (NZCOM, 2015). This includes a statement of philosophy, definition of midwifery scope of practice, a code of ethics, detailed standards of practice and decision points for midwifery care (see Ch. 13).

Section 88 specifications

The Section Notice in general:
- specifies all aspects of services to be provided by LMCs—it outlines all expected services from the woman's first contact with the maternity services until discharge and referral of her baby to the Well Child services. If the LMC cannot provide any aspect of care, they must ensure that others provide the care
- identifies expectations of practitioners to participate in professional quality assurance mechanisms such as the College's Midwifery Standards Review
- sets out prices and payment rates—the Notice has a comprehensive and integrated pricing structure that recognises factors such as miscarriage, place of birth, and rural and travel requirements

Box 2.1   Section 88 specifications

The service specifications of the Section 88 notice provide that:

- LMCs receive written authorisation from the Ministry of Health to provide maternity services, as authorised practitioners, in order to be able to work under the conditions of the notice.
- Payment is made to authorised practitioners via HealthPAC, the business unit of the Ministry of Health, which administers payment for primary care services.
- Each women chooses an LMC, who works with the woman to assess, plan and provide her primary maternity care, coordinate and arrange access to additional care as required. This allows for continuity of carer throughout the maternity care episode.
- An LMC can be either a midwife, a GP with a diploma in obstetrics, or an obstetrician.
- Care is from the woman's registration with an LMC to 4–6 weeks postpartum according to clinical need. There are four modules of care, with the expectation that all four will be provided by the same carer.

- The payment structure is modular and each module of care is capped at a set price but there are a variety of mechanisms to enable LMC work to be recompensed if it falls outside these module definitions.
- Childbirth education other than the usual information provided by the woman's individual LMC also has a separate budget,
- A woman can have only one LMC at a time but there is provision for her to change at any time.

The choice of LMC depends to some extent on where a woman lives, as the full range of options is not available in all areas. There is a nationwide government-subsidised service provided by the New Zealand College of Midwives called 'Find your midwife' that gives women information on LMCs available in their area (https//www.findyourmidwife.co.nz). A full copy of the Maternity Advice Notice is accessible from the Ministry of Health website (http://www.moh.govt.nz) and more information about midwifery practice in New Zealand is available from the NZCOM website (http://www.midwife.org.nz).

LMC = lead maternity carer.

- requires the use of the referral guidelines—these guidelines were drawn up by all maternity providers and professionals in 1996 and have been reviewed regularly with little substantial change. At the time of writing they are under review again. They are a comprehensive set of guidelines on conditions/circumstances that require referral to be discussed with the woman in a three-way conversation between her and her family, the LMC and the obstetrician or specialist to whom she is being referred or transferred. A primary referral is optional and can be with a GP, another midwife or allied health professional; a consultation referral requires the LMC to recommend to the woman that she consult a specialist; and a transfer referral requires an LMC to recommend to a woman that there is a transfer of clinical responsibility to specialists at the secondary or tertiary service. An emergency referral is where an emergency necessitates the immediate transfer of clinical responsibility to the most appropriate practitioner available
- requires the LMC to have an access to hospital facilities agreement—this is an agreement between the hospital facility and the LMC on the conditions under which the LMC can access the hospital for her (over 99% of midwives are women) clients
- requires claimants to provide information on the service they provided, including outcomes, in order to claim their fees.

Women and their families have a range of LMC choices (Fig. 2.4), including the following:

1. *Self-employed community midwife*—midwives specialise in attending women and their family for 'normal' or

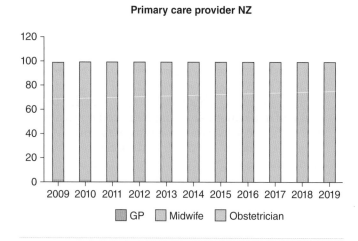

Primary care provider NZ

FIGURE 2.4 The choices women make regarding LMC in New Zealand
(Source: https://minhealthnz.shinyapps.io/Maternity_report_webtool/)

physiological pregnancy and birth. They can provide all care during pregnancy, labour, birth and postpartum. Care may be in the woman's home or in the midwife's clinic rooms. Midwives can also provide care for women with complicated maternity conditions alongside a specialist in either the public or the private health system. In 2019, 94.8% of LMCs were midwives (MOH, 2021).

2. *Community caseloading employed LMC midwives*—very few maternity hospitals now offer primary LMC services compared with the early years of the midwifery LMC model development. Most maternity hospitals

do not compete with self-employed midwives by forming teams from primary care. They are increasingly working to support the community-based model provided by LMCs as this is what most women have come to expect. Primary midwifery teams, where they do exist, are more likely to reflect the inability of the maternity hospital to attract midwife LMCs to the area. In such models, women receive care from a small team of midwives—generally no more than three or four, but possibly up to six.

Regretfully, very few maternity hospitals offer full continuity of midwifery care to women with complex conditions (e.g. women with diabetes). When they do the continuity is generally provided by midwives in the antenatal and postnatal periods. Women give birth at the hospital attended by core midwives on duty.

3. *Family doctor or GP*—GPs can also provide care for normal pregnancy and birth. Some also provide care for women with some existing medical problems that may complicate pregnancy, such as diabetes or asthma. GPs provide care in their practice rooms/surgery, attend labour when needed and are present for the birth with a self-employed midwife or a core/staff midwife. They share postnatal care with hospital- or self-employed midwives. In 2019 some 0.1% of LMCs were GPs (MOH, 2021).

4. *Hospital specialists*—hospital specialists provide care for women whose pregnancies and births involve complications. Other hospital staff (such as midwives, registrars and house surgeons) will be involved in the care. Pregnancy care is usually provided by the hospital team at hospital antenatal clinics but is often also in collaboration or a shared care arrangement with the LMC midwife or GPs in the community, particularly if the woman lives rurally. Care during labour and birth is provided by hospital staff or a self-employed midwife under the supervision of the specialist who is on duty at the time.

5. *Private obstetrician*—obstetricians specialise in complications during pregnancy and birth but can also provide medical care for women experiencing a normal pregnancy. They attend labour as needed and are present for the birth with a core/staff or self-employed midwife. They share care with hospital or self-employed midwives. Care provided by private obstetricians usually involves a cost to the woman. Overall in New Zealand, obstetricians make up 4.9% of LMCs (MOH, 2021) with most private obstetric services situated in Auckland. In Auckland National Women's Hospital, 18.3% of women who gave birth were registered with an obstetrician LMC (Auckland District Health Board, 2020).

6. *Core or hospital staff midwives*—if women are having their babies in a hospital with their own LMC, their LMCs rely on core midwives to facilitate the experience for them as they move from a community to hospital service. The core midwife is on rostered duties for either 8 or 12 hours depending on hospital employment practices. She develops the knowledge and expertise to work with women who often have complex conditions requiring a variety of ongoing monitoring and obstetric management. Women with these complex conditions continue to require midwifery support and midwifery care (Currie & Barber, 2016). The hospital midwife provides support and back-up for the LMC midwife and full midwifery care for women with medical LMCs.

LMC midwives have a range of experience. Some will continue to provide care in all situations and some will transfer the care of the woman to the hospital obstetric team because of the woman's need for more intensive obstetric care. The core midwife can then provide the secondary or tertiary midwifery services for those women, with the LMC midwife remaining if appropriate.

Section 88 funding levels

In August 2015 the New Zealand College of Midwives took a claim against the government to the high court under the NZ Bill of Rights, citing gender discrimination against midwifery. The antecedent for this case was static fees for a number of years, during which the requirements on midwife LMCs had increased considerably, as had the costs of providing a community-based service. The case was adjourned in favour of mediation in September 2016. The Human Rights Commission mediated and over a period of several months the parties reached agreement on some funds for emergency locum relief and pay increases of 8.5% as a short-term adjustment while the whole payment and funding system was redesigned. The parties (the Ministry of Health and the New Zealand College of Midwives) agreed that a co-design process involving both parties would be used to arrive at the most appropriate funding model for LMC midwifery services. In a letter to College members on 5th April 2017, the College team explained that the agreement specified that any new model 'needs to remain free for women, support high quality, accessible and acceptable care, should eliminate gender discrimination and ensure equity and fairness for midwives in line with the government's workforce equity principles'. These principles were won in a historical pay equity case taken by the aged care workers in 2016. The co-design process between the Ministry of Health and the College was based on these pay equity principles and sought to address the historic underfunding of LMC midwifery. The co-design team agreed on a preferred funding model which blended the best of fee-for-service and salaried-time approaches while retaining the right of midwives to be self-employed. The self-employed midwifery model is key to midwifery autonomy and to women's control over their pregnancy and birth choices. The co-design team proposed that, for the first time, midwives will have their on-call and business costs met and that additional funding will be available when extra time and travel is required. Unfortunately, in spite of a legally binding agreement which committed the Ministry of Health to progress the implementation of the new model, this did not occur. Some elements of the model were implemented in 2018, including a Second Midwife fee being added to Section 88 and an annual Business Contribution payment (a contribution towards the costs of self-employment). The Ministry acknowledged that it had breached the agreement with a public apology, and a new agreement between the parties was reached in December 2018. This agreement committed the Ministry to having the new contract model in place by July 2020. However, the New Zealand government's Health and Disability System Review has proven to be a major barrier to the new contract model being implemented. In July 2020, instead of a new contract, a large increase of funds were allocated into Section 88 (enabling fee increases) and the terms and conditions of the Notice were revised. This is intended as an interim measure, while the New Zealand health system is reconfigured over the coming years. Since 2015 to 2021 due to the College's initial court case and subsequent mediation agreements, Section 88 fees have increased by nearly 40%. In addition, the terms and conditions of the Section 88 Notice have improved, with midwives now being able to claim a Second Midwife fee, and for elements of care which have been previously under-funded or even unfunded. In spite of these improvements, the Ministry has twice breached its legally binding agreement to implement a new contract model. The College is pursuing further legal action at the time of writing.

New Zealand midwifery workforce

Understanding the funding and contractual nature of the service is essential to understanding how New Zealand's midwife-led and woman-centred maternity service successfully developed to the model in existence today.

Midwifery was New Zealand's first health workforce 'redesign'—that is, the first non-medical discipline in New Zealand to achieve full practice autonomy, full prescribing rights, referral to diagnostics and access to hospital facilities and government fees for services. This integrated service is the result not only of the professional changes enabled by the 1990 Nurses Amendment Act, which reinstated midwifery autonomy, but also of the health reforms of the 90s that changed the way in which maternity services were funded.[a]

Midwives today have many work options including self-employed LMC practice, employed roles as core midwives, specialist midwives (e.g. diabetes) educators, administrators and managers, professional advisors and researchers. Overall numbers of practising midwives have increased from 2107 in 2002 to 3274 in 2020 (Midwifery Council of New Zealand (MCNZ) Te Tatau o te Whare Kahu, 2020). The proportion of midwives identifying caseload midwifery as their primary work situation have remained fairly stable at 39.9% in 2002 and 38.1% in 2020 (MCNZ Te Tatau o te Whare Kahu, 2020). So too have the numbers of midwives for whom core midwifery is the main work type: 52.9% in 2002 and 49.0% in 2020 (MCNZ Te Tatau o te Whare Kahu, 2020; Nursing Council of New Zealand, 2004). The flexibility of midwifery is evident through the numbers who practise part time (46.4% reported working 32 or fewer hours per week in 2020) and those who have more than one work type (21.0% in 2020). The numbers of midwives with practising certificates who work in other roles remain low in 2020, with 3.0% in administration, 2.1% in tertiary education, 1.2% in DHB education, 0.4% in research and 0.6% in professional advice and policy (MCNZ Te Tatau o te Whare Kahu, 2020).

Midwives must meet both regulatory and professional requirements and the midwifery profession has established a number of structures that support midwives in their roles as LMC or core midwives (see Ch. 13).

Workforce challenges

Workforce shortages cause many hospitals to use the LMC system as a mechanism to cost-shift expensive secondary care services onto the community LMC workforce without any supportive systems for collaborative care.

Outcomes of midwifery care in New Zealand

The move to continuity of midwifery care that started in the 1990s (with the amendment to the Nurses Act) has meant that hundreds of thousands of New Zealand women have received continuity of care from a midwife. It is now known that continuity of care contributes to improved short-, medium- and long-term outcomes for mothers and babies (Sandall et al., 2016) but this evidence was not available during the 1990s, resulting in ongoing surveillance and critique of the New Zealand maternity system and midwifery. New Zealand has developed robust data collection systems, based on the claiming data from LMCs, and maternity data from the District Health Boards and population data from Statistics New Zealand.

An independent report commissioned in 2012 by the Ministry of Health on comparisons of New Zealand maternity services with the maternity services of six other countries (Australia, Canada, Ireland, the Netherlands, the United Kingdom and the United States) found that New Zealand has similar or better outcomes across a wide range of measures, such as maternal and neonatal mortality, consumer satisfaction and accessibility of services (Rowland, 2012). It also found that the role of GPs within these countries had changed as midwifery was strengthened to fill workforce shortages. They found that the strengths of the NZ system were:

- universal access to maternity care (both primary and secondary) and well-established referral guidelines
- a strong midwifery workforce and stable maternity service
- the LMC model as the foundation for strong community-based care, continuity of care and public health
- strong advocacy for the different professions and improved relationships between these groups
- high levels of consumer satisfaction
- established and effective reporting and review of all maternity-related mortality through the Perinatal and Maternal Mortality Review Committee (PMMRC).

These findings highlight the social and public health benefits that can be achieved with continuity of care and autonomous midwifery as well as effective clinical outcomes for women and their babies.

Increasing demand and complexity

New Zealand has led the world in supporting continuity of care and access to midwifery services for all women during childbirth (Grigg et al., 2013); however, years of inadequate funding leading to midwifery workforce shortages, increasing demand for midwifery care and the social determinants of health also have the potential to influence maternity outcomes.

The demands of the health system continue to grow, with the majority of women registering in the first trimester with midwives as their Lead Maternity Carer, making this the foundation of maternity care in New Zealand (Fig. 2.5).

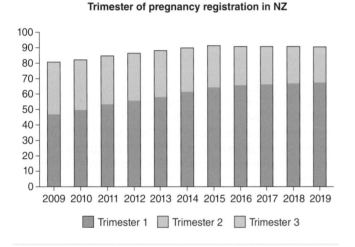

Trimester of pregnancy registration in NZ

■ Trimester 1 ■ Trimester 2 □ Trimester 3

FIGURE 2.5 The percentage of women giving birth with an LMC, 2009–18: registrations by trimester
(Source: https://www.health.govt.nz/system/files/documents/publications/report_on_maternity_further_information.pdf)

There has been a concerted effort within the health sector to encourage women to register before 10 weeks of gestation to support assessment and optimising of health in early pregnancy. The last decade has seen some positive shifts in first trimester LMC registration, with higher increases among groups with lower access. Between 2009 and 2018 the rate of first trimester LMC registration doubled for Pacific women, and increased by 64% for Māori, 82% for Indian women, 62% for Asian women and 31% for European / other ethnicity women. The number of young women (<20 years old) registering in the first trimester increased by 50% over the decade, and the proportion of women living in deprivation quintile 5 increased by 69%. Significant inequities remain, with the system continuing to work best for higher resourced, older and Pākehā women. Facilitating equitable access to care and responding to te Tiriti responsibilities is a key focus for the New Zealand College of Midwives as it works with the Ministry and DHBs on how the projected health reforms will support the diversity of New Zealand's maternity population.

Changing demographics of women

The proportion of women who smoke during pregnancy has reduced from 13.7% in 2009 to 8.4% in 2019. During this time obesity has increased from 22.1% in 2009 to 28.1% in 2019. Ethnic diversity has changed with an increasing proportion of women identifying as Asian, and within this group Indian ethnicity has increased from 2.9% to 7.6% (MOH, 2021; see Figs 2.6 and 2.7).

Interventions during birth

Over the years, the proportion of women having labour augmented reduced from 28.7% in 2009 to 20.5% in 2019,

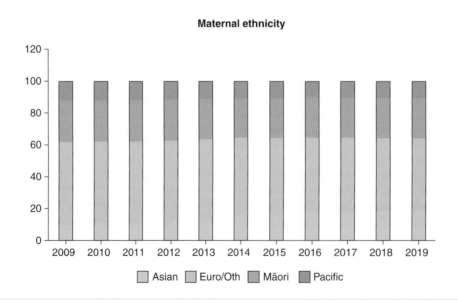

Maternal ethnicity

□ Asian □ Euro/Oth ■ Māori ■ Pacific

FIGURE 2.6 Maternal ethnicity in New Zealand 2009–19
(Source: https://www.health.govt.nz/system/files/documents/publications/report_on_maternity_further_information.pdf)

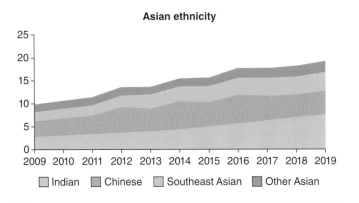

Asian ethnicity

□ Indian □ Chinese □ Southeast Asian ■ Other Asian

FIGURE 2.7 Asian ethnicity in New Zealand
(Source: https://www.health.govt.nz/system/files/documents/publications/
report_on_maternity_further_information.pdf)

but the proportion having their labour induced increased from 19.6% to 27.1% (Fig. 2.8). Women who identified as Indian or Pacific ethnicity had the highest proportions of labour induction (37% and 31.2% respectively). There has also been an increase in the proportion of women using an epidural during labour from 24.8% in 2009 to 27.1% in 2019 with 42.4% of these women primiparous. Women of Indian and Asian ethnicity had a higher proportion of epidural use (42.1% and 34.5% respectively) (MOH, 2021).

Type of birth

The proportion of women who had a vaginal birth has reduced from 67% in 2009 to 59.8% in 2019 (Fig. 2.9).

Women who identified as Māori (70.9%) and Pacific (64.4%) ethnicity had a higher proportion of spontaneous vaginal birth than those of other ethnicities. Women who identified as Indian (42.6%) or Asian (51.0%) ethnicity had the lowest proportion of spontaneous vaginal birth. The proportion of women who had a caesarean section increased from 24.2% in 2009 to 29.1% in 2019 while the assisted birth rate has remained relatively unchanged.

Other outcomes

The majority of women receive between 11 and 15 visits during their pregnancy, which supports the building of the partnership relationship, and 71.5% receive between six and nine home visits for postnatal assessment of the mother and baby (NZCOM, 2016).

The preterm birth rate has been static over the last ten years at 7.7% in 2019, although this is higher for women over 40 years of age (10%), women of Māori (9.1%) and Pacific (8.1%) ethnicity, and women living in socioeconomic deprivation (9.3% deprivation group 5) (MOH, 2021). Exclusive breastfeeding at 2 weeks has been relatively static at 68.3%, with 17% of women partially breastfeeding and 6.8% artificial milk feeding.

The proportion of babies whose birthweight was under 2.5 kg is another statistic that has been static over the last ten years (6.3%) but this again varies depending on age (higher for those under 20 and over 40 years), ethnicity (higher for women of Indian ethnicity) and socioeconomic deprivation (higher for women living in deprivation levels 4 and 5).

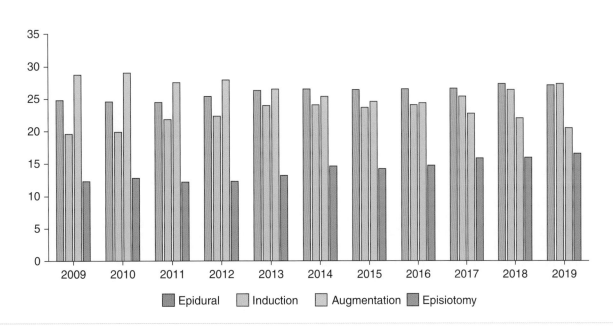

■ Epidural □ Induction □ Augmentation ■ Episiotomy

FIGURE 2.8 The changing rate of interventions in birth in New Zealand 2009–18
(Source: https://www.health.govt.nz/system/files/documents/publications/report_on_maternity_further_information.pdf)

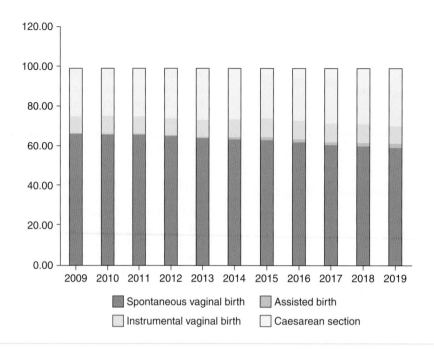

FIGURE 2.9 Mode of birth in New Zealand 2009–19
(Source: https://www.health.govt.nz/system/files/documents/publications/report_on_maternity_further_information.pdf)

International comparisons

Comparison of some key outcomes provides a better understanding of the similarities and differences between the New Zealand, Australian (Australian Institure of Health and Welfare, 2020) and United Kingdom (UK) maternity services (DOH, 2019). New Zealand (Fig. 2.10) is comparable in terms of early pregnancy registration, and low birthweight babies. However, New Zealand has proportionately more women with a BMI > 30, yet a lower caesarean section and induction of labour rate. Australia has higher rates of caesarean section and induction of labour, lower BMI but similar first trimester registration and low birth weight (< 2.5 kg) rates to the UK.

A review of the frequency of caesarean sections globally found a doubling of caesarean section births between the years 2000 and 2015 (Boerma et al., 2018). Some countries / regions reported rates of 44% (Latin America and Caribbean). Caesarean sections are often a lifesaving intervention for the woman and her baby when medically indicated, but the optimal rate remains unclear and overuse has not demonstrated benefit but can increase harms (Betrán et al., 2018).

The short and long-term effects of caesarean section involve increased maternal mortality and morbidity when compared to vaginal birth, as well as increased risk for subsequent pregnancies of uterine rupture, abnormal placentation, ectopic pregnancy, stillbirth and preterm birth (Sandall et al., 2018). Understanding the reasons for caesarean section is necessary to ensure that benefits outweigh the harms, with a range of strategies being used globally to reduce unnecessary caesarean section (Betrán et al., 2018). These include external cephalic version for

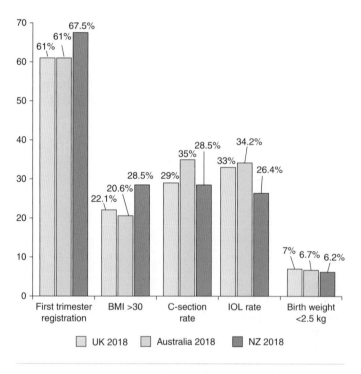

FIGURE 2.10 Comparison of some key outcomes between the New Zealand, Australian and the UK maternity services
(Source: https://www.health.govt.nz/system/files/documents/publications/report_on_maternity_further_information.pdf)

breech presentation, vaginal breech births where appropriate, and support for women to have a vaginal birth after caesarean section. Other strategies include labour support and midwife-led care. Caseload midwifery has been found to be the most cost-effective strategy when compared to auditing each case or routine induction of labour at 39 weeks (Callander et al., 2019).

Determinants of health — challenges in maternity care

In New Zealand there are increasingly complex health issues that can affect the health of pregnant women, such as increasing BMI and diabetes, as well as complexities in the social determinants of health and wellbeing that can increase the time midwives need to spend with women (New Zealand Institute of Economic Research, 2020). An increasing public health role (more screening requirements and health advice / referrals) coupled with women's increasingly complex health and social needs (mental health support, material deprivation) and inequity of access to resources, have resulted in increased workloads for midwives wherever they work.

Maternal health inequity continues to grow in New Zealand despite attempts to address the problem (Neely et al., 2021). Providing care for women and families living with socioeconomic disadvantage is complex and demanding. Midwives report that they frequently provide care to women who are transient, homeless, or living in poor-quality accommodation, with 26.2% of the women that midwives care for living with material deprivation (level 5; MOH, 2021), and often having insufficient funds for food, transport and communication, placing them at a further disadvantage. These women are often unable to attend appointments, unable to pay the co-payment for scans and the additional essential items they may need for the baby (Dixon et al., 2020).

Continuity of care is therefore only one factor in reducing unnecessary intervention. Determinants of health, access to care and changes to primary and public health services all influence clinical practice and social expectations at a population-based level.

Women's satisfaction with maternity care

Since 1999 the Ministry of Health has contracted (every 3–4 years) a Maternity Consumer Survey to explore women's views on the New Zealand maternity services. Although there has been a gap since 2014, a consumer survey is currently being undertaken. Women's satisfaction with maternity services increased over three national surveys (MOH, 1999, 2003, 2008), as did the intensity of that satisfaction. This level of satisfaction compared favourably with other international models of care with 96% satisfied with the overall service (MOH, 2008).

In 2011 and 2014 the format and questions of the consumer survey were changed so that results were not directly comparable with previous reports (MOH, 2012b, 2015). The 2014 survey of 4000 women found high levels of satisfaction. During the antenatal period, 90% of women were satisfied or very satisfied with their care and reported feeling that they were well informed (91% satisfied or very satisfied), felt listened to (90% satisfied or very satisfied), and that it was easy to get the care they needed while pregnant (90% satisfied or very satisfied). During labour, 87% felt satisfied or very satisfied with the care they received from their LMC or midwife during labour and birth. The majority (92%) reported being satisfied with the way in which their background, culture, beliefs and values were respected and felt confident with the skills of the people caring for them (90% satisfied or very satisfied). During the postnatal period, 80% felt satisfied or very satisfied with the care received in the hospital or birthing unit after the birth, with 89% satisfied / very satisfied with the care received in the first weeks following the birth (Research New Zealand, 2014).

The intangible effects of positive experiences on women are hard to quantify (Sawyer et al., 2013). It is not unreasonable to postulate that healthy, informed and happy women are also empowered women and that empowerment has a positive influence on both women's mothering and society in general (Guilliland, 2005).

CRITICAL THINKING EXERCISE

1. How can women's voices be heard within the maternity service in general and by the midwifery profession specifically? What influences do you think society itself brings to bear on the way birth is experienced and midwifery is practised?

2. Do you think the way maternity services are funded can influence the practice of midwifery? If so, how can we ensure this influence is used in a positive way? Imagine you are a self-employed midwife about to set up practice. What can you do to ensure you utilise your income potential while providing optimal care?

SIMILARITIES AND DIFFERENCES IN HEALTH FUNDING: AUSTRALIA AND NEW ZEALAND

Some similarities exist today between the health systems of Australia and New Zealand. For example, both countries meet the cost of publicly funded health through taxation rather than social insurance; government provides for both secondary and tertiary care. GPs act as 'gatekeepers' to control access to general medical secondary services, and specialist staff work in both the public and the private sphere (Davies & Hindle, 1999). However, major differences have also emerged between Australia and New Zealand in the funding of the health systems, and these have influenced the way in which maternity services can be provided (see Fig. 2.3 and Fig. 2.11). New Zealand has a unique constitutional relationship between the Crown and the Māori people — the Treaty of

Government expenditure on health care is about 67% of the total

FEDERAL GOVT funds 100% of public hospital stays (administered through each state and territory through ABF funding).

Medicare Australia Is responsible for administering Medicare, which provides subsidies for health services. It is primarily concerned with the payment of doctors and nursing staff, and the financing of state-run hospitals.

- OVERALL Funds 70% of overall medical charges

   - 80% of primary care services

   - Part of Specialist charges (vary/around 70–80% coverage)

Pharmaceutical Benefits Scheme (PBS) provides subsidised medications to patients.

National Immunisation Program Schedule—immunisations free of charge.

Australian Organ Donor Register, national register of organ donors.

Therapeutic Goods Administration regulates medicines and medical devices in Australia.

Australian Quarantine and Inspection Service (border control).

Australian Institute of Health and Welfare (AIHW) national agency for health statistics.

Food Standards Australia New Zealand.

Australian Radiation Protection and Nuclear Safety Agency.

FEDERAL FUNDS

Responsible for the operation of public hospitals (through Federal funding).

Healthcare Initiatives such as breast cancer screening programs, Aboriginal youth health programs or school dental health.

STATES

Australian Red Cross Blood Service collects blood donations and provides them to Australian Healthcare Providers.

Medical imaging (MRI and so on) is often provided by private corporations, but patients can still claim from the government if they are covered by the Medicare Benefits Schedule.

National Health and Medical Research Council (NHMRC) funds competitive health and medical research, and develops statements on policy issues.

NON-GOVERNMENT AGENCIES

Private healthcare Insurance is available in Australia but it is extremely regulated.

Remainder of health costs - **out of pocket costs or copayment** - are paid by the patient. Services not covered by **Medicare** may be covered, in whole or in part, by **private health Insurance.**

FIGURE 2.11 The current Australian model of health funding

Waitangi, signed in 1840 (see Ch. 11). No such treaty exists in Australia between the Aboriginal and Torres Strait Islander people and the Crown. The Treaty of Waitangi has, over time, fostered innovative approaches to healthcare, resulting in greater autonomy for indigenous people over their own healthcare and lowering disparities in health status (Davies & Hindle, 1999). There are other important differences:

1. New Zealand has a unitary national system of funding, whereas Australia divides responsibilities between the state and Commonwealth governments.
2. Private health insurance in New Zealand is not subsidised or regulated by government, as it is in Australia.
3. While New Zealand's publicly owned hospitals are constrained in their ability to deliver other health services to private patients, this does not apply to a maternity service where the LMC is a private obstetrician.

HEALTH FUNDING IN AUSTRALIA

Responsibility for healthcare in Australia is shared between the Commonwealth government—responsible for subsidising medical services, pharmaceuticals, private health insurance and aged care—and the states, which are responsible for public hospitals, although the Commonwealth provides grants to the states which cover about 40% of the costs of public hospitals (Fig. 2.11). The dual responsibility and the revenue squeeze on the states have resulted in disagreements and accusations of cost shifting between the Commonwealth and state governments over the share of public hospital costs met by the Commonwealth government. These exchanges have dominated the Australian healthcare debate and led to cost and blame shifting (Duckett, 2018).

One of every five dollars paid in Australian tax goes to health. It is a major component of the national economy, at around 10% of the Australian gross domestic product (GDP) (Duckett, 2017).

Medicare

All Australians are covered by the universal, national, tax-financed health insurance scheme **Medicare**, which provides rebates against the cost of medical fees. This Commonwealth-funded health insurance scheme was introduced on 1 February 1984, following the passage of the *Health Legislation Amendment Act 1983*. It ensures that all Australians have access to free or low-cost care while being free to choose private health services and, in special circumstances, allied health. Medicare covers three healthcare areas:

1. Inpatient services in public hospitals, with zero cost to the patients.
2. For private hospital care, Medicare pays 75% of the Medicare schedule fee, with the balance met by private health insurance (if purchased) (Biggs, 2013). Out-of-pocket costs occur for private inpatient services

depending on the fees charged by the specialists and the level of private health insurance held by the patient.

3. Medicare pays part (or all, if the service is bulk billed) of eligible out-of-hospital services such as GP visits, specialists' consultations, pathology and diagnostic imaging services (Biggs, 2013; Van Gool et al., 2009).

About 80% of GP visits incur no out-of-pocket costs because the bill is paid directly by the government (bulk billed). But doctors are allowed to charge what they like, with no real cap on fees. Consequently 'out-of-pocket costs' remain a significant problem (Duckett, 2017).

A distinguishing characteristic of Australian healthcare is the strong role played by the private sector in hospital provision. The business of private hospitals is underpinned by private health insurance, which is in turn subsidised by the Commonwealth government (Duckett, 2018). Under half of all Australians have private hospital insurance, which provides cover towards the cost of private hospital treatment and attendance fees for privately practising clinicians. The Commonwealth government provides a subsidy of up to 27% of the cost of insurance premiums for low-to-middle-income people under 65, and imposes tax penalties on middle-to-high-income people who do not have private health insurance.

One of the newest innovations in health funding in Australia concerns public hospital funding. Public hospital care is now paid for systematically across states and territories using 'activity-based' funding (ABF), where a price is set for each type of care based on the patient's condition, diagnosis and procedures—using a diagnosis-related classification—called a diagnosis-related group (DRG). State governments, in their role as 'system managers' for public hospitals, distribute the ABF they receive from the Commonwealth and oversee planning, regulation and the governance of public hospitals.

In 2009 the National Health and Hospitals Reform Commission (NHHRC) recommended that ABF should be the principal mode of funding for public and private hospitals (NHHRC, 2009). This recommendation was made in the context of health expenditure estimates that showed hospitals to be one of the fastest growing areas of health spending over the next few decades. Spending on hospital services was projected to triple from $25.9 billion in 2002–03 to $81.4 billion in 2032–3 (Goss, 2008).

Following the recommendations of the reform commission the Independent Hospital Pricing Authority, an independent Commonwealth agency, was established under Commonwealth legislation on 15 December 2011. It forms part of the National Health Reform Agreement (NHRA) reached by the Council of Australian Governments (COAG) in August 2011. The Independent Hospital Pricing Authority (IHPA) was charged with determining the National Efficient Price and the National Efficient Cost for public hospital services, allowing for the national introduction of ABF for Australian public hospitals. Although this does nothing to ameliorate the cost shifting between the states and Commonwealth, it does ensure a consistency of funding for acute hospital services that includes funding for public hospital maternity care. The IHPA sets a national price for each type of care, for public inpatient and eligible outpatient care across Australia.)

The split between Commonwealth and state/territory health funding

It is widely recognised that the division of responsibilities between Commonwealth and state governments continues to contribute to a fragmented and uncoordinated health system structure. Several reviews have identified that existing structural arrangements have contributed to waste, duplication and cost shifting between states and territories with separate institutional 'silos' around funding and service provision creating significant barriers to individuals receiving integrated healthcare with the optimal mix of service components (Commonwealth of Australia (C of A), 2006; NHHRC, 2009).

In single-payer systems, such as New Zealand, governments generally have the capacity and the will to regulate and control budget outlays and to keep overall costs under control. In multipayer systems, no one is in charge and no single agency has the power to control total expenditures. Funders are usually interested in their own costs, not the costs of the system as a whole. Under these circumstances, the easiest way of reducing costs is to shift them to other payers. Cost shifting replaces cost control, with expensive and regressive results (Gray, 2004).

In Australia two levels of government have overlapping responsibilities in the area of funding healthcare. The states and territories are responsible for delivering public health services, public acute and psychiatric hospital services and community services such as school health, dental health, maternal and child health, and environmental health programs. The Commonwealth funds public hospital services, most medical services out of hospital via the Medical Benefits Schedule (MBS) and Medicare, and the Pharmaceutical Benefits Schedule (PBS) in addition to most health research. The Commonwealth also finances and regulates care for older people and the disabled. In 2010 the Commonwealth introduced a body to oversee the national regulation for health practitioners through the Australian Health Practitioners Regulatory Authority (AHPRA).

Hospital funding policies operate under two assumptions based on economic theory: firstly that money will motivate individuals to change their behaviour and secondly that behavioural change will result in improvements in quality (Baxter et al., 2015). This thinking underpins the policy of ABF in Australia, which offers hospitals a fixed amount of money for patients with clinical similarities based on their diagnoses and classified through DRGs. ABF systems were implemented in Australia as in other jurisdictions with the intent of achieving a variety of different policy objectives, the most common being to increase productivity, enhance transparency and increase efficiency while decreasing costs (Baxter et al., 2015).

Funding midwifery

In Australia, as in other resource-rich nations, childbirth accounts for the highest number of occupied bed days (IHPA, 2017); however, the current structure and funding of the public maternity system makes it challenging to deliver value for money. Financing arrangements based on traditional long-standing approaches to public hospital funding direct maternity care into the acute care setting where specialist obstetric care is prioritised while limiting the role of midwives. Maternity care is unique because the services support predominantly healthy women through a natural life event that does not always require a doctor-led intervention (Redshaw et al., 2015).

Until the 1990 reforms in New Zealand, midwifery in both countries ran parallel. More than a decade after the reforms in New Zealand, which placed a greater emphasis on the autonomy and practice of midwifery, changes in Australia began to occur. In June 2008 the Minister for Health and Ageing, Hon. Nicola Roxon, called for a review into the delivery of maternity services in Australia. The Maternity Services Review (the Review) attracted more than 900 submissions from a range of stakeholders including health professionals, researchers, non-government organisations, representative organisations and individuals.

The Review report, released in February 2009, noted that Australia is one of the safest countries in the world in which to give birth or to be born. At the same time, maternity care was seen not to be meeting the needs of all women (C of A, 2009a). Despite the review team's claims to expand birthing choices to women and prioritise safe, evidence-based care (C of A, 2009a), home birth as an option for women and privately practising midwives in Australia was not recognised or supported by the Review. It appears that home birth was considered by the Review to be politically 'too hot to handle' and by dismissing it as a minority issue the government sought to avoid dealing with home birth, calling it a 'sensitive and controversial issue' (Dahlen et al., 2011).

Although the 2009 Commonwealth Budget heralded a bright future for Australian midwifery in terms of access to the Pharmaceutical Benefits Scheme (PBS) and the Medical Benefits Scheme (MBS) for what the health minister described as 'eligible' midwives (now known as 'endorsed' midwives), sadly the minister explicitly excluded the option of home birth in the new package. In response to this omission, the largest home-birth rally Australia has ever seen was held outside the Federal Parliament House on 7th September 2009. Fig. 2.12 captures the mood that day. Three thousand men, women and children converged from every corner of Australia on to the lawn in front of Parliament House to protest in support of home birth. (For more information on endorsed midwives in Australia, see https://www.midwives.org.au/endorsement-medicare).

Following these long-awaited reforms in Australia, the reality has been bitterly disappointing. One positive report

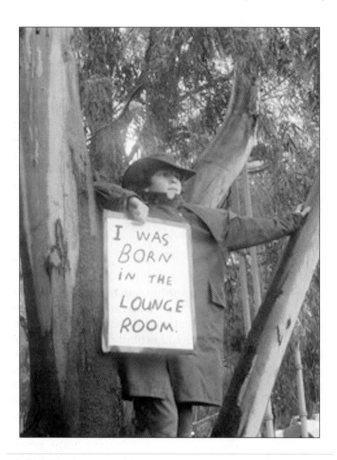

FIGURE 2.12 'The mother of all marches'—home-birth protest, Canberra, 7 September 2009
(Photo: Sue Kruske)

has emerged, however, in a paper published in 2015 discussing the legislative and regulatory changes affecting midwifery practice, and describing Australia's first private midwifery practice with visiting rights to hospital for labour and birth care, and the maternal and neonatal outcomes of this service (Wilkes et al., 2015). The reforms paved the way for women to receive primary maternity care in a community setting from a privately practising midwife. Under the reforms, privately practising midwives (with visiting access) may admit and care for women as private patients during labour and birth in a public or private hospital. Securing hospital visiting rights for private practice midwives is essential for women to experience continuity of midwifery care in hospital; but to date very few midwives practising outside Queensland have managed to secure visiting rights to hospitals to provide care for women in labour (Wilkes et al., 2015). The maternal and newborn outcomes reported by Wilkes et al. (2015) are very favourable when compared with the national core maternity indicators. The caesarean section rate of 22% for the all-risk group receiving care through the private midwifery practice was similar to the rate reported in the M@NGO trial, which reported 21% for all-risk women receiving continuity of midwifery care through hospital-based caseload care (Tracy et al., 2013). These rates are similar to those

in New Zealand where the majority of women receive continuity of midwifery-led care. In those circumstances, midwives do not need to be employees of the public hospital system as they are in Australia.

Although there are small pockets of successful models under the 'endorsed midwife' model in Australia such as the one described above (Wilkes et al., 2015), on the whole women do not have the opportunity to choose a midwife universally under the new legislation as they do in New Zealand.

Continuity-of-care models exist primarily in the public hospital system where midwives are salaried and employed and remain unaffected by the reforms to Medicare and the PBS. District health services draw up **annualised salary agreements** for the midwives based in the Midwifery Group Practices and their funding continues to come out of the acute services budget for public hospitals. In addition to this, there is not an agreed Midwifery Group Practice model of care, or an agreed 'salary' for midwives offering these **midwifery models** of care. Salary packages differ in 'on-call' costs between 25% and 29% both between and within states (e.g. between South Australia (SA) and New South Wales (NSW), and between areas within NSW). There are also different levels of base rates, again between and within states. For example, some Midwifery Group Practitioners are paid a base rate for Level 8 midwifery and others a Clinical Midwifery Consultant base rate (2018, personal communication with SKT). The industrial body that oversees working conditions and wages (the Australian Nursing Federation (ANF)) sets stringent rules for the time midwives can be 'on duty' providing midwifery care to women in the public hospital system. Consequently many variations on the theme of rosters and 'on call' have emerged which may not serve the best interests of women or midwives. Australia continues to categorise midwives as nurses in all but title in many jurisdictions. The governments in Australia have been very slow to recognise women's choice of home birth. The only concession offered to women who would like to give birth at home is to enrol in hospital-based home-birth programs where they are insured by the state treasury-managed funds indemnity cover, or enrol with an endorsed midwife and give birth at home uninsured. The Australian government has not yet managed to agree on an indemnity package to cover women who choose to give birth at home. Some private health insurance companies are currently reviewing their policies to possibly include home birth within the next couple of years (private health insurance companies 2018, personal communication). Professional indemnity cover for independently practising midwives in Australia ceased in July 2001. Since this time women who give birth at home are not covered by professional indemnity cover unless they are part of the publicly funded hospital home-birth program.

(For more information on the cost and funding of midwifery in Australia see Scarf et al. (2021) and Eklom et al. (2021) in Further reading at the end of the chapter).

REFLECTIVE THINKING EXERCISE

Consider whether the current support and funding for midwives in your jurisdiction could be better managed through funding reform or policy reform. Do midwives have the ability to undertake a full scope of practice? Is the best evidence around continuity of care fully supported? Could changes to funding mechanisms make a difference to the way midwives practice?

Hospital-based home birth in Australia

Since the reforms of 2009, in order to meet the demand for safe and affordable home-birth care, a number of publicly funded home-birth programs have been established in association with Australian public hospitals (Coddington et al., 2017).

The number of women accessing home birth through these publicly funded models remains very small, mainly owing to the restrictive risk screening that occurs and the lack of midwives willing to work from the hospital out to the community through the public group practice models.

In summary, the reforms of 2009 had the potential to allow Australian midwives to access Medicare provider numbers, so that women could choose for themselves to have a midwife caregiver for pregnancy, labour and birth. Sadly the government Determination that regulates the provision of care by the 'endorsed midwife' hit huge resistance from all sectors of the Australian medical profession (Australian Medical Association (AMA), 2012). An attempt to modify the Determination in 2012–13 has not significantly increased the accessibility of midwifery care funded through Medicare, or the access to home birth. Until midwives in Australia have the same status as their medical counterparts offering the same service in maternity care, they will not achieve equal pay for equal work, and pregnant women will not have the same midwifery care opportunities as their counterparts in New Zealand. The guiding principles of Medicare as the universal taxpayer-funded health insurance system are equal access to equal care for equal need. For pregnant women in Australia the model of maternity care available is often a function of income, locality and/or private health insurance status rather than need.

A comment on the Maternity Services Review (2009) (a report tabled by the Centre for Health, Economics Research and Evaluation (CHERE) at the University of Technology, Sydney) in 2009 spelt out the tensions that exist (and remain) in the maternity system in Australia (Van Gool, 2009). It stated:

There are considerable tensions between midwives and obstetricians about what constitutes appropriate models of care. The tensions are underlined by the way Australia funds maternity services. Most obstetricians receive a substantial part of their income by providing services to wealthier sections of the community on a fee-for-services basis. Midwives, on the other hand, are most often salaried and employed by public hospitals and provide care to public patients.

Importantly, obstetrician services are eligible for reimbursement under Australia's Medicare program—whereas midwife services generally are not. This has meant that doctors providing obstetric services have access to uncapped public funding whereas funding for services provided by midwives are by-and-large capped.

(Van Gool, 2009, pp. 3, 4)

Hospital-based caseload continuity in Australia

For women wanting the option of continuity of midwifery care in the Australian context there is growing support for caseload care offered in public hospitals. The COSMOS and the M@NGO randomised controlled trials (McLachlan et al., 2012; Tracy et al., 2013) and the continued success of small but significant Midwifery Group Practices in many of the secondary and tertiary teaching hospitals in Australia offer a ray of hope that women will have the opportunity to book with a midwife and have more continuity of midwifery care in Australia in the public hospital system.

Midwifery-led models of care are associated with an increased likelihood of maternal satisfaction across antenatal, intrapartum and postnatal care (McLachlan et al., 2016). Caseload midwifery is a complex intervention because it has a number of interacting components that act both independently and interdependently. These complex networks can have powerful and pervasive effects on how systems actually perform and function (Braithwaite et al., 2009; Medical Research Council (MRC), 2008; Newton et al., 2016).

In the case of the M@NGO trial (Tracy et al., 2013), performance and function were affected by factors such as enhanced senior management support, clear governance structures and communication, clinical engagement and 'give and take' between professionals (MacFarlane et al., 2011). Both the M@NGO and the COSMOS trials contributed Australian data to the latest Cochrane review of midwifery-led care (Sandall et al., 2016). In addition to this, one of the most compelling outcomes of the COSMOS trial (McLachlan et al., 2012) was the reduction of caesarean section amongst low-risk women receiving caseload midwifery (19.4% versus 24.9%; risk ratio (RR) 0.78; 95% confidence interval (CI) 0.67–0.91; $p = 0.001$). The researchers found the difference was primarily related to a reduction in unplanned caesareans. This was in contrast to the M@NGO trial where the statistically significant difference in caesarean sections was amongst elective caesarean sections (before labour) (69 (8%) versus 94 (11%); odds ratio (OR) 0.72; 95% CI 0.52–0.99; $p = 0.05$) (Tracy et al., 2013).

Both trials found a significantly higher rate of unassisted vaginal birth. The M@NGO trial reported a reduction in overall caesarean section rate from the base rate of 29% at the beginning of the trial to 22% in the standard group and 21% in the trial group (Tracy et al., 2013). This may have been due to the Hawthorne effect, given that more than one-third of women in the tertiary teaching hospital were receiving the intervention; the restructuring of midwifery care to caseload midwifery might have positively affected clinical practice in the standard care model, particularly within the birth environment. Nevertheless the decrease in caesarean sections in both trials represented more than a 25% reduction compared with Australian national rates in 2012. (In the 5 years since the M@NGO trial ended the Caesarean section rate has remained at 21%–23% in the caseload groups while those receiving standard rostered care have a caesarean section rate of 31% at present (Personal communication, Directors of Obstetric Services, Royal Hospital for Women, Sydney, 2018). These results are similar to the cohort study of caseload midwifery care published in 2014 (Tracy et al., 2014) which highlighted serious unexplained clinical variation and different outcomes for a similar demographic of women receiving one of the three models of maternity care offered in Australia: caseload versus standard care versus private obstetric care in the public hospital.

Preliminary findings from the follow-up studies planned for long-term outcomes of midwifery-led care have shown some promising moderating effects on maternal stress during birth (Kildea et al., 2018).

Cost of continuity

There are few studies that compare the cost of birth setting. A recent systematic review concluded that there needs to be a better understanding of the cost of birth setting so as to inform policy makers and service providers (Scarf et al., 2016).

Two papers that measured the cost of providing continuity of care in Australia have been published. The M@NGO randomised controlled trial (2013) found that the two groups had similar outcomes in terms of the health of the mother and baby; however, women who were cared for by the same midwife in a caseload model throughout their pregnancy, during labour and after birth saved the public health system around $566.74 per woman, and $271.43 per infant. In a second paper examining cost of care in one tertiary hospital, the same authors found that, from the public hospital perspective, over one financial year the average cost of care for a woman having a first baby and receiving continuity of care from a caseload midwife was $1375.45 less per woman than for those receiving private obstetric care and $1590.91 less per woman than standard hospital care ($p < 0.001$). Similar differences in cost were found in favour of Midwifery Group Practice for all women in the study who received caseload care (Tracy et al., 2014).

A cost reduction from a reorganisation of the way in which care is delivered in the public hospital system could play a major part in reducing public health expenditure. In the case of the M@NGO trial (Tracy et al., 2013),

small differences in most clinical outcome measures in favour of caseload midwifery accounted for the lower median cost for caseload midwifery than for standard care. In the caseload group, higher proportions of women with spontaneous onset of labour, unassisted vaginal birth and using less pharmacological analgesia for labour, and fewer women having a postpartum blood loss greater than 500 mL, combined with one fewer antenatal visit and a significant reduction in the postnatal stay in hospital in the caseload group, led to a significant reduction in cost per woman for caseload midwifery. Amongst the neonates there were fewer babies admitted to the NICU (neonatal intensive care unit) from the caseload group. Given that 1 day in the NICU can cost in excess of $2000, fewer admissions amount to large savings.

Research by Tracy & Tracy (2003) into the antecedents of operative birth showed through cost modelling that the introduction of interventions during labour for women who were otherwise 'low risk' increased the expenditure incrementally in association with the introduction of each labour intervention. The incremental difference in the cost ratios is as relevant in 2023 as it was twenty years ago (Fig. 2.13).

Having a baby in Australia is by any standards a safe event. Consequently, the measure of a safe and effective outcome for childbirth in Australia (as in other affluent industrialised countries) has shifted its focus from a measure of maternal mortality to measures of perinatal morbidity. Notwithstanding, there are some women—Aboriginal women, those of culturally and linguistically diverse backgrounds, and those living in remote and rural areas—who are more likely to experience poorer outcomes in terms of both maternal and perinatal mortality than the community generally (Graham et al., 2007; Kildea et al., 2017).

The Australian Commission for Safety and Quality in Health Care (ACSQHC) in its 2014 paper *Exploring Healthcare Variation in Australia* noted that 'Australia has a high rate of caesarean section compared to the OECD average', with 322.3 caesareans per 1000 live births reported in 2011 (ACSQHC, 2014). This included, for example, a four-fold unexplained and potentially modifiable variation in casemix-adjusted caesarean section rates by hospitals in New South Wales (Lee et al., 2013), and across Australia in women aged 20–34 years there was a threefold variation in caesarean section rates. Australia has a higher rate of caesarean section than the OECD-reported average (ACSQHC, 2017). The rate continues to increase in both the public and private sectors in Australia, showing a significant degree of unexplained clinical variation (Lee et al., 2013; Nippita et al., 2015, 2016) and a substantially higher rate in the private sector than in the public sector (Dahlen et al., 2012; Lee et al., 2013; Roberts et al., 2000).

In addition to the potential long-term morbidity following caesarean section (Cardwell et al., 2008; Hyde et al., 2012; MacKay et al., 2010), operative birth costs more (C of A, 2009b). Many countries have responded to the perceived inevitability of a rising caesarean rate and are looking at ways to address the issue (Declercq et al., 2011).

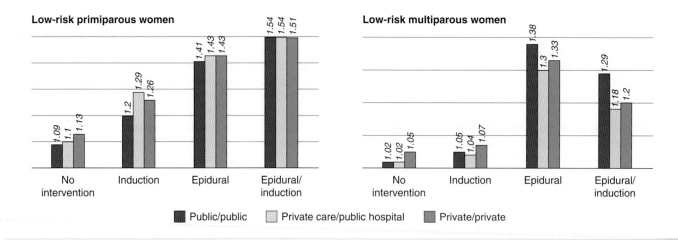

FIGURE 2.13 Costing the cascade of interventions. A model of the cost units per woman that are incurred with the introduction of interventions in labour, Australia 1996–7
(Based on Tracy & Tracy 2003)

Public health policies designed to promote a lower rate of operative birth and increase the rate of normal vaginal birth have been implemented in many countries including Australia. In the US, the *Healthy People 2020* report contained a national objective to reduce caesarean births among low-risk first-time mothers at full term by 10% to 23.9% over the next 10 years (US Department of Health and Human Services, 2010). Similar policies have been promoted in the UK (*Better Births—the National Maternity Review* released by the NHS in 2016). In many states in Australia such as New South Wales, the 'Towards Normal Birth' policy directive was launched with the explicit aim of increasing the vaginal birth rate and decreasing the caesarean section rate (New South Wales Health, 2011).

International comparisons show Australia to have among the highest rates of obstetric intervention in labour and birth compared with those in other resource-rich nations. The caesarean section rate appears to be rising markedly in comparison with the New Zealand rate, which appears to have reached a plateau over the past 5 years (Fig. 2.10).

Obstetric intervention is life saving when serious complications arise during pregnancy or labour. However, previous population-based research from Australia (Dahlen et al., 2012) showed that private obstetric care in Australia was a stronger risk factor for intervention in childbirth than either age or risk status. When women are offered interventions in labour, such as induction and epidurals, they may not be informed of the cascade of interventions in birth that inevitably follow (Tracy et al., 2007). There is a possibility that if women have information on the extent of the association between interventions in labour and birth this may ultimately influence their choice of caregiver and place of birth. Morbidity is costly in monetary, social and emotional health terms, for both families and funders of healthcare.

Roberts et al. (2000) found that as the proportion of low-risk primiparous women with private health insurance increases the rate of normal birth decreases.

This decline has continued over the past decade (Dahlen et al., 2012). Homer (2002) argued that Australian government policy has encouraged large numbers of women of childbearing age to enter private health insurance and that this increased uptake of private health insurance affects the rate of normal birth, caesarean section and the costs of providing maternity care for low-risk primiparous women in NSW. Private providers and hospitals are heavily subsidised by government and so the additional costs are costs to the Australian community, not merely additional costs to women and their families (Homer, 2002, p. 36).

Postnatal re-admission to hospital—the silent cost

One of the silent costs to the health system relates to the re-admission to hospital following childbirth. In Australia this may be one of the most compelling reasons to re-examine the extent and quality of routine postnatal care currently offered to women. Women may be re-admitted to hospital during the postnatal period for a variety of reasons (see Table 2.1) The leading cause of re-admission was infection, with the high-volume principal diagnoses being 'puerperal sepsis', 'infection of obstetric surgical wound' and 'infections of the breast associated with childbirth'. For newborns, the leading cause of re-admission was neonatal jaundice. Table 2.1 shows the mode of birth (by DRG) in relation to the proportion of women re-admitted to hospital following birth in Australia during 2013–14.

Recent history

Currently the division of state and Commonwealth funding in health service provision in Australia acts as a disincentive to providing more community-based midwifery services. Cash-strapped district health boards are keen to promote more medical (Commonwealth-funded through

Table 2.1 Postnatal re-admission to hospital showing mode of birth by diagnosis-related group, Australia, 2013–14

Diagnosis related group	Total
001A—Caesarean delivery, major complexity	7%
001B—Caesarean delivery, intermediate complexity	5%
001C—Caesarean delivery, minor complexity	3%
002A—Vaginal delivery with operating room procedures, major complexity	6%
002B—Vaginal delivery with operating room procedures, minor complexity	3%
060A—Vaginal delivery, major complexity	5%
060B—Vaginal delivery, intermediate complexity	3%
060C—Vaginal delivery, minor complexity	2%
Total	3%

(Source: IHPA Final report. *Bundled Pricing for Maternity Care*, 2017: https://www.ihpa.gov.au/sites/g/files/net4186/f/bundled_pricing_for_maternity_care_-_final_report.pdf)

Medicare) services rather than replace these with midwives working in group practices in the community.

Bundled pricing for maternity care

One of the most promising reforms to be investigated in Australia in 2016 was the plan for *bundled pricing* in maternity care (IHPA, 2017). Bundled pricing is where a single price is determined to cover a full package of care over a defined period of time, spanning multiple events and settings of care. The intention is for resources and funding to be easier for hospitals to manage, to allow financial flexibility to encourage improved models of care and drive better service delivery in the long run, which should lead to better patient outcomes and lower costs. The plan was to provide hospitals with a single price for the cost of treating a pregnant woman across the continuum of her pregnancy care. It was hoped that by introducing bundled pricing into maternity care the managers and policy leaders would be able to better promote Midwifery Group Practice care within the public hospital system. However, after more than 15 months deliberation the IHPA identified significant barriers to the implementation of the bundled pricing model. The primary barrier to implementation was the absence of unique patient identifiers in the national data collections. It is hoped that this will be addressed by Australian governments in the future.

Maternity care service volumes and outcomes are relatively predictable and there is huge potential for savings. Bundled payments for maternity care are the norm in New Zealand. A review of comparable statistics provided by the Organisation for Economic Co-operation and Development (OECD) indicates that Australia, New Zealand and Canada have similar perinatal outcomes overall (OECD, 2015). The lower rate of growth in interventions in New Zealand (caesarean section, instrumental births, induction and epidurals) and higher levels of satisfaction have been linked to the introduction of the midwife-led contracting model (MOH, 2017).

DATA RETRIEVAL

Maternity systems in Australia and New Zealand rely on adequate and appropriate data retrieval and analysis in order to evaluate processes, outcomes and costs in relation to maternity care. Systems for the collection of a minimum dataset are in place in both countries, although the data retrieved are not uniform across all states and territories in Australia and some states are not included at all across a wide range of outcomes. New Zealand data now cover 95% of all women who give birth.

A National Minimum Dataset (NMDS) is a core set of data elements agreed to and endorsed by the health departments of each country for mandatory collection and reporting at a national population level. An NMDS depends on national agreements to collect uniform data. A perinatal NMDS includes data items relating to the mother, including demographic characteristics and factors relating to the pregnancy, labour and birth, and data items relating to the baby, including birth status, sex and birth weight.

The Australian National Perinatal Data Collection (NPDC) is a collection of national data based on notifications to the perinatal data collection in each state and territory. Midwives and other staff using information obtained from mothers and from hospital and other records complete notification forms for each birth in each state and territory. Information is included in the NPDC for all births of at least 400 grams birth weight or at least 20 weeks gestation. Each year the AIHW produces a report using the NPDC known as the *Australia's Mothers and Babies* report (https://www.aihw.gov.au/reports/mothers-babies/australias-mothers-babies-2015-in-brief/contents/table-of-contents). Other government statistics are also available online at: https://www.aihw.gov.au/reports-statistics.

National maternity data has been collected in New Zealand for some years. The Maternal and Newborn Information System (MNIS) was established in 1999 to collect perinatal information amalgamating data from both the LMC payment claims through Health PAC and the data collected at hospital discharge through the NMDS. It has now been renamed the **National Maternity Collection**. When New Zealand established this dataset it was based on the Australian NPDC in order to facilitate comparison between both countries; it also includes data for all births of at least 400 grams birth weight or at least 20 weeks gestation. The quality relies on data being accurately entered by LMC practitioners and hospital coders. The *Report on Maternity* is published annually by the Ministry of Health.

In both countries it takes approximately two years to analyse each year's data and therefore the most recent reports available for both countries is based on data collected two years previously.

Each perinatal data collection has the potential to inform both women and practitioners about the results of practice.

PERINATAL STATISTICS FOR AUSTRALIA AND NEW ZEALAND

Given that the death of newborns and children is a proxy measure for society's health, it is clear to see that it is comparatively very safe to be born in both Australia and New Zealand. However, variations in the precise definition of perinatal and neonatal deaths make it confusing to try and compare perinatal outcomes across countries (Table 2.2). The World Health Organization (WHO) defines *perinatal mortality* as the 'number of stillbirths and deaths in the first week of life per 1000 live births, the perinatal period commences at 22 completed weeks (154 days) of gestation and ends seven completed days after birth'. Both New Zealand and Australia define *perinatal mortality rate (PMR)* as the number of deaths (fetal deaths and neonatal deaths) of babies of at least 400 grams birth

weight or, if birth weight is unavailable, a gestational age of at least 20 weeks, up to 28 completed days after birth per 1000 live births during a given period. Both New Zealand and Australia publish their respective mortality rates on government websites for each country.

Both Australia and New Zealand have the same definition for a *stillbirth*: a "still-born child" means a dead fetus that—(a) weighed 400 grams or more when it issued from its mother; or (b) issued from its mother after the 20th week of pregnancy' (*NZ Births, Deaths and Marriages Registration Act, 1995*). Variations in definition occur in Australia, New Zealand, the United States, Canada and Latin America, where a gestational age of ≥ 20 complete weeks is used to define a birth. In contrast, there is marked variability in the definition of birth among European countries. For some countries (e.g. Norway, France and Finland) the inclusion criteria for a birth is a gestational age of ≥ 22 complete weeks, whereas for others the gestational age is either ≥ 24 in the United Kingdom, or ≥ 28 weeks in Sweden and Denmark (Sullivan et al., 2013) (Fig. 2.14).

New Zealand's Perinatal and Maternal Mortality Review Committee was established in 2007 and reports annually. This is a high case ascertainment, reliable database with one-on-one case review of all deaths. The

Table 2.2 Differing definitions of mortality and death of babies

	Perinatal deaths		
	Fetal deaths		
Institution	Birth weight (grams)	Gestational age (only if birth weight is unavailable) (weeks)	Neonatal deaths (days)
WHO—international comparisons	1000	28	<7
WHO—national reporting	500	22	<7
ABS	400	20	<7
NHDD & NPDC	400	20	<28

ABS = Australian Bureau of Statistics; NHDD & NPDC = National Health Data Dictionary and National Perinatal Data Collection; WHO = World Health Organization. (Adapted from PMMRC, *Reporting Mortality 2010*. Sixth Annual Report of the Perinatal and Maternal Mortality Review Committee. Wellington, NZ: Health Quality and Safety Commission, 2012)

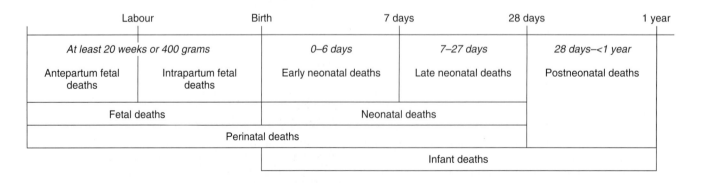

FIGURE 2.14 Perinatal and infant death periods
(Source: PMMRC, 2017, p. 205; adapted from New Zealand Health Information Service, 2007 and MOH, 2010b)

2021 report (Perinatal and Maternal Mortality Review Committee (PMMRC), 2021) indicated that:

- since 2007 there is evidence of a statistically significant decrease in perinatal-related mortality and a significant reduction in fetal and early neonatal deaths
- death dues to fetal anomaly are the leading cause of death
- women living in the most deprived areas were more likely to lose a baby from stillbirth, neonatal death and perinatal-related death
- babies of Māori, Pacific and Indian women are over-represented within the mortality data.

In 2018 the perinatal-related mortality rate was 10.1 / 1000 births.

Statistics from NZ (2008, 2017) show that New Zealand's infant mortality rate has been steadily declining since 1962 and that Australia, Scotland, England and Wales have similar rates, although some Scandinavian and European countries have slightly lower rates. The infant mortality rate continues to decline and has reduced from 5.2 per 1000 live births in 2009 to 3.9 per 1000 live births in 2019 (https://www.statista.com/statistics/807063/infant-mortality-in-new-zealand/) (see Fig. 2.15). Deprivation and smoking during pregnancy have been major factors keeping the perinatal mortality rate from falling further and contributing to inequalities of outcomes between European and Māori statistics. However, New Zealand is now beginning to see a significant reduction in smoking among young people and women.

Maternal mortality

The death of a mother or a baby has significant lifelong impacts on both the family and the wider community. The World Health Organization estimates that 303,000 women died in pregnancy and childbirth in 2015, with 99% of these deaths occurring in low-income countries (WHO, 2015).

A *maternal death* is defined as the death of a woman while pregnant or within 42 days of termination of pregnancy (miscarriage, termination or birth), irrespective of the duration and site of the pregnancy, from any cause related to or aggravated by the pregnancy or its management. It does not include accidental or incidental causes of death of a pregnant woman.

The incidence of maternal death is expressed as a *maternal mortality ratio (MMR)*. The MMR is the number of deaths due to complications of the pregnancy (direct deaths) or aggravation of existing disease processes by the pregnancy (indirect deaths) per 100,000 women giving birth. The calculation does not include deaths from unrelated causes that occur in pregnancy or the puerperium (incidental deaths) and deaths that occur more than 42 days after the end of a pregnancy.

Maternities are all live births and all fetal deaths at 20 weeks or beyond or weighing at least 400 g if gestation is unknown.

The most common causes of maternal death in both New Zealand and Australia—infection, abortion and pre-eclampsia—have been replaced by maternal cardiovascular disease and psychosocial health. Of the six most prominent causes of maternal death between 1973 and 2012, psychosocial death is the only group where the MMR is rising; the incidence of maternal death due to cardiovascular disease, obstetric haemorrhage, thromboembolism, hypertensive disorders and sepsis are all decreasing.

Most of the deaths classified as psychosocial deaths are due to suicide, although some are related to fatal complications of substance misuse and homicide in domestic

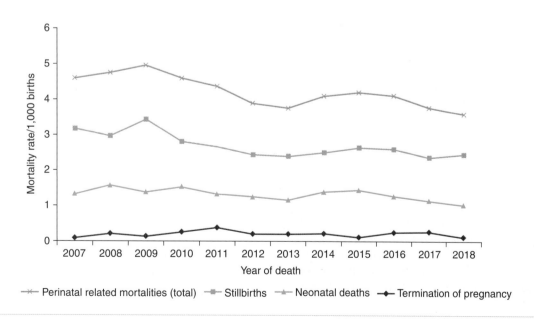

FIGURE 2.15 Perinatal related mortality annual rates (per 1,000 births) using international definitions by year 2007–18
(Source: https://www.hqsc.govt.nz/assets/PMMRC/Publications/14thPMMRCreport/report-pmmrc-14th.pdf)

Deaths per 1,000,000
women giving birth

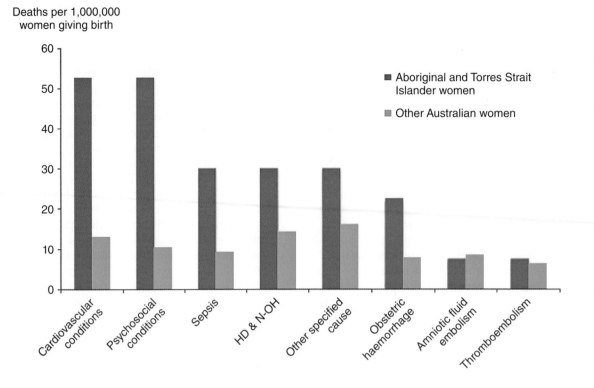

FIGURE 2.16 Cause of maternal death among Aboriginal and Torres Strait Islander women and other Australian women, 2000–12 HD&N-OH = hypertensive disorders and non-obstetric haemorrhage
(Source: AIHW, 2015)

situations. Death by suicide is the leading cause of maternal death in New Zealand (44% of direct causes of maternal death since 2006), with a statistically significant higher rate of maternal mortality for wāhine Māori. Although there is a downward pattern in maternal death, this has not yet achieved statistical significance. There has been a correlation between increasing deprivation and maternal death.

It is important to separate out the rise in maternal deaths that are due to better ascertainment and reporting from the actual rise in mental health conditions that end in maternal deaths. It appears from the Australian data we have that a significant portion of late maternal deaths are related to suicide; however, without a clear review of the cases by multidisciplinary committees, the relationship between pregnancy and suicide more than 42 days after the end of pregnancy remains speculative. It is not clear whether the incidence of suicide in association with pregnancy is more or less common than in comparable non-pregnant women. Nevertheless, the apparently increasing incidence of psychosocial maternal death is a matter of concern. Of even more concern is the disparity between the Aboriginal mothers in Australia and other Australian mothers with cause-specific mortality due to these causes (see Fig. 2.16).

In the period 2008–12 the MMR in Australia was 7.1 (Humphrey et al., 2015).

In New Zealand every maternal death is examined by the Maternal Mortality Committee of the PMMRC. The MMR over the rolling three years for 2016–18 was 11.6/100,000 maternities. The single largest cause of maternal death in New Zealand between 2006 and 2018 has been suicide (30 deaths, 23.8%) followed by amniotic fluid embolism (14 deaths, 11.1%) (PMMRC, 2020).

Cautionary note

Maternal death is one of the few defined core sentinel events in healthcare. In Australia, a significant portion of maternal deaths are not subjected to a root cause analysis or similar review. The application of a systematic review to identify gaps in hospital systems and healthcare processes which are not immediately apparent and may have contributed to the occurrence of an event should be applied to all maternal deaths, whether occurring in public or private health systems. Currently the question of the presence or absence of contributory factors is now being actively pursued by some state and territory maternal mortality review committees, and similar questions are also being raised internationally. New Zealand has paved the way in this area finding that, over the years 2006 to 2015, contributory factors were identified in 62% of maternal deaths, and 39% of the deaths were potentially avoidable (Farquhar et al., 2011; PMMRC, 2017).

Conclusion

In Western societies such as Australia and New Zealand, women expect to receive maternity care that is of a high standard where midwives are available for all. There is strong evidence that a midwife-led maternity service and stand-alone primary units provide a safe service and meet the needs of women and their families (Homer et al., 2014; Sandall et al., 2016). In midwifery, the widely adopted 'partnership model' characterises the relationship as one of trust, shared control and responsibility, and shared meaning through mutual understanding (Guilliland & Pairman, 2010b)—a 'professional friendship' (Pairman, 2000).

Researchers who have explored women's experiences of their Midwifery Group Practice care to determine how women conceptualised midwifery-led care found that women had a positive experience of birth with caseload care (Allen et al., 2017, 2019, 2020; Forster et al., 2016; McCourt et al., 1998; Redshaw et al., 2015), and with caseload midwifery students (Kelly et al., 2014), and continued to have a positive birth experience if their midwife provided continuity of care in collaboration with obstetricians if the woman's risk status changed (Lewis et al., 2016).

In 1990, the New Zealand Government took an unprecedented lead in making women the central focus of its maternity services reform. A comparison of the rates of access to midwifery care between Australia and New Zealand demonstrates the potential of such reform. In the years since 1990, midwives in New Zealand have been funded to provide a primary care service, to provide care for the entire maternity experience, and to provide the majority of care by being present during labour and birth. In 2017 approximately 5% of women booked with a midwife in Australia compared with 93.8% of New Zealand women who booked with a known LMC, over 94.8% of whom were midwives (MOH, 2021).

The funding mechanisms that govern the provision of maternity care in Australia are based on a fee-for-service model that does not enhance the use of midwifery care to the same extent as in New Zealand.[b] Where caseload midwifery models have been implemented in Australia and evaluated, the outcomes show they are of benefit to women and babies (Homer et al., 2000; Kenny et al., 1994; McLachlan et al., 2012; Rowley et al., 1995; Thiele & Thorogood, 1998, 2001; Tracy & Hartz, 2005; Tracy et al., 2013, 2014). Until funding encourages a restructuring of midwifery services and non-intervention by providers, probably through some form of capped prospective allowance for each woman attended, mothers and babies will continue to be disadvantaged by not having access to proven practices of safety and comfort in childbirth. Such a system is based on 'collaboration' and 'cooperation' across all levels of service provision (Beasley et al., 2012).

The service itself must cross both acute hospital and community boundaries to achieve a balance between hospital-based and community-based care. This, coupled with funding an LMC through a capped maternity allowance allocated in terms of a maternity benefit for every pregnant woman, is known to contribute significantly to the welfare of childbearing populations.

New Zealand leads the world in its access to, and the skilful use of, midwifery services for women in childbirth (Grigg et al., 2013). However, over the last 10–15 years the inadequate funding of LMC and hospital midwifery services is seriously undermining the ability of midwives to sustain NZ's unique model of care—again highlighting how important the structural and funding supports are for midwifery to provide continuity of care.

Australian maternity reforms promise significant changes in future. With the new National Register of Health Practitioners, the government-subsidised indemnity insurance for eligible midwives and the path clear for PBS and MBS access for midwives, Australia remains poised on the brink of a new era for midwifery while New Zealand waits to see whether the health sector reassesses the value of midwifery for future women.

Review questions

1. Define the terms 'lead maternity carer' and 'continuity of care'.
2. Identify the key mechanism by which New Zealand's maternity service funding supports midwifery professional autonomy.
3. How does Australia's maternity service funding support midwifery professional autonomy?
4. Identify four main differences between the maternity services and maternity service funding mechanisms in Australia and New Zealand.
5. How do funding mechanisms affect maternity outcomes for mothers and babies?
6. Does private obstetric care pose a risk to women and babies?
7. Why is the collection of data important for midwifery?
8. What is the best way to collect information about birth outcomes?
9. How would you describe the most cost-effective maternity services in New Zealand and Australia?
10. What role do women (consumers) play in the design and delivery of maternity services in New Zealand or Australia?

NOTES

a. For more on the New Zealand health reforms and changes to maternity services funding see *Women's Business: The Story of the New Zealand College of Midwives 1986–2010* by Karen Guilliland and Sally Pairman.

b. As this chapter highlights, there is no universally agreed model of maternity care. Most health systems in most countries have not achieved a model of care that fully recognises and adapts to the needs of women and their babies in a way that allows all women and their babies to meet their health and wellbeing potential. Nor is there a model that completely enables midwives to practise in an environment that strengthens their potential to keep birth normal.

Scrutiny of the antecedents of normal birth will possibly reveal that women should be encouraged to birth in units where intrathecal and epidural opioids and other invasive technology are not routinely on hand and are not used unless the condition of the mother and baby require intervention.

Online resources

Australian Government Department of Health. Private health insurance: https://www.health.gov.au/health-topics/private-health-insurance.

'Find your midwife' is a website service created by the New Zealand College of Midwives with funding from the Ministry of Health to help women to choose a midwife who suits them: https://www.findyourmidwife.co.nz.

House of Commons Health Committee 2003. Choice in maternity services. Ninth Report of Session 2002–03. Volume I: https://publications.parliament.uk/pa/cm200203/cmselect/cmhealth/796/79602.htm.

International Consortium for Health Outcomes Measurement. Pregnancy and Childbirth Standard Set and Reference Guide. 2016: http://www.ichom.org/medical-conditions/pregnancy-and-childbirth/.

Maternity Choices Australia. Primary Maternity Care: https://www.maternitychoices.org/about.

Midwifery Council of New Zealand (MCNZ): https://www.midwiferycouncil.health.nz/.

Ministry of Health (MOH) 1999. Report on Maternity series: https://www.health.govt.nz/nz-health-statistics/health-statistics-and-data-sets/report-maternity-series.

Ministry of Health (MOH) 2002. Section 88 Maternity Notice: https://www.health.govt.nz/publication/primary-maternity-services-notice-2007.

National Center for Health Statistics. Vital statistics data from: http://www.cdc.gov/nchs/data_access/VitalStatsOnline.htm.

National Health and Hospital Reform Commission Discussion papers 2009: https://www.aph.gov.au/About_Parliament/Parliamentary_Departments/Parliamentary_Library/pubs/rp/rp0809/09rp24.

National Institute for Health and Clinical Excellence (NICE) 2004. National Collaborating Centre for Women's and Children's Health. *Caesarean Section*. Clinical guidelines 13 (commissioned by the National Institute for Clinical Excellence). 2nd ed. 2011: https://www.rcog.org.uk/.

New South Wales Health: NSW Mothers and Babies 2015: http://www.health.nsw.gov.au/hsnsw/Publications/mothers-and-babies-2015.pdf.

New Zealand Baby Friendly website: https://www.babyfriendly.org.nz.

New Zealand College of Midwives: http://www.midwife.org.nz.

World Health Organization (WHO). Sexual and reproductive health and research: https://www.who.int/teams/sexual-and-reproductive-health-and-research-(srh)/overview.

References

Allen J, Kildea S, Hartz DL, et al. The motivation and capacity to go 'above and beyond': Qualitative analysis of free-text survey responses in the M@NGO randomised controlled trial of caseload midwifery. *Midwifery*. 2017;50:148–156.

Allen J, Tracy SK, Kildea S, et al. The impact of caseload midwifery, compared to standard care, on women's perceptions of antenatal care quality: survey results from the M@NGO randomised controlled trial for women of any risk. *Birth*. 2019; 439–449. doi:10.1111/birt.12436.

Allen J, Jenkinson B, Tracy SK, et al. Women's unmet needs in early labour: Qualitative analysis of free-text survey responses in the M@NGO trial of caseload midwifery. *Midwifery*. 2020;88:102751. doi:10.1016/j.midw.2020.102751.

Auckland District Health Board. *National Women's Health 2020 Pūronga Haumanu ā tau Annual Clinical Report*. Auckland: Auckland District Health Board; 2020. Online: https://www.nationalwomenshealth.adhb.govt.nz/healthprofessionals/annual-clinical-report/national-womens-annual-clinical-report/.

Australian Commission for Safety and Quality in Health Care (ACSQHC). *Exploring Healthcare Variation in Australia: Analyses Resulting from an OECD Study*. Sydney: ACSQHC; 2014. Online: https://www.safetyandquality.gov.au/publications/exploring-healthcare-variation-in-australia/.

Australian Commission for Safety and Quality in Health Care (ACSQHC). *Second Australian Atlas of Healthcare Variation*. Sydney: ACSQHC; 2017. Online: https://www.safetyandquality.gov.au/search/Atlas.

Australian Institute of Health and Welfare (AIHW). *Maternal Deaths in Australia 2008–2012*. 2015. Online: https://www.aihw.gov.au/getmedia/07bba8de-0413-4980-b553-7592089c4c8c/18796.pdf.aspx?inline=true.

Australian Institute of Health and Welfare (AIHW). *Australia's Mothers and Babies 2015*. 2017. Online: https://www.aihw.gov.au/reports/mothers-babies/australias-mothers-babies-2015-in-brief/contents/table-of-contents.

Australian Institute of Health and Welfare (AIHW). *Australia's health 2020*. 2020. Online: https://www.aihw.gov.au/reports-data/australias-health.

Australian Medical Association (AMA). *Medical Supervision Key to Safe Maternity Services*. Barton, ACT: AMA; 2012.

Baxter P, Hewko S, Pfaff KA, et al. Leaders' experiences and perceptions implementing activity-based funding and pay-for-performance hospital funding models: a systematic review. *Health Policy (New York)*. 2015;119(8):1096–1110. doi:10.1016/j.healthpol.2015.05.003.

Beasley S, Ford N, Tracy SK, et al. Collaboration in maternity care is achievable and practical. *Aust N Z J Obstet Gynaecol*. 2012;52:576–581.

Beehive.govt.nz. The official website of the New Zealand Government. *Major reforms will make healthcare accessible for all NZrs*. 2021. Online: https://www.beehive.govt.nz/release/major-reforms-will-make-healthcare-accessible-all-nzers.

Betrán A, Temmerman M, Kingdom C, et al. Interventions to reduce unnecessary caesaran sections in healthy women and babies. *Lancet.* 2018;13(392):1358–1368. doi:10.1016/S0140-6736(18)31927-5.

Biggs A. *Health in Australia: A Quick Guide.* Commonwealth of Australia; 2013. Online: https://www.aph.gov.au/About_Parliament/Parliamentary_Departments/Parliamentary_Library/pubs/rp/rp1314/QG/HealthAust.

Births Deaths and Marriages Registration Act 1995 [NZ]. Online: http://www.legislation.govt.nz/act/public/1995/0016/latest/DLM359369.html.

Boerma, T, Ronsmans, C Melesse, D, et al. Global epidemiology of use of and disparities in caesarean sections. *Lancet.* 2018;13(392):1341–1348. doi:10.1016/S0140-6736(18)31928-7.

Braithwaite J, Runciman WB, Merry AF. Towards safer, better healthcare: harnessing the natural properties of complex sociotechnical systems. *Qual Saf Health Care.* 2009;18(1):37–41.

Callander E, Creedy D, Gamble J, et al. Reducing caesaran delivery: An economic evaluation of routine induction of labour at 39 weeks in low-risk nulliparous women. *Paediart Perinat Epidemial.* 2019;3–11. doi:10.1111/ppe.12621.

Cardwell CR, Stene LC, Joner G, et al. Caesarean section is associated with an increased risk of childhood-onset type 1 diabetes mellitus: a meta-analysis of observational studies. *Diabetologia.* 2008;51(5):726–773.

Coddington R, Catling C, Homer C. From hospital to home: Australian midwives' experiences of transitioning into publicly-funded homebirth programs. *Women Birth.* 2017;30:70–76.

Commonwealth of Australia (C of A). *The Blame Game: Report on the Inquiry Into Health Funding. House of Representatives Standing Committee on Health and Ageing.* Canberra: Commonwealth of Australia; 2006.

Commonwealth of Australia (C of A). *Improving Maternity Services in Australia: The Report of the Maternity Services Review.* Canberra: Commonwealth of Australia; 2009a. http://www.health.gov.au/internet/main/publishing.nsf/Content/maternityservicesreview-report.

Commonwealth of Australia (C of A). *Midwife Professional Indemnity (Commonwealth Contribution) Scheme Bill 2009.* Canberra: Commonwealth of Australia; 2009b. Online: http://www.aph.gov.au/hansard.

Council of Australian Governments (COAG). *National Health Reform Agreement.* Canberra: COAG; 2011.

Currie J, Cornsweet Barber C. Pregnancy gone wrong: Women's experiences of care in relation to coping with a medical complication in pregnancy. *NZCOM J.* 2016;52:35–40. Online: http://dx.doi.org/10.12784/nzcomjnl52.2016.5.35–40.

Dahlen H, Schmied V, Tracy SK, et al. Home birth and the National Australian Maternity Services Review: too hot to handle? *Women Birth.* 2011;24:148–155.

Dahlen HG, Tracy S, Tracy M, et al. Rates of obstetric intervention among low-risk women giving birth in private and public hospitals in NSW: a population-based descriptive study. *BMJ Open.* 2012;2:e001723. doi:10.1136/bmjopen-2012-001723.

Davies P, Hindle D. Editorial. Health policy and management across the Tasman. *Aust Health Rev.* 1999;22(4):3–7.

Declercq E, Young R, Cabral H, et al. Is a rising cesarean delivery rate inevitable? Trends in industrialized countries, 1987 to 2007. *Birth.* 2011;38(2):99–104.

Department of Health (DOH). *The Australian health system.* 2019. Online: https://www.health.gov.au/about-us/the-australian-health-system.

Dixon L, Neely E, Eddy A, et al. Maternal socio-economic disadvantage in Aotearoa New Zealand and the impact on midwifery care. *J N Z Coll Midwives.* 2020;56:26–34. Online: https://doi.org/10.12784/nzcomjnl56.2020.4.26-34.

Duckett S. *Australia's health system is enviable, but there's room for improvement.* 2017. Online: https://theconversation.com/australias-health-system-is-enviable-but-theres-room-for-improvement-81332.

Duckett S. Expanding the breadth of Medicare: learning from Australia. *Health Econ Policy Law.* 2018;1–25. doi:10.1017/S1744133117000421.

Farquhar C, Sadler L, Masson V, et al. Beyond the numbers: classifying contributory factors and potentially avoidable maternal deaths in New Zealand, 2006–2009. *Am J Obstet Gynecol.* 2011;205:331.

Forster D, McLachlan H, Davey MA, et al. Continuity of care by a primary midwife (caseload midwifery) increases women's satisfaction with antenatal, intrapartum and postpartum care: results from the COSMOS randomised controlled trial. *BMC Pregnancy Childbirth.* 2016;16:28. doi:10.1186/s12884-016-0798-y.

Goss J. *Projection of Australian Health Care Expenditure by Disease, 2003–2033*, Cat. No. HWE 43. Canberra: Australian Institute of Health and Welfare; 2008.

Graham S, Pulver LR, Wang YA, et al. The urban–remote divide for Indigenous perinatal outcomes. *Med J Aust.* 2007;186(10):509–512.

Gray G. *The Politics of Medicare.* Sydney: UNSW Press; 2004.

Grigg CP, Tracy SK. New Zealand's unique maternity system. *Women Birth.* 2013;26(1):e59–e64.

Guilliland KM. A decade in review; midwives and the New Zealand maternity system. *O&G Magazine.* 2005;7(3):37–39.

Guilliland KM, Pairman S. *Women's Business. The Story of the New Zealand College of Midwives 1986–2010.* Christchurch: New Zealand College of Midwives; 2010a.

Guilliland KM, Pairman S. *The Midwifery Partnership: A Model for Practice.* 2nd ed. Christchurch: New Zealand College of Midwives; 2010b.

Health Legislation Amendment Act 1983. No. 54,1983 updated in 2003 with the Health Legislation Amendment (Medicare and Private Health Insurance) Bill 2003.

Health Legislation Amendment (Midwives and Nurse Practitioners) Bill 2009. Bills Digest no. 11 2009–10. Commonwealth of Australia. Online: https://www.aph.gov.au/Parliamentary_Business/Bills_Legislation/bd/bd0910/10bd011.

Homer C. Private health insurance uptake and the impact on normal birth and costs: a hypothetical model. *Aust Health Rev.* 2002;25(2):32–37.

Homer CS, Friberg IK, Dias MA, et al. The projected effect of scaling up midwifery. *Lancet.* 2014;384(9948):1146–1157.

Homer CSE, Davis GK, Brodie P, et al. Collaboration in maternity care: a randomised controlled trial comparing community-based continuity of care with standard hospital care. *BJOG.* 2000;108:16–22.

Humphrey MD, Bonello MR, Chughtai A, et al. *2015 Maternal Deaths in Australia 2008–2012* (AIHW Cat. No. PER 70; Maternal Deaths Series No. 5). Canberra: Australian Institute of Health and Welfare; 2015.

Hunter M, Pairman S, Benn C, et al. Do low risk women actually birth in their planned place of birth and does ethnicity influence women's choices of birthplace? *NZCOM J.* 2011; 44:5–11.

Hyde MJ, Mostyn A, Modi N, et al. The health implications of birth by caesarean section. *Biol Rev Camb Philos Soc.* 2012;87(1):229–243. doi:10.1111/j.1469-185X.2011.00195.x.

Independent Hospital Pricing Authority (IHPA). *Final Report—Bundled Pricing for Maternity Care.* Darlinghurst, NSW: Independent Hospital Pricing Authority; 2017.

Kelly J, West R, Gamble J, et al. 'She knows how we feel': Australian Aboriginal and Torres Strait Islander childbearing women's experience of Continuity of Care with an Australian Aboriginal and Torres Strait Islander midwifery student. *Women Birth.* 2014;27:157–162.

Kenny P, Brodie P, Eckermann S, et al. *Westmead Hospital Team Midwifery Project Evaluation. Final Report*. Westmead, NSW: Centre for Health Economics Research and Evaluation; 1994.

Kildea S, Gao Y, Rolfe M, et al. Risk factors for preterm and low birth weight babies among Aboriginal Women from remote communities in northern Australia. *Women Birth*. 2017;30(5):398–405. doi:10.1016/j.wombi.2017.03.003.

Kildea S, Simcock G, Liu A, et al. Continuity of midwifery carer moderates the effects of prenatal maternal stress on postnatal maternal wellbeing: the Queensland flood study. *Arch Womens Ment Health*. 2018;21(2):203–214. doi:10.1007/s00737-017-0781-2.

Lee YYC, Roberts CL, Patterson JA, et al. Unexplained variation in hospital caesarean section rates. *Med J Aust*. 2013;199(5):348–353.

Lewis L, Hauck YL, Crichton C, et al. An overview of the first 'no exit' midwifery group practice in a tertiary maternity hospital in Western Australia: outcomes, satisfaction and perceptions of care. *Women Birth*. 2016;29:494–502.

McCourt C, Page L, Hewison J, et al. Evaluation of one-to-one midwifery: women's responses to care. *Birth*. 1998;25(2):73–80.

Macfarlane F, Greenhalgh T, Humphrey C, et al. A new workforce in the making? A case study of strategic human resource management in a whole-system change effort in healthcare. *J Health Organ Manag*. 2011;25(1):55–72.

MacKay DF, Smith GCS, Dobbie R, et al. Gestational age at delivery and special educational need: retrospective cohort study of 407,503 schoolchildren. *PLoS Med*. 2010;7(6):e1000289. doi:10.1371/journal.pmed.1000289.

McLachlan HL, Forster DA, Davey MA, et al. Effects of continuity of care by a primary midwife (caseload midwifery) on caesarean section rates in women of low obstetric risk: the COSMOS randomised controlled trial. *BJOG*. 2012;119:1483–1492.

McLachlan HL, Forster DA, Davey MA, et al. The effect of primary midwife-led care on women's experience of childbirth: results from the COSMOS randomised controlled trial. *BJOG*. 2016;123(3):465–474.

Medical Research Council (MRC). *Developing and Evaluating Complex Interventions: New Guidance*. London: MRC; 2008.

Mein Smith P. *Maternity in Dispute. New Zealand 1920–1939*. Wellington, NZ: Department of Internal Affairs, Historical Publications Branch; 1986.

Midwifery Council of New Zealand (MCNZ) Te Tatau o te Whare kahu. *2016 Midwifery Workforce Survey*. 2020. Online: https://www.midwiferycouncil.health.nz.

Ministry of Health (MOH). *Report on Maternity: Maternal and Newborn Information*. Wellington, NZ: Ministry of Health; 1999.

Ministry of Health (MOH). *Maternity Services. Notice Pursuant to Section 88 of the New Zealand Public Health and Disability Act 2000*. Wellington, NZ: Ministry of Health; 2000.

Ministry of Health (MOH). *Media Release, 21 January 2003. Ministry Releases Maternity Services Consumer Survey*. Wellington, NZ: Ministry of Health; 2003.

Ministry of Health (MOH). *Report on Maternity: Maternal and Newborn Information 2005*; 2008.

Ministry of Health (MOH). *Maternity Services Consumer Satisfaction Survey Report*. Auckland: Health Services Consumer Research; 2008b. Online; https://www.health.govt.nz/system/files/documents/publications/hospital-based-maternity-events-2007a_0.pdf.

Ministry of Health (MOH). *New Zealand Maternity Standards: A Set of Standards to Guide the Planning, Funding and Monitoring of Maternity Services by the Ministry of Health and District Health Boards*. Wellington: Ministry of Health; 2011. Online: https://www.health.govt.nz/system/files/documents/publications/nz-maternity-stds-sept2011.pdf.

Ministry of Health (MOH). *Maternity Consumer Survey 2011*. Wellington: Ministry of Health; 2012b. Online: http://www.health.govt.nz/publication/maternity-consumer-survey-2011.

Ministry of Health (MOH). *Maternity Consumer Survey 2014*. 2015. Online: http://www.health.govt.nz/publication/maternity-consumer-survey-2014.

Ministry of Health (MOH). *Report on Maternity 2015*. 2017. Online: https://www.health.govt.nz/system/files/documents/publications/report-on-maternity-2015-updated_12122017.pdf.

Ministry of Health (MOH). *Report on Maternity 2019*. 2021. Online: https://minhealthnz.shinyapps.io/report-on-maternity-web-tool/.

National Health and Hospitals Reform Commission (NHHRC). *A Healthier Future for All Australians: Final Report*. Canberra: NHHRC; 2009.

Neely E, Dixon L, Bartle C, et al. Providing maternity care for disadvantaged women in Aotearoa New Zealand: The impact on midwives. *Women Birth*. 2021;35(2):S1871–5192. doi: 10.1016/j.wombi.2021.03.014.

New South Wales (NSW) Health. *Maternity—Towards Normal Birth in NSW PD2010_045*. Sydney, Australia: NSW Health; 2011.

New Zealand College of Midwives (NZCOM). *Midwives Handbook for Practice*. 4th ed. Christchurch, NZ: NZCOM; 2015.

New Zealand College of Midwives (NZCOM). *Report on New Zealand's MMPO Midwives Care Activities and Outcomes*. Christchurch, NZ: NZCOM; 2016.

New Zealand College of Midwives (NZCOM). *Midwives Handbook for Practice*. 5th ed. Christchurch, NZ: NZCOM; 2018.

New Zealand Health Information Service (NZHIS). *Fetal and Infant Deaths 2003 & 2004*. Wellington, NZ: MOH; 2007. Online: http://www.health.govt.nz/system/files/documents/publications/fetal200304.pdf.

New Zealand Institute of Economic Research. *Sustainable midwifery supporting improved wellbeing and greater equity*. 2020. NZIER report to New Zealand College of Midwives. Auckland

Newton MS, McLachlan HL, Forster DA, et al. Understanding the 'work' of caseload midwives: a mixed-methods exploration of two caseload midwifery models in Victoria, Australia. *Women Birth*. 2016;29:223–233.

Nippita TA, Lee YY, Patterson JA, et al. Variation in hospital caesarean section rates and obstetric outcomes among nulliparae at term: a population-based cohort study. *BJOG*. 2015;122:702–711.

Nippita TA, Trevena JA, Patterson JA, et al. Interhospital variations in labor induction and outcomes for nullipara: an Australian population-based linkage study. *Acta Obstet Gynecol Scand*. 2016;95:411–419.

Nursing Council of New Zealand (NCNZ). *New Zealand Registered Nurses, Midwives and Enrolled Nurses: Workforce Statistics 2002*. Wellington, NZ: Nursing Council of New Zealand; 2004.

OECD. *Health at a Glance 2015: OECD Indicators*. Paris: OECD Publishing; 2015. Online: http://apps.who.int/medicinedocs/documents/s22177en/s22177en.pdf.

OECD. *OECD Health Statistics 2021*. 2021. Online: https://www.oecd.org/els/health-systems/health-data.htm.

Pairman S. Women-centred midwifery: partnerships or professional friendships? In: Kirkham M, ed. *The Midwife-Mother Relationship*. London: Macmillan; 2000:207–226.

Pairman S. *Workforce to Profession: An Exploration of New Zealand Midwifery's Professionalising Strategies from 1986 to 2005 (Doctoral thesis)*. Sydney: University of Technology; 2005.

Pairman S. Educating midwives for autonomous practice. In: Guilliland K, Pairman S, ed. *Women's Business. The Story of the New Zealand College of Midwives 1986–2010*. Christchurch, NZ: New Zealand College of Midwives; 2010:480–563.

Parkes CM. The impact of the medicalization of New Zealand's maternity services on women's experiences of childbirth, 1904–1937. In: Bryder L, ed. A Healthy Country. *Essays on the Social History of Medicine in New Zealand*. Wellington, NZ: Bridget Williams Books; 1991:165–180.

Perinatal and Maternity Mortality Review Committee (PMMRC). *Reporting Mortality 2010*. Sixth Annual Report of the Perinatal and Maternal Mortality Review Committee. Wellington, NZ: Health Quality and Safety Commission; 2012.

Perinatal and Maternal Mortality Review Committee. *Eleventh Annual Report of the Perinatal and Maternal Mortality Review Committee: Reporting Mortality and Morbidity 2015*. Wellington, NZ: Health Quality & Safety Commission; 2017. Online: https://www.hqsc.govt.nz/assets/PMMRC/Publications/2017_PMMRC_Eleventh_Annual_Report.pdf.

Perinatal and Maternal Mortality Review Committee (PMMRC). *Fourteenth Annual Report of the Perinatal and Maternal Mortality Review Committee | Te Pūrongo ā-Tau Tekau mā Whā o te Komiti Arotake Mate Pēpi, Mate Whaea Hoki: Reporting mortality and morbidity 2018 | Te tuku pūrongo mō mate me te whakamate 2018*. Wellington: Health Quality & Safety Commission; 2021. Online: https://www.hqsc.govt.nz/resources/resource-library/fourteenth-annual-report-of-the-perinatal-and-maternal-mortality-review-committee-te-purongo-a-tau-tekau-ma-wha-o-te-komiti-arotake-mate-pepi-mate-whaea-hoki/.

Redshaw M, Henderson J. *Safely Delivered: A National Survey of Women's Experience of Maternity Care, 2014*. Oxford UK: National Perinatal Epidemiology Unit; 2015.

Research New Zealand. *Maternity Consumer Survey 2014*. Wellington, NZ: Ministry of Health. Online: https://www.health.govt.nz/publication/maternity-consumer-survey-2014.

Roberts CL, Tracy S, Peat B. Rates for obstetric intervention among private and public patients in Australia: a population based descriptive study. *BMJ*. 2000;321:137–141.

Rowland T, McLeod D, Freese-Burns N. Comparative study of maternity systems. In: *Malatest International Consulting and Advisory Services*. Wellington, NZ: Ministry of Health; 2012.

Rowley M, Hensley M, Brinsmead M, et al. Continuity of care by a midwife team versus routine care during pregnancy and birth: a randomised trial. *Med J Aust*. 1995;163(9):289–293.

Sandall J, Soltani H, Gates S, et al. Midwife-led continuity models versus other models of care for childbearing women. *Cochrane Database Syst Rev*. 2016;(4):CD004667, doi:10.1002/14651858.CD004667.pub5.

Sandall J, Tribe R, Avery L, et al. Short-term and long-term effects of caesaran section on the health of women and children. *Lancet*. 2018;13(392):1349–1357. doi:10.1016/S0140-6736(18)31930-5.

Sawyer A, Ayers S, Abbott J, et al. Measures of satisfaction with care during labour and birth: a comparative review. *BMC Pregnancy Childbirth*. 2013;13:108.

Scarf V, Catling C, Viney R, et al. Costing alternative birth settings for women at low risk of complications: a systematic review. *PLoS ONE*. 2016;11(2):e0149463. doi:10.1371/journal.pone.0149463.

Streat S, Munn S. Health economics and health technology assessment: perspectives from Australia and New Zealand. *Crit Care Clin*. 2012;28:125–133.

Sullivan EA, Wang YA, Norman RJ, et al. Perinatal mortality following assisted reproductive technology treatment in Australia and New Zealand, a public health approach for international reporting of perinatal mortality. *BMC Pregnancy Childbirth*. 2013;13:177.

Thiele B, Thorogood C. *Evaluation of the Community Based Midwifery Program*. Fremantle WA: Community Midwifery WA; 1998.

Thiele B, Thorogood C. *Evaluation of the Community Midwifery Program*. Fremantle WA: Community Midwifery WA; 2001.

Tracy SK, Hartz D. *Final Report: The Quality Review of Ryde Midwifery Group Practice, September 2004 to October 2005*. Gosford, NSW: Northern Sydney and Central Coast Health; 2005.

Tracy SK, Tracy MB. Costing the cascade: estimating the cost of increased intervention in childbirth using population data. *BJOG*. 2003;110(8):717–724.

Tracy SK, Wang A, Black D, et al. Associating birth outcomes with obstetric interventions in labour for low risk women. A population based study. *Women Birth*. 2007;2:41–48.

Tracy SK, Hartz DL, Tracy MB, et al. Caseload midwifery care versus standard maternity care for women of any risk: M@NGO, a randomised controlled trial. *Lancet*. 2013;382:1723–1732.

Tracy SK, Welsh A, Hall B, et al. Caseload midwifery compared to standard or private obstetric care for first time mothers in a public teaching hospital in Australia: a cross sectional study of cost and birth outcomes. *BMC Pregnancy Childbirth*. 2014;14:46. doi:10.1186/1471-2393-14-46.

US Department of Health and Human Services. *Healthy People 2020*. Washington DC: US Department of Health and Human Services; 2010.

Van Gool K. *Maternity Services Review: Australia*. Health Policy Monitor; April, 2009. Online: http://www.hpm.org/au/a13/1.pdf.

Wilkes E, Gamble J, Adam G, et al. Reforming maternity services in Australia: outcomes of a private practice midwifery service. *Midwifery*. 2015;31:935–940.

World Health Organization. *Trends in Maternal Mortality: 1990 to 2015. Estimates by WHO, UNICEF, UNFPA, World Bank Group and the United Nations Population Division*. Geneva: WHO; 2015.

Further reading

Centre for Health Economics Research and Evaluation (CHERE). *Funding of Public Hospitals*. Sydney: CHERE; 2000.

Chernichovsky D. Health system reforms in industrialised democracies: an emerging paradigm. *Milbank Q*. 1995;73(3):339–372.

Chernichovsky D. Pluralism, public choice, and the state in the emerging paradigm in health systems. *Milbank Q*. 2002; 80(1):5–39.

Church A, Nixon A. *An Evaluation of the Northern Suburbs Community Midwifery Program*. Adelaide: Department of Human Services; 2002.

Commonwealth of Australia. Senate Community Affairs References Committee. *First Report—Public Hospital Funding and Options for Reform*. 2000. Online: https://www.aph.gov.au/Parliamentary_Business/Committees/Senate/Community_Affairs/Completed_inquiries/1999-02/pubhosp/report/index.

Eklom B, Tracy SK, Callander E. An exploration of potential output measures to assess efficiency and productivity for labour and birth in Australia. *BMC Pregnancy Childbirth*. 2021. 21:703. Online: https://doi.org/10.1186/s12884-021-04181-x.

Guilliland KM. *Demographic Profile of Self-employed / Independent Midwives in New Zealand and Their Birth Outcomes (MA thesis)*. Wellington, NZ: Victoria University of Wellington; 1998.

Guilliland KM. Autonomous midwifery in New Zealand: the highs and lows. *Birth Issues*. 1999a;8(1):14–20.

Guilliland KM. Shared care in maternity services: with whom and how? *Health Manager*. 1999b;6(2):4–8.

Guilliland KM. *Do women want midwives? Midwives and the New Zealand maternity system in 2005*. Proceedings, International Confederation of Midwives Conference, Brisbane (CD-ROM). 2005.

Guilliland KM, Pairman S. *The Midwifery Partnership: A Model for Practice*. Monograph Series 95 / 1. Wellington, NZ: Department of Nursing and Midwifery, Victoria University; 1995.

Kohn LT, Corrigan JM, Donaldson MS, ed. *Committee on Quality of Health Care in America, Institute of Medicine. To Err is Human:*

49

Building a Safer Health System. Washington DC: National Academy Press; 2000. Online: https://www.nap.edu/catalog/9728/to-err-is-human-building-a-safer-health-system.

Pairman S. Towards self-determination: the separation of the midwifery and nursing professions in New Zealand. In: Papps E, ed. *Nursing in New Zealand: Critical Issues, Different Perspectives*. Auckland: Pearson Education; 2002:14–27.

Pairman S, Guilliland K. Developing a midwife-led maternity service: the New Zealand experience. In: Kirkham M, ed. *Birth Centres. A Social Model for Maternity Care*. London: Books for Midwives; 2003:223–237.

Scarf V, Yu S, Viney R, et al. Modelling the cost of place of birth: a pathway analysis. *BMC Health Serv Res.* 2021;21:816. Online: https://bmchealthservres.biomedcentral.com/articles/10.1186/s12913-021-06810-9.

CHAPTER 3

Human rights in childbirth

Bashi Kumar-Hazard

LEARNING OUTCOMES

Learning outcomes for this chapter are:

1. To describe what human rights are and how they apply to the provision of maternity care
2. To outline human rights issues affecting the provision of maternity healthcare in Australia, New Zealand and around the globe
3. To report on how, and the reasons why, violations of women's human rights can and have become a normalised, accepted practice in maternity healthcare
4. To present evidence around the impact of human rights violations on maternal and infant health in rich and poor countries
5. To discuss the way in which the practice of medicine and medical law institutionalises human rights violations against women
6. To list the strategies and resources midwives can use to support and defend the human rights of women in pregnancy and childbirth.

CHAPTER OVERVIEW

This chapter has been written to bring the importance of human rights in pregnancy and childbirth to the forefront of student midwives' thinking. This chapter provides an overview of human rights issues for childbearing women and midwives, with a particular focus on Australia and New Zealand. We explore the impact of human rights violations on maternal and infant health. Strategies and resources that midwives will find helpful in supporting human rights in childbirth are provided.

KEY TERMS

autonomy
disrespect and abuse (D&A)
equality

fetal rights
human rights
information asymmetry

informed consent

INTRODUCTION

Human rights are fundamentally important to the development, provision and practice of midwifery-led care. By its very nature, the quality education and training that midwives now receive in Australia and New Zealand, which focus on the provision of woman-centred care and continuity of carer, constitute the core elements required for the provision of quality maternity healthcare through a human rights lens. No other healthcare professional is trained to provide care through a human rights lens. As a midwife, you are in a position of privilege, but also responsibility, as you support not just the birth of a baby but also the creation of a mother who, under your care will become the heart and soul of her family and her community. You have the power to build, or destroy, those family bonds with the type of care you give your clients.

WHAT ARE HUMAN RIGHTS?

Human rights are a set of moral and legal principles that promote and protect the recognition and use of fundamental human and humane values in our interactions with each other. We are all born with human rights, regardless of race, ethnic origin or socioeconomic status. We cannot alienate, trade or extinguish them.

All human rights lie at the heart of our common, social values as human beings, even if they are not covered by specific national laws. They can be:

1. civil and political rights (e.g. the freedom of speech)
2. economic or social rights (e.g. the right to health and education), or
3. collective rights (e.g. the right to live in a healthy environment or indigenous persons' rights) (Australian Human Rights Commission (AHRC), 2016; New Zealand Human Rights Commission (NZHRC), 2014).

Some rights are written into the Constitution and legislation in Australia, such as the right to vote and the right to a fair trial.

Human rights are a powerful tool for preserving universal values, such as dignity and respect, in all areas of human activity and interaction. They are used to develop a framework for advocacy, particularly in circumstances where rules and policies can affect an individual. They are used by courts to interpret national laws in ways that hold governments accountable for their actions.

Human rights *should* serve as a reminder of the fundamental moral protections that apply to every human being in Australia and New Zealand. We emphasise the word 'should' because the ability to turn human rights into everyday reality depends on us, and sadly, too many of us forget their importance in our dealings with each other. We each have the power to know, respect and defend the human rights of all, particularly in relation to the people who are vulnerable and voiceless, with limited recourse to accountability. When we ignore or dismiss the significance of all our rights, we start to doubt the existence of rights with implications for all of us (Dean, 2017; Meredith, 2015). This is especially true in the provision of maternity healthcare.

WHY HUMAN RIGHTS?

Around the world, a technocratic approach to the planning and implementation of maternity health services is becoming increasingly popular, with a focus on the low-cost dissemination of medical treatment and resources. This has been fuelled by a global push to create standardised institutional maternity care as a quick, cheap and easy fix to maternal and newborn mortality. It has come at the expense of the human rights of mothers and babies (Beogo et al., 2017; Clark, 2016; Haque & Waytz, 2012; McIntosh, 2012; Odent, 2002; Sacks, 2017).

The 2016 *Lancet Maternal Health Series* highlights the dangerous realities of the global technocratic pursuit as a standard of care. Maternity healthcare is characterised as either 'too little too late' (inequitable and/or insufficient access to care) or 'too much too soon' (excessive medicalisation), or even a disastrous mix of both (Miller et al., 2016). Despite these warnings, excessive medicalisation and inequitable access remain prevalent with the World Health Organisation predicting that, *on average*, one third of births will likely be by caesarean section by 2030 (Betran et al., 2021). The pursuit of this technocratic approach highlights the disconnect between the way we frame problems and push for solutions without regard for the lived realities of mothers and babies (Freedman, 2016; Walsh, 2009). The result is to cause greater harm and long term disruptions to good health than were intended by careproviders. The success of systematic and medically standardised care has come at the expense of health and human rights for women and children.

The problem: putting process before people

Many low- and medium-income nations have failed to realise the basic survival needs of mothers and babies, decades after many of those needs were identified. The costs of providing fragmented, poorly timed and highly medicalised care focused on identifying and treating pathology can be unduly burdensome. Low- and middle-income countries are influenced by the institutional set ups of medically driven maternity healthcare in high-income countries, even where it proves to be financially prohibitive and unsustainable in the long term. Precious resources are spent on equipment, diagnostics and medical treatment at the expense of equally life-saving improvements in maternity healthcare, such as the provision of woman-centred midwifery care.

It is therefore not surprising that the United Nations Population Fund (UNFPA) and the World Health Organization (WHO) have for the last decade advocated strongly for the introduction of quality, trained midwifery care as integral to the improvement of maternity healthcare services for all countries, rich and poor (Australian Health Ministers' Conference, 2011; UNFPA, 2011; UNFPA, International Confederation of Midwives, WHO et al., 2010). The Working Group on the Health and Human Rights of

Women, Children and Adolescents was also established by both the WHO and the Office of the High Commissioner on Human Rights in 2016 to identify practical recommendations to better operationalise human rights, in order to achieve the targets in *The Global Strategy for Women's, Children's and Adolescents' Health (2016–30)* (WHO, 2015). At the launch of the Working Group's first report in 2017, Co-chair Hina Jilani said:

> *Many promises have been made but still millions of women, children and adolescents are denied their fundamental human rights, leading to preventable deaths, injury, physical and mental illness and other harm. Despite medical breakthroughs and scientific advances, societies continue to undervalue the health and dignity of women, children and adolescents, undermining their rights and dismissing their rightful claims.*
>
> (WHO, 22 May 2017)

In high-income countries like Australia and New Zealand, the problem of over-servicing and practice of defensive medicine is endemic. This is caused, in part, by a pervasive belief that, in order to get the highest quality of care, pregnancy and birth must be overseen in hospital by a senior medical clinician with immediate access to high-cost, high-technology medical resources (Mello et al., 2010). In Australia, women with private insurance choose a private hospital because they believe that a 'nicer' environment, a private room and a known clinician will support their needs in labour, birth and postpartum (Willis & Lewis, 2016). They are rarely advised of the higher incidence of medical interventions, the fragmented care they receive at the hospital *during* labour or the tendency for practitioners in the private sector to overtreat, which many women perceive as a risk and a cause of significant distress (Einarsdóttir 2012a; 2012b). By contrast, women in the public sector are unaware and rarely informed that the care they receive is fragmented, based on uniform, standardised protocols with limited flexibility and aimed at producing a live mother and baby as cheaply and as quickly as possible. Both private and public systems are enabled by 'information asymmetry' (explained below) and a lack of choice. The incidence of women rejecting institutionalised maternity healthcare is significantly higher amongst those who have experienced it (Dahlen et al., 2020).

Institutional care is designed around provider convenience, insurance policy constraints and medical liability laws, but not around human rights. (Tarzia et al., 2018). Practice is not informed by the right to **informed consent**, the right to **equality** and freedom from discrimination, and the right to the highest attainable level of health (Béhague et al., 2002). So much so, that many maternity healthcare providers do not even realise that they are violating these human rights in practice. For example, despite very high investment and costs associated with childbirth (Truven Health Analytics, 2013), the USA reported the highest maternal mortality ratios amongst high-income countries in 25 years (Main & Menard, 2013). That mortality and acute morbidity is overwhelmingly affecting the African American community in the USA, the group most likely to experience highly medicalised care (Giscombé & Lobel, 2005; Howell et al., 2016). Induction, epidurals, caesarean deliveries and other childbirth interventions have escalated in use over the past few decades without apparent improvement in outcomes, and without informed consent (Arrieta, 2011; Baker, 2010; Dahlen & Kruske, 2012; Declercq 2012, 2015; Declercq et al., 2013; Diniz & Chachamb, 2004; Dumas, 2016; Ghosh, 2017; Hyderi, 2017; Iyengar, 2017; Mayor, 2016; Mossialos et al., 2005; Shah, 2015; Vedam, 2003; Weiner, 2016).

In Australia, there is strong evidence of the reported harms arising from, and the higher risks associated with, interventions such as caesarean section, induction, preterm delivery, excessive use of forceps and episiotomies, for both mother and baby (Coxon et al., 2016; Dahlen et al., 2014; Chen et al., 2017). Studies also highlight the limited understanding of the meaning and application of informed consent and bodily autonomy amongst care providers (Hall et al., 2011; Kruske et al., 2013). When women refuse to consent to unwanted interventions, care providers use a range of strategies akin to bullying and abuse to pursue their goals (Jenkinson, 2015; Jenkinson et al., 2017; Waters, 2011).

The reported harms significantly affect the lived experiences of marginalised groups from immigrant, refugee and indigenous backgrounds who already struggle to navigate the vast, complex, typically fragmented and often racially discriminatory maternity healthcare systems (Rogers et al., 2020; Humphrey et al., 2015; Kildea et al., 2016; Kruske et al., 2006, 2013; Rigg et al., 2017).

By contrast, the rights of all health consumers in New Zealand are enshrined under the *Health and Disability Commissioner Act 1994 (NZ)*. Under that Act, the Commissioner is required to establish and implement a Code of Rights for health services consumers which imposes obligations on healthcare providers to take reasonable actions to give effect to those rights and to comply with their duties under the Code. The Code of Rights (Health and Disability Commissioner, 2018) sets out the following basic rights in the provision of healthcare:

1. The right to be treated with respect
2. The right to freedom from discrimination, coercion, harassment and exploitation
3. The right to dignity and independence
4. The right to services of an appropriate standard
5. The right to effective communication
6. The right to be fully informed
7. The right to make an informed choice and give informed consent
8. The right to support
9. Rights in respect of teaching and/or research
10. The right to complain.

While this may not always prevent violations of human rights in New Zealand, particularly against vulnerable groups of women, such clear expectations are an important, differentiating factor shaping quality in the provision of maternity healthcare in New Zealand.

The solution: putting people before process

The development and discussion of human rights in maternity healthcare is an alarm bell for all of us—a signal that there is a quality and accountability crisis affecting the way in which maternity healthcare is delivered. These quality and accountability crises will be discussed further below.

Equally, the that access to high-quality continuity of midwifery care can protect the human rights of mothers and babies has grown exponentially around the world. A Cochrane systematic review showed that positioning midwives as primary carers in pregnancy and birth promotes a sense of normalcy, which is strongly reaffirming for mothers and has significant health benefits for newborns (Sandall et al., 2016). The New Zealand and Netherlands maternity healthcare systems, built on a woman-centred care framework and focused on continuity of care for all women, are fine examples of maternity healthcare delivered through a human rights lens.

In the rest of the chapter, we discuss some of the human rights that affect the provision of maternity healthcare and the typical practices that violate those rights.

WHICH HUMAN RIGHTS ARE VIOLATED IN MATERNITY CARE?

The human rights to dignity and respect, equal treatment and freedom from discrimination, bodily autonomy and privacy are the most relevant rights affecting the provision of maternity health services. Each of these is discussed below.

(a) The human right to dignity and respect

Article 1 of the *Universal Declaration of Human Rights* provides is the ideal overarching moral framework for developing appropriate standards of provider behaviour in maternity healthcare (Box 3.1).

Dignity and *respect* are fundamental to the realisation of all human rights. They are afforded when individuals are free to make personal decisions without interference from the state in an area as important and intimate as sexual and reproductive health. The importance of treating a woman with dignity and respect in front of her spouse or family cannot be overstated. Remember that, with the authority you have as a midwife, you are publicly modelling behaviours that signal how women—as mothers—should be treated in your community.

Many of the systemic violations discussed in the rest of this chapter are the product of poor-quality care, now called **disrespect and abuse (D&A)** of pregnant and birthing women in health facilities (Bohren et al., 2015; Goldwin, 2013; Harvard School of Public Health and University Research, 2010; Hill, 2017; Madeira et al., 2017; Mane, 2015; Sadler et al., 2016; Schuiling, 2016). Women are speaking out and reporting violations of their fundamental right to dignity and respect in childbirth. They describe medical neglect, verbal and physical abuse, crude and aggressive attacks on women's sexuality and invasions of privacy when they are at their most vulnerable (White Ribbon Alliance, 2017; Dahlen et al., 2020). This mistreatment is now legally referred to as 'obstetric violence' and is discussed in detail below (Borges, 2018; Kukura, 2018).

In Australia, mistreatment by care providers is driven by structural or systemic stressors, even in highly resourced or privately funded maternity health facilities (Dahlen et al., 2012, 2020; Declercq et al., 2013. Employment obligations can force midwives to choose between the provision of woman-centred care and employer-mandated protocols. The pressure on a midwife to cope with this obvious conflict of interest can result in mistreatments such as the use of emotional blackmail, bullying and badgering, threats of calling child protection services, shroud waving (i.e. telling a woman that she or her baby is going to die if she doesn't do as she is told) and neglect to obtain compliance (Cooper et al., 2021).

Compliance is not consent. In Australia, mandated protocols include the imposition of strict time limits on stages of labour, routine inductions, routine vaginal examinations, prioritising caesarean section deliveries and episiotomies to support provider convenience, physically restraining women or forcing them into stirrups for delivery, refusing access to food and water during labour, unnecessary invasions of privacy and threatening to remove or discipline doulas or spouses for non-compliance. Women are rarely informed about these practices and protocols before they attend hospital, even when they request this information.

It is interesting to note that women who are transferred from a birth centre or home birth to a tertiary hospital also report experiencing structural and systemic disrespect and abuse. By comparison with Australia, New Zealand midwives operating as independently practising profesionals have utilised the Code of Rights for debriefing, lodging complaints and developing strategies for subsequent births that mitigate the impact of transfer on their clients Women. As Australia has no equivalent Code, independent midwives have not been able to hold hospital staff to account in the same way.

> ### Box 3.1 The moral framework
>
> *All human beings are born free and equal in dignity and rights. They are endowed with reason and conscience and should act towards one another in a spirit of brotherhood.*
>
> (Article 1, Universal Declaration of Human Rights (UN, 1948))

Dignity and respect matter in childbirth. In Australia, mothers report that the trauma in childbirth is compounded by the fact that no one seemed to recognise or care about their fear and suffering. They didn't know or understand what was happening to them or why and, if they asked questions, were dismissed, derided or further mistreated (Hackenberg, 2017). This is consistent with Lancet findings on the global phenomenon of mistreatment in childbirth:

> *Blind-spot is indeed an appropriate metaphor for the way that disrespectful and abusive treatment (D&A) of women during childbirth in facilities has evaded the attention of the global health community and of national and local health authorities, including those governing midwifery and other health professions, in countries worldwide, both rich and poor. But it has not evaded the attention of women themselves: women choose where to deliver based in large part on their perceptions of the way they will be treated in the facilities available to them.*
>
> (Freedman & Kruk, 2014, e42)

A woman must be able to turn to her care providers when something doesn't feel right during childbirth, and she needs to feel respected and heard. As we saw in the Victorian Department of Health's probe into the avoidable deaths of seven newborns in 2013 and 2014 at the Bacchus Marsh and Melton Regional Hospital, not listening doesn't just injure dignity—it can kill mothers and their babies (Box 3.2). Every woman who lost an infant described heartbreaking instances of having their concerns dismissed and belittled by their care providers (Dobbin-Thomas, 2015).

Some women try to protect themselves from mistreatment by choosing to birth at home, even in high-risk situations (Sassine, 2021). A growing number of women are choosing to 'freebirth', which is to give birth without the assistance of a skilled provider (Rigg, 2020; Dahlen et al., 2020). In Australia, women are socially vilified and publicly shamed through our coronial systems and the media for making the decision to protect themselves from mistreatment (Bodkin, 2012; *Inquest into the Death of Roisin Fraser*, 2012; Kurz et al., 2017; Gartry & Arrow, 2015). Needless to say, healthcare providers who abuse freebirthing mothers serves no purpose other than to alienate them further.

Box 3.2   Not listening': a common problem in the provision of maternity healthcare

Hospital staff did not listen to me, didn't trust me to know my body. Dismissed me as a first time mother who was over reacting. In actual fact I dilated from 0 to 6 in just over an hour. The hospital midwives told me that I was just feeling the period pain associated with early labour and induction …

(Reed et al., 2017, p. 4)

RESEARCH ACTIVITY

In the context of the significant medical resources allocated to, and advancements associated with, maternal health in Australia and New Zealand, is the goal of 'live mother live baby' at the end of labour and birth enough or an appropriate standard of care?

For mothers and babies who suffer unrecognised (or unacknowledged) maternal and infant trauma, who is responsible for their injuries? Who should take responsibility for their injuries? If those injuries remain unrecognised, how are they to be treated? If they are not treated and/or efforts are not taken to prevent trauma, can we hold mothers who neglect or struggle to care for their infants responsible or accountable?

(b) The human right to equal treatment

The human right to equality and equal treatment or, to put it differently, the right to be free from discrimination means that all people are entitled to exercise the full range of human rights without facing differential treatment on the basis of personal characteristics. Discriminating against someone on the basis of race, skin colour, gender, age, pregnancy, indigenous heritage, sexual preferences or parental status is a violation of their human right to equality and equal treatment.

Between and within nations, minority groups are at a significantly increased risk of dying in childbirth and of seeing their babies die in childbirth compared with privileged or controlling groups. Some of this inequality occurs at a systemic level through problems associated with poverty, nutrition and access to healthcare. Some of it occurs at an individual level when women and their infants are treated as 'the others' or 'less than …' by their providers who consciously or unconsciously associate that woman with a socially undesirable or disliked status or category (e.g. *Alyne da Silva Pimentel v Brazil*, 2011; *Laxmi Mandal v NCT Delhi*, 2009; Mayra & Kumar-Hazard, 2020).

The practice of profiling women to determine what medical interventions they may require in advance of birth can violate the human right to equality and equal treatment. Examples include performing a greater number of caesarean sections on immigrant and refugee women (Trinh et al., 2020), using algorithms to promote racial bias in maternity health management (Obermeyer et al., 2019), using language barriers to assert power and control (MRWHP, 2018); using race to determine the risk profile of individual women (Reddy et al., 2017), threatening child removal for non-compliant Indigenous and migrant mothers (Aubusson, 2017) and forcing electronic fetal monitoring (EFM) for fetal assessment during labour on women deemed to be high risk because of age, racial heritage or body weight (Alfirevic et al., 2017).

Playing the 'dead baby card'

In maternity health services, discrimination on the basis of pregnancy occurs when care providers profess to speak on behalf of the fetus to secure compliance for treatment, (De Costa & Robson, 2012; MacKenzie Bryers & van Teijlingen, 2010). Examples include the following:

- A Muslim refugee does not want a male obstetrician to attend her. There is a female doctor in the labour ward. Despite that, a male visiting medical officer storms into the birthing suite and says 'A baby died in this room yesterday! We don't want that to happen again, do we? Let's focus on delivering this baby right now. I would like to perform a vaginal examination—now!'
- A woman asks for more time before agreeing to a C-section. Her midwife says 'Baby is getting tired now … if you don't make a decision now, you will be putting your baby at risk.'
- A woman refuses CTG monitoring. Her midwife says 'You don't want your baby to die, do you?'

Asserting the 'dead baby card' or professing to defend the interests of the fetus against its mother is based on the **'fetal rights** doctrine'. This is where care providers act on the mistaken belief that an unborn fetus has equal and opposite rights and interests to its mother. Through the use of technological aids like ultrasound and cardiotocography (CTG), care providers gather limited information which they use to pitch a mother against her unborn infant and dictate treatment terms to women who resist or question medical recommendations (McLean & Petersen, 1996; Weigel, 2017). When a mother resists or questions the recommendations of the care provider, overriding her decision is based on two assumptions:

1. that the mother's interests are in conflict with the interests of the infant
2. that the care provider has the right to speak for the infant or assume the role as advocate for the fetus, in order to justify overriding the wishes of the mother.

Both these assumptions are wrong. The decision to override the wishes of a pregnant person on the basis of the pregnancy, however well intentioned, constitutes discrimination.

Australian and New Zealand common (or judge-made) laws do not recognise the doctrine of fetal rights. The oft-used legal principle used to defend against this doctrine is referred to as the 'born-alive rule'. Under this legal principle, a fetus does not have separate legal status until and unless it is born alive and physically separated from its mother. That means the only person who can make decisions on behalf of a fetus is its mother. In law, this means a healthcare provider's duty of care must be to the woman who is pregnant, not the fetus.

There are very good reasons why the common law has historically imposed and maintained the born-alive rule of law. Every time the spectre of fetal rights is raised, we are imposing legal and moral obligations on pregnant women which we do not impose on any man or a woman who is not pregnant (McLachlan, 2017; Minkoff & Paltrow, 2004; Samuels et al., 2007). Treating a person or group of persons less favourably on the basis of certain personal characteristics, such as pregnancy, race or age, is a form of direct discrimination.

This form of discrimination also offends another common law protection known as the 'Good Samaritan' legal principle. In accordance with this principle, the law cannot and does not compel any of us to be a 'Good Samaritan', whether it be to give blood or to share our bodily organs in order to save another's life. The US Court in *McFall v Shimp* (1978) put it best when it said:

> … *for our law to compel [the] defendant to submit to an intrusion of his body would change every concept and principle upon which our society is founded.*

Imposing fetal rights to discriminate against pregnant women can be socially and politically dangerous for many reasons. First, there is substantial evidence to show that the added duty and burden on pregnant women subjugates them, socially and legally, to a subservient class of person in violation of their fundamental human right to equity and equality (*Barrett v Coroner's Court of South Australia*, 2010; Savell, 2006). In the USA, particularly in states where religious influences have a significant impact on government, fetal rights have been used to override the rights of pregnant women and force them to submit to medical interventions, coercion (with or without court orders) even where the fetus is not viable or where submission could compromise the health of the mother (Cudahy, 2015; Paltrow & Flavin, 2013). Like medical negligence laws, it only takes one court to put the fetus before the mother to create a snowball effect of similar cases which increasingly erode women's sexual and reproductive rights (Ehrlich, 2007; Vanderwalker, 2008). Use of court processes to force women to submit to medical treatment in pregnancy and childbirth occurs in the USA, Brazil, Argentina, Peru, Hungary and Slovakia. In the UK, Australia, New Zealand and Canada, health services are more likely to use reports (actual and threatened) to child services to coerce women into submission. The decision to treat a class of persons as subservient, in violation of their human rights, is not a matter for healthcare practitioners. who face no accountability for their actions. It is a matter for our elected officials who can be held accountable at the ballot box.

Giving unaccountable healthcare providers power over pregnant women can have severe health consequences for women and their families. In Ireland, constitutional laws giving doctors the power to treat the unborn fetus as having rights over its mother resulted in the tragic and untimely death of 23-year-old Savita Halapavannar (Arulkumaran et al., 2013). In that case, despite the fact that Ms Halapavannar's miscarriage was causing clear signs of sepsis, doctors refused her and her family's request for a termination on the remote possibility that the fetus would survive. In its Inquiry Report, the HSE noted that:

> *The investigation team is satisfied that concerns about the law, whether clear or not, impacted on the exercise of clinical professional judgement.*

> (Arulkumaran et al., HSE Inquiry, 2013, p. 69)

Following the tragic deaths of Ms Halapavannar and others, the people of Ireland voted, in overwhelming numbers, to change the constitutional laws which, in substance, discriminated against women on the basis of pregnancy.

In Australia and New Zealand, the spectre of fetal rights equally impacts the clinical judgment of care providers. Studies in Australia point to a similar confusion over fetal rights (Jenkinson et al., 2017; Kruske et al., 2013). Confusion has led to the assumption that women do not have the right to make decisions that, in a care provider's opinion, put their fetus at risk:

> When women share their birth stories, the language they use speaks volumes about how little they understand regarding their rights, and/or how poorly their rights were respected … 'I wasn't allowed to go more than two weeks overdue', 'They wouldn't let me try for a vaginal birth', 'They told me I had to be monitored continually on the CTG machine.'
> (Sargent & Sargent, *Voice for Parents* blog, 10 Aug 2017)

To be clear, no care provider has the power to decide whether a patient is competent, or choose or impose a treatment option on a patient. That is the law. At best, the imposition of fetal rights masks the personal interests of care providers, whether motivated by fear of litigation or loss of employment or reputation (Minkoff & Paltrow, 2004; Samuels et al., 2007). At worse, the imposition of fetal rights is at odds with women's human and legal rights to equality and autonomy. Benevolence, or the belief that you are saving or helping someone in spite of their wishes, cannot justify the violation of a human being's right to bodily autonomy. Such behaviour, in extremes, can amount to torture, assault or battery.

(c) The human right to bodily autonomy

The human right to bodily **autonomy** and self-determination is about the right to decide what happens to your body, under any circumstances, and includes both the right to informed consent and the right to refuse medical treatment (Article 1, Declaration of the Elimination of Violence Against Women (UN, 1994); Article 1, International Covenant on Economic, Social and Cultural Rights (OHCHR, 1976); Article 5, Universal Declaration on Bioethics and Human Rights (UNESCO, 2005); Article 9.1, 18.2, International Covenant on Civil and Political Rights (OHCHR, 1966); Kotaska, 2017).

Common law jurisdictions in the UK and Australia are, at the highest judicial levels, very clear about the importance of patient autonomy, a position best illustrated in relation to pregnant women by the UK Court of Appeal's unanimous judgment in *Re MB*:

> A competent woman who has the capacity to decide may, for religious reasons, other reasons, for rational or irrational reasons or for no reason at all, choose not to have medical intervention, even though the consequence may be the death or serious handicap of the child she bears, or her own death.

> In that event the courts do not have the jurisdiction to declare medical intervention lawful and the question of her own best interests objectively considered, does not arise.
> (*Re MB (Caesarean Section)* [1997] EWCA Civ 1361, para 30)

A similar judicial stance was adopted by the highest appellate courts in the USA (*Society of N.Y. Hosp. v Schloendorff*, 1914), Australia (*Secretary, Department of Health and Community Services v JWB and SMB (Marion's case)*, 1992) and Canada (*Mallette v Shulman*, 1990).

Unfortunately, confusion amongst care providers about pregnant people's rights to decide what happens to their bodies is caused by inconsistent lower court and coronial court findings, in circumstances where well-meaning judges go to extraordinary lengths to deliver what they perceive to be justice. They do so by indirectly implementing the fetal rights doctrine, in violation of a woman's right to determine what happens to her body (*Chavkin & Diaz-Tello*, 2017; *N.J. Div. of Youth & Family Servs. v V.M.*, 2009). In the USA, Rinat Dray, an Orthodox Jewish woman, engaged a physician who agreed to support her attempts at a vaginal birth after two caesarean sections (VBAC2) because of legitimate concerns about her rising risk of mortality and morbidity from having several caesarean sections (Nisenblat et al., 2005). When she arrived at the hospital in labour, her chosen physician was not available. The substitute physician immediately pushed her to have another caesarean section without clinical indication. When she declined, he threatened to call child services and to get a court order forcing her to submit to the treatment. With the agreement of the hospital lawyer, the physician falsely asserted that a court order had been obtained and used this false claim to forcibly perform a caesarean section delivery. She sued the hospital for obstetric malpractice, but the Court dismissed her claim in the first instance, using the fetal rights doctrine to state that when:

> [an] individual's conduct threatens injury to others, the State's interest is manifest and the State can generally be expected to intervene.
> (*Dray v Staten Island Univ. Hosp.*, 2014)

The Court's initial dismissal has been appealed by human rights advocates concerned about the implications of this case for all women, which are serious. According to this lower court, the current legal position is that Mrs Dray's normal bodily function of going into labour and delivering her infant can be viewed as 'conduct capable of harming another', and that 'another' will be none other than her own fetus that she has physically carried and nurtured for 9 months. The decision also erroneously aligns the interests of a private hospital with that of the state, even though the hospital never obtained a court order in the first place (Diaz-Tello, 2016).

In Australia, the coroner's court has been used to undermine the human right to bodily autonomy and women's rights to self-determination. In coronial inquiries concerning infant deaths, findings and determinations have, in effect:
(a) eroded the born-alive rule
(b) legitimised provider justifications for overriding consent

(c) elevated medical paternalism over patient autonomy
(d) reinforced gender-based stereotypes by positioning birthing women as either irresponsible or misguided victims
(e) called on women to be compliant to and grateful for medical intervention irrespective of the significant personal cost, shame and stigma they have already endured
(f) dismissed claims that women experienced mistreatment, disrespect and abuse in hospitals
(g) ignored or derided womens' decision making that was influenced by prior evidence of mistreatment in facility- based childbirth
(h) recommended disciplinary and criminal investigations against anyone who purports to support women who reject medical recommendations (Sassine & Dahlen, 2020; Rigg, 2020; Kumar-Hazard, 2020).

While coroners genuinely believe they are acting in the public interest, the implications of such findings are deeply concerning because they effectively undermine women's human rights to equality. They can slowly, but surely, undermine the public perception of what constitutes the right to equality and equal treatment. After all, if our healthcare providers—do not believe that consent is necessary if acting with good intentions, why should a marital partner, or a parent, or an employer, or a priest? This is not just theoretical argument. At the time of writing this chapter, Australia is battling an epidemic of gender-based violence against women and girls. Reproductive coercion is internationally recognised as a subset of gender-based violence (Fay & Yee, 2018). It remains to be seen whether Australia acknowledges that reality.

The doctrine of informed consent

The following international instruments define and oblige the implementation of the doctrine of informed consent in Australia and New Zealand. In General Recommendation No. 24 on the core obligations of States parties under article 12 of the Convention (women and health), the Committee on the Elimination of Discrimination Against Women (CEDAW, 1999) stated:

States parties should also report on measures taken to ensure access to quality health-care services, for example, by making them acceptable to women. Acceptable services are those that are delivered in a way that ensures that a woman gives her fully informed consent, respects her dignity, guarantees her confidentiality and is sensitive to her needs and perspectives.
(para 22)

In addition, Article 6 of the Universal Declaration on Bioethics and Human Rights 1997 provides that:

any preventive, diagnostic and therapeutic medical intervention is only to be carried out with the prior, free and informed consent of the person concerned, based on adequate information.

The human right to make autonomous decisions about one's own body is enshrined in legal protections such as the doctrine of informed consent and the right to refuse medical treatment (Kotaska, 2017). These rights

are not nullified because a woman is also making decisions for her unborn baby (*Draper v Jasionowski*, 2004). The person giving birth is the person best positioned to weigh her needs and options in combination with the needs of her unborn child.

Informed consent, at its simplest, can be thought of as two sides of the same coin: (a) the duty to inform; and (b) the right to consent. In *I. V. v. Bolivia* (2014, para 186), the Inter-American court stated, in relation to the sterilisation of a pregnant refugee without consent:

the informed consent of the patient is a sine qua non condition for the medical intervention, which is based on respect for the patient's personal autonomy and freedom to choose her life plans without interference.

The practitioner's duty to inform

The practitioner carries the duty or obligation to inform, which must:
- explain the risks, benefits and alternative options to undertaking any procedure
- be given in a timely manner so the patient has time to consider her options
- take into account and understand the patient's individual needs and circumstances
- be free of threats, coercion or punitive actions.

There remains substantial misunderstanding amongst practitioners as to the scope and application of their duty to afford informed consent. This is due, in part, to a limited understanding by lawyers and the courts in medical negligence litigation of the implications of attaching greater significance to injuries to an infant over injuries to a woman. It is also due to a watering down, in medical liability laws, of the obligation to afford informed consent to the weaker, easier practitioner's duty to warn of material risks (Field, 2008; *Rogers v Whitaker*, 1992). To protect themselves and their clients from liability, insurers encourage governments and practitioners to practise within the limited confines of the duty to warn of material risks. This has all but eroded the skill and capacity of providers to fully inform women of their options in maternity healthcare. In turn, governments and hospitals are supplementing the limited and poor communication skills of providers with an excessive reliance on technology and hospital protocols and policies. Technological surveillance and hospital protocols and policies to standardise practice, when used to monitor and control women are, in themselves, a form of intervention that *should* trigger the obligation to inform because they inevitably force women to accept certain treatment options they did not realise they had to accept when they agreed to either the surveillance or to concede to hospital protocols. For example, women are not aware that:
- agreeing to CTG surveillance is more likely to lead to a caesarean section (Alfirevic et al., 2017)
- routine inductions are more likely to require interventions such as the use of forceps or caesarean section (Ryan & McCarthy 2019)
- risk of infection and bladder irritation can be caused by routine vaginal examinations (Dahlen et al., 2013).

Asking women to sign consent forms they cannot read and/or without explanation does not satisfy the obligation to obtain informed consent. In a case (the *Montgomery case*) concerning a pregnant woman with gestational diabetes who wanted, but was not offered, a caesarean section, the UK Supreme Court found that the doctor's duty to inform was not fulfilled by bombarding the woman with technical information that she could not reasonably be expected to grasp. In addition, the duty cannot be satisfied by routinely demanding the patient's signature on a consent form (*Montgomery v Lanarkshire Health Board (Respondent) (Scotland)*, 2015, para 90).

There has been a perverse tendency to interpret the *Montgomery case* as creating a duty to warn women about the risks associated with physiological birth or natural bodily functions (Black, 2016; Downe, 2016). The issue before the UK Supreme Court was whether a care provider could ignore or dismiss a patient's legitimate request to know more about her treatment options during childbirth. The court was not concerned with whether she had a physiological birth or a caesarean section. The court took exception to the doctor's belief that she knew better than her ignorant and naive patient.

The patient's right to consent

The patient's right to consent must be:
1. freely given
2. affirmative (a 'maybe' is not a 'yes')
3. specific (required for each intervention, every time)
4. informed (but does not require explanation or justification)
5. reversible.

Practitioners are not comfortable dealing with patients who refuse recommended medical treatments in pregnancy and childbirth. They manage their discomfort by deploying a range of measures aimed at securing compliance, such as engaging in discussions that intimidate, threaten or bully, neglect and co-opting family members. (Niles et al., 2021). Care providers appear unaware that a patient is entitled to refuse a recommendation, regardless of the consequences to her or her unborn baby. If a provider has explained the risks, documented the discussion and the patient still refuses, any further action by the provider can, and in most cases will, amount to coercion and/or assault. This is, in itself, a form of mistreatment in the provision of healthcare.

The rising emphasis in maternity healthcare on questioning the competence and the capacity of a pregnant woman to make decisions, particularly in the face of conflict with her care provider, is also the result of poor provider communication skills which are informed by harmful gender stereotypes about women and motherhood. A refusal of recommended medical treatment does not have to be informed or acceptable to the provider to meet the provider's understanding of 'competence'. Informed consent rests upon an assumption that, despite the esoteric nature of medical knowledge, ordinary people can assess their medical options and make decisions about them. From the woman's perspective, decision making in healthcare is a personal process that incorporates her history, cultural and spiritual values, and family values. These do not have to be seen as rational or appropriate from a care provider's point of view to be respected. There is no obligation on the patient to justify or explain their decisions.

Providers are also using competence to control and discipline providers, who seek to protect a person's human rights. Hospital staff use it as a basis for pursuing disciplinary complaints against independent midwives. For example, independent midwives will only transfer care to a hospital with their client's consent. This can result in transfer delays which trigger the disapproval of hospital staff and complaints to AHPRA. Complaints about independent midwives typically proceed on two grounds. The first ground assumes that a competent woman, if properly counselled about the risks, would not have resisted either the transfer or hospital care. The complaint will proceed on the grounds that the independent midwife failed to advise the woman of the risks. Alternatively, the second ground assumes that the client was not competent and needed to be coerced into compliance as is usually done in hospital. Both complaints rest on erroneous assumptions about competence. Those assumptions are based on harmful gender stereotypes about women as either victims or irresponsible mothers. If staff conclude that the woman was an irresponsible mother (for example, outspoken women or persons with Indigenous heritage, addictions or 'alternate' or 'hippy' views), they may also notify child protection services. (Hunter et al., 2020; Jenkinson & Fox 2020; Kuliukas et al., 2016; Sosa et al., 2018).

There is a legal presumption that adults are competent. To challenge that presumption, care providers must obtain both a psychiatric opinion and a court order to override an adult patient's decisions about treatment.

There is growing international recognition that the failure to afford informed consent constitutes 'obstetric violence' or the mistreatment and abuse of women in maternity healthcare facilities. In 2019, the UN *Special Rapporteur on violence against women, its causes and consequences* (UN, 2019) cited a failure to afford informed consent as driving mistreatment and violence in childbirth. The root causes of that mistreatment and violence are harmful gender stereotypes about motherhood and women's subordinate role in society, and the unequal power dynamic within provider-patient relationships.

In 2020, the Committee for the Elimination of Discrimination against Women determined in *S.F.M v Spain* (2020) that Spain had used gender-based stereotyping to perpetuate 'obstetric violence' against S.F.M. in childbirth. In a separate statement issued through the UN Human Rights Committee, the Vice-Chair of the Committee stated:

> *This woman has had a normal pregnancy but then was subjected to interventions that deeply affected her physical and mental health and the health of her baby …*
>
> *It's time to stop obstetric violence. Women shouldn't experience abusive or discriminatory treatment during childbirth …*

I trust that Spain will take the recommendations made in the decision very seriously, and that the decision's wide dissemination will promote substantial changes in health care protocols in many countries.

(OHCHR, 2020)

It is worth noting that Australia has a maternity health system that is very similar to that in Spain.

The UN Special Rapporteur also expressed concern over the abuse of the doctrine of medical necessity. This is where care providers claim an emergency to justify overriding the patient's right to give consent, usually as a justification following the event. This justification is regularly raised in Australia following unplanned and unwanted interventions such as episiotomies, forceps use and caesarean sections. Except in cases of a genuine emergency, care providers in Australia and New Zealand must seek the approval of a court of law to override the bodily integrity or autonomy of any adult. A woman in labour is presumed competent and is not considered to be in a genuine emergency.

(d) The human right to privacy

The right to choose your care provider and to determine the circumstances of your birth is protected under Article 8 of the European Convention of Human Rights . Article 8 protects the right to respect for private and family life. (see *Ternovszky v Hungary* (2010); *S.F.M v Spain* (2020)).

Choice is fundamental to maintaining quality in healthcare. Choice gives consumers the ability to 'vote with their feet' and acts as a powerful and effective antidote to abusive or unethical business practices or monopolies, and boosts consumer-friendly changes on the supply side of the market. While Australia and New Zealand have strong, effective consumer protection laws, maternity healthcare systems and its providers appear to have enjoyed an informal immunity from consumer feedback and competition (Cook et al., 2010; Davis & Hoey, 2017; Diaz-Tello, 2015).

This immunity is primarily due to the lack of available and accessible information on important quality measures such as differences in models of care, options in childbirth, and care provider preferences and performance. These quality measures matter to maternity healthcare consumers. It is highly unlikely, for example, that women who do not want to have major surgery will agree to attend a hospital or engage a provider which they know has high caesarean section rates. In addition, those who do receive experience unwanted treatments will never truly know, *even after receiving the treatment,* whether treatment was needed or performed with the requisite skill. Without information, consumers are forced to depend, not on independent inquiry, but on information supplied by the same providers who stand to benefit financially and professionally from either overservicing or increasing prices. These goods are referred to as 'credence goods', unique because it is not possible to assess the value or quality of the good either before or after consuming those services. Other types of credence goods include

> ### Box 3.3 Medical treatment is a 'credence good'
>
> *With a credence good, consumers are never sure about the extent of the good they actually need. Therefore, sellers act as experts determining the customers' requirements. This **information asymmetry** between buyers and sellers obviously creates strong incentives for sellers to cheat on services.*
>
> (Emons, 1997, p. 107)

legal and mechanical services. (Box 3.3). Without information, consumers are rendered powerless and providers can position themselves as the experts who decide the type and quantity of service the consumer pays for (Lewis et al., 2017). Strictly speaking, maternity healthcare providers and hospitals are no different to any other supplier of goods and services, and are subject to the same consumer protection laws affecting any other business or supplier. Efforts are being undertaken to provide consumers with better information so they can either exercise choice or hold providers to account.

A growing number of women are opting out of hospital care and choosing to birth at home, with or without support, following a negative hospital experience. (Dahlen et al., 2011; Lee et al., 2016; *Switzer v Rezvina et al.,* 2015). Maternal satisfaction and choice, factors of significance to women, unfortunately do not feature in news reports about home birth. Women's home-birth experiences are usually described, by a medical professional, as a dangerous 'indulgence', followed by statements that reinforce the importance of using hospitals maternity services only. These claims are usually met with the ire of home-birth advocates. Unfortunately, the controversy is nearly always resolved in favour of the medical hegemony (Box 3.4). (Catling-Paull et al., 2013; Coddington et al., 2017; Ieraci & Tuteur, 2013; Olsen & Clausen, 2012).

Debates about home birth need to be economically and historically contextualised to be properly understood. A lot of effort is spent arguing about the relative safety of a practice utilised by just 0.3% of the birthing population in Australia and approximately 4% in New Zealand. This may seem like a wasted effort if the argument is purely about home birth. The conflict, however, is not over home birth. It is over the independence of the midwifery profession. The medical obstetric profession has, for over a century, successfully controlled the provision of maternity health services. A profession historically dominated by men, they have protected themselves by operating as a guild and forging close ties with government. In exchange for public health management and monitoring of women and infants, they received government-funded resources and facilities. As the independent practice of midwifery was made a crime, nurses were brought into health facilities and trained to provide

Box 3.4   Medical hegemony

Hegemony is defined as the preponderant influence or authority over others, the social, cultural, ideological, or economic influence exerted by a dominant group. Medical hegemony is the dominance of the biomedical model, the active suppression of alternatives as well as the corporatization of personal, clinical medicine into pharmaceutical and hospital centered treatment.

(Weber, 2016, p. 65)

care under the supervision and tutelage of obstetric medical providers (Lane & Reiger, 2009; McIntyre et al., 2011; McIntoxh, 2012).

Today, midwifery has been reestablished as a profession and is asserting its independence. Independent midwives do not need health facilities or access to high-end technology to care for women. They prefer to be embedded in a community where they can attend women, instead of making women come to them. They offer a suite of services that extend beyond pregnancy, from infant care to family planning, which are well received by women (Lane & Reiger, 2009; McIntyre et al., 2011; McIntosh, 2012).

Home birth is a representation of the conflict between medical providers and midwives. It signals the end of medical hegemony in childbirth. It also signals the rise of a profession once thought redundant. It challenges the notion that maternity health services cannot be safely provided without a hospital. From a consumer and economic perspective, it represents choice.

News reports covering debates about home birth struggle to address these complexities. The general public have a limited understanding of the relative powerlessness of midwives, not just from a historical and economic perspective but also from their subordinate social standing as women. News reports rely on sensationalist content that sells news and this is easily achieved by stereotyping women as victims or evildoers, whether they are midwife or mother. The well-resourced and experienced public relations machines of medical professional associations are skilled at using news reporting as a 'blunt instrument to bludgeon' the credibility and professionalism of independently practising midwives (MacColl, 2007). Ultimately, midwives need to appreciate that incumbent actors in maternity care with market share, social prestige, government support and advertising dollars (together referred to as the medical hegemony, see Box 3.4) can strategically use these advantages to dominate and shape public perceptions on home birth. To publicly disparage independent midwives without regard for the difficult socioeconomic context in which all midwives practise is to disparage the midwifery profession as a whole, for little gain. This is not to say that a midwife cannot or should not raise concerns about a colleague. Regulators and professional bodies provide a discrete process to both address quality concerns and protect the reputation of the profession as a whole. Professional collegiality is important to ensuring the independence and longevity of the midwifery profession is maintained.

From a human rights perspective, whether or not a woman can birth at home should not be determined by stakeholders who are financially affected by that choice. Access to choices in childbirth, systemic recognition and support for those choices, and the provision of easily accessible information to facilitate that choice is the responsibility of governments. Our elected representatives can, and should, be held accountable for failing to offer these choices in violation of a woman's right to privacy and choice, including in relation to the circumstances of her birth. It is truly that simple.

REFLECTIVE CASE STUDY

What does the right to the highest attainable level of health mean to you? Is it the right to:

- be alive?
- be alive and physically intact?
- be alive, physically intact but mentally traumatised?
- be alive, physically intact and mentally well?
- be alive and thrive?

(As you are thinking about the above options, you may want to consider the following: in 2015 the World Health Organization launched its revised *Global Strategy for Women's, Children's and Adolescents' Health (2016–30)* with the social targets of 'Survive, Thrive, Transform' (WHO, 2015). The Global Strategy presents a roadmap for achieving the highest attainable standard of physical and mental health by prioritising human rights to, and through, health. The roadmap aims to set the path to a world in which each woman, child and adolescent in every setting can realise their rights to physical and mental health and wellbeing, has social and economic opportunities, and is able to participate fully in shaping prosperous and sustainable societies.)

Now ask yourself: how many women do you know who have realised their rights to physical and mental health and wellbeing, and are able to participate fully in shaping prosperous and sustainable societies, after giving birth at the hospital in which you work?

CRITICAL THINKING EXERCISE

Read the following passage, then answer the questions below.

In 2010, the European Court of Human Rights recognised that the right to privacy, the foundation of reproductive rights in Europe and the United States, applies to childbirth. In the case of *Ternovszky v Hungary* (2010), the Court held that, as a woman has the right to choose whether to give birth to a child, she also has the right to choose the circumstances in which she gives birth. The Court held that the state violates this human right if it fails to legitimise the choice for home birth through regulation, and if it criminally sanctions birth professionals, in particular midwives, for supporting women in that choice by attending them at home. The Court noted that, when the law circumscribes women's birth choices instead of supporting them, it makes birth less safe, not more. In considering Anna Ternovszky's claim, the Court examined the state's obligations around childbirth, the mistreatment of pregnant women in health facilities and the prevailing medical monopoly over the provision of maternity health services in Hungary. The court expressed concern that, under the Hungarian maternity health system, pregnant women are expected to submit to medical hegemony, passively absorb and accept the doctor–patient power imbalance and comply with all instructions. At the heart of the case is the story of Agnes Gereb, an obstetrician-turned-midwife who was being criminally prosecuted for supporting several high-risk home births, at least two of which resulted in stillbirths. Gereb was known for challenging Hungary's medical hegemony over maternity health services, which resulted in the removal of her licence to practise obstetric medicine. Gereb became a midwife and ran an oversubscribed birth centre which was eventually shut down for transferring women needing medical assistance to hospitals without the approval of hospital staff. Following that, Gereb supplied home-birth services.

For midwives, a concerning aspect of the case is the prosecution of a health professional for doing their job. To achieve a conviction in criminal law, motive or intention to do the wrongful act or criminally reckless behaviour must be proven beyond reasonable doubt. In her defence, Gereb denied an intention to hurt the women or infants in her care. She submitted that she acted out of benevolence, because no one else would support her clients' choices, and had applied due skill and care when providing services. Her defence was dismissed even where her clients gave evidence in support of her claims.

A similar prosecution was attempted, albeit without success, in Australia. The similarities between the two cases were uncanny. Inquests prior to the prosecutions promoted the same harmful stereotypes as in Hungary: the midwife faced criminal sanctions, health systems were lauded for imposing restrictions on pregnant women and the women who home birthed were portrayed as victims of deception. From a human rights perspective, the inquests and prosecution in both countries did not improve the delivery of maternity health services. They did, however, increase the monitoring and policing of pregnant women and new mothers, in further violation of their right to privacy (Soderberg, 2016).

1. Should midwives be criminally prosecuted for supporting women who pursue home birth against medical advice?

2. Should anyone be criminally prosecuted for doing their job?

Conclusion

How much would change if it were really clear to everybody in the birth room that the birthing woman is the only person with the right to make all the decisions?

How much would change if law and practice aligned to reflect the human right to choose the circumstances of childbirth, and to uphold every pregnant woman's right to make supported decisions for her body and her baby?

For decades, the industrialisation of childbirth, birthing room power dynamics and the social and legal policing of women have combined to create the perfect storm that has become the maternity healthcare experience of all but a small percentage of fortunate pregnant women. Women are often systematically and systemically excluded from decision making in maternity healthcare. The disrespect and abuse of pregnant people in violation of their human rights is undermining the health and wellbeing of mothers and babies. The vilification of women who resist reproductive coercion compounds dangerous stereotypes casting women as either victims or irresponsible mothers. The subordination of midwives within a medicalised maternity system violates principles of equity and equality. Intimidating medical and midwifery providers who seek to defend women's human rights in pregnancy and childbirth undermines and limits opportunities to reform a health system through a human rights lens. This is making maternity healthcare practices less safe for everyone.

But the storm is breaking. More and more, women are calling on judges, lawyers and policy makers to challenge the medical, social and legal norms that violate their human rights and limit their access to services they actually want. It is time for all women to take this journey—an important step in realising the full spectrum of women's human and reproductive rights—for all of us. There will come a time when it will not be possible to ignore us any longer.

Review question: are you bearing witness to these human rights violations?

In 2011, the White Ribbon Alliance, together with the World Health Organization, International Confederation of Midwives, USAID, Centre for Reproductive Rights, the National Advocates for Pregnant Women and many other stakeholders collaboratively developed the charter of the universal rights of childbearing women, based on the human rights that were discussed above. (See the White Ribbon Alliance, 2017, https://www.whiteribbonalliance.org/wp-content/uploads/2017/11/RMC_Brochure.pdf.)

Table 3.1 summarises the violations that have been reported to Human Rights in Childbirth by women, care providers and family members over the last 5 years. The consistency and similarities in the reports indicate that these practices have become normal, everyday healthcare practices in maternity hospitals around the world.

- As you review these practices, ask yourself the following question: How many times a day have you been a silent witness to such conduct?

Table 3.1 Violations reported to Human Rights in Childbirth		
Disrespect and abuse	Everyday healthcare practices	Corresponding human rights violation
Physical abuse	Non-consented force, restraints, unnecessary procedures such as cord clamping and episiotomies, failure to provide pain relief or using pain relief as a coercion tool	The right to liberty, autonomy and self-determination
Disrespect	Verbal abuse, bullying, blaming, humiliating, body shaming, reprimands, 'shroud waving' or playing the 'dead baby card'	The right to dignity, and to be free of violence and ill treatment
Non-confidential care	Unauthorised revelation of personal details (particularly in staff rooms), physical exposure	The right to privacy and confidentiality
Non-consented care	Procedures performed without adequate information or dialogue to enable autonomous decision making, undue pressure to make specific clinical choices, imposition of time limits or restrictions for hospital convenience	The right to bodily integrity and self-determination
Misinformed care	Biased, non-transparent clinical information, disabling women from giving true informed consent, for e.g. breech birth and VBAC	The right to information, informed consent and the right to refuse medical treatment
Depersonalised/ dehumanised care	Inflexible application of institutional policy, failure to take into account women's individual circumstances, including around companionship of choice	The human right to dignity and respect
Discriminatory care	Unequal treatment based on personal attributes such as age, race, disability, sexual preferences, marital status	The right to equality, freedom from discrimination, and equitable care
Abandonment of care	Refusal to provide care owing to inability to pay or birth choices outside guidelines	The right to healthcare and the highest attainable level of health

VBAC=vaginal birth after caesarean.
(Source: White Ribbon Alliance, 2017)

Online resources

Australian Human Rights Commission: https://www.humanrights.gov.au.

Australian Institute of Health and Welfare (AIHW). Maternal Deaths in Australia 2008–2012: https://www.aihw.gov.au/getmedia/07bba8de-0413-4980-b553-7592089c4c8c/18796.pdf.aspx?inline5true.

GIRE. Obstetric violence report: https://www.gire.org.mx/en/wp-content/uploads/sites/2/2015/11/ObstetricViolenceReport.pdf.

Health and Disability Commissioner. The code and your rights. 2018: https://www.hdc.org.nz/disability/the-code-and-your-rights.

HeinOnline—an online database containing more than 140 million pages and 125,000 titles of legal history and government documents: http://heinonline.org.

Office of the High Commissioner for Human Rights (OHCHR). International Covenant on Civil and Political Rights: http://www.ohchr.org//EN/ProfessionalInterest/Pages/CESCR.aspx.

United Nations (UN). Declaration of the Elimination of Violence Against Women: https://www.ohchr.org/en/professionalinterest/pages/violenceagainstwomen.aspx.

United Nations Educational, Scientific and Cultural Organization (UNESCO). Universal Declaration on Bioethics and Human Rights: http://portal.unesco.org/en/ev.php-URL_ID=31058&URL_DO=DO_TOPIC&URL_SECTION5201.html.

References

Alfirevic Z, Gyte GML, Cuthbert A, Devane D. Continuous cardiotocography (CTG) as a form of electronic fetal monitoring (EFM) for fetal assessment during labour. *Cochrane Database of Sys Rev.* 2017;(2):CD006066, doi: 10.1002/14651858.CD006066.pub3.

Alyne da Silva Pimentel v Brazil (Communication No. 17/2008). (*UN Committee on the Elimination of Discrimination Against Women*). 2011. Online: https://www.escr-net.org/caselaw/2011/alyne-da-silva-pimentel-v-brazil-communication-no-172008.

Arrieta A. Health reform and cesarean sections in the private sector: the experience of Peru. *Health Policy (New York).* 2011;99(2):124–130. doi:10.1016/j.healthpol.2010.07.016.

Arulkumaran S, McCaughan C, Molloy C, et al. *Investigation of Incident 50278 from time of patient's self referral to hospital on the 21st of October 2012 to the patient's death on the 28th of October, 2012.* Dublin: Health Service Executive; 2013. Online: https://www.hse.ie/eng/services/news/nimtreport50278.pdf.

Aubusson, Kate, Healthcare News, "Terrified they will take their babies": Aboriginal midwives break cycle of distrust in health services, *Sydney Morning Herald* (online, 23 April 2017, 12.15am)

Australian Human Rights Commission (AHRC). *Rights and freedoms: right by right*; 2016. Online: https://www.humanrights.gov.au/rights-and-freedoms-right-right-0.

Baker H. We don't want to scare the ladies: an investigation of maternal rights and informed consent throughout the birth process. *CUNY Law Rev*. 2010;538:594. Online: http://heinonline.org.

Barrett v Coroner's Court of South Australia, SASCFC 70 (Sth Aust Sup Court, Full Court 2010).

Béhague DP, Victora CG, Barros FC. Consumer demand for caesarean sections in Brazil: informed decision making, patient choice, or social inequality? A population based birth cohort study linking ethnographic and epidemiological methods. *BMJ*. 2002;324(7343):942–945.

Beogo I, Mendez Rojas B, Gagnon M. Determinants and materno-fetal outcomes related to cesarean section delivery in private and public hospitals in low- and middle-income countries: a systematic review and meta-analysis protocol. *Syst Rev*. 2017; 6(1). doi:10.1186/s13643-016-0402-6.

Betran, AP, Ye J, Moller A-B, et al. Trends and projections of caesarean section rates: global and regional estimates. *BMJ Global Health*. 2021;6(6), e005671. doi:10.1136/bmjgh-2021-005671.

Black M. *Vaginal birth comes with risks too—so should it really be the default option?* The Conversation. 2016. Online: https://theconversation.com/vaginal-birth-comes-with-risks-too-so-should-it-really-be-the-default-option-62855.

Bodkin P. *'Free birth' delivery led to baby's death, coroner rules*. Daily Telegraph. 2012; June 28. Online: https://www.dailytelegraph.com.au/news/national/coroner-declares-free-birth-advocate-janet-frasers-decision-to-deliver-third-child-roisin-without-nurse-or-midwife-led-to-babys-death/news-story/84c086460a64001c2c8156e5070ab58c.

Bohren M, Vogel J, Hunter E, et al. The mistreatment of women during childbirth in health facilities globally: a mixed-methods systematic review. *PLoS Med*. 2015;12(6):e1001847. doi:10.1371/journal.pmed.1001847.

Borges MTR. A Violent Birth: reframing coerced procedures during childbirth as obstetric violence. *Duke Law Journal* 2018; 67(4): 827.

Catling-Paull C, Coddington R, Foureur M, et al. Publicly funded homebirth in Australia: a review of maternal and neonatal outcomes over 6 years. *Med J Aust*. 2013;199(11):743. doi:10.5694/mja13.11003.

Chavkin W, Diaz-Tello F. When courts fail: physicians' legal and ethical duty to uphold informed consent. *Col Med Rev*. 2017; 1(2):6–9.

Chen HH, Lai JC, Hwang SJ, et al. Understanding the relationship between cesarean birth and stress, anxiety, and depression after childbirth: A nationwide cohort study. *Birth (Berkeley, Calif)* 2017; 44(4): 369–76.

Clark J. The global push for institutional childbirths—in unhygienic facilities. *BMJ*. 2016;i:1473. doi:10.1136/bmj.i1473.

Coddington R, Homer C, Catling C. From 'homebirth sceptics' to 'homebirth champions': the influence of Australian publicly-funded homebirth programs on care provider's attitudes. *Women Birth*. 2017;30:16. doi:10.1016/j.wombi.2017.08.041.

Committee on the Elimination of Discrimination Against Women (CEDAW). *General recommendation No. 24.* 1999. Online: https://tbinternet.ohchr.org/Treaties/CEDAW/Shared%20Documents/1_Global/INT_CEDAW_GEC_4738_E.pdf

Cook R, Cusack S, Dickens B. Unethical female stereotyping in reproductive health. *Int J Gynaecol Obstet*. 2010;109(3): 255–258. doi:10.1016/j.ijgo.2010.02.002.

Cooper M, McCutcheon H, Warland J. 'They follow the wants and needs of an institution': Midwives' views of water immersion. *Women Birth*. 2021;34(2):e178–e187. doi: 10.1016/j.wombi.2020.02.019. Epub 2020 Mar 3.

Cox K, Bovbjerg M, Cheyney M, et al. Planned home VBAC in the United States, 2004–2009: outcomes, maternity care practices, and implications for shared decision making. *Birth*. 2015; 42(4):299–308. doi:10.1111/birt.12188.

Coxon K, Homer C, Bisits A, et al. Reconceptualising risk in childbirth. *Midwifery*. 2016;38:1–5. doi:10.1016/j.midw.2016.05.012.

Cudahy S. *Update: Augusta Co. jury rules in favor of doctor in C-section case*. NBC29. 2015. Online: http://www.nbc29.com/story/30455784/update-augusta-co-jury-rules-in-favor-of-doctor-in-c-section-case.

Dahlen H, Downe S, Duff M, et al. Vaginal examination during normal labor: routine examination or routine intervention? *International Journal of Childbirth* 2013; 3(3): 142–52.

Dahlen H, Jackson M, Stevens J. Homebirth, freebirth and doulas: casualty and consequences of a broken maternity system. *Women Birth*. 2011;24(1):47–50. doi:10.1016/j.wombi.2010.11.002.

Dahlen HG, B Kumar-Hazard and V Schmied, eds, *Birthing Outside the System: The Canary in the Coalmine*. Routledge Research in Nursing and Midwifery; 2020.

Dahlen H, Kruske S. *Forget too posh to push: doctors are behind the rise in C-sections. The Conversation*. 2012;20 January. Online: https://theconversation.com/forget-too-posh-to-push-doctors-are-behind-the-rise-in-c-sections-4986.

Dahlen H, Tracy S, Tracy M, et al. Rates of obstetric intervention and associated perinatal mortality and morbidity among low-risk women giving birth in private and public hospitals in NSW (2000–2008): a linked data population-based cohort study. *BMJ Open*. 2014;4(5):e004551. doi:10.1136/bmjopen-2013–004551.

Dahlen H, Tracy S, Tracy M, et al. Rates of obstetric intervention among low-risk women giving birth in private and public hospitals in NSW: a population-based descriptive study. *BMJ Open*. 2012;2(5):e001723. doi:10.1136/bmjopen-2012-001723.

Davis S, Hoey W. Publicly funded homebirth in Western Australia. *Women Birth*. 2017;30:44–45. doi:10.1016/j.wombi.2017.08.118.

De Costa C, Robson S. *MJA Insight*. 2012. Online: https://www.doctorportal.com.au/mjainsight/2012/25/caroline-de-costa/.

Dean R. The beauty and fun of Identity Politics. *The Daily Telegraph*. 2017; May 15.

Declercq E. The politics of home birth in the United States. *Birth*. 2012;39(4):281–285. doi:10.1111/birt.12001.

Declercq E. Childbirth in Brazil: challenging an interventionist paradigm. *Birth*. 2015;42(1):1–4. doi:10.1111/birt.12156.

Declercq E, Sakala C, Corry M, et al. *Listening to Mothers III: Pregnancy and Birth*. 3rd ed. New York: Childbirth Connection; 2013. Online: http://transform.childbirthconnection.org/wp-content/uploads/2013/06/LTM-III_Pregnancy-and-Birth.pdf.

Diaz-Tello F. When the invisible hand wields a scalpel: maternity care in the market economy. *CUNY Law Rev*. 2015;197:228.

Diaz-Tello F. Invisible wounds: obstetric violence in the United States. *Reprod Health Matters*. 2016;24(47):56–64. doi:10.1016/j.rhm.2016.04.004.

Diniz S, Chachamb A. "The cut above" and "the cut below": the abuse of caesareans and episiotomy in Sao Paulo, Brazil. *Reprod Health Matters*. 2004;12(23):100.

Dobbin-Thomas M. *Mother knows best: why hospitals should always respect maternal instinct. The Age*. 2015. Online: http://www.theage.com.au/victoria/mother-knows-best-why-hospitals-should-always-respect-maternal-instinct-20151019-gkcpdr.html.

Downe S. *It's no wonder women opt for caesareans over natural birth when they are not given a real choice*. The Conversation. 2016.

Online: https://theconversation.com/its-no-wonder-women-opt-for-caesareans-over-natural-birth-when-they-are-not-given-a-real-choice-63736.

Draper v Jasionowski (NJ Supr.Ct.App.Div 2004). Online: https://law.justia.com/cases/new-jersey/appellate-division-published/2004/a3697-03-opn.html.

Dray v Staten Island Univ. Hosp., No. 500510/2014 (N.Y. Sup. Ct. Kings County 2014).

Dumas SG. *Erdoğan banned caesarean sections, so why does Turkey have the highest rates in the OECD?* The Conversation. 2016;26 Sept. Online: https://theconversation.com/erdogan-banned-caesarean-sections-so-why-does-turkey-have-the-highest-rates-in-the-oecd-65660.

Ehrlich J. Breaking the law by giving birth: the war on drugs, the war on reproductive rights, and the war on women. *Rev Law Soc Change*. 2007;32(3):381. Online: https://heinonline.org/HOL/LandingPage?handle=hein.journals/nyuls32&div=16&page=.

Einarsdóttir K. *Private hospitals, health insurance and the rise of caesarean births*. 2012a. The Conversation. Online: https://theconversation.com/private-hospitals-health-insurance-and-the-rise-of-caesarean-births-9348.

Einarsdóttir K, Kemp A, Haggar FA, et al. Increase in caesarean deliveries after the Australian private health insurance incentive policy reforms. *PLoS ONE*. 2012b;7(7):e41436. doi:10.1371/journal.pone.0041436.

Emons W. Credence goods and fraudulent experts. *Rand J Econ*. 1997;28(1):107–119.

Fay K, Yee L. Reproductive Coercion and Women's Health. *J Midwifery Womens Health* 2018.

Field A. 'There must be a better way': personal injuries compensation since the 'crisis in insurance'. *Deakin Law Rev*. 2008;13(1):67. doi:10.21153/dlr2008vol13no1art153.

Freedman L. Implementation and aspiration gaps: whose view counts? *Lancet*. 2016;388(10056):2068–2069. doi:10.1016/s0140-6736(16)31530-6.

Freedman L, Kruk M. Disrespect and abuse of women in childbirth: challenging the global quality and accountability agendas. *Lancet*. 2014;384(9948):e42–e44. doi:10.1016/s0140-6736(14)60859-x.

Gartry L, Arrow B. *"Women ignoring medical advice on homebirth 'selfish': peak medical body says"*. ABC News. 2015. Online: http://www.abc.net.au/news/2015-06-18/women-choosing-home-births-selfish-peak-medical-groups-says/6555662.

Ghosh S. *Make it mandatory for all hospitals to declare number of caesarean deliveries #SafeBirth*. Change.org. 2017. Online: https://www.change.org/p/make-it-mandatory-for-all-hospitals-to-declare-number-of-caesarean-deliveries-safebirth?recruiter=312942865&utm_source=share_petition&utm_medium=copylink.

Giscombé C, Lobel M. Explaining disproportionately high rates of adverse birth outcomes among African Americans: the impact of stress, racism, and related factors in pregnancy. *Psychol Bull*. 2005;131(5):662–683. doi:10.1037/0033-2909.131.5.662.

Goldwin C. *Libby didn't know whether her newborn baby was alive for SIX HOURS and needs post-traumatic stress counselling over the birth experience … so what IS going wrong in Britain's labour wards? Daily Mail UK*. 2013. Online: http://www.dailymail.co.uk/femail/article-2270941/Birth-trauma-Libby-ORourke-Toni-Harman-Julie-Hainsworth-traumatic-labours-Britains-hospital-wards.html.

Hackenberg H. *Birth trauma doesn't mean I'm not grateful for my healthy child*. Kidspot. 2017. Online: http://www.kidspot.com.au/birth/labour/real-life/birth-trauma-doesnt-mean-im-not-grateful-for-my-healthy-child/news-story/dd4396b-6026429f2e9fbea10519a80d0.

Hall W, Tomkinson J, Klein M. Canadian care providers' and pregnant women's approaches to managing birth. *Qual Health Res*. 2011;22(5):575–586. doi:10.1177/1049732311424292.

Haque O, Waytz A. Dehumanization in medicine: causes, solutions, and functions. *Perspect Psychol Sci*. 2012;7(2):176.

Harvard School of Public Health and University Research Co. *Exploring Evidence for Disrespect and Abuse in Facility-Based Childbirth: Report of a Landscape Analysis*. Washington DC: Harvard School of Public Health and University Research; 2010.

Health and Disability Commissioner (HDC). *The code and your rights*. 2018. Online: https://www.hdc.org.nz/disability/the-code-and-your-rights/.

Hill M. *The sad truth about having a baby: 'cattle' care is now the norm. Guardian*. 2017; https://www.theguardian.com/commentis-free/2017/jan/17/having-a-baby-cattle-midwives-report. Online.

Howell E, Egorova N, Balbierz A, et al. Black-white differences in severe maternal morbidity and site of care. *Am J Obstet Gynecol*. 2016;214(1):122.e1–122.e7, doi:10.1016/j.ajog.2015.08.019.

Humphrey M, Colditz P, Ellwood D, et al. *Maternal and perinatal mortality in Queensland. Queensland Maternal and Perinatal Quality Council Report*. 2015. Online: https://www.health.qld.gov.au/__data/assets/pdf_file/0037/437986/qmpqc-report-2015-full.pdf.

Hunter J, Dixon K, Dahlen HG. The experiences of privately practising midwives in Australia who have been reported to the Australian Health Practitioner Regulation Agency: A qualitative study. *Women Birth*. 2020.

Hyderi M. *Caesarean delivery rates rise up to a shocking 80% in Kashmir government hospitals. Inuth*. 2017. Online: http://www.inuth.com/india/jammu-and-kashmir/caesarean-delivery-rates-rise-upto-a-shocking-80-in-kashmir-government-hospitals/.

Ieraci S, Tuteur A. Publicly funded homebirth in Australia: a review of maternal and neonatal outcomes over 6 years. *Med J Aust*. 2013;199(11):742. doi:10.5694/mja13.10863.

Re MB (Caesarean Section), EWCA Civ 1361 (UK 1997).

Inquest into the death of Roisin Fraser (Coroners Court NSW 2012).

I. V. v. Bolivia, Report No. 72/14. Merits, Inter-American Commission on Human Rights, Case 12.655 (August 15, 2014).

Iyengar R. *Making profits through unnecessary Caesareans: the dark underbelly of India's healthcare industry. Indian Express*. 2017. Online: http://indianexpress.com/article/opinion/web-edits/making-profits-through-unnecessary-caesareans-this-is-the-dark-underbelly-of-indias-healthcare-industry/.

Jenkinson B. When 'no' means 'no': supporting women's rights to informed consent and refusal. *Women Birth*. 2015;28:S20. doi:10.1016/j.wombi.2015.07.072.

Jenkinson B, Kruske S, Kildea S. The experiences of women, midwives and obstetricians when women decline recommended maternity care: a feminist thematic analysis. *Midwifery*. 2017;52:1–10. doi:10.1016/j.midw.2017.05.006.

Jenkinson R, Fox D. Maternity care plans and respectful homebirth transfer. In: Dahlen HG, Kumar-Hazard B, Schmied V, eds. *Birthing Outside the System: The Canary in the Coalmine*. London: Routledge Research in Nursing and Midwifery; 2020: Chapter 15.

Kildea S, Tracy S, Sherwood J, et al. Improving maternity services for Indigenous women in Australia: moving from policy to practice. *Med J Aust*. 2016;205(8):374–379. doi:10.5694/mja16.00854.

Kotaska A. Informed consent and refusal in obstetrics: a practical ethical guide. *Birth*. 2017;44(3):195–199. doi:10.1111/birt.12281.

Kruske S, Kildea S, Barclay L. Cultural safety and maternity care for Aboriginal and Torres Strait Islander Australians. *Women Birth*. 2006;19(3):73–77. doi:10.1016/j.wombi.2006.07.001.

Kruske S, Young K, Jenkinson B, et al. Maternity care providers' perceptions of women's autonomy and the law. *BMC Pregnancy Childbirth*. 2013;13(1):84. doi:10.1186/1471-2393-13-84.

Kukura E. Obstetric Violence. *Georgetown Law Journal*. 2018; 106: 721.

Kuliukas LJ, Lewis L, Hauck YL, Duggan R. Midwives' experiences of transfer in labour from a Western Australian birth centre to a tertiary maternity hospital. *Women Birth*. 2016; 29(1): 18–23.

Kumar-Hazard B. The role of the coroner in Australia: listen to or ignore the canary? In: Dahlen HG, Kumar-Hazard B, Schmied V, eds. *Birthing Outside the System: The Canary in the Coalmine.* London: Routledge Research in Nursing and Midwifery; 2020: Chapter 14.

Kurz E, Browne J, Davis D. Trial by media; the vilification of home-birth. *Women and Birth.* 2017; 3: 15–16.

Lane, K., & Reiger, K. Risk and homebirth: what's at stake? *On Line Opinion.* 2009.

Laxmi Mandal v NCT Delhi (Supreme Court of India 2009). Online: https://docs.escr-net.org/usr_doc/HRLN_Summary_-_Laxmi_Mandal_v_Deen_Dayal_Hospital.pdf.

Lee S, Ayers S, Holden D. Risk perception and choice of place of birth in women with high risk pregnancies: a qualitative study. *Midwifery.* 2016;38:49–54. doi:10.1016/j.midw.2016.03.008.

Lewis S, Collyer F, Willis K, et al. Healthcare in the news media: the privileging of private over public. *J Sociol.* 2017; 144078331773332. doi:10.1177/1440783317733324.

MacColl, M.-R. (2007). *The birth wars. Griffith Review.* Retrieved from https://www.griffithreview.com/articles/the-birth-wars at 40.

MacKenzie Bryers H, van Teijlingen E. Risk, theory, social and medical models: a critical analysis of the concept of risk in maternity care. *Midwifery.* 2010;26(5):488–496. doi:10.1016/j.midw.2010.07.003.

Mayra, K., & Kumar-Hazard, B. Why South Asian women make extreme choices in childbirth. In H. G. Dahlen, B. Kumar-Hazard, & V. Schmied, eds. *Birthing Outside the System: The Canary in the Coalmine.* London: Routledge Research in Nursing and Midwifery; 2020, Chapter 9.

McFall v Shimp, 10 Pa.D & C.3d 90 (Allegheny County Ct 1978).

McIntosh TA. *Social History of Maternity and Childbirth.* London: Routledge; 2012.

McIntyre, MJ, Francis, K, & Chapman, Y. Shaping public opinion on the issue of childbirth; a critical analysis of articles published in an Australian newspaper. *BMC Pregnancy & childbirth.* 2011; 11(47), 1–10.

McLachlan H. *There is no moral imperative for women to give birth in hospital. The Conversation.* 2017. Online: https://theconversation.com/there-is-no-moral-imperative-for-women-to-give-birth-in-hospital-22732.

McLean S, Petersen K. Patient status: the foetus and the pregnant woman. *Aust J Hum Rights.* 1996;2(2):229.

Madeira S, Pileggi V, Souza J. Abuse and disrespect in childbirth process and abortion situation in Latin America and the Caribbean—systematic review protocol. *Syst Rev.* 2017; 6(1):152. doi:10.1186/s13643-017-0516-5.

Main E, Menard M. Maternal mortality. *Obstet Gynecol.* 2013; 122(4):735–736. doi:10.1097/aog.0b013e3182a7dc8c.

Mallette v Shulman, 67 DLR (4th) 321 (1990).

Mane P. Some thoughts on disrespect and abuse in childbirth in response to FIGO's Mother-Baby Friendly Birthing Facilities Initiative. *Int J Gynaecol Obstet.* 2015;130(2):115. doi:10.1016/j.ijgo.2015.05.004.

Mayor S. Lack of consultant obstetrician is not associated with worse outcomes in babies, UK study shows. *BMJ.* 2016;353:i2242. doi:10.1136/bmj.i2242.

Mello M, Chandra A, Gawande A, et al. National costs of the medical liability system. *Health Aff (Millwood).* 2010;29(9):1569–1577. doi:10.1377/hlthaff.2009.0807.

Meredith C. *Humanity despairs as the Daily Express and Mail Celebrate the end of human rights.* HuffPost UK. 2015. Online: http://www.huffingtonpost.co.uk/2014/10/03/daily-mail-daily-express-human-rights-twitter-reaction_n_5925540.html.

Miller S, Abalos E, Chamillard M, et al. Beyond too little, too late and too much, too soon: a pathway towards evidence-based, respectful maternity care worldwide. *Lancet.* 2016;388(10056): 2176–2192. doi:10.1016/s0140-6736(16)31472-6.

Migrant and Refugee Women's Health Partnership (MRWHP). *Enhancing health literacy strategies in the settlement of migrant and refugee women.* Cultural Diversity in Health Report; 2018.

Minkoff H, Paltrow L. Melissa Rowland and the rights of pregnant women. *Obstet Gynecol.* 2004;104(6):1234–1236. doi:10.1097/01.aog.0000146289.65429.48.

Montgomery v Lanarkshire Health Board (Respondent) (Scotland), UKSC 11 (UK House of Lords 2015). Online: https://www.supremecourt.uk/decided-cases/docs/UKSC_2013_0136_Judgment.pdf.

Mossialos E, Allin S, Karras K, et al. An investigation of Caesarean sections in three Greek hospitals. *Eur J Public Health.* 2005;15(3):288–295. doi:10.1093/eurpub/cki002.

New Zealand Human Rights Commission (NZHRC). *Te Kāhui Tika Tangata Statement of Intent 2014/15–2017/18.* Wellington: NZHRC; 2014.

Niles PM, Stoll K, Wang JJ, et al. "I fought my entire way": Experiences of declining maternity care services in British Columbia. *PLoS One.* 2021; 16(6): e0252645.

Nisenblat V, Barak S, Ohel G, et al. Maternal morbidity associated with multiple cesarean deliveries. *Am J Obstet Gynecol.* 2005;193(6):S127. doi:10.1016/j.ajog.2005.10.456.

N.J. Div. of Youth & Family Servs. v V.M. (In re J.M.G.), 974 A2d 448 (NJ Sup Ct, App Div 2009).

Obermeyer Z, Powers B, Vogeli C, et al. Dissecting racial bias in an algorithm used to manage the health of populations. *Science.* 2019; 366(6464): 447–453.

Odent M. *The Farmer and the Obstetrician.* London: Free Association Books; 2002.

Office of the High Commissioner for Human Rights (OHCHR). *International Covenant on Civil and Political Rights (ICCPR).* Geneva: OHCHR; 1966. Online: http://www.ohchr.org/Documents/ProfessionalInterest/ccpr.pdf.

Office of the High Commissioner for Human Rights (OHCHR). *International Covenant on Economic, Social and Cultural Rights (ICESCR).* Geneva: OHCHR; 1976. Online http://www.ohchr.org/Documents/ProfessionalInterest/cescr.pdf.

Office of the High Commissioner for Human Rights (OHCHR). *Thematic Report on Discrimination Against Women in Health and Safety.* Geneva: OHCHR; 2016. Online: http://www.ohchr.org/EN/Issues/Women/WGWomen/Pages/GoodpracticesintheeliminationofDAW.aspx.

Office of the High Commissioner for Human Rights (OHCHR). *Spain needs to combat obstetric violence – UN experts.* Geneva: OHCHR; 2020. Online: https://www.ohchr.org/en/press-releases/2020/03/spain-needs-combat-obstetric-violence-un-experts?LangID=E&NewsID=25688.

Olsen O, Clausen J. Planned hospital birth versus planned home birth. *Cochrane Database Syst Rev.* 2012;(9):CD000352, doi:10.1002/14651858.CD000352.pub2.

Paltrow L, Flavin J. Arrests of and forced interventions on pregnant women in the United States, 1973–2005: implications for women's legal status and public health. *J Health Polit Policy Law.* 2013;38(2):299–343. doi:10.1215/03616878-1966324.

Reddy M, Wallace EM, Mockler JC, et al. Maternal Asian ethnicity and obstetric intrapartum intervention: a retrospective cohort study. *BMC Pregnancy Childbirth.* 2017;**17**(1):3.

Rigg E. The Rise of the Unregulated Birth Worker in Australia: The Canary flees the coal mine. Ibid.: In: Dahlen HG, Kumar-Hazard B, Schmied V, eds. *Birthing Outside the System: The Canary in the Coalmine.* London: Routledge Research in Nursing and Midwifery; 2020: Chapter 5.

Rigg E, Schmied V, Peters K, et al. Why do women choose an unregulated birth worker to birth at home in Australia: a qualitative study. *BMC Pregnancy Childbirth.* 2017;17:99.

Rogers HJ, Hogan L, Coates D, et al. Responding to the health needs of women from migrant and refugee backgrounds – models of maternity and postpartum care in high-income countries: a systematic scoping review. *Health Soc Care Community.* 2020.

Rogers v Whitaker, 175 CLR 479 (High Court of Australia 1992).

Ryan RM, McCarthy FP. Induction of labour. *Obstetrics, Gynaecology & Reproductive Medicine.* 2019; 29(12): 351–8.

Sacks E. Defining disrespect and abuse of newborns: a review of the evidence and an expanded typology of respectful maternity care. *Reprod Health.* 2017;14(1):66. doi:10.1186/s12978-017-0326-1.

Sadler M, Santos M, Ruiz-Berdún D, et al. Moving beyond disrespect and abuse: addressing the structural dimensions of obstetric violence. *Reprod Health Matters.* 2016;24(47):47–55. doi:10.1016/j.rhm.2016.04.002.

Samuels T, Minkoff H, Feldman J, et al. Obstetricians, health attorneys, and court-ordered cesarean sections. *Womens Health Issues.* 2007;17(2):107–114. doi:10.1016/j.whi.2006.12.001.

Sandall J, Soltani H, Gates S, et al. Midwife-led continuity models versus other models of care for childbearing women. *Cochrane Database Syst Rev.* 2016;(4):CD004667, doi:10.1002/14651858. CD004667.pub5.

Sargent C, Sargent J. *The top 3 reasons your 'good' birth left you feeling so broken.* Voice For Parents. 2017. Online: http://www.voiceforparents.co.nz/blog/2017/8/6/the-top-3-reasons-your-good-birth-left-you-feeling-so-broken.

S.F.M v Spain, CEDAW/C/75/D/138/2018 reported in 2020.

Sassine H, Dahlen H. Identifying the poisonous gases seeping into the coal mine: what women seek to avoid in choosing to give birth at home. In: Dahlen HG, Kumar-Hazard B, Schmied V, eds. *Birthing Outside the System: The Canary in the Coalmine.* London: Routledge Research in Nursing and Midwifery; 2020: Chapter 6.

Sassine H, Burns E, Ormsby S, et al. Why do women choose homebirth in Australia? A national survey. *Women Birth.* 2021;34(4): 396–404. doi:10.1016/j.wombi.2020.06.005.

Savell K. Is the 'born alive' rule outdated and indefensible? *Syd Law Rev.* 2006;28:625.

Schuiling K. Disrespect and abuse of women during childbirth: a significant factor in the efforts to reduce maternal and perinatal morbidity and mortality. *Int J Childbirth.* 2016;6(1): 2–4. doi:10.1891/2156-5287.6.1.2.

Secretary, Dept of Health and Community Services v JWB and SMB (Marion's case), FLC 92 (Federal Law Court 1992).

Shah N. *Are hospitals the safest place for healthy women to have babies? An obstetrician thinks twice. The Conversation.* 2015; 4 June. Online: https://theconversation.com/are-hospitals-the-safest-place-for-healthy-women-to-have-an-obstetrician-thinks-twice-42654.

Society of N.Y. Hosp. v Schloendorff, 211 NY 125 (1914).

Soderberg V. More than receptacles: an international human rights analysis of criminalising pregnancy in the United States. *Berkley J Gender, Law and Justice.* 2016;299:351.

Sosa GA, Crozier KE, Stockl A. The experiences of midwives and women during intrapartum transfer from one-to-one midwife-led birth environments to obstetric-led units. *Midwifery.* 2018; 65: 43–50.

Switzer v Rezvina et al., Docket No L-3697-14 (NJ Sup Ct 2015). Online: http://www.healthymothersmattertoo.com/uploads/6/5/3/3/65336197/lindsay_switzer_deposition_02_06_15.pdf.

Tarzia L, Wellington M, Marino J, et al. "A huge, hidden problem": Australian health practitioners' views and understandings of reproductive coercion. *Qual Health Res.* 2018; 29(10): 1395–407.

Ternovszky v Hungary, App. No. 67545/09 (Eur Ct Human Rights 2010).

Truven Health Analytics. *The cost of having a baby in the United States.* New York: Childbirth Connection; 2013. Online: http://transform.childbirthconnection.org/wp-content/uploads/2013/01/Cost-of-Having-a-Baby1.pdf.

Trinh LTT, Assareh H, Achat H, et al. Caesarean section by country of birth in New South Wales, Australia. *Women Birth.* 2020; 33(1): e72–e8.

United Nations (UN). *Universal Declaration of Human Rights.* Geneva: UN; 1948. Online: http://www.un.org/en/universal-declaration-human-rights/.

United Nations (UN). General Assembly. *Declaration of the Elimination of Violence Against Women.* Geneva: UN; 1994. Online: http://www.un.org/documents/ga/res/48/a48r104.htm.

United Nations Educational, Scientific and Cultural Organization (UNESCO). *Universal Declaration on Bioethics and Human Rights.* Geneva: UNESCO; 2005. Online: http://portal.unesco.org/en/ev.php-URL_ID=31058&URL_DO=DO_TOPIC&URL_SECTION=201.html/.

United Nations Population Fund (UNFPA), International Confederation of Midwives, WHO, et al. *A Global Call to Action: Strengthen Midwifery to Save Lives and Promote Health of Women and Newborns.* Washington DC: UNFPA; 2010.

United Nations Population Fund (UNFPA). *The State of The World's Midwifery 2011: Delivering Health, Saving Lives.* New York: UNFPA; 2011.

United Nations. Special Rapporteur on violence against women, its causes and consequences. *Report on a human rights-based approach to mistreatment and violence against women in reproductive health services with a focus on childbirth and obstetric violence* [UN Doc. A/74/137]. 2019. Online: https://www.ohchr.org/EN/Issues/Women/SRWomen/Pages/Mistreatment.aspx

Vanderwalker I. Taking the baby before it's born: termination of the parental rights of women who use illegal drugs while pregnant. *NYU Rev Law Soc Change.* 2008;32(3):423. Online: http://heinonline.org/HOL/Page?handle=hein.journals/nyuls32&div=15&g_sent=1&casa_token=&collection=journals.

Vedam S. Home birth versus hospital birth: questioning the quality of the evidence on safety. *Birth.* 2003;30(1):57–63. doi:10.1046/j.1523-536x.2003.00218.x.

Walsh D. Childbirth embodiment: problematic aspects of current understandings. *Sociol Health Illn.* 2009;32(3):486–501. doi:10.1111/j.1467-9566.2009.01207.x.

Waters J. In whose best interest? New Jersey Division of Youth and Family Services V. V.M. and B.G. and the next wave of court-controlled pregnancies. *J Law Gender.* 2011;34:81.

Weber D. Medical hegemony. *Int J Complement Alt Med.* 2016; 3(2):65. doi:10.15406/ijcam.2016.03.00065.

Weigel M. *How ultrasound helped advance the idea that a fetus is a person.* The Atlantic. 2017. Online: https://www.theatlantic.com/health/archive/2017/01/ultrasound-woman-pregnancy/514109/.

Weiner J. *'Don't cut me!': Discouraged by experts, episiotomies still common in some hospitals.* Kaiser Health News. 2016. Online: http://khn.org/news/dont-cut-me-discouraged-by-experts-episiotomies-still-common-in-some-hospitals.

White Ribbon Alliance. *Respectful Maternity Care: The Universal Rights of Childbearing Women.* Washington DC: White Ribbon Alliance; 2017. Online: https://www.whiteribbonalliance.org/wp-content/uploads/2017/11/RMC_Brochure.pdf.

Willis K, Lewis S. *Which are better, public or private hospitals?* The Conversation. 2016;March 18. Online: https://theconversation.com/which-are-better-public-or-private-hospitals-54338.

World Health Organization (WHO). *The Global Strategy for Women's, Children's and Adolescents' Health (2016–30).* Geneva: WHO; 2015. Online: http://www.who.int/life-course/partners/global-strategy/globalstrategyreport2016-2030-lowres.pdf.

World Health Organization (WHO). *Stand up for human rights to—and through—health, experts urge Governments (Press release).* Geneva: WHO; 22 May 2017. Online: http://www.who.int/life-course/news/launch-hhrwg-report/en.

Further reading

American College of Obstetricians-Gynecologists (ACOG). Episiotomy: clinical management guidelines for obstetrician-gynecologists. ACOG Practice Bulletin no. 71. *Obstet Gynecol.* 2006;107(4):957–962.

Australian Health Ministers' Advisory Council (AHMAC). *National Framework for Maternity Services Project—Fact Sheet 1 (Nov 2016).* Canberra: Australian Health Ministers' Advisory Council; 2016. Online: http://www.coaghealthcouncil.gov.au/Portals/0/ National%20Framework%20for%20Maternity%20Services% 20Project_Fact%20Sheet%20Nov2016.pdf.

Australian Health Ministers' Conference. *National Maternity Services Plan.* Canberra: Commonwealth of Australia; 2011.

Australian Institute of Health and Welfare (AIHW). *Maternal Deaths in Australia 2008–2012. 2014.* Canberra: AIHW. Online: http://www.aihw.gov.au/WorkArea/DownloadAsset. aspx?id=60129551117.

Commonwealth of Australia (COA). *Improving Maternity Services in Australia: Report of the Maternity Services Review.* Canberra: AGS Publications; 2009.

Eunice Kennedy Shriver National Institute of Child Health and Human Development, NIH, DHHS. *Prematurity Research at the National Institute of Child Health and Human Development (NA).* Washington DC: US Government Printing Office; 2008.

General Purpose Standing Committee No. 2. Answers to questions on notice, Alliance for Family Preservation and Restoration. NSW: NSW Parliament; 2017.

Hall M, Ahmed A, Swanson S. Answering the millennium call for the right to maternal health: the need to eliminate user fees. *Yale Hum Rights Dev Law J.* 2009;12(62).

Human Rights in Childbirth India Conference, Mumbai; 2017. Online: http://www.humanrightsinchildbirth.org/event/in-dia-2017.

National Federation of Women's Institute & National Childbirth Trust. *Support Overdue UK/Wales: NFWI.* 2017. Online: https:// www.thewi.org.uk/__data/assets/pdf_file/0009/187965/NCT-nct-WI-report-72dpi.pdf.

NSW Parliament Legislative Council. *Inquiry into Child Protection Report No. 46.* NSW: General Purpose Standing Committee No. 2; 2017.

Office of the High Commissioner for Human Rights (OHCHR). *Report of the Special Rapporteur on Torture and Other Cruel, Inhuman or Degrading Treatment or Punishment.* Geneva: OHCHR; 2017. Online: http://www.ohchr.org/EN/Issues/Torture/ SRTorture/Pages/SRTortureIndex.aspx.

CHAPTER 4

Fear, risk and safety in maternity care

Hannah G Dahlen

LEARNING OUTCOMES

Learning outcomes for this chapter are:

1. To explain the concept of risk and the scientific and sociocultural contexts in which risk is manifest
2. To present the place that fear plays in midwifery
3. To highlight the centrality of the relationship with the woman in the provision of safe care
4. To discuss the importance of skilled midwifery care and the place of accountability for the use or misuse of midwifery skills
5. To discuss the place of referral and the importance of collaborative relationships
6. To acknowledge the complexity of the environment in which safe midwifery care is provided.

CHAPTER OVERVIEW

This chapter focuses on why risk is such an important concept in maternity care. It begins by presenting some of the key theoretical approaches and how these are related to midwifery, and it makes clear that understanding and managing risk and fear are not simple matters. However, the concerns related to risk need not always engender fear and anxiety. The chapter then looks at the role that fear plays in maternity care and it finishes with a framework that the midwife can use to support safe, effective and life-affirming care within this risk environment. The framework acknowledges the complex and often paradoxical nature of midwifery practice and provides a way for the midwife to put the management of risk into practice and into perspective.

KEY TERMS

accountability
fear
normality

referral
risk
safety

technorational discourse
values

INTRODUCTION

The management and interpretation of **risk** impact daily on healthcare provision (Heyman et al., 2010; Taylor-Gooby, 2006; Scamell et al., 2019). The assessment of risk and the promotion and protection of safe childbirth are key elements in the provision of maternity care. Many midwives who promote birth as a normal physiological process often don't effectively challenge the current risk management approaches (Scamell, 2011; Scamell & Alaszewski, 2012) or become complicit in them. Safe practice minimises and 'manages' risk; risks are assessed, avoided or managed in order to provide a safe environment in which to give birth. Risk affects the lives of midwives, both in the assessment of risk in the childbearing woman and in the management of their own risk within the medicolegal context. Yet there is something about how risk is currently constructed, not only in maternity care but also throughout the Western world, that reflects rising levels of anxiety and fear (Dahlen, 2014).

Midwifery academics Scamell et al. (2019) argue there are three interlinked propositions that need to be considered when looking at risk and birth practices:

1. the operations of the technorational approach to risk are not as self-evident as they appear and they do not necessarily coincide with evidence-based approach practice
2. the contemporary understanding of risks in maternity care are linked to the increased application of technology
3. critical evaluation and analysis of how risk operates in maternity care provides a unique opportunity to re-frame birth as a trustworthy physiological process worthy of protection (Scamell et al., 2019).

Writers in this area have described a risk culture (Beck, 1992; Füredi, 2006) or risk epidemic in healthcare (Skolbekken, 1995). This increased anxiety about risk is reflected in maternity care and is occurring despite a growing understanding of the causes, incidence and prevention of negative outcomes. This has been accompanied by increasing levels of intervention, **accountability** and surveillance, with significant implications for the way midwifery is practised (Skinner, 2003). It challenges the model of birth as a normal part of human life and thus presents challenges for midwives attempting to enact in practice this model of **normality**. Midwives are faced with a significant paradox in attempting to work a 'birth is normal' perspective within a 'birth is risky' context (Copeland et al., 2014). Working in this context requires the midwife to have a sophisticated understanding of the meanings of risk aversion and of safe practice. Without such understanding, risk overwhelms normality (Dahlen, 2014; Scamell & Alaszewski, 2012). We also know that many midwives feel a sense of professional powerlessness and distress when dealing with the fear-laden environments in which they work (Dahlen & Caplice, 2014).

There is also an important distinction between taking risks and being 'at risk' (Heyman & Titterton, 2012). There is little acceptance that taking risks is not only a normal part of life but is also essential. Without it, humans do not develop. We can miss valuable and life-changing opportunities. In order to achieve **safety** we might sometimes put ourselves at risk of unforeseen and unknown risks. Sometimes one has to take risks to be safe, yet safe action may have unforeseen negative outcomes. Complete safety cannot be assured and there is no such thing as a risk-free birth. Risk in the current environment has become associated with the possibility of negative outcome rather than with the possibility of positive experience (Tulloch & Lupton, 2003). It is the fear of a negative outcome that is most often expressed. One rarely (if ever) reads reports of the risks of a positive outcome of a planned action. For example, how often is it expressed that if a woman plans a home birth she risks having a birth with no intervention? Women have told us also that they have broader and more nuanced interpretations of risk, seeing emotional, psychological, spiritual and cultural risks as important, not just the physical risks on which mainstream maternity care is focused (Dahlen et al., 2020).

It is important, then, for the midwife practising in this environment to have an understanding of how and why risk has become so prominent, to understand the fear that this can engender and to have some tools to deal with the reality of how this affects safe and fulfilling practice.

WHAT IS RISK AND HOW DO WE WORK WITH IT?

The first place to investigate, and the one that holds the dominant position in current risk discourse, is the technorational or scientific approach. It is here that we see research dominated by epidemiology and by the randomised controlled trial (RCT), and the use of this research in informing practice. These approaches to risk are focused on the mathematical calculations of risk associated with the probability of events occurring. Their main concerns are in the measurement of physical risks and effects. These approaches provide valuable information for the midwife in the provision of safe care and are an essential part of her knowledge base. For example, the meta-analysis of the RCTs on continuous fetal monitoring (CFM) indicates that, for low-risk women, CFM increases the risk of unnecessary intervention (Alfirevic et al., 2017; Small et al., 2019). However, the application of the scientific evidence in the management of risk and the promotion of safety are seldom simple. Any midwife working in a mainstream obstetric unit would see CFM used much more than it should be. There are several challenges that midwives face in assessing and managing risk from a science- or evidence-based framework.

For the individual healthcare practitioner there is a fundamental difficulty in extrapolating knowledge from large studies and applying it to individual situations. The early identification of risk can be notoriously imprecise in predicting adverse outcomes for the individual. Once the complexity of the individual situation is identified, the ability to know the quantified risks of an adverse event occurring are further eroded. The quantification of risk must take into account not only the rate of adverse outcome but also the possible benefits, and must ensure that there is some consistency in how the risks are framed (Dahlen & Gutteridge, 2015).

Van Wagner interviewed 50 Canadian midwives, doctors and nurses involved in maternity care to uncover the 'how' and 'whys' of differing interpretations and uneven application of evidence (Van Wagner, 2016). She found professionals tried to mitigate risk by comparing childbirth risk to everyday risks and using words and pictures to describe numbers. Figs. 4.1 and 4.2 from this paper demonstrate this attempt by health workers to keep risk in perspective, and could help midwives when trying to discuss risk with women in a tangible and accessible way. Using words instead of numbers is another way to discuss risk, as is the use of absolute risk.

The identification of risk is also tied up with control. Heyman (1998) contends that, where healthcare practitioners claim to predict the probability of an outcome for individuals, there is a tendency to attempt to make decisions on their behalf. He states: 'The health professionals' crystal ball, although providing only cloudy, probabilistic glimpses of possible futures, through the methodology of epidemiology, leads them into attempting to manage risks on behalf of their clients' (Heyman, 1998, p. 22). Skilled, clinical assessment and effective communication therefore remain core competencies for the midwife in assisting a client in decision making around safe care. The scientific evidence is one important tool to inform this practice.

The technorational model of maternity care also has particular implications for the understanding of what is normal and so has a special importance for midwifery, which claims the expertise in 'normal' birth. Understandings of what is risky and what is normal both dominate

Risk	Word
1 in 1	Certain
1 in 2	Likely
1 in 10	Common
1 in 100	Uncommon
1 in 1,000	Rare
1 in 10,000	Very rare
1 in 100,000	Negligible
1 in one million	Theoretical

FIGURE 4.2 Words instead of numbers
(Source: Van Wagner, 2016)

and delineate midwifery practice and yet are often seen as juxtaposed positions. Normality has changed from being a social to a scientific concept, as we have come to accept the idea that one can't know something unless it can be measured (Hacking, 1990). As Scamell (2011) wrote in her study on midwifery risk in the UK: 'There is low risk and there is high risk, but there is no such thing as no risk'. If 'being normal' has come to mean having no measurable risk factors it is little wonder that fewer and fewer women are having births without intervention even when they are low risk (Dahlen et al., 2014).

This search for measurable regularity and thus quantifiable normality has given rise to rules about childbirth that have not undergone in-depth analysis (Murphy-Lawless, 1998). An example of this is the decision about

Numbers and more than numbers	Avoiding risk and using risk	'Risk talk' as a work in progress
Comparing to everyday risks	Avoiding the word risk	Understanding power and limitations
Using words	Accounting for maternal altruism	Taking time to build confidence
Using visual aids	Including long term outcomes	'Both/and' permission giving
Using absolute risk	Listening versus listing	Sharing uncertainty
Using numbers needed to treat	Leaning towards normal	Awareness/humility
	Risks, benefits and alternatives	

FIGURE 4.1 Keeping risk in perspective
(Source: Van Wagner, 2016)

what constitutes a normal labour. This needed to be measurable, so statistical data on the length of labour have been applied to individual women's progress. Deviations from the measurable, statistically assessed norm are then seen as needing to be managed and controlled. In essence, then, science in the guise of medicine has re-created and redefined 'normal' and has seen pregnancy as normal only in retrospect (Cartwright & Thomas, 2001; Wagner, 1998). Recently, understanding of progress in labour has once again been turned on its head, with established labour defined as not occurring for most women until 6 cm and beyond (Zhang et al., 2010). This has resulted in leading obstetric organisations such as the American College of Obstetricians (ACOG) changing their approach to progress of labour (American Congress of Obstetricians and Gynecologists, 2014). This has led more recently to the WHO changing their recommendations on labour progress (WHO, 2018). Just looking at various editions of textbooks will show that definitions of the length of labour have changed over decades because of how labour has been managed, not because of changes in the physiology of women (Dahlen et al., 2013).

It is within this dominant **technorational discourse** that midwifery stays firm in its claim of expertise in normal childbearing. It is a precarious position to take, given who is defining normality and who is defining risk. The challenge for midwifery is to look beyond the technorational definitions of normal and to claim midwifery definitions. Midwifery sees birth as a normal process, not only physiologically but also socially, culturally and spiritually (Australian College of Midwives (ACM), 2017; New Zealand College of Midwives (NZCOM), 2008). This is reflected in the commitment that midwifery has to partnership and to women-centred care. One of the risks of this perspective, however, is the possibility of decreased emphasis on the physical aspects of what we currently call normal birth—that is, birth with no intervention.

The technorational approach has also tended to turn the concept of safety into a commodity, one that professionals are meant to be able to provide. Symon (1998), in his study of midwives' and obstetricians' attitudes to litigation, found that both midwives and obstetricians agreed that women had been given the impression that science (in the form of obstetric intervention) can achieve more than it actually can (Symon, 1998). The technorational model focuses on making danger visible (technology) and measurable (epidemiology) (Cartwright & Thomas, 2001). However, this is not always possible and there is an 'unsafeness' that is unknown (Smythe, 2000). Some things can appear unannounced, suddenly and without warning. The normal and the abnormal can 'mimic' each other. Smythe (2000) also comments that being safe or being unsafe (being at risk) is, in a sense, already there. Some women could give birth safely with no professional input and others will not give birth safely even with all the help that professionals can provide. So the midwife is there not to 'sell' a safe birth as some sort of objective, measurable commodity but rather to support safety and to uncover, as much as she can, the risks

that might threaten this safety. This unknowable nature of risk and safety means that the midwife must be skilled and vigilant.

The technorational approach also implies that decision making should be made by rational experts rather than by the 'insignificant others' (Stapleton, 1997). Davis-Floyd (2001) describes this approach as technocratic; based on the pre-eminence of technology and of mind–body separation, the technocratic approach, she says, treats the 'patient' as object and sees responsibility and authority as being held by the practitioner. This approach also presupposes that both the assessment of risk and the experts themselves are objective and rational and that people will make rational decisions about what is risky and what is safe (Lupton, 1999). It is based on assumptions that the evidence provides clear answers so that choices will also be clear and self-evident. However, this is not often the case.

Beck (1999), a prominent sociologist in risk theory, has proposed that we now live in a 'risk society' (Beck, 1999). Modern life, he asserts, has been based on the idea that technology and science can provide the answers to our problems. Progress and controllability have been fundamental beliefs in the search for safety and security. The success of modernity, as represented by science and technology, has led to globalisation and thus to a growing understanding of the multiple ways of living and viewing the world. Modernity has also led to individualisation and a sense of self-determination. This in turn has challenged traditional social understandings, including the role of women and the place of the family, leading to increasing uncertainty. This uncertainty is also reflected in the undermining of faith in science and technology: by the growing understanding that not only does technology not solve all our problems, but actually creates some of them.

The uncertainty about societal roles and loss of faith in technology have led to a generalised fear and anxiety, along with a loss of faith in professionals and in technology. We are in a state of being 'in between', where we have not yet created social and cultural forms that replace the tenets of modernity. We are, according to Beck (1999), not yet postmodern but are living in what he calls 'late modern' society, where we live with, among other things, the paradox of losing faith in experts while at the same time still expecting that their work will be free of negative outcomes. The levels of anxiety that are produced become counterproductive. In terms of maternity care, this reflexive culture means that maternity practitioners can be constantly questioned, challenged and increasingly restricted in their practice. The accountability that results causes fear and stress not only in the practitioners but also in the consumers of maternity care, as they themselves are required to make choices with risks attached that are difficult or impossible to quantify.

Ironically, this desire to avoid or control all risk in itself creates its own problems. Annandale (1996) comments that the consumerism and managerialism that have emerged as part of the risk society have tended to further increase the levels of anxiety and, paradoxically, to undermine the quality of care that is provided. It is this combination of managerialism in the form of protocols and guidelines, and consumerism in the form of informed choice and consent, that provides the current background for midwifery practice. One needs only to reflect on the increase in caesarean section rates in light of the 'risk society' to see how this can be applied to maternity care and to midwifery. In the effort to control for all risk, both for the mother and baby and for the maternity practitioner, caesarean sections are an increasingly used intervention. Yet this intervention comes with its own risks. The dilemma for the midwife is to work in this increasingly constrained environment while providing care that is flexible and truly women-centred—and all this in an environment focused on risk aversion.

The risk society as manifest in maternity care reflects the tension between the acceptance and the rejection of modern biomedicine. Davis-Floyd (2001) accepts the valuable knowledge that biomedicine has provided but also contests its dominance. The anxiety associated with risk and safety can be seen, then, as having its origins in the movement beyond an uncritical acceptance of biomedicine. The resurgence of midwifery and the increase in the valuing of humanistic or holistic care could be seen as part of the movement towards a new, more postmodern way of viewing the world. We certainly seem to be in a state of transition.

Another way to view risk and safety is to take a *cultural view*. Cultural perspectives attend not so much to the way in which current social forms are reflective of risk (as in Beck's 'risk society'), but rather to the way in which societal forms themselves affect the way decisions about risk are made. One of the most influential thinkers in this field is the anthropologist Mary Douglas (Douglas, 1992; Douglas & Wildavsky, 1982). Douglas (1992) points to the lack of uniformity in opinions about what makes something risky, how risky it might be and what should be done about it. She rejects both a scientific, objectivist approach and an individual rational choice approach to risk decision making. Instead, she proposes that risks are decided upon according to the cultural meaning associated with them, and is critical of experts' attempts to get to the objective truth of risk by protecting it from the 'dirty' side of politics and morals. People, she proposes, do not make decisions about risk according to individualised circumstances and beliefs, but rather are culturally conditioned to prefer some types of decisions over others. Their beliefs and actions are therefore culturally constructed. Within any culture there will be subgroups and communities who have varied value bases and ethical systems. These ethical systems too are culturally constructed and may vary. This variety is not related to any misguided perception, as objectivists would propose, but to different political, moral and aesthetic positions (Lupton, 1999).

Values and uncertainties are an integral part of these choices, and Douglas proposes that the choices between risky alternatives are not value free. Choice in the end, therefore, is essentially based on social rather than scientific knowledge. This decision-making process can also be seen as political. Who should make decisions, and who and what should matter, are related to whose knowledge is regarded as authoritative. Douglas's position does acknowledge that dangers and risks are real but proposes that it is impossible to rank them in any rational sense; there are simply too many of them (Douglas & Wildavsky, 1982). A cultural approach therefore helps us to see risk decision making as a result of community consensus, rather than rational individual choice. It is this community consensus that gives preference to some risks over others. We see this clearly in the decision-making processes around birth. Take, for example, a woman's decision to deliver her breech baby without intervention, compared with an obstetrician's wish to deliver that baby by caesarean section; or a woman's choice to have an elective epidural anaesthetic despite her midwife's commitment to normal birth. How do the women's decisions reflect their cultural and community perspectives? Whose knowledge is authoritative? How is fear being expressed? And, of course, who is at risk?

Both the social and the cultural interpretations of the current risk discourse speak to how *blame* is apportioned. Both see blame as a reflection of societal and cultural forms that have some basis in controllability. Where adverse outcomes eventuate, someone must be held accountable for the mismanagement of risk. Blame, then, is a deflection onto someone else. Accountability for adverse outcomes is required and is usually punitive. This is reflected in the 'name, blame and shame' approach that is manifest not just in maternity care or even just in healthcare but increasingly in every sphere of life. This has significant implications for healthcare practitioners in the risk of litigation. Healthcare practitioners, including those in maternity care, express considerable anxiety related to this risk of litigation (Symon, 1998).

Risk and safety, then, can be seen not only as core business for the midwife but also as having been made even more dominant in current maternity care by the 'risk society' in which we now live and work. The technorational approach to maternity care still dominates despite a growing understanding of the place of values and cultural understandings of risk and safety. The midwife must provide care that incorporates these different ways of knowing, and acknowledges and deals with the complex and often conflicting perspectives inherent in these approaches. Alongside this the midwife must understand the role of anxiety and fear in the provision of care and be able to put this into perspective.

REFLECTIVE THINKING EXERCISE

Take some time to reflect on your own perspective on risk and safety. What is the level of tolerance for risk in your own life? How do you think this affects the way you practise, especially the way you communicate risk and safety to the woman? What are your tactics when risk becomes evident? How do you balance the evidence of risk with the woman's values?

HOW DOES FEAR INFLUENCE MIDWIFERY AND OBSTETRIC PRACTICE?

Fear runs as an undercurrent through birth. Fear is ruining birth and it's ruining life. Fear is robbing women of power. A future based on fear is no future at all.

(Dahlen, 2006, p. 7)

It is impossible to talk about risk and safety without exploring **fear**, as this motivates us to avoid danger and seek safety. Fear and concepts of risk and safety are inextricably entwined and it is important we look at what it is that midwives fear and how this can shape the care they give.

There is a certain irony that, in the developing world at a time of scientific advancement, longer life expectancy and greater prosperity, we are faced with the fact that people are increasingly fearful. There has been increased interest in women's fear of childbirth over the past decade and how this contributes towards rising intervention rates and the dominant risk agenda. Research does indicate that the fear of childbirth affects a large number of women and past negative birth experiences play a big role in this (Dencker et al., 2019). Research from the UK indicates that this fear may have increased over recent years, along with an increased willingness to accept medical intervention during childbirth (Green & Baston, 2007). However, key questions need to be asked—such as whose fear is this really, are women simply reflecting health providers' fear, is health providers' fear impacting on the care they give and is this care causing fear in women (Dahlen, 2010)? Where relationships of trust are developed between women and midwives and birth environments enable women to feel safe and powerful, fear can be reduced (Dahlen et al., 2008) and it appears the risk agenda can be ameliorated.

The limited literature available about how healthcare providers' fears can impact on women and childbirth suggests there is a link (Regan & Liaschenko, 2007; Saisto & Halmesmaki, 2003). In Powell Kennedy & Shannon's (2004) qualitative study examining midwives' beliefs about normal birth, some of the midwives reported that when they became fearful when caring for women giving birth they were less able to care effectively for the women and they felt their anxiety may have impacted negatively on the birth outcome. A study undertaken by Regan & Liaschenko (2007) in the US showed that nurse midwives viewed birth through a lens of risk, with three categories found: birth as a natural process, birth as a lurking risk and birth as a risky process. The authors found the nurses' beliefs about birth could influence their care and associated interventions and caesarean section rates.

Styles et al. (2011) found that midwives in Scotland working under different health boards made specialist **referrals** at different times during labour, and the authors suggest that highly publicised adverse events in that health service might be making midwives more conservative in their practice, suggesting negative recent events could impact on midwives' perception of fear and risk and thus impact on their practice (Styles et al., 2011). Morris describes an atmosphere of anxiety and lost confidence in midwives as impacting on their ability to facilitate normal births (Morris, 2005). She argues that, while midwives are less likely to be the direct cause of birth trauma that results in litigation, they are encouraged to practise within a *just-in-case* framework and spend much of their time in documenting and justifying their decisions. Other writers report anecdotally on the fear that governs midwives' practice and how this shapes practice and feeds the current risk agenda in maternity care (Crabtree, 2008; Dahlen, 2010).

Likewise there is evidence that obstetric practice may be influenced by particular beliefs. A commonly cited study, where 31% of female London obstetricians indicated that they would opt for a caesarean for their own births (Al-Mufti et al., 1997), is used to argue that this indicates choices made by 'an informed cohort of women' (Thornton & Lubowski, 2006). However, it is equally interesting to look at other less-cited studies from countries such as Norway, Denmark and the Netherlands where the caesarean section rate is low compared with other resource-rich countries. Here similar surveys indicate that small numbers (1.1%–2%) of obstetricians would choose caesarean section for themselves or partners (Backe et al., 2002; Bergholt et al., 2004). Rather than being 'an informed cohort', it appears that when obstetricians work in environments where the rate of caesarean is high, so too are the personally perceived benefits (Homer & Dahlen, 2007).

A study conducted in a major teaching hospital in Sydney examined the risk of morbidity that nulliparous pregnant women would be prepared to accept before requesting an elective caesarean section and then compared their views with those of clinicians (Turner et al., 2008). Pregnant women in this study were willing to accept higher risks than clinicians for all 17 complications presented to them. The views of midwives were closest to those of pregnant women—urogynaecologists and colorectal surgeons being the most risk adverse, with 42% and 41% respectively stating that they would request an elective caesarean section for themselves or their partners.

When does advice around risk become coercion?

Andrew Kotaska (2017) wrote recently that risk is personal and subjective, using the example of the NASA space program, where the death rate of astronauts was 14 out of 789 astronauts who flew in the program (a rate of 1.8%) and this is deemed acceptable, yet women who want to have a vaginal birth after caesarean (VBAC) with a 0.05% fetal risk have had court orders to force them to have repeat caesarean sections. He argues that astronauts face 40 times the risk but we celebrate them and no one seeks a court order to ground them. In this scenario the fetus is the focus. There is little consideration about the lifetime risk to the mother, and emotional and psychological considerations of safety are completely ignored. Kotaska exposes coercion as taking several forms in maternity care under the guise of risk management:

1. magnifying risk estimates to dissuade a patient from an option
2. exaggerating benefits or withholding risks of a recommended treatment
3. demeaning a woman for putting her fetus at risk
4. asserting that a woman's decision makes her a 'bad parent' and threatening to involve child protection services
5. threatening to withdraw care if a woman refuses medical advice.

Kotaska goes on to provide guidance for clinicians faced with women who accept or choose additional risk:

1. Clearly recommend against the 'risky' course of action.
2. Have a second practitioner counsel the patient, if possible.
3. Document informed refusal, using a preprinted form if desired.
4. Reassure her that she will continue to receive courteous, professional care.

There is no place for coercion in modern maternity care and continuing to take a coercive approach will only drive women to potentially more risky options such as free birth (Dahlen et al., 2020).

What do Australian and New Zealand midwives fear?

So what do Australian and New Zealand midwives fear, and how could this fear shape their practice? Dahlen & Caplice (2014) ran a series of workshops across Australia and New Zealand through CAPERS from 2009 to 2011. In total, 17 workshops were held around Australia and New Zealand, supporting over 700 midwives with skills to keep birth normal and manage common obstetric emergencies. A session on fear was held during these workshops. Midwives were asked to write their greatest fear on a piece of paper and return it to the presenters; 739 fears were recorded (some wrote more than one fear) and only one midwife reported she had no fear. In total there were 667 midwives, 72 student midwives and 10 obstetric registrars who recorded fears for us. The top fears of midwives were: death of a baby ($n = 177$), causing harm ($n = 176$), obstetric emergencies, in particular shoulder dystocia and PPH ($n = 114$), maternal death ($n = 83$), being watched and criticised ($n = 68$), being the cause of a negative birth experience ($n = 52$), dealing with the unknown and not being prepared ($n = 36$), and losing passion and confidence around normal birth ($n = 32$). Student midwives were more concerned about knowing what to do, whereas home-birth midwives were mostly concerned with being blamed if something went wrong. Ten obstetric registrars were also involved and were almost entirely concerned with the death of a baby and mother (Dahlen & Caplice, 2014).

So how could the fears that midwives hold impact on women's fear and the risk agenda that is now so pervasive in maternity care? Physiologically, fear appears to leave indelible memory traces, with researchers telling us that, even after a fear-inducing conditioned stimulus has been extinguished, the brain retains a changed pattern of neuronal firing in response to that stimulus (LeDoux et al., 1989; Quirk et al., 1995). This means that midwives working in environments where there are high levels of fear are potentially being physiologically and psychologically reshaped and primed to be even more fearful. So what is it that creates this fear? Is it the size of a hospital, the model of care, the place of birth or the personal philosophy of the care provider that actually makes a difference in the intervention rates we see in maternity care today, and does fear have a role to play?

The fundamental difference between a medical and midwifery philosophy is in the view taken of pregnancy and birth: normal healthy life event, or potential ill health that requires prevention and cure. However, it is quite clear that midwives struggle to hold onto this belief and be authentic to it in practice. Blaaka & Schauer (2008) describe this in a paper titled 'Doing midwifery between different belief systems'. They describe how midwives struggle to merge midwifery knowledge and judgment based on intuition and observation with the dominant logical biomedical model (Blaaka & Schauer, 2008). Other studies have shown that there is a significant amount of conflict between how midwives believe they should provide care and obstetric units' medically orientated practices that dictate decision making, which may not sit comfortably with this belief (Keating & Fleming, 2007). Walsh (2006) found in his study on free-standing birth centres, where there was less surveillance by management and more autonomy, that lower intervention rates are the result. It is also quite clear that, where there is a healthy collaborative culture in a large maternity unit, continuity of midwifery care brings extraordinary results in terms of safety and quality (Sandall et al., 2016). It also appears that, when working in continuity of care where collaboration is strong, midwives do not feel a sense of subordination or feel undervalued by their medical colleagues (Moore, 2009). So midwives' practice is clearly influenced by the environments they work in and relationship they have with women, medical staff and their managers.

Is fear all bad?

The dilemma we face is that both fear and trust are essentially critical for our survival—so how can we get the balance right? Our focus as health professionals should be on reducing manufactured fear and building responsive trust, but also we should focus on listening to fear and being aware that wishful thinking is not the same as trust. The very small number of midwives who believe fervently that birth is always a normal and natural process may not recognise and act on warning signs because of this strongly held view (Dahlen, 2010).

It is important not to demonise fear as it serves to protect us. Some Darwinians believe that the early humans who were most afraid were most likely to survive. The result, says De Becker (1997, p. 278) is 'the emergence of man as we know him: a hyperanxious animal who constantly invents reasons for anxiety even when there are none'. The human psyche it appears is skewed to the negative (Klein, 2002). Of the six main emotions we have (fear, anger, distrust, sadness, happiness, surprise), four are negative. These authors argue that in relative terms it has not been long since we crawled out of the cave and felt safe enough to interact. We have evolved in an age of immense adversity. As a result, people lean towards tragedy. Losses inflict hurt more than their equivalent gains bring joy. Bad news in the paper gets a bigger headline than good news. More people believe now that life is getting worse rather than getting better, despite the contrary being true (Dahlen, 2010).

Grayling (2002, p. 54) points out that what we fear comes to pass more rapidly than what we hope mainly because we make it so. This means we can in fact create a reality that wasn't even there in the first place. De Becker argues in *The Gift of Fear*: 'True fear is a gift. It is a survival signal that sounds only in the presence of danger. Yet unwarranted fear has assumed a power over us that it holds over no other creature on Earth. It need not be this way' (De Becker, 1997, p. 227). It need not be this way in childbirth either. We can differentiate between the fear that is real and protects us and the fear that is manufactured and constrains us (Box 4.1).

The 0.1% doctrine or the 99.9% response

Every day we make choices that increase our risks dramatically and think nothing of it. After the September 11th terrorist attacks in the USA, a fear of flying meant more people travelled by car. In the 3 months that followed the attacks, US road fatalities jumped by 1000 (Allard, 2007). This illogical fear was best summed up in the book *The One Percent Doctrine* (Suskind, 2006). This was inspired by Dick Cheney's famous comment following September 11th, 'If there is even a 1% chance of a terrorist act occurring we must treat that as if it were a certainty.' We all now live today with the ramifications of this thinking (Dahlen, 2010).

This 1% doctrine has in fact become the 0.1% doctrine in maternity care or the '1 : 1000 club' as coined by Canadian obstetrician, Andrew Kotaska (2008). Kotaska says we live in a culture of risk magnification—the media does it; researchers do it; clinicians do it. As research methods advance, we are able to determine ever-smaller increments of risk and, in some cases, interventions to avoid them. With large trials, we now are able to determine very small amounts of risk, but we do not have a common

---

> ### Box 4.1 Tips for midwives for dealing with fear
>
> - Identify the fear.
> - Take responsibility for it (it's your fear).
> - Do an obstetric emergency course.
> - Don't forget to breathe.
> - Practise visualisation.
> - Watch the self-talk and practise thought stopping.
> - Talk to someone about how you feel.
> - Move (take a break from the situation, ask someone else's opinion).
> - Have a cup of tea.
> - Knitting at birth can reduce adrenaline (epinephrine) and keep anxious hands out of mischief.
> - Write about how you are feeling and reflect on it.
> - Get some evidence to support or refute your fear.
> - Centre yourself with affirmations such as 'trust in birth'.
> - If the fear will not go away or gets stronger then take note: it may be real. While birth should be trusted it also needs to be respected.
> - Shed the fear and do not carry it into the next birth.
>
> (Source: Dahlen & Caplice, 2010)

---

vernacular to discuss these levels of risk with each other or our clients.

Kotaska describes the '1 : 1000 club' as leading to a lot of intervention in childbirth (e.g. the increased risk of stillbirth between 41 and 42 weeks gestation, the excess risk of perinatal death with cautious selective vaginal breech delivery versus caesarean). Yet even by talking about 1 in 1000 we place the emphasis on the one adverse event, thus subconsciously focusing on it as a certainty. Why do we not say 999 : 1000 and talk about the fact that 999 times out of 1000 things will be okay? This shifts us from the 0.1% doctrine to the 99.9% response. What obstetrics frames as 1 : 1000, midwifery frames as 999 : 1000. While this is the same thing the impact is massively different. We have moved from the 0.1% doctrine to the 99.9% doctrine. The concept of certainty would seem to apply much more accurately to this statistic. Fundamentally our belief systems around birth and around the concepts of risk and safety are reflected in our language and our language impacts on the choices women make (Dahlen, 2010, 2011).

Dancing in the grey zone between normality and risk

I argue in a paper I wrote called 'Dancing in the grey zone between normality and risk' that childbirth is

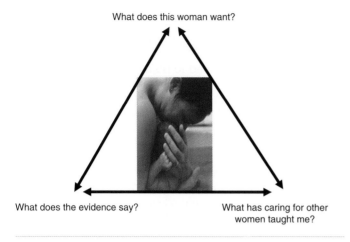

What does this woman want?

What does the evidence say?

What has caring for other women taught me?

FIGURE 4.3 The triangle of wisdom
(Source: Dahlen, 2016)

mainly grey (Dahlen, 2016). The most straightforward of births can lead to unexpected, heart-stopping moments and the highest-risk woman can, despite our fears, give birth without any of the imagined horrors being realised. As midwives we can choose to be paralysed with fear over this, or to be responsive to and respectful of such an amazing process. Most of the time as midwives we 'waltz' with women and they lead and we follow, but sometimes we dance the 'tango' and the rhythm is intense and the footwork complicated. There are times we 'hip hop' with women where we dodge and negotiate policies, delay interventions and sidestep expectations. Whatever form of dancing in the grey zone we take, midwives need to remember to stay in the 'triangle of wisdom' (Fig. 4.3).

Box 4.2 represents midwifery practice as a three-legged 'birth stool'.

Box 4.2 Working with risk and fear: a birth stool for the midwife

Joan Skinner

How do midwives ever manage to provide effective care that is both safe and satisfying in this risk context? One answer was provided in a piece of research conducted in New Zealand (Skinner, 2005). The framework represents midwifery practice as a simple three-legged stool (Fig. 4.4). It is a birth stool—not this time for the woman, but rather for the midwife. It is a tool that she can take with her and use wherever she practises.

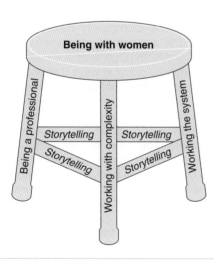

Being with women

Being a professional

Storytelling

Storytelling

Working with complexity

Storytelling

Storytelling

Working the system

FIGURE 4.4 A birth stool for the midwife

The seat of the stool: being 'with women'

The most important part of a stool is of course the seat. The seat of this stool is called 'being with women'. It represents the centrality of the midwife–woman relationship and the

importance of being alongside the woman in her journey to motherhood. It is the quality both of the relationship and of the communication that is the critical factor in the maintenance of safe and appropriate care (Edwards, 2000; Symon & Wilson, 2002; Wilkins, 2000). Relationships matter. It is within this relationship that trust is formed, information is shared, options are offered and decisions are made. Being 'with women' provides the space and time for the midwife to know the woman, to understand her perspectives and to anticipate her needs. Partnership is incorporated into the seat, yet this on its own is not sufficient in helping to understand the complex and challenging work of midwifery. It is, in a sense, a seat without legs. It doesn't lift the midwife off the ground or support her enough. The legs of the stool provide the other aspects of practice that are vital in the provision of safe care in the current sociocultural context. Being a professional, knowing how to work the system and understanding and working with complexity provide the stability required to stay 'with women' and to work towards partnership with them. These are the legs of the midwife's birth stool that give support; the legs help to lift the midwife above the 'messy swamp' of practice (Schon, 1983).

First leg of the stool: being a professional

The first leg of the stool is called 'being a professional'. It includes being both a skilled and an accountable practitioner. Midwifery incorporates knowledge from many different sources. It comes from within its own discipline and from other fields such as physiology, pharmacology, epidemiology and medicine. It also sources knowledge from the humanities, such as sociology and psychology. This knowledge then informs practice in the provision of safe care. A safe midwife is attentive to sound research and seeks answers to problems. A skilled midwife is also a skilled communicator and listener, attentive not only to the physical factors of the

Continued

Box 4.2   Working with risk and fear: a birth stool for the midwife—cont'd

woman but also to her social and cultural milieu. She seeks to understand what the woman and her family value and thus to understand how they themselves see risk. She communicates her own understanding of risk in a way that promotes the woman's autonomous decision making and minimises unnecessary fear and anxiety. She is reflective of her own position and attempts to provide care that is not dominated by it. Communication with the woman and her family is based on the quality of the relationship that she develops. It is fundamental to her 'being with' the woman.

Current constructions of professional practice are also very attentive to accountability.

There are several ways in which the midwife can minimise her own risk in this context. Accurate and complete documentation will provide evidence of the care that was provided. This should include documentation of the decision-making processes, including noting the information that was provided. The midwife needs to understand and implement her professional code of ethics and the standards for care. Safety for the midwife includes attending to the whole of practice, to all the parts of this midwife's birth stool. It remains based in the sound development of the relationship with the woman, in providing skilled care, and also in an understanding of and connection with the systems that are in place. It is supported by an understanding of, and negotiation between, the complex and often contradictory environment in which she works.

Second leg of the stool: working the system

The next leg of the stool has been called 'working the system' and is an important part of providing safe care—care that continues to be based on staying connected with the woman and her experience. It is called 'working the system' as it is a reminder that the focus remains on being 'with women'. Midwives work the system in order to meet the needs of the woman. This leg reminds us that we do not provide care in isolation. We provide care within a system, and it is important not only to understand how the system works but also to participate in it.

Three aspects of knowing the system are important: the development and maintenance of successful collaborative relationships with others in the system; understanding and working with the processes that the system puts in place, participating in organisational risk management and clinical governance processes (Cooper, 2000); and managing the power disparities.

In order to manage risk and safety, then, the midwife must learn to 'work the system'. She should keep connected and keep involved, actively participating in building collaborative relationships and in the planning of guidelines and policy. Safe practice is connected practice. Midwives need to build solid and collaborative relationships and to be involved in policy making and in research. They need to be active members of their professional organisation and develop a system for their own practice that is safe

and sustainable. They need to both claim and share their power, and challenge power systems that are unjust. When midwives work in isolation, they put themselves and the women for whom they care at risk.

Third leg of the stool: working with complexity

Complexity is such an integral part of midwifery care that it deserves a leg of the birth stool of its own. In being alongside women, things are often complex and unclear. The midwives in my study, in reflecting on how they managed risk, frequently talked about working in the 'grey areas', not only in the physical processes of birthing but also in the relationships that they developed with women, with medicine and with the system. There was a good deal of unknowing and uncertainty. The more-experienced midwives described how these grey areas of practice became even bigger the more experienced they became. Yet as they became more experienced they also became more comfortable. Uncertainty and complexity became less disturbing. They accepted that risk and uncertainty were normal parts of practice. They accepted the need to understand and accommodate many different perspectives reflecting the differing underlying cultural and value systems in which both they and the women lived.

Dealing with risk, then, is complex and challenging work, done in the context of the primacy of 'being with the woman' and alongside astute, professional care. If it is so complex, how might the midwife go about it? Understanding some of the theory about how complex systems work might be of assistance. Complexity theory tells us that tension and paradox are natural phenomena. Problems are often not resolvable through simple cause-and-effect processes. Instead, they occur in ways that are non-linear. Unpredictability is inherent in complex systems, although patterns emerge through inherent self-organisation. There always remain things that are unknowable (Plsek & Greenhalgh, 2001). Paradox and uncertainty, however, are not necessarily negative. They can be used as sources of change and improvement. Complexity theory rejects the machine model of the human body and of healthcare systems, where the whole is broken down into smaller and smaller parts for treatment or intervention. Action, then, requires a holistic approach, accepting unpredictability yet building on the emergent forces and processes that become evident. It requires careful observation and the application of astute, involved, creative and intuitive care.

The struts in the stool: storytelling

The last part of the birth stool is the struts. Struts connect the legs with each other and with the seat, and help to hold the stool together firmly. These struts are named 'storytelling'. Midwives are great storytellers. We tell stories to share and connect with each other. The stories can be both healing and sense making. Stories express and create the norms of practice. We tell stories in our documentation and

Box 4.2   Working with risk and fear: a birth stool for the midwife—cont'd

in our formal practice review. We tell stories to the women we care for, and sometimes we have to tell the story to the disciplinary bodies and to our professional organisation. Storytelling is probably the most valuable tool in the teaching and development of midwifery, as it is in storytelling that the messy and real complexity of practice is revealed and understood. Sharing stories keeps us connected with each other, helps us to understand the complexities of practice and provides a way of understanding what is expected. Stories can both challenge us and affirm us. Storytelling keeps us mindful and reflective. It brings to our attention those things that we may have let go of, and offers us other possibilities for action. It helps to keep our practice connected and safe.

Although these parts of the stool are described separately, they are not separate at all. You will find that the themes are interconnected and are found embedded in the whole stool.

In this way the stool embraces the complex and messy world of practice. The realities of real-world midwifery mean that we seldom, if ever, have a perfect stool. However, the good thing about a three-legged stool is that it remains stable even if it is a bit 'out of kilter'. The legs do not have to be exactly the same shape and size to be secure and sturdy. For example, where the relationship with the woman is challenging and difficult, strong, well-connected legs will support it. Where the new practitioner is still developing her skills and expertise, her relationship with the woman and the connections and involvement she develops with the system will ensure that she is supported. Where deficiencies in the system challenge the ability of the midwife in her work, an astute midwife who understands the power dynamics and the variety of apparent worldviews, and who is skilled and accountable in the context of a strong relationship with the woman, can still provide safe care.

REFLECTIVE THINKING EXERCISE

Use each part of the birth stool to reflect on the following stories.

- Suzy is 34 and is expecting her first baby, conceived by in vitro fertilisation (IVF). She works as a program manager for a computer company and her husband is a lawyer. On her first visit with you she asks you whether she could have a home birth and how safe it would be. How would you approach this question?

- Karen is expecting her second baby and is now a week past her due date. She had a long labour with her first baby and had an epidural and a forceps delivery. Although this pregnancy is normal she has become increasingly anxious about the birth, and when you visit her she states that she wants an induction and another epidural, as she has heard that babies sometimes die when they are overdue. How do you manage these concerns and how do you negotiate and support Karen's final decision?

- Marg is expecting her fourth baby. She has had three normal births before and is relaxed and confident about this birth, although the baby is currently a breech presentation. She was shocked to be told by the obstetrician that she should have a caesarean section and is determined to have a vaginal birth with no intervention. She says she will just have you and not the doctors. How do you manage this?

- Beth is in labour with her first baby. She is now at the birthing unit and has been actively pushing for 2 hours. Although progress has been slow, Beth is coping well and the baby's heart rate has been stable. You can just see the baby's head appearing but the fetal heart rate is beginning to drop during contractions. What do you do and what do you say to Beth and her family?

CRITICAL THINKING EXERCISE

Fear is an increasing problem affecting maternity care and women appear to be getting more fearful about birth as are health professionals.

- In your practice what are the things you see that trigger this fear?

- As a midwife what can you do to help reduce this fear in women?

- How as a midwife do you work on keeping your own fear in check?

--- Conclusion ---

Midwives are in the perfect place to make sense of risk. We work with, understand and indeed embrace the complexity and uncertainty of our work. The challenges of working in a world where fear about risk has become paramount can be partly overcome by our unique connectedness with women, our astute knowledge of the science, the context and of our own place in the picture. It can support us to open up to the possible rather than close down with the risky. It can put fear into perspective.

--- Review questions ---

1. How are the concepts of risk and safety related?
2. How has the technorational or scientific approach to birth affected the way risk is perceived?
3. How can one consider normality when risk is identified?
4. How does the 'risk society' affect the provision of maternity care?
5. How does fear impact on care?
6. What role do cultural values play in risk decisions?
7. How does the quality of the relationship that the midwife has with the woman support safe practice?
8. What else in the midwife's practice supports safe care?
9. What role does accountability play?
10. How does the midwife ensure her own safety?
11. Why is it important to have good collaborative relationships with other healthcare providers?

Acknowledgements

With acknowledgement to Joan Skinner, who co-authored with Hannah Dahlen Chapter 5 'Risk, fear and safety' in the 3rd edition of this text, upon which this chapter is largely based.

Online resources

Australian Commission on Safety and Health Care: https://www.safetyandquality.gov.au.
Australian Institute of Health and Welfare: https://www.aihw.gov.au/.
How Fear Works: http://science.howstuffworks.com/life/fear.htm.
Psychology Today: http://www.psychologytoday.com/basics/fear.

References

Al-Mufti R, McCarthy A, Fisk NM. Survey of obstetricians' personal preference and discretionary practice. *Eur J Obstet Gynecol Reprod Biol.* 1997;73(1):1–4.

Alfirevic Z, Devane D, Gyte GML, et al. Continuous cardiotocography (CTG) as a form of electronic fetal monitoring (EFM) for fetal assessment during labour. *Cochrane Database Syst Rev.* 2017;(5):CD006066. doi:10.1002/14651858.CD006066.pub2.

Allard T. The terror factory. *Sydney Morning Herald.* 2007;9 June:27.

American Congress of Obstetricians and Gynecologists. *Safe Prevention of the Primary Cesarean Delivery.* USA: ACOG; 2014.

Annandale E. Working on the front-line: risk culture and nursing in the new NHS. *Sociol Rev.* 1996;44(3):416–436.

Australian College of Midwives (ACM). *Midwife means 'with woman': this underpins midwifery's philosophy, work and relationships.* 2017. Online: https://www.midwives.org.au/midwifery-philosophy.

Backe B, Salvesen KA, Sviggum O. Norwegian obstetricians prefer vaginal route of delivery. *Lancet.* 2002;359(9306):629.

Beck U. *Risk Society: Towards a New Modernity.* London: Sage; 1992.

Beck U. *World Risk Society.* Cambridge: Polity; 1999.

Bergholt T, Ostberg B, Legarth J, et al. Danish obstetricians' personal preference and general attitude to elective caesarean section on maternal request: a nation-wide postal survey. *Acta Obstet Gynecol Scand.* 2004;83:262–266.

Blaaka G, Schauer T. Doing midwifery between different belief systems. *Midwifery.* 2008;24:344–352.

Cartwright E, Thomas J. Constructing risk: maternity care, law and malpractice. In: DeVries R, Benoit C, Teijlingen ER, et al, eds. *Birth by Design. Pregnancy, Maternity Care, and Midwifery in North America and Europe.* New York: Routledge; 2001:218–228.

Cooper IG. Clinical risk management. In: Fraser D, ed. *Professional Studies for Midwifery Practice.* Edinburgh: Churchill Livingstone; 2000:143–158.

Copeland F, Dahlen HG, Homer CE. Conflicting contexts: midwives interpretation of childbirth through photo elicitation. *Women Birth.* 2014;27(2):126–131. doi:10.1016/j.wombi.2013.11.004.

Crabtree S. Midwives constructing normal birth. In: Downe S, ed. *Normal Childbirth: Evidence and Debate.* Edinburgh: Elsevier; 2008:97–113.

Dahlen H. Midwifery at the edge of history. *Women Birth.* 2006;19(1):3–10.

Dahlen H. Undone by fear? Deluded by trust? *Midwifery.* 2010;26(2):156–162.

Dahlen H. Perspectives on risk or risk in perspective? *Essentially MIDIRS.* 2011;2(7):17–21.

Dahlen HG. Managing risk or facilitating safety? *Int J Childbirth.* 2014;4(2):66–68.

Dahlen HG. Dancing in the grey zone between normality and risk. *Pract Midwife.* 2016;19(6):18–20.

Dahlen H, Caplice S. *Keeping birth normal.* CAPERS Workshop; 2010.

Dahlen H, Caplice S. What do midwives fear? *Women Birth.* 2014;27(4):266–270. doi:10.1016/j.wombi.2014.06.008.

Dahlen H, Gutteridge K. Stop the fear and embrace birth. In: Byrom S, Downe S, eds. *The Roar Behind the Silence: Why Kindness, Compassion and Respect Matter in Maternity Care.* London: Pinter & Martin; 2015 [Ch. 15].

Dahlen H, Barclay L, Homer C. The novice birthing: theorising first time mothers' experiences of birth at home and in hospital in Australia. *Midwifery.* 2008;26(1):53–63.

Dahlen H, Downe S, Duff M, et al. Vaginal examination during normal labour: routine examination or routine intervention? *Int J Childbirth.* 2013;3(3):142–152.

Dahlen H, Tracy S, Tracy MB, Bisits A, Brown C, & Thornton C. (2014). Rates of obstetric intervention and associated perinatal mortality and morbidity among low-risk women giving birth in private and public hospitals in NSW (2000–2008): a linked data population-based cohort study. *BMJ Open*. 2014;4:e004551. doi:10.1136/bmjopen-2013-004551.

Dahlen, H., Kumar-Hazard, B., & Schmied V (eds.). *Birthing Outside the System: The Canary in the Coal Mine*. New York: Routledge; 2020.

Davis-Floyd R. The technocratic, humanistic, and holistic paradigms of childbirth. *Int J Gynaecol Obstet*. 2001;75(1):S5–S23.

De Becker G. The Gift of Fear. London: Bloomsbury; 1997.

Dencker A, Nilsson C, Begley C, et al. Causes and outcomes in studies of fear of childbirth: A systematic review. *Women Birth*. 2019; 32(2): 99–111.

Douglas M. *Risk and Blame: Essays in Cultural Theory*. London: Routledge; 1992.

Douglas M, Wildavsky A. *Risk and Culture: An Essay on the Selection of Technical and Environmental Dangers*. Berkeley: University of California Press; 1982.

Edwards NP. Women planning homebirths: their own views on their relationships with midwives. In: Kirkham M, ed. *The Midwife–Mother Relationship*. London: Macmillan; 2000:55–84.

Füredi F. *Culture of Fear Revisited*. New York: Continuum; 2006.

Grayling AC. *The Meaning of Things: Applying Philosophy to Life*. London: Phoenix; 2002.

Green JM, Baston HA. Have women become more willing to accept obstetric interventions and does this relate to mode of birth? Data from a prospective study. *Birth*. 2007;34(1):6–13.

Hacking I. *The Taming of Chance*. Cambridge: Cambridge University Press; 1990.

Heyman B. *Risk, Health and Healthcare*. London: Arnold; 1998.

Heyman B, Titterton M. Introduction. In: Heyman B, Shaw M, Alaszewski A, et al., eds. *Risk, Safety and Clinical Practice*. New York: Oxford University Press; 2012:37–58.

Heyman B, Alaszewski A, Shaw M. *Risk, Safety and Clinical Practice: Health Care Through the Lens of Risk*. New York: Oxford University Press; 2010.

Homer C, Dahlen H. Obstetric-induced incontinence: a black hole of preventable morbidity? An alternative opinion. *Aust N Z J Obstet Gynaecol*. 2007;47:89–90.

Keating A, Fleming V. Midwives' experience of facilitating normal birth in an obstetric-led unit: a feminist perspective. *Midwifery*. 2007;25(5):518–527.

Klein S. *The Science of Happiness*. New York: Avalon; 2002.

Kotaska A. Normalising birth in the 21st century. Paper presented at the Breathing New Life into Maternity Care: Working Together for Normal Birth, Surfers Paradise; 2012.

Kotaska A. Informed consent and refusal in obstetrics: a practical ethical guide. *Birth*. 2017;44(3):195–199. doi:10.1111/birt.12281.

LeDoux JE, Romanski L, Xagoraris A. Indelibility of subcortical memories. *J Cogn Neurosci*. 1989;1(3):238–243. doi:10.1162/jocn.1989.1.3.238.

Lupton D. *Risk*. London: Routledge; 1999.

Moore A. *Pioneering a New Model of Midwifery Care: A Phenomenological Study of a Midwifery Group Practice*. Melbourne: Australian Catholic University; 2009.

Morris S. Is fear at the heart of labour? *MIDIRS Midwifery Digest*. 2005;15(4):508–511.

Murphy-Lawless J. *Reading Birth and Death: A History of Obstetric Thinking*. Bloomington and Indianapolis: Indiana University Press; 1998.

New Zealand College of Midwives (NZCOM). *Midwives Handbook for Practice*. Christchurch: NZCOM; 2008.

Plsek PE, Greenhalgh T. The challenge of complexity in healthcare. *BMJ*. 2001;323(7313):625.

Powell Kennedy H, Shannon M. Keeping birth normal: research findings on midwifery care during childbirth. *J Obstet Gynecol Neonatal Nurs*. 2004;33(5):554–560.

Quirk GJ, Repa JC, LeDoux JE. Fear conditioning enhances short-latency auditory responses of lateral amygdala neurons: parallel recordings in the freely behaving rat. *Neuron*. 1995;15: 1029–1039.

Regan M, Liaschenko J. In the mind of the beholder: hypothesized effect of intrapartum nurse's cognitive frames of childbirth caesarean section rates. *Qual Health Res*. 2007;17(5):612–634.

Saisto T, Halmesmaki E. Fear of childbirth: a neglected dilemma. *Acta Obstet Gynecol Scand*. 2003;82:201–208.

Sandall J, Soltani H, Gates S, et al. Midwife-led continuity models versus other models of care for childbearing women during pregnancy, birth and early parenting. *Cochrane Database Syst Rev*. 2016;(4):CD004667, doi:10.1002/14651858.CD004667.pub5.

Scamell M. The swan effect in midwifery talk and practice: a tension between normality and the language of risk. *Sociol Health Illn*. 2011;33(7):987–1001.

Scamell M, Alaszewski A. Fateful moments and the categorisation of risk: midwifery practice and the ever-narrowing window of normality during childbirth. *Health Risk Soc*. 2012;14(2):207–221.

Scamell M, Stone N, Dahlen HG. Risk, safety, fear and trust in childbirth. In S. Downe & S. Byrom, eds *Squaring the Circle: Normal Birth Research, Theory and Practice in a Technological Age*. UK: Pinter Martin; 2019; 100–110.

Schon DA. *The Reflective Practitioner*. New York: Basic Books; 1983.

Skinner J. The midwife in the 'risk' society. *NZCOM J*. 2003;28(1):4–7.

Skinner J. *Risk and the Midwife: A Descriptive and Interpretive Examination of the Referral for Obstetric Consultation Practices and Attitudes of New Zealand midwives (Doctoral thesis)*. 2005. Victoria University of Wellington. Online: http://researcharchive.vuw.ac.nz/xmlui/handle/10063/56.

Skolbekken JA. The risk epidemic in medical journals. *Soc Sci Med*. 1995;40:291–305.

Small K, Sidebotham M, Fenwick J, et al. Intrapartum cardiotocograph monitoring and perinatal outcomes for women at risk: Literature review. *Women Birth*. 2019. doi:10.1016/j.wombi.2019.10.002.

Smythe L. Being safe in childbirth; what does it mean? *NZCOM J*. 2000;22:18–21.

Stapleton H. *Choice in the Face of Uncertainty*. London: Ballière Tindall; 1997.

Styles M, Cheyne H, O'Carroll S, et al. The Scottish trial of refer or keep (the Stork study): midwives' intrapartum decision making. *Midwifery*. 2011;27:104–111.

Suskind R. *The One Percent Doctrine: Deep Inside America's Pursuit of its Enemies Since 9/11*. New York: Simon & Schuster; 2006.

Symon A. *Litigation; The Views of Midwives and Obstetricians*. Cheshire: Hochland & Hochland; 1998.

Symon A, Wilson J. The way forward: clinical competence, co-operation and communication. In: Symon A, Wilson J, eds. *Clinical Risk Management in Midwifery. The Right to a Perfect Baby*. Oxford: Books for Midwives; 2002:153–165.

Taylor-Gooby P. Trust, risk and health care reform. *Health Risk Soc*. 2006;8(2):97–103.

Thornton MJ, Lubowski DZ. Obstetric-induced incontinence: a black hole of preventable morbidity. *Aust N Z J Obstet Gynaecol*. 2006;46:468–473.

Tulloch J, Lupton D. *Risk and Everyday Life*. London: Sage; 2003.

Turner CE, Young JM, Solomon MJ, et al. Vaginal delivery compared with elective caesarean section: The views of pregnant women and clinicians. *BJOG*. 2008;115(12):1494–1502. doi:10.1111/j.1471-0528.2008.01892.x.

Van Wagner V. Risk talk: using evidence without increasing fear. *Midwifery*. 2016;38:21–28.

Wagner M. The public health versus clinical approaches to maternity services: the emperor has no clothes. *J Public Health Policy.* 1998;19(1):25–35.

Walsh D. Subverting the assembly line: childbirth in a free-standing birth centre. *Soc Sci Med.* 2006;62(6):1330–1340.

WHO. World Health Organisation. WHO recommendations: intrapartum care for a positive childbirth experience. Geneva, Switzerland: WHO; 2018.

Wilkins R. Poor relations; the paucity of the professional paradigm. In: Kirkham M, ed. *The Midwife–Mother Relationship.* London: Macmillan; 2000:28–54.

Zhang J, Landy HJ, Branch DW, et al. Contemporary patterns of spontaneous labor with normal neonatal outcomes. Consortium on Safe Labor. *Obstet Gynecol.* 2010;116:1281–1287.

Further reading

Beck U. *Risk Society: Towards a New Modernity.* London: Sage; 1992.

De Becker G. *The Gift of Fear.* London: Bloomsbury; 1997.

Symon A. *Risk and Choice in Maternity Care: an International Perspective.* London: Churchill Livingstone; 2006.

CHAPTER 5

Sustainability and ecosystem approach to health

Lorna Davies and Tricia Thompson

LEARNING OUTCOMES

Learning outcomes for this chapter are:

1. To describe the concept of sustainability and identify the main tenets and how they interrelate
2. To demonstrate an understanding of the effects of climate change on human health
3. To describe the importance of self-sustainability in midwifery
4. To discuss social sustainability in relation to midwifery practice
5. To explain what sustainable midwifery looks like within the scope of your own practice.

CHAPTER OVERVIEW

This chapter is a new addition to the textbook, although sustainability has been incorporated into other chapters in previous editions. This reflects the increasing significance of sustainability literacy in health generally and in midwifery specifically, and the importance of being able to relate to both current and future challenges that our profession faces in relation to things such as climate change and wealth distribution inequalities. This chapter will introduce the broad principles concerning environmental, economic and social sustainability, and continue to apply these to the healthcare setting and finally to midwifery practice.

KEY TERMS

climate change
COVID-19
environmental sustainability
healthy ecosystems

midwife as social connector
moment of revelation
oxygen analogy
self-sustainability

social sustainability
sustainability
sustainability voice

INTRODUCTION

The term 'sustainability' has an almost ubiquitous presence in many areas of contemporary life, including in healthcare. Most definitions of sustainability, including those in healthcare, now address concern for ecology and the environment but also embed concerns for economic development and social equity. As a society we are reliant on a healthy environment around us; **healthy ecosystems** and environments are required to provide resources including food, and services within a social and economic context. Sustainability can therefore be viewed as a key health-related issue concerned with the maintenance of health and wellbeing of the human population. Healthcare professions have comprehended that there are significant global environmental threats to human health resulting from climate change (Davies, 2017), although it is acknowledged that different areas of healthcare will have a different focus on issues that have greater relevance to their own areas of practice. In this chapter we set out to explore what sustainability means in the context of midwifery care and to consider how the midwifery profession can address the real-life issues relating to the existential crisis that we are currently facing. We will begin the chapter by introducing the concept of sustainability, the tenets that it incorporates and the challenges that overuse of global resources has led to. This will be linked to issues relating to social justice and inequities resulting from a significant inequality in global wealth distribution. The COVID-19 pandemic will be viewed in relation to what has been described by Aotearoa New Zealand's prime minister as a climate emergency, and how we can use the lessons learnt from the pandemic to futureproof against climate-related events and economic and social crises. Consideration of healthcare as an ecosystem will be introduced and self-sustainability in terms of our own health and wellbeing examined. The final section focuses on social sustainability, women and birth where the threads are drawn together in terms of the part that midwives can play in creating a sustainable ecosystem of birth.

THE CONCEPT OF SUSTAINABILITY

The concept of **sustainability** may once have been associated simply with environmental concerns, however, for decades now it has been clear that sustainability must also encompass economic and sociocultural factors. These three tenets of sustainability—environmental, economic and sociocultural—cannot be considered in isolation as they are in so many ways interwoven and interdependent. Thus sustainability is described as an interweaving of the '3 Ps' of people, planet and prosperity (Purvis et al., 2019).

In terms of the *planet*, within the scientific community it is now well understood that without good environmental management and science, the Earth's resources cannot be sustained in the long term and that action is needed as a matter of urgency if a global catastrophe is to be avoided. But globally, we won't achieve **environmental sustainability** without having *people* committed to achieving that cause. The balance point is *prosperity*; currently some people have 'too much' while others do not have enough. People's human needs must be met and people want to live a good life, but this must occur within the limits of nature. Since the 1970s humanity's demand for ecological resources and services has exceeded what our planet can regenerate in any given year. This is known as 'ecological overshoot' and means that we are in debt environmentally; 'living off our ecological credit card' is one way of describing it. Eventually, at current consumption rates, the renewable resources will be depleted, and the carbon dioxide waste that is produced is trapped and will not be able to be absorbed. Already there are stresses evident on Earth's biodiversity and ecosystems.

While carbon dioxide is naturally present in the atmosphere there have been increasing amounts of anthropogenic or manmade carbon dioxide released into the atmosphere that comes primarily from burning fossil fuels—coal, natural gas and petroleum—for energy use and transport. The Intergovernmental Panel on Climate Change (IPCC) has found that emissions from fossil fuels are the dominant cause of global warming. In 2018, 89% of global CO2 emissions came from fossil fuels and industry processes. The remainder comes mostly from methane, ozone, nitrous oxide and chlorofluorocarbons (CFCs). This excessive concentration of gases traps the sun's heat in the Earth's atmosphere and has the effect of acting like a 'greenhouse' in creating a warmer environment.

The environment is changing; in particular the climate is changing. The US National Aeronautics and Space Administration (NASA) explain that **climate change** is a change in the usual weather found in a place (Stillman & Green, 2017). They go on to outline that local climate change could be a change in how much rain a place usually gets in a year, or it could be a change in a place's usual temperature for a month or a season. Climate change is also a change in the Earth's climate. This could be a change in Earth's usual temperature, or a change in where rain and snow usually fall. The Earth's climate is always changing; there have been times in history when Earth's climate has been warmer than it is now; there have been times when it has been much cooler. While weather can change in just a few hours, the climate takes hundreds or even millions of years to change and the change is very gradual—at least, it has been in the past.

There is evidence to show that in the last 100–150 years, since the industrial revolution, Earth's climate has changed much more rapidly than it had in the millennia before. Earth's climate is getting warmer; in 2015, Earth's temperature had gone up by 1°C above pre-industrial temperatures for the first time, making it the warmest year in more than 11,000 years (Climate Analytics, 2015). This may not seem like much, but very small changes in the Earth's temperature can have very big effects. Some effects are already happening; warming of Earth's climate has caused snow and ice to melt; the warming has also caused oceans to rise. This process is often called global warming, but it is better to think of it as climate change. This is because it is likely to change other aspects of the climate as well as the temperature, and also bring about more extreme climate events such as floods, storms, cyclones and droughts.

As these effects of climate change become more evident it is increasingly clear that something must change if we are to avert continued and worsening climate disaster. There is also the looming prospect of generational inequality, with future generations being left to pay for the environmental decisions—and lack of decisions—of the past and of today.

But because of the complex interweaving described earlier, climate change does not just affect the environment; it also has economic costs and affects social determinants of health such as clean air, safe drinking water, sufficient food and secure shelter. The World Health Organization (WHO) estimates that climate change is expected to cause many additional deaths per year, and that will lead to increased direct health costs (WHO, 2018). Of course, areas of the world with weak health infrastructure, mostly in developing or resource-poor countries, will be least able to prepare and respond to such changes without assistance.

Climate change has been described as the biggest global health threat of the 21st century. The health effects are within three possible pathways: direct, indirect and diffuse (Table 5.1).

At the same time as we confront the global crisis of climate change, society also faces changing social, cultural and economic concerns. Both Australia and New Zealand have a growing wealth and income inequality, and this has led to increased social and health inequities. In the Oxfam 2017 report, data showed that the two wealthiest billionaires in Australia had the same amount of wealth as the poorest 20% of the adult population, and in New Zealand the disparity was even greater, where it was equivalent to the wealth of the poorest 30%.

While it may be argued that some level of inequality is inevitable, inequality matters because it is associated with poor long-term social outcomes. It can be a barrier to participating fully in society, and that disadvantage can be intergenerational. When adults lack wealth to own their own home, for example, their children have increased health risks from being raised in crowded, damp and unhealthy homes. When children fall behind at school because of ill health or transience of housing due to an unaffordable rental market, those children do not reach their educational potential. That contributes to ongoing cycles of lower income, lower education and lower wealth. These are some of the interwoven problems that threaten the world we each inhabit as citizens and as midwives. The women and families we care for also face these issues. The science is known; the problems are known; but there are solutions, and they also are known.

It can be easy to be overwhelmed and feel that the problem of climate change is too big to solve. People can

Table 5.1 Ways climate change affects health	
Three causal pathways	Effects may include
Direct or primary pathway	• Physical injury or death due to extreme weather events such as floods, storms, and fires. • Heat stroke due to more hot days. • Direct biological consequences of heat waves, extreme weather events, and temperature-enhanced levels of urban air pollutants.
Indirect or secondary pathway Health effects that happen when a changing climate alters biological processes. These changes in biophysical and ecological processes or systems affect food, water, and infectious disease vectors particularly.	• Food scarcities due to changing rainfall patterns and higher temperatures affecting what food can be grown. • Food poverty and food insecurity [particularly for the poorest]. • Water-borne diseases—gastroenteritis due to changing rainfall patterns and higher temperatures affecting quality of drinking water [and recreational / swimming water]. • Salmonella and other infectious diseases due to higher temperatures affecting food safety. • Respiratory problems due to higher temperatures extending pollen and allergen season, as well as respiratory effects of smoke from wildfires leading to increased asthma and other respiratory illnesses. • Increase in vector-borne diseases—mosquito-borne infectious diseases, due to changing temperature and rainfall patterns increasing geographical distribution of mosquitoes of concern.
Diffuse or tertiary pathway Health effects that happen when people need to substantially change their lives as a result of climate change.	• Mental health issues, particularly when the change affects whole communities such as in failing farm communities or having to leave your home or nation due to sea level rises [climate refugees], or other displaced groups, as well as disadvantaged, indigenous and minority ethnic groups. • Consequences of tension and conflict owing to climate change related declines in basic resources such as water, food, timber, shelter.

(Source: Environmental Health Indicators New Zealand (EHINZ) (2021); McMichael, 2013: Royal Society Te Apārangi, 2017; US Global Change Research Program, n.d.; WHO, 2018).

then feel immobilised, switch off or be side-tracked by 'trivial' pursuits (Macy & Johnstone, 2013). Inertia can make progress towards solutions seem very slow. A multi-layered approach is needed for genuine change to occur. Individuals need to take actions in their own lives and homes, and in the choices they make—what to buy or not to buy, what services to use—and midwives can help families in this by promoting sustainable values and role-modelling a more sustainable approach within their practice. But collective action will also need to be taken. Big businesses and corporations are reluctant to take action that may interfere with profits; collective action from consumers will be needed to pressure businesses to change policies and business practices. Governments are reluctant to take actions that may cost money or make them unpopular; collective action is needed from voting citizens to push governments to take action and make binding changes, both nationally and internationally.

It is easy to say that the solution to these large problems facing us—globally, nationally, individually—is to have more sustainable development; some speak of the need for more resilience. Are they the same thing, sustainability and resilience? The terms are frequently used to mean the same thing, but, while they are connected, they are actually two different concepts. Spacey (2016) describes sustainability as the practice of reducing or eliminating environmental impact and improving the quality of life for communities, whereas resilience is the practice of designing things to endure physical, social and economic shocks and stresses.

> Resilience is the capacity of a system, be it an individual, a forest, a city or an economy, to deal with change and continue to develop. It is about how humans and nature can use shocks and disturbances like a financial crisis or climate change to spur renewal and innovative thinking.
>
> (The Stockholm Resilience Centre, 2015, p.1)

The Paris Agreement on Climate Change, along with the 2030 Agenda with the Sustainable Development Goals, forming 'the most comprehensive blueprint to date for eliminating extreme poverty, reducing inequality, and protecting the planet' (UNSSC, 2020), were seen as the way ahead to developing the global sense of balance which is required.

What is it that would propel individuals and groups to change and take the actions needed to help bring about a more sustainable world?

Some groups and filmmakers seem to believe that if they tell us more about what is wrong environmentally or socially, we will act differently. But in fact, sometimes having more information (especially in the absence of clear messages about actions you can take) can cause people to disengage. Macy & Johnstone (2013) suggest that rather than more facts, it is hope and 'moral imagination' that gives people the strength to take action that will improve the situation for future generations.

When describing agents of positive social, economic and environmental sustainability change amongst leaders within business, one writer reflects that they are people who have undergone an inner journey alongside their external path (Confino, 2012). When the ego is thus put aside, a personal **'moment of revelation'** is possible, when there is more clarity and the leadership and action required for change can occur—when they find their **sustainability voice**. That concept, of an inner journey alongside the day-to-day reality, is something that midwives understand very well. At every labour and birth both midwives and parents face that potential trigger moment for change. When you witness or experience the amazing journey of a woman surrendering to the power of labour and birth, when you witness the miracle of birth, those are moments of awe that inspire hope and action towards making the world a better place. Those moments of awe also affirm a midwife in her role as guardian of normal birth.

Many individuals play an individual role, in their own lives, in the choices they make every day to help contribute towards 'making the world a better place' and such individual actions are important. Even more important is collective action, because that can help create more 'noise' and visibility and therefore create more pressure on governments and corporations to also make the bigger changes that need to be made.

In his new book *Regeneration: Ending the Climate Crisis in One Generation*, noted environmentalist Paul Hawken (2021) offers a positive and visionary approach to bringing people together to undertake actions and push for policy to transform current climate, environmental and human injustices.

One person standing up can set an example. Who can forget the example of one young student, Sweden's Greta Thunberg, speaking her truth? That has inspired tens of thousands of school strikers to take to the streets around the world demanding a solution to the climate emergency facing their world. They certainly found their sustainability voice. It was cultural anthropologist Margaret Mead who said 'Never doubt that a small group of thoughtful, committed, citizens can change the world. Indeed, it is the only thing that ever has.' It may be that the sight of those 'future generations' fighting for their future will shock their elders into taking action, too.

Why do some individuals feel a desire or a responsibility to make a difference in the world, and improve the state of the world in its environmental and social crises, and others don't? (Or perhaps they do, but don't know what to do about it?) Prakash (2017) argues that it is related to a basic feeling of connection to others, to the community, both locally and globally. She argues that connection comes from 'care, connection, and a degree of selflessness' (para. 3) and that extending our circle of connection and taking action for others can not only make us happy but also empowered.

At governmental level, with such a huge climate crisis facing the entire planet, national and international response should be swift and decisive. Yet progress by governments around the world has been achingly slow. Many commitments have been set to reduce carbon emissions, but few are binding, and targets frequently missed.

In Paris in 2015 at the COP 21 (Conference of the Parties) meeting, world leaders from 197 countries pledged to put people first and reduce their countries' greenhouse gas emissions. The Paris Agreement had the aim of limiting global warming to well below 2°C and ideally to 1.5°C. Yet in 2021 the United Nations Framework Convention on climate change (UNFCCC) reports that nations must re-double their efforts and make more ambitious national climate action plans if they are to achieve that goal. UN Secretary-General António Guterres stated: '2021 is a make or break year to confront the global climate emergency. The science is clear, to limit global temperature rise to 1.5C, we must cut global emissions by 45% by 2030 from 2010 levels' (Climate Action, 2021).

However imperfectly and slowly, nations and global agencies had plans in place to both achieve the 17 Sustainable Development Goals (SDGs) and to limit global temperature rise by 2030 … when along came a global pandemic!

Many governments met the threat of the **COVID-19** pandemic with unprecedented funding and immediate action plans. Suddenly individuals, communities, businesses and governments could all rally around and most could make sacrifices for the greater good. Many people could work from home after all. Money could be found to support those who could not. Essential workers were suddenly seen as important and valued. Families walked and biked in their neighbourhoods; carbon emissions dropped as traffic largely came to a standstill. Midwives and other health professionals worked out new ways to take care to where it was needed in women's homes and their communities; more women chose to birth in the security of their own home when it suddenly seemed safer than birthing in an institutional setting. The pandemic has provided some opportunity for 'post traumatic growth', Taylor (2020) describes, saying that when people have gone through something stressful together they often become better people, appreciating the little things, and having a greater appreciation for family, friends and community. Of course, everything was not perfect; Berkhout et al. (2021) in their recent Oxfam International report 'The Inequality Virus' describe that, apart from the millions of deaths globally, 'this virus has exposed, fed off, and increased existing inequalities of wealth, gender and race' (p.1).

The environmental crisis demands a similar emergency response. Huge investment will be needed, beyond what is being considered or delivered anywhere in the world. But as Atwoli et al. (2021) outline, such investments will produce positive outcomes for both the economy and population health. That would include high-quality jobs, reduced air pollution, increased physical activity, and improved housing and diet. They observe that better air quality alone would realise health benefits that easily offset the global costs of emissions reductions.

Despite the world's necessary preoccupation with COVID-19, Atwoli and others (2021) put out an urgent call to world leaders prior to the September 2021 UN General Assembly, in their 'Call for emergency action to limit global temperature increases, restore biodiversity, and protect health', saying that 'we cannot wait for the pandemic to pass to rapidly reduce emissions' since health is already being harmed by global temperature increases and the destruction of the natural world; the science is unequivocal.

ECOSYSTEM APPROACH: SUSTAINABILITY AND HEALTH

What is an ecosystem?

An ecosystem or ecological system in nature is a biological community with a complex set of relationships among all aspects of that environment. In nature, that includes the habitat, as well as the plants, trees, animals, fish, birds, microorganisms, water, soil—and the humans who interact with it. Natural ecosystems are dynamic self-organising systems that humans have evolved within, and the ecosystem must remain healthy if the humans too are to thrive.

Natural ecosystems vary in size and in the elements that make them up, but what they have in common is that everything that lives in that ecosystem is dependent on all the other species and elements in that ecological community—they are all linked. If one part is damaged or disappears it has an impact on every other aspect of the ecosystem.

A more modern use of the term 'ecosystem' is as a description of any complex network or interconnected system. Thus, taking an ecosystem approach is to use a framework which has an underlying principle that the complex interactions and links between all aspects of the system need to be understood. Using the term 'ecosystem approach' reminds us of the complexity of the issues as well as the interconnectedness of the systems.

Human health and healthcare cannot be discussed, or planned for, in a vacuum if we understand that we are only a part of a complex ecosystem. An ecosystem approach to sustainability and health therefore acknowledges the complexity of the issues, and the links and interdependence between health, the environment, the economy and social and cultural wellbeing. Holistic approaches are called for, ones that recognise the fundamentally interdependent nature of health and other societal, developmental and ecosystem-related factors in human communities (Asakura et al., 2015). An ecosystem approach to human health can be referred to as 'eco-health'.

CRITICAL THINKING EXERCISE

What is health?

List any ideas that you have for how you would define health. What would you include as important aspects of what it is to be healthy?

The ancient Latin phrase '*Mens sana in corpore sano*', which translates as 'a healthy mind in a healthy body', has contributed to a rather old-fashioned view of health as encompassing physical and mental health. The World Health Organization (WHO) when it formed in 1948 adopted in their constitution a definition of health as being 'a state of complete physical, mental and social well-being and not merely the absence of disease or infirmity' (WHO, 1948).

Today, a more nuanced understanding of health would include that it is dynamic and changes over time, and would also include a sense of wellbeing, which is a complex concept that includes how satisfied people are with their life as a whole, their sense of purpose, and how in control they feel. Measures of wellbeing might include measures of life satisfaction, of happiness or contentment, of connectedness or social isolation, and participants' perceptions of whether the things they did were worthwhile to them. 'Wellbeing can be understood as how people feel and how they function, both on a personal and a social level, and how they evaluate their lives as a whole' (New Economics Foundation, 2012).

Health is affected by social determinants such as poverty, education, gender, genetics, social supports and physical environment. Contributing factors to health and wellbeing include external factors such as income, housing and social networks, and internal factors such as optimism, resilience, and self-esteem.

While the above discussion of human health and wellbeing includes many important aspects, if we took an ecosystem approach to health then we could not see our human health as separate from the health of the ecosystem in which we live—and on which we rely for life. The health consequences of environmental degradation, for instance, must affect us and our wellbeing. Asakura et al. (2015) argue that the 'increasing interconnectedness of ecosystems in a globalizing world requires an ethical approach that considers human responsibility for the global biosphere' (p.1). They go on to suggest that eco-health could be 'a countervailing force to our excessive concentration on economy and technology' of the modern world.

Rachel Carson in her iconic 1962 book *Silent Spring* said, 'Those who contemplate the beauty of the earth find reserves of strength that will endure as long as life lasts. There is something infinitely healing in the repeated refrains of nature—the assurance that dawn comes after night, and spring after winter' (Howard, 2020). There are many today who recommend time in nature for its health benefits; for example, the Japanese practice of *Shinrin yoku* or 'forest bathing' is being recommended in Western countries also (Aubrey, 2017; Livni, 2019; Plevin, 2019) as a way to boost immunity and improve mood.

Unfortunately, in modern times an increasing proportion of the population are urban dwellers who may be quite disconnected from nature. Without a connection to it people no longer have a sense of protection for nature and become alienated from it. The term 'nature-deficit disorder' is credited to American journalist and author Richard Louv from his 2008 book *Last Child in the Woods*. While it is not a clinical diagnosis, others have subsequently used this term to describe the effect on both children's and adults' physical, mental and social health as increased screen time, stress and time pressures affect health and wellbeing, and evidence shows that a 'dosage of nature' can promote health (Driessnack, 2009; Kuo, 2013; McGuire, 2016; Peters, 2015; Warber et al., 2015).

When humans have a connection with nature and understand themselves as a part of nature they are also more likely to actively work to protect the planet. Sanchez et al. (2017) suggest that this is because 'they realize that there is an intimate connection between the well-being of humanity and the well-being of nature as a whole' (para 2).

The deterioration of the environment and the simultaneous deterioration of human health are partially linked, Kjaegard et al. (2014) believe. The authors explain that many health problems and sustainability problems emerge because of the intensification (for example, of agriculture and food production) and overuse of natural resources, and that there needs to be more integration between local, regional and international health promotion strategies and sustainable development strategies and policies so that there are not inadvertent negative effects in either direction. They conclude that 'from a duality perspective, integration means conceiving sustainability from a health perspective and health from a sustainability perspective' (Kjaegard et al., 2014, p. 558).

This dual perspective is also seen in the 2020 *WHO Global Strategy on Health, Environment, and Climate Change*, with the subtitle of this strategy document being 'The transformation needed to improve lives and wellbeing sustainably though healthy environments'.

The WHO describe this strategy as aiming to 'provide a vision and way forward on how the world and its health community need to respond to environmental health risks and challenges ... and to ensure safe, enabling and equitable environments for health by transforming our way of living, working, producing, consuming, and governing' (WHO, 2020, p. 3).

Specifically applying the concept of sustainability to health care, a health care system would need to be financially viable, have fair and timely access for all (Fischer, 2015; Prada, 2012), and '... improve, maintain or restore health, while minimizing negative impacts on the environment and leveraging opportunities to restore and improve it, to the benefit of the health and well-being of current and future generations' (WHO European Office, 2017, p. v).

As midwives wanting to be part of a sustainable healthcare system we must consider whether our practice meets the needs of all of our ecosystem. For our midwifery care to be sustainable we need to review whether we are considering the environment, as well as paying attention to the economic and sociocultural aspects of our care.

An indigenous perspective

Indigenous groups customarily have a world view that is far more integrated than the reductionist Western perspective (Dockry et al., 2015). This is borne of survival strategies that have evolved over centuries and which was traditionally embodied in localised knowledge about the environment and how it supports both the people and other species who share the environment. However, this harmonious relationship has by and large been marginalised as Western values and behaviours took precedence in the lands that indigenous people inhabited (Klein, 2014). Australian First Nations people have lived in a sustainable way for countless generations to 'nurture country, nurture their bodies, nurture their spirits and culture' (Sydney Environment Institute, 2018). In Aotearoa New Zealand, Mātauranga Māori (Māori knowledge) has been defined as 'the knowledge, comprehension, or understanding of everything visible and invisible existing in the universe' (Williams, 1989), which is as holistic as is possible.

There is a clear synergy between some indigenous concepts and midwifery concepts. The traditional Māori view of kaitiakitanga embodies a number of beliefs that connect environmental, physical, social, cultural, economic and spiritual aspects of Māori, and midwifery philosophy aligns well with this. Midwifery views the childbearing continuum through a holistic lens that hinges on relationships and encompasses all of the elements that matter to the woman and her pēpi (baby) and whānau (family), including those relating to the culture and the spiritual beliefs of the woman. A current review of the Health and Disability System in Aotearoa New Zealand is currently underway. The review aims to address inequity in health outcomes achieved including those in the maternity sector, to improve outcomes for Māori wāhine (women) and their whānau by ensuring that Te Tiriti o Waitangi (the Treaty of Waitangi) is embedded in health governance arrangements. This could lead to a more sustainable outlook for those both working in and accessing the maternity system.

SUSTAINING THE SELF

When health is absent
Wisdom cannot reveal itself, art cannot manifest, strength
Cannot fight, wealth becomes useless, and intelligence cannot
be applied.

(Herophilus, 300 B.C.)

As we have already established in this chapter, sustainability is about a commitment to surviving, growing and prospering within supportable limits. In the same vein, **self-sustainability** means that we are able to sustain our own health and wellbeing in order to survive, grow and prosper. It is about being able to recognise our own limitations by developing an awareness of our own specific psychosocial, emotional, spiritual and physical resources and knowing how to maintain them. Self-sustainability is about choosing behaviours that create balance between our emotional and physical stressors. It is also about learning to self-soothe or calm our physical and emotional reactions to dis-stress. If we do not or cannot care

for ourselves and maintain these precious resources then dis-stress and burnout can result.

The term 'self-care' is no doubt more commonly recognised than 'self-sustainability', but we feel that it would be prudent to use a degree of caution when using this term. The concept of self-care has developed a close relationship with market forces and the notion of individualism and in recent decades has developed into an industry built on the principles of consumerism. The self-care industry is now estimated to be a 'vast $450 billion self-care marketspace' where retailers and manufacturers are urged to 'keep up or risk missing tremendous growth opportunities' (MMR, 2021). Such a market-driven approach could philosophically challenge the notion of sustainability. 'Self-compassion' is another similar expression which may have greater affiliation with healthcare. Byrom & Menage (2020) describe self-compassion as treating yourself as someone who you care for and respect and for whom you are responsible. They suggest that self-compassion means 'recognising and attending to your own needs in order to maximise self-sustainability'. It is important to remember that language frames the worlds that we inhabit, and consideration of semantics is therefore, in our view, important.

When the World Health Organization (WHO) first defined the concept of self-care in 1983, it was described as a far-reaching concept that encompassed socioeconomic as well as environmental concerns. The WHO analysis also identified that the core principles of self-care would include concepts such as self-reliance, empowerment, autonomy, personal responsibility and self-efficacy, identifying personal responsibility. The inclusion of such values could be said to emphasise the responsibility of the individual to self-provide when it comes to their health and wellbeing. However, the WHO also emphasised that community participation, community involvement and community empowerment were important considerations in relation to self-care. This definition therefore recognises the importance of community in relation to caring for self, which is closely linked with caring for others.

These concepts are discussed further in Ch. 16.

REFLECTIVE THINKING EXERCISE

What does self-sustainability mean to you?

Self-sustainability in healthcare practice

A strong sustainable healthcare system is reliant on a sustainable workforce. In recent years there has been a burgeoning in the number of research studies, articles and resources relating to self-care in this area. It is recognised

Table 5.2 Stress and burnout	
Stress	Burnout
The body's response to the perception of threat, with resulting anxiety, discomfort, emotional tension, and difficulty in adjustment. (Fink, 2017)	A psychological condition in which an individual responds to chronic professional stressors with pathologic levels of: *emotional exhaustion* *depersonalization/cynicism* *a sense of lack of personal accomplishment/efficacy.* *(Maslach et al., 2001)*
Indicators of stress	Indicators of burnout
Typified by over-engagement	Typified by disengagement
Emotionally overreactive	Emotionally blunted
Manifests urgency and hyperactivity	Manifests helplessness and hopelessness
Causes decreased levels of energy	Causes decrease in motivation, ideals and hope
May result in anxiety disorders	May result in detachment and depression
Main damage is physical	Main damage is emotional
May cause premature death	May make life not seem like living
(Adapted from Smith et al. Burnout prevention and treatment. *HelpGuide.* 2021.)	

that the potential for stress-related consequences and burnout in healthcare is considerable (Lyndon, 2015). The terms 'burnout' and 'stress' are often used interchangeably but there are some key differences between the two. Table 5.2 defines the concepts of stress and burnout and outlines the signs and symptoms of both. Health work is emotionally and psychologically challenging, taking on the complex needs of those facing a range of diverse biopsychosocial problems. Pines & Aronson (1988) identify three characteristics which are the classic antecedents of stress-related burnout in human service careers; performing emotionally taxing work; presenting certain personality traits, such as empathy, and sharing a client-centred orientation. These are characteristics that can be considered to be synonymous with midwifery.

Burnout can be seen as the consequence of unresolved issues relating to stress and so it is important that we are able to activate our own internal 'stress awareness monitor' in order to keep track of where we are with regard to stress levels. There are many stress inventories online that may help with this and the links for some of these can be found in the Online resources at the end of the chapter. The bottom line is, that as primary carers, if we do not look after ourselves then we may be challenged when it comes to caring for others. An analogy sometimes used to illustrate self-care in this context is the **'oxygen analogy'**, that of the globally adopted airline instructions for functioning adults to put their own oxygen mask in place before applying on a child or other person requiring additional support. We may struggle to give care to our clients, family and friends if we don't take care of ourselves. We must think of self-care as fundamental and life-enriching rather than indulgent and egotistic. This means looking beyond the marketing messages and really reflecting on what sustains us at a deeply personal and professional level.

Self-sustainability in midwifery

Working within an area of healthcare practice that is built around relationality and that represents a significant time in the life course of its client group, it is imperative that midwives are able to care for themselves in order to provide effective and authentic care and to flourish. This involves nurturing and monitoring emotional and psychological wellbeing as well as observing any physical demands of the role. The impact of stress and burnout within the sphere of midwifery practice has been explored in many different settings and countries in recent years (Creedy et al., 2017; Dixon et al., 2017; Donald, 2014; Eaves & Payne, 2019; Hildingsson et al., 2013; Mollart et al., 2013; Suleiman-Martos et al., 2020; Yoshida & Sandall, 2013). Geraghty et al. (2018) identified some of the stressors that midwives viewed as affecting their working environment and these included finances, interprofessional interface, unsocial hours and multifarious social changes. When these factors present individually, they may well be manageable, but when two or more present simultaneously, the result of conflicting demands may become untenable.

A significant study from Australasia, the Whelm Study (Dixon et al., 2017) elucidated that of almost 2000 participating midwives, one-third scored moderate and above for stress, anxiety and depression, and two-thirds recorded moderate and above for work-related burnout. In this extensive study, burnout appeared to be more prevalent for those aged under 40, those performing hospital-based shift work and those with a disability of any kind. An interesting outcome of the study was that the data challenged the popular belief that continuity of care (CoC) models lead to increased levels of stress and burnout in midwifery practice. The study concluded that, unless they are working without any level of support on their own, then CoC midwives in New Zealand demonstrate less burnout than their employed counterparts even if they are working unpredictable and longer hours. Certainly, there is supporting evidence that CoC midwives thrive on the demands of a caseload model (McAra-Couper et al., 2014) although other researchers have concluded that for some it is unsustainable and can result in burnout. (Young, 2011).

CRITICAL THINKING EXERCISE

List what you consider to be some of the barriers to self-sustainability in your professional context.

Now consider some of the enablers.

Self-sustainability literacy

Some of the barriers to self-sustainability identified within the literature are the divergent demands of time, busyness, lack of planning / prioritising, unsupportive working environment, inadequate boundaries between work and home and low self-worth / esteem. This is not a definitive list and there are likely to be many others. Midwives and student midwives alike therefore need to be able to develop strategies that enable them to weather the storm and to both identify and ameliorate the effects of stress in practice.

The inclusion of education content in midwifery programs around self-sustainability may assist in preparing the next generation of midwives for the realities of practice as well as providing tools to assist them when the going gets tough. Interestingly, a small study carried out in the South Island of New Zealand concluded that student midwives had to be able to integrate the element of self-sustainability before they could see sustainability in a more general way that related to the midwifery profession (Davies et al., 2020). This introduction of self-sustainability could be extended to the provision of workshops and courses for qualified midwives in the workplace.

An important aspect of 'self-sustainability literacy' is an understanding of the neurohormonal mechanisms that regulate our physical and emotional responses. A recognition that our bodies and minds connect to create the world that we experience physically, emotionally and psychologically is the starting point of this approach. Understanding the effects of excessive catecholamine production on our reactive states or how melatonin may be able to heal deep emotional wounds as well as helping us sleep (Davies, 2017) can change the way that we function both personally and professionally.

Once we understand the mechanism of the fight / flight / freeze effect of the sympathetic nervous system versus the rest / digest / repair response of the parasympathetic nervous system, we understand that what we do, say and feel influences what happens within our bodies and, more importantly, that we have considerable control over how that works. By taking just two deep diaphragmatic breaths we can change our physiology from 'fast to slow' in just six seconds.

The inclusion of self-sustainability literacy in any curricula must additionally focus on reciprocity and relationality and not just practical ideas for self-care. The value of compassion as a key value in healthcare can be seen to be currently undergoing a renaissance. As Byrom & Menage (2020) identify, 'an act of compassion towards another has reciprocal benefits and is therefore an act of compassion towards self'.

Sustaining self as a part of life

Taking time in a busy world to look after ourselves is key to maintaining and sustaining ourselves as midwives. The focus of this should be on 'small actions that restore a sense of balance in our hectic lives'. This may include eating nutritious food on a regular basis, sleep health, meditating, engaging with the natural environment or spending quality time with our families. The potential list is extensive and needs to relate to our individual needs and requirements.

REFLECTIVE THINKING EXERCISE

List the things that you already do in order to sustain yourself.

Now consider others that you may like to incorporate.

It may be easier to practise some of these if we purposefully schedule them into our lives. Just like other important tasks and appointments, perhaps we should diarise a time of meditation in the morning, for example, or a walk in the park at the end of the day, to ensure it happens. Sustaining self is not something that happens overnight after a brief introduction. It has to be an ongoing process that reinforces positive behaviours with repetition of those behaviours.

A lot of focus in recent years has been about goal-setting in life. Having meaningful goals is important and it can be argued that goals help to support our overall health and wellbeing (Bandura, 1998). However, we do need to remind ourselves that life is often a balancing act with competing goals calling on our time and energy and it is easy to feel that we have failed in some way if our planned goals are not fulfilled. In the context of midwifery, we need to learn to manage these competing goals and accept that not all goals are achievable. This will help to develop an adaptive self-regulating approach that will help to pave the way to enhancing health and wellbeing.

Self-sustainability is strongly linked with community sustainability as the WHO noted several decades ago. Within a social model of childbirth, midwives are expected to support the emotional, psychological, cultural and spiritual aspects of the wellbeing of women. This means dealing with social conditions and stress-related factors that may impact on them. Facilitating connections with women and other groups and agencies is therefore an essential part of the role. Midwives have been described as '**social connectors**' (Davies & Crowther, 2020) because the midwife and her practice are inherently founded on sociability. The social connecting role extends to engaging with colleagues within the profession. Meeting with colleagues for social events regularly, sharing journal groups, secret buddy-type activities and finding a way to share social time within the day are just some of the possibilities that will foster this enjoyable aspect of the job. After all, the need for social connection is a fundamental human motive (Hutcherson et al., 2008).

REFLECTIVE THINKING EXERCISE

List any ideas that you have for increasing your engagement with your midwifery community that would contribute both to community and self-sustainability.

Self-sustainability in midwifery practice calls for the adopting of ways of living and working that facilitate the maintaining of our mental, emotional and physical capacity. We need to learn to be responsive and to know how to move from one state of being to another with ease and, if necessary, with a sense of urgency. We therefore need to recognise that self-sustainability is not an abstract theoretical construct but a crucial survival strategy in healthcare.

SOCIAL SUSTAINABILITY, WOMEN AND BIRTH

In this section of the chapter, the particular focus is on the social sustainability issues of and for women who birth, and of birth itself. Any discussion of the concept of sustainability in relation to birth must include some critical analysis of the role of the media, including social media, in the social construction of women's perceptions of and fears about birth. Another key concern is how the increasing intervention rates in birth nationally and globally are already affecting, or may in future affect, the sustainability of birth. As midwives, we need to reflect on the role of the midwife in strengthening the sustainability of birth.

REFLECTIVE THINKING EXERCISE

If a general definition of **social sustainability** is the ability of a social system, such as a country, to function at a defined level of social wellbeing indefinitely …

- Could 'birth' as a social system be substituted instead of 'a country'?
- Could 'midwifery' be substituted?

What do you think?

1. Is *birth* able to function at a defined level of social wellbeing indefinitely?
2. Is *midwifery* able to function at a defined level of social wellbeing indefinitely?
3. What would contribute to birth and midwifery being socially sustainable?
4. What inhibits or disempowers that sustainability?

Social determinants of health (SDH) are the non-medical factors that affect health, the economic and social conditions and their distribution among the population that influence individual and group differences in health status. Thus the issue of social determinants of health is important to consider in assessing the woman for whom care is being provided by midwives. SDH are the conditions in which people are born, grow, live, work and age, and the forces that shape their daily lives (Health Navigator, 2021). These circumstances are shaped by the distribution of money, power and resources at global, national and local levels. This is what is largely responsible for health inequities—the unfair and avoidable differences in health status seen within and between countries, and between sectors within society, within a country or a community.

Social sustainability of maternity services

As well as assessing the environmental footprint of maternity services, when considering whether or not any system is sustainable one must also consider the economic and sociocultural impacts of that system. As discussed earlier in this chapter, one important aspect of social sustainability of maternity care would be to assess whether the service is accessible to all of the potential users of that system.

REFLECTIVE THINKING EXERCISE

1. What are the implications of the following statement for the maternity system in your country? In your local area?

   One important aspect of social sustainability of maternity care would be to assess whether the service is accessible to all of the potential users of that system.

2. Are all aspects of the maternity system accessible for all women?

3. Who are the women for whom all aspects of maternity care are most easily accessible, and for whom are they least accessible, or least easily accessible?

4. Considering the social determinants of health, what are the implications of that?

5. What does this mean for midwifery, and for midwives in your location?

In their 2015 study in New Zealand Bartholomew et al. (2015) outline that the vast majority of pregnant women in the country enrol for care early in their pregnancy and are happy with the options of care available to them. But the research findings go on to say that 'despite high overall satisfaction, there were persistent inequalities between ethnicities, age groups and socioeconomic status with regard to the timeliness and uptake of maternity services, and the choice women experience when looking for a lead maternity carer (LMC)'.

Social perceptions of pregnancy and birth

As a species, humans are social beings who live in company with other humans, organise in various social groupings; and who work, trade, play and interact with each other. Socialisation and social behaviours change over time, and the patterns of human society can be different from era to era, and across cultures.

One focus of this change in social behaviour and attitude is seen in relation to social perceptions of pregnancy and birth, both in terms of what is 'normal' and in attitudes to and beliefs about birth. Childbirth is both a biological and a cultural phenomenon; there are also political, social and gendered aspects.

Some have argued that if women want what society values, and if a modern technocratic society places higher value on technology than on nature, then that will follow through in childbirth also (Klein et al., 2006). Is this a version of the 'nature deficit disorder' that was discussed earlier in the chapter?

In one ethnographic study exploring social attitudes to birth, researchers particularly focused on beliefs, values and traditions, and in learning about women's preferred mode of birth today, whether vaginal or caesarean (Roudsari et al., 2015). Although this study was based in Iran, which may have some cultural differences to society in Australasia, universal themes were raised including discussion on the social and cultural influences which contributed to women's decisions about birth. Hearing negative and unpleasant birth stories, and negative social media were named as points of concern. While on the one hand normal birth could be viewed as a symbol of women's power and ability, it was also seen by some as a 'low-cost type of delivery' compared to the more 'prestigious' caesarean section which indicated higher social class.

Sharing birth stories

Ina May Gaskin (2011) asserts that when women are no longer able to hear the birth stories of women who gave birth vaginally, most will eventually believe that a caesarean is normal. Is it just idealisation, to imagine that before the medicalisation of childbirth young women heard stories about women's strength and power in birthing, not just about difficulty and suffering? Philby (2015) debates the effect of young women today hearing mainly negative birth stories and concludes that 'knowledge is not always power. Not if it leaves you feeling more fearful, less capable of building up the internal resolve needed for labour'. Suzanne Arms (1992) described the inheritance of young women today as a 'toxic legacy of attitudes about childbirth' (p. 26). She believed that distinction between attitudes towards childbirth in the past and the present is attributed to a loss of familiarity with the birth process, the loss of community with other women, and the loss of traditional feminine wisdom.

A positive effect of shared birth stories is that because birth stories contain vast amounts of information and are grounded in real-life experience, they may offset the medical model of birthing as the ideal.

When positive birth stories are shared, special messages are conveyed that describe the courage and power of women as birth givers, the integrity of the birth process, and the sanctity of the family; thus, the beauty and delicacy of the maternal newborn interactions are conveyed. These stories have the potential to change the beliefs of those who become vicarious learners.

(Davis-Floyd, 1992, 2003)

Fears and attitude towards childbirth

In a cross-cultural study between Australia and Sweden, Haines et al. (2012) set out to explore whether women's fears and attitudes towards childbirth influenced both the outcomes of their birth and the maternity care they received. After interviews during pregnancy the women in the study were divided into three different groupings, according to their attitude towards birth. They were classified as one of the following:

- *self-determiner*: possessing clear attitudes about birth, including seeing it as a natural process, with no childbirth fear
- *'take it as it comes'*: having no fear of birth and low levels of agreement with the attitude statements given by the researchers
- *fearful*: afraid of birth, with concerns for the personal impact of birth, including pain and control, safety concerns and low levels of agreement with attitudes relating to women's freedom of choice or birth as a natural process.

Perhaps unsurprisingly, the study found that those in the 'fearful' cluster were more likely to have had: a negative effect on their emotional health during pregnancy; increased likelihood of a negative birth experience; greater likelihood of having had an elective caesarean; greater likelihood to have had an epidural if they laboured; and / or greater likelihood to experience their labour pain as more intense, than women in the other clusters.

REFLECTIVE THINKING EXERCISE

1. Do you recognise those three categories as described by Haines et al. (2012)—*self-determiner*, *take it as it comes* and *fearful*—in yourself, your friends and / or the women whose care you are involved with as a student midwife?

2. Would you proffer any new or alternative categories?

3. Can you think of any impact or implications for you and your future work as a midwife?

4. Currently, do you observe that attitudes and fears are asked about or discussed, as a part of pregnancy care?

5. Do you think they should be?

6. Do you think the midwifery care approach should be, could be, individualised depending on women's fears and attitudes towards childbirth?

Pregnancy is a major physical, psychological and social event for every woman who experiences it. While having a baby is generally a joyful experience, some concern or worry about the unknown may be normal. Most women are able to overcome or deal with it through self-help measures and support; it is only a small minority for whom the fear may become pathological and require treatment. This profound fear has been termed 'tokophobia'; this has been described as *primary* when it is suffered by those who are not pregnant, have not been pregnant, or who may be avoiding pregnancy because of the extent of this condition of fear; and *secondary* if it is a fear of childbirth developed after a traumatic event in a previous pregnancy or birth.

In various studies in the past, while 20% to almost 80% of pregnant women reported some fears, 6% described 'a fear that is disabling' and 13% of non-pregnant women reported fear of childbirth so strong they postpone or avoid pregnancy (Hofberg & Ward, 2003). Fear in primigravida women is often linked to a perceived lack of control, and lack of belief in the body's ability to give birth safely; and for multiparous women the fear may be as a result of previous negative and / or traumatic birth experiences (Fenwick et al., 2013).

In a study of the attitudes of young people who had never been pregnant, 3616 young people across 8 countries (including Australia and New Zealand), were asked online questions to identify how many women would prefer caesarean section (CS) in a hypothetical healthy pregnancy; if so, why they preferred CS; and whether they report knowledge gaps or misperceptions about pregnancy and childbirth that could inform educational interventions (Stoll et al., 2017). The researchers found that 1 in 10 young women in the study preferred CS, including 18.4% in Australia. The major reasons given were fear of labour pain, and fear of physical damage. The researchers also found that as the level of confidence in women's knowledge of pregnancy and birth increased, both fear of childbirth and preferences for CS declined. The authors concluded that improving knowledge through means such as social media, hearing stories, and face-to-face education could increase young women's understanding of labour and birth and thus reduce those fears.

Two central factors reported in various studies (Araji, 2020; Fisher et al., 2015; Hassanzadeh et al., 2020; Rondung, 2018) as helping to reduce women's fear of childbirth are (1) positive relationships with their midwife and (2) the support received from their social network including partners and in educational contexts such as antenatal classes. Some women also found psycho-educative therapies such as cognitive behavioural therapy (CBT) and hypnotherapy or hypnobirthing helpful.

Fear in childbirth, as any fear, can trigger a high-cortisol, high-adrenaline environment, which is unhelpful for the positive childbirth hormones of oxytocin and endorphins; this can have a negative impact on the progress of labour and birth, including increased interventions.

Sustainability of birth

The use of medical interventions such as caesarean section (CS) including elective CS, epidural analgesia, electronic fetal monitoring, and induction of labour has dramatically increased in recent years. In 1990, worldwide, 7% of babies were born by CS but now that figure is 21%—or 29.7 million births annually (Boerma et al., 2018; WHO, 2021). The rise is unequal, however. Statistics for 2015 show rates ranging from a concerningly low 4.1% in west and central Africa, indicating a likely lack of access to CS as a lifesaving intervention, up to 44.3% in Latin America and the Caribbean, indicating massive overuse of CS (Boerma et al., 2018).

Within regions there can be rather unequal distribution of CS rates. As an example, the CS rate in 2018 for Oceania was 21.4%, which is about the same as the average world rate (21.1%). However, that masks the fact that for the grouping of Melanesia, Micronesia and Polynesian the CS rate was 3.6% while for the grouping of Australia and New Zealand it was 33.5% (WHO, 2021).

Within countries there are also disparities, with five times higher rates amongst the wealthiest quintile of the population, and in private hospitals compared to public facilities (Boerma et al., 2018). They also estimate that there are about six million unnecessary CSs done each year, half of them in just two countries, Brazil and China. Although the reasons for this rapid rise are complex it is suggested that they are often for non-medical or social reasons, such as 'advanced maternal age', maternal request, fear of labour and birth, or to select an auspicious date (Nagy & Papp, 2020; Shi et al., 2021). If this trend of increase continues, by 2030 some regions of the world would reach a CS rate of up to 63%, and the rate for Australia and New Zealand would be 45%, the research suggests (WHO, 2021).

This disparity has both economic and social equity issues. Although CS is in general a safe procedure it can lead to short- and long-term health consequences and complications for women, children and future pregnancies (Chien, 2021; Nagy & Papp, 2020). In some parts of the world women face mortality and morbidity associated with unmet need for CS (Boerma et al., 2018), but in other regions overuse of the surgical procedure drains national health resources and adds avoidable morbidity and mortality (Betran et al., 2021). If the Sustainable Development Goals are to be achieved, comprehensively addressing the CS issue is a global priority (Betran et al., 2021).

How can such high rates of operative birth be sustainable; and what do these rising intervention rates mean for midwifery? One midwife author suggests that the increasing interventions challenge 'those things that have traditionally been at the heart of childbirth: the ability of the woman to birth and the clinical skills of the health professional' (McAra-Couper, 2007, ix).

It is important for the sustainability of normal birth, and indeed of midwifery, that we question the growing intervention rates. Yes, there are women who need secondary- or tertiary-level collaborative care due to related health or medical factors, and they need midwives as part of a complex care team. But it is important for women, for midwives and for society that women who have normal pregnancies remain within primary care, and that midwives provide normal midwifery care. If birth and midwifery are to remain sustainable, then women and midwives must affirm and continue to believe in women's innate ability to give birth normally.

An unexpected outcome of the COVID-19 pandemic has been a preference expressed for 'out-of-hospital' birth due to psychological processes related to risk perception. Suddenly the perceived risks of home or birth centre birth were outweighed by fears of being isolated from partner and family in a hospital setting, and / or of the hospital being seen as a place of potential infection risk (Gildner & Thayer, 2021; Pries et al., 2021). If this preference continues, it could be a saving to health system resources due to an increase in normal vaginal birth rates and a decreased caesarean section rate (Callander et al., 2021).

Will it turn out that an unexpected side effect of the global pandemic will be an increased understanding of the benefits of midwifery care in the community, and a renewed belief in community birth settings and normal vaginal births for normal low-risk women? That would be a positive!

Conclusion

In this chapter we have demonstrated that sustainability is a systemic concept that influences society environmentally, economically, socially, culturally and even spiritually. An awareness of the need for greater sustainability has increased exponentially in the last decade. It would seem that the world has begun to awaken to the existential threat of climate change, and we are beginning to see action to address at least some of the many related issues now affecting the planet, our lifestyles and our workplaces.

Healthcare has an important part to play in building sustainability into every level at which it operates. Midwifery is an area of health practice that has sustainability built into its very fabric by virtue of its resilience across millennia and as a low-tech, high-touch healthcare profession. Midwifery therefore has the potential to inform and lead future developments in the field of healthcare wherever sustainability needs to be highlighted and addressed.

Review questions

1. What would you identify as your own ecosystem, working your way from the inside with your microbiome to your external environment?

2. As we are confronted with more reports and experiences of natural disasters, do you think that the media adequately addresses the issue of climate change from the perspective of human health?

3. What do you see in indigenous communities in your locality or globally that can teach us more about our responsibility to the environment?

4. How do you think midwifery education could be used to improve levels of sustainability literacy and, ultimately, improve sustainable practice?

5. Identify a self-care strategy and consider how it can contribute to your health and wellbeing.

6. How would you describe your attitude towards childbirth? Would you categorise yourself in one of these groups: (a) seeing it as a normal event and having no particular fears, (b) having a 'take it as it comes' attitude, or (c) feeling fearful of the pain, lack of self-control, or safety of birth?

7. When you see representations about childbirth in the media or social media, does it reflect your attitude? Does the attitude of the author affect how childbirth is represented publicly?

8. Can you think of some ways that as a midwife you could help women to feel empowered by their birth story, whatever the outcome of the birth?

9. In what ways do you interact with nature on a regular basis? Does your connection with nature or natural things have an effect on your health?

10. Why do you think self-care could be seen as an essential professional responsibility for midwives and all health professionals?

11. What are the criticisms of the concept of resilience and how might these relate to midwifery?

12. Identify who you count on as your close connections, your community. In what ways has the COVID-19 pandemic helped strengthen your connection with these people? Are there ways in which the pandemic has caused stress in those connections?

Online resources

all4maternity.com. Why does self-care matter to midwives?: https://86e81b25b3bd830d509e-6dcaed68ce9607bb74994a568d9fea63.ssl.cf3.rackcdn.com/2021/8/490b0760-1ce9-11ec-9306-000000000000/all4maternity.com-Why%20does%20self-care%20matter%20for%20midwives.pdf

Are disposable hospital supplies trashing the planet?: https://healthydebate.ca/2016/08/topic/hospital-medical-waste/.

Holmes and Rahr Stress Inventory: https://www.stress.org/holmes-rahe-stress-inventory.

Mind Tools: https://www.mindtools.com/pages/main/newMN_TCS.htm.

Self-care questionnaire: https://wellness.sfsu.edu/sites/default/files/documents/Self-Care%20Questionnaire%20and%20Contract%20%281%29%28Accessible%29.pdf.

The Lancet article by KJ Wabnitz, S Gabrysch, R Guinto, et al.: A pledge for planetary health to unite health professionals in the Anthropocene: https://www.thelancet.com/article/S0140-6736(20)32039-0/fulltext.

References

Araji S, Griffin A, Dixon L, et al. An overview of maternal anxiety during pregnancy and the post-partum period. *J Ment Health Clin Psychol.* 2020;4(4):47–56. Online: https://www.mentalhealthjournal.org/articles/an-overview-of-maternal-anxiety-during-pregnancy-and-the-post-partum-period.pdf.

Asakura T, Mallee H, Tomokawa S, et al. The ecosystem approach to health is a promising strategy in international development: lessons from Japan and Laos. *Globalisation Health.* 2015;11(3). doi:10.1186/s12992-015-0093-0.

Atwoli L, Baqui AH, Benfield T, et al. Call for emergency action to limit global temperature increases, restore biodiversity, and protect health. *Lancet.* 2021;398(10304): 939–941. doi:10.1016/S0140-6736(21)01915-2.

Aubrey A. *Forest bathing: A retreat to nature can boost immunity and mood.* NPR Morning Edition; 2017. Online: https://www.npr.org/sections/health-shots/2017/07/17/536676954/forest-bathing-a-retreat-to-nature-can-boost-immunity-and-mood.

Bandura, A. Health promotion from the perspective of social cognitive theory. *Psychol Health.* 1998;13:623–649.

Bartholomew K, Morton SMB, Atatoa Carr PE. Provider engagement and choice in the Lead Maternity Carer system: Evidence from the Growing up in New Zealand study. *Aust New Zeal J Obstet Gynaec.* 2015;55(4),323–330.

Berkhout E, Galasso N, Lawson M, et al. *The inequality virus.* Oxfam International; 2021. Online: https://www.oxfam.org/en/research/inequality-virus.

Betran AP, Ye J, Moller AB, et al. Trends and projections of caesarean section rates: global and regional estimates. *BMJ Global Health.* 2021;6(6). Online: http://dx.doi.org/10.1136/bmjgh-2021-005671.

Boerma T, Ronsmans C, Melesse DY, et al. Global epidemiology of use of and disparities in caesarean sections. *Lancet.* 2018;392(10155):1341–1348. doi:10.1016/s0140-6736(18)31928-7.

Byrom S, Menage D. Sustained by compassion. In: Davies L, Daellenbach R, Kensington M, eds. *Sustainability, Midwifery and Birth.* Routledge; 2020.

Callander EJ, Bull C, McInnes R. The opportunity costs of birth in Australia: hospital resource savings for a post-Covid-19 era. *Birth.* 2021;48(2):274–282. doi:10.1111/birt.12538.

Chien P. Global rising rates of caesarean sections. *BJOG.* 2021;128(5):781–782. doi:10.1111/1471-0528.16666.

Climate Action. *UNFCCC: Climate commitments 'not on track' to meet Paris Agreement Goals.* 2021. Online: https://www.climateaction.org/news/unfccc-climate-commitments-not-on-track-to-meet-paris-agreement-goals.

Climate Analytics. *Global warming reaches 1°C above preindustrial, warmest in more than 11,000 years.* [Climate Analytics Briefings]; 2015, November. Online: https://climateanalytics.org/briefings/global-warming-reaches-1c-above-preindustrial-warmest-in-more-than-11000-years/.

Confino J. *Moments of revelation trigger the biggest transformations.* The Guardian; 2012; 9 November. Online: https://www.theguardian.com/sustainable-business/epiphany-transform-corporate-sustainability.

Creedy D, Sidebotham M, Gamble J. Prevalence of burnout, depression, anxiety and stress in Australian midwives: A cross-sectional survey. *BMC Pregnancy Childbirth.* 2017;17:13. doi:10.1186/s12884-016-1212-5.

Davies L. *Midwifery: A model of sustainable healthcare practice?* Unpublished Thesis. 2017. Online: https://ir.canterbury.ac.nz/bitstream/.../Davies,%20Lorna%20final%20PhD%20thesis.pdf.

Davies L, Harré N, Kara K. A values based approach to sustainability literacy in a Bachelor of Midwifery Programme. In: Davies L, Daellenbach R, Kensington M, eds. *Sustainability Midwifery and Birth.* Routledge; 2020.

Davies L, Crowther S. The midwife as social connector. In: Davies L, Daellenbach R, Kensington M, eds. *Sustainability Midwifery and Birth.* Routledge; 2020.

Davis-Floyd, RE. *Birth as an American Rite of Passage.* Berkeley, CA: Universtiy of California Press; 1992.

Davis-Floyd, RE. *Birth as an American Rite of Passage.* 2nd ed. Berkeley, CA: Universtiy of California Press; 2003.

Dixon L, Guilliland K, Pallant J, et al. The emotional wellbeing of New Zealand midwives: Comparing responses for midwives in caseloading and shift work settings. *N Z Coll Midwives J.* 2017; 53:5–14.

Dockry MJ, Hall K, Van Lopik W et al. Sustainable development education, practice, and research: an indigenous model of sustainable development at the College of Menominee Nation, Keshena, WI, USA. *Sustain Sci.* 2015;1–12. doi:10.1007/s11625-015-0304-x.

Donald H, Smyth L, McAra-Couper J. Creating a better work-life balance. *NZCOM J.* 2014;49:5–10. Online: http://156.62.60.45/bitstream/handle/10292/12753/Creating%20a%20better%20work%20life%20balance.pdf?sequence=2&isAllowed=y.

Driessnack M. Children and nature-deficit disorder. *J Spec Pediatr Nurs.* 2019;14(1):73–75. doi:10.1111/j.1744-6155.2009.00180.x 2009.

Eaves JL, Payne N. Resilience, stress and burnout in student midwives. *Nurse Educ Today.* 2019;79:188–193. doi:10.1016/j.nedt.2019.05.012.

Environmental Health Indicators New Zealand (EHINZ). *Vulnerability to climate change.* [Factsheet]. Environmental Health Indicators Programme, Massey University. 2021; Online: https://www.ehinz.ac.nz/assets/Factsheets/Released-2019/ClimateChangeVulnerability-released032019.pdf.

Fenwick J, Gamble J, Creedy DK, et al. Study protocol for reducing childbirth fear: a midwife-led psycho-education intervention. *BMC Pregnancy Childbirth.* 2013;13:190. doi:10.1186/1471-2393-13-190.

Fink G. Stress: concepts, definition and history. In: *Reference Module in Neuroscience and Biobehavioral Psychology.* Elsevier; 2017.

Fisher C, Hauck Y, Fenwick J. How social context impacts on women's fears of childbirth: a Western Australian example. *Soc Sci Med.* 2015;63(1):64–75. doi:10.1016/j.socscimed.2005.11.065.

Fischer M. Fit for the future? A new approach in the debate about what makes health care systems really sustainable. *Sustainability.* 2015;7(1):294–312.

Geraghty S, Speelman C, Bayes S: Fighting a losing battle: Midwives experiences of workplace stress. *Women Birth.* 2018. doi:10.1016/jwombi.2018.07.012.

Gildner TE, Thayer ZM. Maternity care preferences for future pregnancies among United States childbearers: the impacts of Covid-19. *Front Sociol.* 2021;6. doi:10.3389/fsoc.2021.611407.

Haines HM, Rubertsson C, Pallant JF, et al. The influence of women's fear, attitudes and beliefs of childbirth on mode and experience of birth. *BMC Pregnancy Childbirth.* 2012;24:12–55. doi:10.1186/1471-2393-12-55.

Hassanzadeh R, Abbas-Alizadeh F, Meedya S, et al. Fear of childbirth, anxiety and depression in three groups of primiparous pregnant women not attending, irregularly attending and regularly attending childbirth preparation classes. *BMC Womens Health J.* 2020;20(180). doi:10.1186/s12905-020-01048-9.

Hawken P. *Regeneration: Ending the Climate Crisis in One Generation.* Penguin Random House; 2021.

Health Navigator. *Social determinants of health.* Online: https://www.healthnavigator.org.nz/clinicians/s/social-determinants-of-health/.

Helpguide Burnout prevention and treatment. 2021. Online: https://www.helpguide.org/articles/stress/burnout-prevention-and-recovery.html.

Hildingsson I, Westlund K, Wiklund I. Burnout in Swedish midwives. *Sex Reprod Health.* 2013;4(3):87–91.

Hofberg K, Ward MR. Fear of pregnancy and childbirth. *Postgrad Med.* 2003;79(503):505–510. doi:10.1136/pmj.79.935.505.

Howard L. *Finding strength in nature.* Paideia Program, University of Pennsylvania; 2020. Online: https://snfpaideia.upenn.edu/finding-strength-in-nature/.

Hutcherson CA, Seppala EM, Gross JJ. Loving-kindness meditation increases social connectedness. *Emotion.* 2008;8(5):720–724. doi:10.1037/a0013237.

Kjaegard B, Land B, Bransholm Pedersen K. Health and sustainability. *Health Promot Int.* 2014;29(3):558–568. doi:10.1093/heapro/das071.

Klein MC, Sakala C, Simkin P, et al. Why do women go along with this stuff? *Birth.* 2006;33(3):245–250. doi:10.1111/j.1523-536X.2006.00110.x.

Klein N. *This Changes Everything: Capitalism vs. the Climate.* London, England: Allen Lane an imprint of Penguin Books; 2014.

Kuo FE. Nature-deficit disorder: Evidence, dosage, and treatment. *J Policy Res Tour Leis Events.* 2013; 5(2):172–186. doi:10.1080/19407963.2013.793520.

Livni E. *There is a word for the trauma caused by distance from nature.* Quartz; 2019. Online: https://qz.com/1557308/psychoterratica-is-the-trauma-caused-by-distance-from-nature/.

Lyndon A. *Burnout among Health Professionals and its effect of patient safety. Patient Safety Network.* Perspectives on Safety. 2015. Online: https://psnet.ahrq.gov/perspective/burnout-among-health-professionals-and-its-effect-patient-safety.

Macy J, Johnstone C. *Active hope: how to face the mess we're in without going crazy.* New World Library; 2013.

Maslach C. What have we learned about burnout and health? *Psych Health.* 2001;16(5):607–611. doi:10.1080/08870440108405530.

Mass Market Retailers (MMR). 2021 MMR Digital Edition. 2021;38(3). Online: https://digitaledition.massmarketretailers.com/publication/?m=65770andl=1.

McAra-Couper J. *What is shaping the practice of health professionals and the understanding of the public in relation to increasing intervention in childbirth (PhD thesis).* Auckland: Auckland University of Technology; 2007.

McAra-Couper J, Gilkison A, Crowther S. Partnership and reciprocity with women sustain lead maternity carer midwives in practice. *N Z Coll Midwives J.* 2014;49:29–33. doi:10.12784/nzcomjnl49.2014.5.29-33.

McGuire T. Nature therapy at work. *Canadian Nurse.* 2016;112(5):34–36.

McMichael AJ. Globalisation, climate change and human health. *N Engl J Med.* 2013;368(14):1335–1343. doi:10.1056/NEJMra1109341.

Mollart L, Skinner VM, Newing C, et al. Factors that may influence midwives work-related stress and burnout. *Women Birth.* 2013; 26:26–32. doi:10.1016/j.wombi.2011.08.002.

Nagy S, Papp Z. Global approach of the cesarean section rates. *J Perinat Med.* 2020;49(1):1–4. doi:10.1515/jpm-2020-0463.

New Economics Foundation. *Measuring Wellbeing: A Guide for Practitioners.* London: New Economics Foundation; 2012.

Oxfam Australia. *An economy for the 99%.* 2017, January. Online: https://www.oxfam.org.au/wp-content/uploads/2017/07/oxfam-An-economy-for-99-percent-oz-factsheet.pdf.

Peters D. From health inequalities to 'nature deficit disorder'. *J Holistic Healthcare.* 2015;12(1):7–10.

Philby, C. *The debate: Should women share negative birth stories?* [Web log post]; 2015, 23 August. Online: http://motherland.net/features/the-debate-should-women-share-negative-birth-stories/.

Pines A, Aronson E. *Career Burnout: Causes and Cures.* New York: Free Press; 1988.

Plevin J. *The healing magic of forest bathing.* Ten Speed Press; 2019.

Prada G. *Sustainability: What does this mean for Canada's health care systems.* In: Proceedings of the Collaborative Meeting of the Conference Board of Canada's Health-Related Executive Networks. 16 April 2012. Online: https://www.conferenceboard.ca/docs/default-source/cashc-public/april2012_presentation_prada.pdf?sfvrsn=0.

Prakash P. *We're all responsible for the state of the world. So why do only some of us care enough to act?* World Economic Forum; 2017. Online: https://www.weforum.org/agenda/2017/10/how-growing-your-connectedness-can-make-a-global-difference/.

Pries H, Mahaffey B, Lobel M. The role of pandemic-related pregnancy stress in preference for community birthing during the beginning of the Covid-19 pandemic in the United States. *Birth.* 2021;48(2):242–250. doi:10.1111/birt.12533.

Purvis B, Mao Y, Robinson D. Three pillars of sustainability: In search of conceptual origins. *Sustain Sci.* 2019;14:681–695. doi:10.1007/s11625-018-0627-5.

Rondung E. Psychological perspectives on fear of birth; heterogeneity, mechanisms and treatment [Doctoral Thesis,

Mid Sweden University]. 2018. Online: https://www.diva-portal.org/smash/get/diva2:1246908/FULLTEXT02.pdf.

Roudsari RL, Zakerihamadi M, Khoei EM. Socio-cultural beliefs, values and traditions regarding women's preferred mode of birth in the north of Iran. *Int J Community Based Nurs Midwifery*. 2015;3(3):165–176.

Royal Society Te Apārangi. *Human health impacts of climate change for New Zealand*. Evidence summary; 2017. Online: https://royalsociety.org.nz/assets/documents/Report-Human-Health-Impacts-of-Climate-Change-for-New-Zealand-Oct-2017.pdf.

Sanchez E, Sullivan M, Dupart L. *In symmetry with nature*. Center for Humans and Nature, Loyola University, Chicago. [Weblog] 2017.

Shi XY, Wang J, Zhang WN et al. Caesarean section due to social factors affects children's psychology and behavior: a retrospective cohort study. *Front Pediatr*. 2021;8. doi:10.3389/fped.2020.586957.

Spacey J. *Sustainability vs resilience*. Simplicable; 2016. Online: https://simplicable.com/new/sustainability-vs-resilience.

Stillman D, Green JC. What is climate change [NASA Knows]; 2017. Online: https://www.nasa.gov/audience/forstudents/k-4/stories/nasa-knows/what-is-climate-change-k4.html.

Stockholm Resilience Centre. *What is resilience? An introduction to social-ecological research*. 2015. Online: https://www.stockholmresilience.org/download/18.2f48c3c31429b6ad0a61cde/1459560221338/SRC_whatisresilience__sida.pdf.

Stoll KH, Hauck YL, Downe et al. Preference for caesarean section in young nulligravid women in 8 OECD countries and implications for reproductive health education. *Reprod Health*. 2017;14:1–9.

Suleiman-Martos N, Albendín-García L, Gómez-Urquiza JL, et al. Prevalence and predictors of burnout in midwives: a systematic review and meta-analysis. *Int J Environ Res Public Health*. 2020;17(2):641. doi:10.3390/ijerph17020641.

Sydney Environment Institute. *Indigenous sustainability practices and processes*. University of Sydney; 2018. Online: https://www.sydney.edu.au/engage/events-sponsorships/sydney-ideas/2018/indigenous-sustainability-practices-and-processes.html.

Taylor S. *The psychology of pandemics*. RNZ Radio interview; 2020. Online: https://www.rnz.co.nz/national/programmes/saturday/audio/2018739528/steven-taylor-the-psychology-of-pandemics.

United Nations Systems Staff College (UNSCC). *UNSCC 2020 online course on the Paris Agreement on Climate Change as a development agenda*. 2020. Online: https://www.preventionweb.net/event/unscc-2020-online-course-paris-agreement-climate-change-development-agenda.

US Global Change Research Program. *Climate change: Impacts on society*. n.d. Online: https://www.globalchange.gov/climate-change/impacts-society.

Warber SL, DeHudy AA, Bialko MF. Addressing 'nature deficit disorder': a mixed methods pilot study of young adults attending a wilderness camp. *Evid Based Complement Alternat Med*. 2015;1–13. doi:10.1155/2015/651827.

Williams CJF. *What Is Identity?* Oxford: Clarendon Press; 1989.

World Health Organization (WHO). *COP24 special report: health and climate change*. 2018. Online: https://apps.who.int/iris/bitstream/handle/10665/276405/9789241514972-eng.pdf?ua=1.

World Health Organization (WHO). *WHO global strategy on health, environment and climate change: The transformation needed to improve lives and wellbeing sustainably though healthy environments*. 2020. Online: https://www.who.int/phe/publications/WHO-STRATEGY-LAY5_fin_red.pdf.

World Health Organization (WHO). *Caesarean section rates continue to rise, amid growing inequalities in access*. 2021. Online: https://www.who.int/news/item/16-06-2021-caesarean-section-rates-continue-to-rise-amid-growing-inequalities-in-access-who.

World Health Organization Regional Office for Europe. *Environmentally sustainable health systems: a strategic document*. 2017. Online: https://www.euro.who.int/__data/assets/pdf_file/0004/341239/ESHS_Revised_WHO_web.pdf.

Yoshida Y, Sandall J. Occupational burnout and work factors in community and hospital midwives: a survey analysis. *Midwifery*. 2013;29(8):921–6. doi:10.1016/j.midw.2012.11.002.

Young C. The Experience of Burnout in Case Loading Midwives (Unpublished thesis). 2011.

Further reading

Business and Economic Research. *Inequality and New Zealand*. Business and Economic Research Ltd; 2020: Online: https://berl.co.nz/our-pro-bono/inequality-and-new-zealand.

Environment and Ecology. *What is sustainability? University of Alberta Office of Sustainability*. 2019. Online: http://environment-ecology.com/what-is-sustainability.html.

Environmental Protection Agency (EPA). *Overview of greenhouse gases*. United States Environmental Protection Agency; 2021. Online: https://www.epa.gov/ghgemissions/overview-greenhouse-gases.

Fitzgerald S. *The secret to mindful travel? A walk in the woods*. National Geographic. 2019. Online: https://www.nationalgeographic.com/travel/article/forest-bathing-nature-walk-health.

Lifset R. Sustainability is more than just the environment, but can we quantify that? [Weblog, Yale School of the Environment]; 2017. Online: https://environment.yale.edu/blog/2017/12/sustainability-is-more-than-just-the-environment-but-can-we-quantify-that/.

National Trust. 'Nature deficit disorder' and its effect on childhood obesity. *Br J Health Care Assistants*. 2013;6(8):414.

World Health Organization (WHO). *What do we mean by self care?* Online: https://www.who.int/reproductivehealth/self-care-interventions/definitions/en/.

CHAPTER 6

Midwifery as primary healthcare

Alison Eddy

LEARNING OUTCOMES

Learning outcomes for this chapter are to:

1. Describe the principles that underpin primary healthcare and how it can be positioned within the healthcare system and its relationship with universal health coverage
2. Describe the relationship between primary healthcare and population health
3. Define primary, secondary and tertiary healthcare
4. Explore the role of the midwife in the primary healthcare setting
5. Explore the midwifery scope of practice in relation to primary healthcare
6. Describe how midwifery as a primary healthcare service can have an impact on outcomes for women
7. Explore the interface between primary and secondary care in relation to the midwifery scope of practice.

CHAPTER OVERVIEW

This chapter provides an overview of primary healthcare and the key concepts which surround it. It discusses the essential nature of primary healthcare within healthcare systems as a means to support the health and wellbeing of individuals and populations. It considers how primary healthcare is positioned within Australia and New Zealand healthcare systems and how primary healthcare can be a focus for preventive and cost-effective care.

The role of midwives as providers of an essential primary healthcare service is then considered and how midwifery can impact on maternal and newborn care in this context. It also explores the interface between primary and secondary maternity services in relation to the midwifery role and scope of practice.

KEY TERMS

primary healthcare
secondary healthcare
tertiary healthcare

public healthcare
primary care
population health

universal health coverage

INTRODUCTION

Primary healthcare (PHC) as a concept

In 1978 the World Health Organization (WHO) issued its declaration in Alma-Ata, Health for All by the Year 2000 (WHO, 1978). This ambitious plan aimed for a worldwide comprehensive system of primary healthcare. As Coreil & Mull (1990) describe it, primary healthcare (PHC) is *essential* healthcare made universally accessible to individuals and families by means acceptable to them, with their full participation, and at a cost that they, their community and the country as a whole can afford. PHC is grounded in the philosophy and practices of the social model of health. The WHO Alma Ata Declaration (1978) set out PHC as a focus for community action to tackle the underlying determinants of health, thus situating PHC within a broader social movement designed to reduce inequities and improve living conditions for whole populations (Baum et al., 2013).

The key elements of PHC were outlined in the 1978 Alma-Ata Declaration. PHC is the first point of contact between people in the community and the healthcare system. However, its scope is greater than simply providing healthcare to individuals when they are ill or injured. It is a philosophical approach to health which seeks not only to treat ill health but also to improve health and wellbeing, promote self-determination and self-care, and increase participation by individuals and communities in healthcare priority setting and planning.

The Ottawa Charter (WHO, 1986)

The Ottawa Charter for Health Promotion (WHO, 1986) further defined primary healthcare in the context of health promotion and public health activities. This Charter still represents consensus agreement on good health promotion practice.

The Charter identifies the prerequisites for health and methods to achieve health promotion as well as five key action areas. The overarching guidance of this charter is the development of strategies according to needs, that when implemented will help to make health choice the easy choice for everyone.

Methods to achieve health promotion are:
- *Advocate*—Good health is a major resource for social, economic and personal development, and an important dimension of quality of life. Political, economic, social, cultural, environmental, behavioural and biological factors can all favour health or be harmful to it. Health promotion action aims at making these conditions favourable through advocacy for health.
- *Enable*—Health promotion focuses on achieving equity in health. Health promotion action aims at reducing differences in current health status and ensuring equal opportunities and resources to enable all people to achieve their fullest health potential. This includes a secure foundation in a supportive environment, access to information, life skills and opportunities for making healthy choices. People cannot achieve their fullest health potential unless they are able to take control of those things which determine their health. This must apply equally to women and men.
- *Mediate*—The prerequisites and prospects for health cannot be ensured by the health sector alone. More importantly, health promotion demands coordinated action by all concerned: by governments, by health and other social and economic sectors, by non-governmental and voluntary organisations, by local authorities, by industry and by the media. People in all walks of life are involved as individuals, families and communities. Professional and social groups and health personnel have a major responsibility to mediate between differing interests in society for the pursuit of health. Health promotion strategies and programs should be adapted to the local needs and possibilities of individual countries and regions to take into account differing social, cultural and economic systems.

The five key action areas for health promotion in the Ottawa Charter are:
1. *build healthy public policy*—requiring all sectors to consider health promotion as they develop policies and each level of government to promote laws that improve health outcomes
2. *create supportive environments for health*—the inextricable links between people and their environment constitutes the basis for a socioecological approach to health
3. *strengthen community action for health*—concrete and effective community action in setting priorities, making decisions, planning strategies and implementing them to achieve better health
4. *develop personal skills*—health promotion supports personal and social development through providing information, education for health, and enhancing life skills
5. *re-orient health services*—the role of the health sector must move increasingly in a health promotion direction, beyond its responsibility for providing clinical and curative services. Health services need to embrace an expanded mandate which is sensitive and respects cultural needs.

Universal health coverage (UHC)

Universal health coverage has been defined by WHO as:

Ensuring that all people have access to needed promotive, preventive, curative, rehabilitative, and palliative health services, of sufficient quality to be effective, while also ensuring that the use of these services does not expose any users to financial hardship.

(WHO, 2019)

Not all countries provide UHC for their populations, making the achievement of UHC as a Sustainable Development Goal (SDG)[a] an important aim. Currently, it is

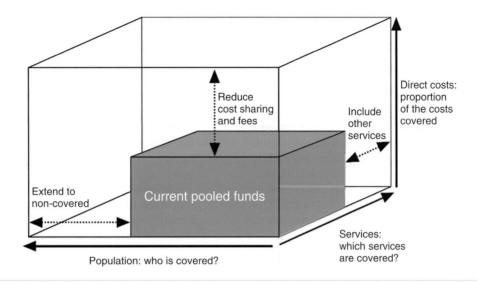

FIGURE 6.1 Three dimensions to consider in progressive realisation of universal health coverage
(Source: Boerma et al., 2014)

estimated that at least half of the people in the world do not receive the health services they need (WHO, n.d.). The contribution UHC makes towards reducing inequities and improving **population health** (which in turn advances a country's overall developmental) is well recognised. Good health allows children to learn and adults to earn, helps people escape from poverty, and provides the basis for long-term economic development (WHO, 2021). The progress towards UHC could be considered as a progressive achievement as the scope of services, the population covered and the proportion of costs covered increases over time (Boerma et al., 2014) (Fig. 6.1).

A strong PHC system is vital to the efficient functioning of the healthcare system as a whole and enables UHC to be achieved, by providing accessible services, particularly for vulnerable populations (Box 6.1) (Blanchet & Makinen, 2016; WHO, 2018). Focusing on preventive care to reduce the need for more costly treatments and preserve health, PHC is cost effective, reduces inequity and improves population health. It is a core, initial step on a country's path towards achieving UHC (WHO, 2018).

Comparison between primary care and primary healthcare

The term 'primary healthcare' (PHC) is commonly and erroneously interchanged with **primary care** even though their philosophies and practices are fundamentally different as they are quite distinct entities. Primary care describes a narrower concept of doctor-led services. It encompasses primary medical (family) practice (perhaps with nurse practitioners) that takes place in the community, but it is not PHC. Primary care is often a patient's first point of entry into the medical (hospital) system. Clinicians' main focus is on illness and cure,

> ### Box 6.1 Contribution of primary healthcare to health and healthcare systems
>
> Strong PHC is associated with
>
> - prevention of illness and death
> - more equitable distribution of health in the population, both within and between countries.
>
> PHC achieves this through
>
> - increasing access of vulnerable populations to healthcare
> - providing comparable or better quality of care than specialists for patients with various chronic diseases, and at lower cost
> - focusing on preventive care
> - avoiding unnecessary specialty care.
>
> (Source: Bourgeault et al., 2015)

timely diagnosis and treatment and, if necessary, referral for medical conditions. More often than not it involves a single service or intermittent management of a person's illness that is typically contained in a time-limited appointment (Muldoon et al., 2006). In contrast primary healthcare is a broader term which derives from core principles articulated by the World Health Organization (1978) and which describes an approach to health policy and service provision that includes a broad range of services (for example primary midwifery or maternity services) delivered to both individuals and populations. Primary care could be considered as one tool or instrument of PHC.

Primary healthcare and public health

PHC responds to individual health needs through the delivery of personalised quality healthcare services *and* population health needs by incorporating many elements of public health. Population-based and individual services are inherently complementary, the impact of each being augmented through integration and coordination with the other. PHC is a vehicle or means for many public health strategies to be realised as many public health programs are provided through the delivery of PHC services and teams (e.g. immunisation, screening programs). The various personal health and public health elements of PHC are defined below (WHO 2018).

A. Personal services
  a. *First contact services* defines primary care as the first point of contact for the large majority of disease prevention activities, as well as for acute and chronic health problems. The availability of quality primary care, particularly at the community level, leads to better outcomes over time (Forrest & Starfield, 1998). For primary care to be effective, a comprehensive array of services needs to be readily available. Arrangements which support access to other levels of care and services, through referral from primary care (gate-keeping), via free or minimal out-of-pocket-cost primary-care services improve continuity and ensure that specialised services are able to maximise their function in the health system, rather than being overused for needs that are better managed in primary care (Forrest & Starfield, 1998).
  b. *Comprehensiveness* refers to the scope, breadth, and depth of care, including the competence to address health issues throughout the life course. The more comprehensive the primary care service, the more likely needs can be met without requiring referral to a higher level of service or care, thus improving accessibility, timeliness and effectiveness of care. Selective PHC describes a different approach, where specific services or programs focusing only on treatment services or a specific program of care (often aimed at high-burden diseases) is generally considered a less effective model (WHO 2018) (see Box 6.1).
  c. *Continuity* of care results from the delivery of seamless care over time across different care encounters and transitions of care (Pereira Gray et al., 2016). Relational continuity (long-term relationship between practitioner(s) and individuals based on mutual trust), management continuity (evidence-based care pathways) and informational continuity (integrated information systems) are linked with improved outcomes (Gray et al., 2018).
  d. *Coordination* across the whole spectrum of health and social care services decreases risks at transition points (from home to clinic and from hospital to clinic) (WHO 2016).

  e. *Person-centredness* describes an approach which takes into account the whole person, in health and in sickness, physical, mental and social circumstances rather than focusing on a specific organ, stage of life or subpopulation.
B. Population-based services
  a. *Health protection* includes enforcement and control of activities for minimising exposure to health hazards in order to protect the population, by ensuring environmental, toxicological, road and food safety.
  b. *Health promotion* enables people to have more control over their own health, through better health literacy and improved ability to provide self-care and care for others.
  c. *Disease prevention* is delivered at both the individual and the population level and in many settings is linked to health promotion and healthcare delivery. Immunisation, screening programs or universal supplementation (e.g. folic acid and iodine) are examples of population-level disease prevention programs delivered at personal health level.
  d. *Surveillance and response* combine monitoring and prevention, using health information at the population and community level.
  e. *Emergency preparedness* Emergency preparedness aims to address unforeseen and catastrophic circumstances that create a surge of demand for health services and strain resources and infrastructure. A strong and well-trained PHC workforce is needed during emergencies to ensure that the health system is responsive and adaptable, and to help with planning, thus helping to avoid the rapid and uncontrolled depletion of health resources.

LEVELS OF HEALTHCARE SERVICES

To place PHC in the context of the wider health system, healthcare services can be loosely categorised as primary healthcare, secondary healthcare, tertiary healthcare and public healthcare. These services do not exist in isolation of each other but, instead, are ideally integrated, enabling seamless transitions between levels for individuals accessing care (MOH Nationwide Service Framework Library, n.d.; AIHW, 2016).

For primary healthcare to maximise its potential it needs to have a central place in the health system, and sufficient resources (such as access to sufficient referral and diagnostic services and workforce) to enable it to be a hub of care provision and coordination.

Systems which enable the transfer of healthcare information between providers to minimise duplication and support ready and timely access to care also need investment in order to maximise the benefits that PHC can offer.

Primary healthcare is a public health strategy and deals with the social determinants of health. It is sometimes described as 'first-level services', meaning it is usually the initial point of contact that people have with the healthcare system. It aims to be universally accessible to individuals and families in the community. Services are coordinated, accessible to all and accessed through a variety of providers (not all of whom are healthcare professionals) who possess the appropriate skills to meet the needs of individuals and the community they serve.

> . . . in the broadest sense, [PHC] may include a range of professionals: medical doctors, nursing, midwifery, allied services such as rehabilitation, physiotherapy and dietetics, and pharmacy, to list a few. It may also involve public health activities such as health promotion, disease monitoring and surveillance, community development, and services aimed at helping patients and communities to achieve various goals. These might be anything from navigating the complexities of the healthcare system and services through to enabling communities to improve their health (WHO, 2008;AIHW 2016). In this way, PHC may integrate aspects of both personal healthcare (seeing a doctor for a health problem) and public health (working with a population with a focus on alleviating conditions—for example, poor housing or inequalities—and reversing behaviours that undermine good health).

(Bourgeault et al., 2015)

Secondary healthcare is healthcare to which people do not have direct access and for which they must be referred from some other part of the health system, such as a primary healthcare practitioner or service. Secondary services are considered specialty services. They are generally provided via hospitals, and may include diagnostic, assessment and treatment services. Within both Australia and New Zealand, secondary healthcare services are also provided in the private sector, which operate outside of hospitals. These services are accessible via referrals from primary healthcare practitioners, such as general practitioners or midwives. Within a maternity context, secondary healthcare in New Zealand and Australia would include services such as obstetric, specialist radiology, physician, gestational diabetes care, anaesthetic, caesarean sections or operative births.

Tertiary healthcare encompasses highly specialised, complex and costly hospital-based inpatient treatment services such as neonatal intensive care. Tertiary healthcare providers are highly specialised and their equipment is usually expensive. Within a maternity context, tertiary healthcare would include services such as neonatal care for extremely premature babies, care for women with complex co-morbidities or fetal maternal medicine services.

Public healthcare encompasses strategies that societies put into place to collectively assure the conditions for people to be healthy are met. These services are generally delivered to populations rather than individuals, although specific public healthcare programs (such as vaccination) can be delivered to individuals by primary healthcare workers.

POSITIONING PRIMARY HEALTHCARE WITHIN THE HEALTHCARE SYSTEM

For much of the 20th century, there has been a disproportionate focus on hospitals, technology and subspecialists ('hospital-centrism') such that they have gained a pivotal role in most health systems. For example, in member countries for the Organisation for Economic Co-operation and Development (OECD), it was reported that the 35% growth in the number of doctors from 1990 to 2005 was driven by rising numbers of specialists (up by nearly 50%, compared with only a 20% increase in general practitioners) (WHO, 2008). This is due to the advancement of technologies and a hospital-centric curative medicine approach. This necessitates immensely costly investment in equipment and technologies which in turn leads to centralisation of services, reducing their accessibility. This disproportionate focus on specialist tertiary care provides poor value for money. Hospital centrism also carries a considerable cost in terms of unnecessary medicalisation and iatrogenesis, as well as reducing the amount of resources that can be invested in primary healthcare

Throughout the world, differences in health outcomes exist, between countries and between populations within the same country. These differences reflect health inequities which result in part from differences in health status or in the distribution of health resources between different population groups, arising from the social conditions in which people are born, grow, live, work and age. Health inequities are unfair and could be reduced by the right mix of government policies. UHC and a strong well-functioning primary healthcare system is a key strategy which, when fully implemented, can reduce these health inequities.

REFLECTIVE THINKING EXERCISE

Consider the ways that primary healthcare provided by midwives and public health policies intersect. For example, think about public health or preventive services that are offered at a population level which midwives might have a role in either directly providing or sharing information with women and their families/whanau about in order to inform healthy choices. Examples might include vaccination, dietary and nutritional education or providing prescriptions for supplementation such as folic acid or iodine.

Selective primary healthcare is a focus on specific services or programs providing treatment services or a specific program of care (often aimed at high-burden diseases).

Comprehensive primary healthcare is an approach that cares for the whole patient and all his or her needs, not just the medical and physical ones. Consider how these public health policies and programs impact on the work of midwives in their primary healthcare role. Could the delivery of public healthcare programs in primary healthcare settings be considered *selective* primary healthcare or *comprehensive* primary healthcare?

How do midwives incorporate public health approaches into their practice whilst maintaining a partnership approach which recognises the individual needs of each woman for whom they are providing care?

REFLECTIVE THINKING EXERCISE

Consider the various elements of personal services and population health. How are midwives or midwifery practice reflected within these elements or how do these elements impact on midwives' practice? List some examples.

In summary, the primary healthcare (social) model of health:

- addresses the broader determinants of health—health is determined by a broad range of social, environmental and economic factors rather than just biomedical risk factors (see also Ch. 9)

- recognises that differences in health status and health outcomes are linked to social factors—including gender, culture, race and ethnicity, socioeconomic status, working conditions, unemployment, housing, location and physical environment—and actively works to address these

- involves intersectoral collaboration—social and environmental determinants of health cannot be addressed by the healthcare sector alone and require close, coordinated collaboration between different public-sector departments and organisations, for example those responsible for employment, housing, education, social welfare, environment and transport as well as the private sector (manufacturers of products or service providers)

- acts to reduce social inequities—equity is a key principle for healthcare service delivery; the social model of health acts to reduce inequities that are related to factors such as gender, culture, race, socioeconomic status, location and physical environment

- empowers individuals and communities—all members of society have the right to participate in decision making about their health and to have equitable access to the skills and resources they need to change factors that influence their health

- acts to enable equitable access to healthcare—healthcare services should be affordable and available according to people's needs; health information should be available to all in accessible and appropriate formats.

Primary healthcare in Australia

For the past 40 years (following the Declaration of Alma Ata), health policy in Australia has been increasingly influenced by the rise and global dominance of a neoliberal economic discourse and its subsequent shaping of public policy choices. Neoliberal economic theory is based on the premise that free markets and minimal government intervention at any level would provide the best outcomes (Baum et al., 2016). This has led in general to health being treated as a commodity rather than a collective good or human right (Baum et al., 2016). Neoliberal policies have shaped Australia's health, education and social security sectors by promoting a market economy that has driven government spending cuts and the privatisation of many public services. According to Baum et al. (2016), with reference to the current state of PHC in Australia:

> Selective PHC, with its 'vertical' emphasis on treating or preventing certain high-burden diseases rather than a 'horizontal' effort to build public health systems, became more entrenched with health reform initiatives of the 1990s and 2000s that were consistent with the core elements of neo-liberalism: cost-containment and efficiency, result-based financing, user fees, managed competition amongst service providers, increased contracting out to private providers, and an emphasis on individual responsibility for maintaining good health.
>
> (Baum et al., 2016, p. 44)

In Australia the provision of primary healthcare services is based on a complex arrangement of Federal and State funding. The Federal government funds private fee-for-service medical and midwifery practice (the Endorsed Midwife) through Medicare; whereas other primary healthcare services are funded by the states. (Further information on health system funding is found in Ch. 2.)

In Aboriginal communities the National Aboriginal Community Controlled Health Organisation (NACCHO) sector (that provides PHC to approximately one-half of all Aboriginal people) was founded on voluntary activism by Aboriginal communities as an expression of self-determination (NACCHO, 2009/10). This represented the truest manifestation of primary healthcare in Australia; however, the government reforms to this model, shaped on the whole by neoliberal policies, fail to recognise adequately either the status of its First Peoples or the impacts of dispossession and colonisation (Dwyer, 2016).

Australia's rural–urban divide

Although one-third of Australia's population lives outside its major cities they are faced with significant health disadvantages as a result of the stark differences between Australia's health system performance in rural and major urban centres (Australian Institute of Health and Welfare (AIHW), 2020). Mortality and illness levels increase with distance from major cities. Moreover, these communities are disadvantaged by reduced access to PHC providers and health services (in part a function of health and medical workforce shortages), leading in turn to lower utilisation rates than in urban areas and consequently poorer health status for rural residents. Access to health practitioners and dentists decreases with remoteness. People living in remote areas have higher rates of hospitalisation and lower pharmacy prescription rates, and are less likely to access disability support services than those living within major cities (AIHW, 2020). In many cases, the inability to access health services when required results in health needs not being adequately met (AIHW, 2020).

In maternity care the market economy has driven decisions to centralise maternity services resulting in the closure of many community-based services. Removing maternity services from rural areas results in a loss of opportunity for PHC to be offered in its full capacity as community care offered close to women's homes and encompassing strategies to enhance and improve health across the spectrum (for an in-depth discussion of primary maternity units see Ch. 2).

Australia is considered to have a high-quality healthcare system and is considered as one of the 'safest countries in which to give birth or to be born' (Australian Government Department of Health (DOH), 2011, p. 3). Regardless of this fact, many women who reside in rural and remote areas, and Aboriginal and Torres Strait Islander women, are not receiving adequate care. Between 1995 and 2005 over 50% (130) of small rural maternity units closed in Australia leaving women without the barest availability of primary level maternity care (Kildea et al., 2015; Longman et al., 2017).

Not only do the closures deprive rural women of primary level maternity care, they are also associated with an increasing and alarming rate of unplanned births of babies being born before arrival at the closest secondary and tertiary level hospitals (Kildea et al., 2015; Longman et al., 2017).

Primary healthcare in New Zealand

Although New Zealand's healthcare system has also been influenced by neoliberal reforms in the 1980s, their impact on PHC has been softened as successive New Zealand governments have recognised the preventive value of primary healthcare as means to contain rising healthcare demands and costs.

New Zealand health system settings have attempted to re-orientate investment towards primary healthcare as a cost-effective strategy which has the potential to reduce the need for and utilisation of more-expensive secondary and tertiary healthcare services, and provide for better health outcomes (Ministry of Health (MOH), 2001, 2011). This has included movement of care and services from secondary or hospital environments into the community or primary healthcare setting and progressively increasing subsidies for general practice care, as a means to improve

accessibility and timeliness of care, and to avoid costly hospitalisation and overtreatment.

Various policy statements have been developed to facilitate this transition, commencing with the Primary Health Care Strategy, which was released in 2001 (MOH, 2001). This strategy set out a vision for the future direction of PHC services, moving from an individual health to a population health focus, from a provider focus to a community and people focus, and from treating ill health to promoting good health and preventing illness. It also recognised the need for services to work more closely together to meet health needs as in many cases no single professional group or single service can meet the needs of every individual, so integration and coordination between service providers is required, both vertical (primary to secondary) and horizontal (primary to primary) (MOH, 2001, 2011a).

In spite of this policy vision, which also included a focus on reducing inequitable health outcomes, particular population groups, including Māori and Pasifika, continue to experience inequities.

Inequity has been defined as '. . . differences in health that are not only avoidable but unfair and unjust. Equity recognises different people with different levels of advantage require different approaches and resources to get equitable health outcomes' (MOH, 2019).

The degree of change and service integration needed to deliver the desired outcomes has not been fully realised. Funding for primary medical care remains a mixture of government subsidy and out-of-pocket payments, resulting in cost being a barrier to access for a significant portion of the population, inequitable access to care and inequitable health outcomes (Jatrana & Crampton, 2009).

In 2020 a government-commissioned review of New Zealand's health and disability system recommended that structural and system culture changes are required to achieve equitable outcomes and a more cohesive system, which incorporates a greater focus on population health outcomes across the entire system. The Review Report has signalled that reorganisation of primary healthcare is needed to realise these aims, including better coordination and integration, more local planning and greater investment (including targeted expansion in public funding of particular services) (HDSR, 2020).

Regardless, maternity care in New Zealand is freely accessible for eligible women, with no co-payments required for women to access midwifery care (MOH, 2011b). This has resulted in almost UHC for primary maternity care in New Zealand, with 92.9% of all women registering with a lead maternity carer (LMC) in 2018 (MOH, 2021). However, like other healthcare services, ethnic, age and geographic inequities exist in maternity care outcomes (MOH, 2021). In 2021, the Section 88 Primary Maternity Services Notice (which funds primary midwifery services) was revised. Changes made enabled the incorporation of targeted funding components which recognise additional care for women with greater medical or social needs to better support more equitable maternity outcomes.

MIDWIFERY AND PRIMARY HEALTHCARE

Countries which have midwives practising in a PHC capacity, across their full scope, working within communities, providing services that are freely available to women, are achieving UHC, at least in relation to maternity services (Nove et al., 2020; SoWMY, 2021; United Nations Population Fund (UNFPA), 2014). Investing in midwifery as a key workforce who are educated and regulated to provide comprehensive primary maternity care has been recognised as a transformative intervention which has the potential to avert maternal and neonatal deaths and stillbirths (Nove et al. 2020; SoWMY, 2021).

For midwives to provide a comprehensive primary maternity care, a supportive and integrated healthcare system is needed to maximise the impact midwifery can make through PHC.

Maternity services hold a unique position in influencing current and future maternal and infant health, and midwives play a pivotal role. Midwives provide care at the most critical times during the childbearing cycle. In New Zealand, midwives are the predominant community-based workforce involved in all aspects of maternity care provision, and their role can make an important contribution to securing the overall health of mothers and babies.

Antenatal care is a key public health strategy both within New Zealand and Australia and globally, and is predominantly provided by midwives. During this time midwives impart a large volume of public health information about food safety, vaccinations during pregnancy and for babies, screening options, healthy weight gain during pregnancy, safe sleeping, promotion and support of breastfeeding, smoking cessation information and referral, drug and alcohol usage and folic acid and iodine prescriptions. Midwifery interventions are effective at supporting women to achieve healthy pregnancies for a range of healthcare issues (East et al., 2021; Haby et al., 2018; Wilcox et al., 2021; Wong Soon et al., 2021; Zinsser et al., 2020).

As PHC practitioners, midwives provide community-based care for individual women in their homes or community clinics with a focus on enhancing and supporting the normal life process of pregnancy and childbirth. PHC interventions that midwives undertake—as well as the better birth outcomes for women having midwifery care (less pre-term birth, etc.)—have a positive flow-on effect for children.

When enabled to work within their full scope of practice, with a direct means to access referral services (e.g. obstetricians, mental health, social services, smoking cessations, housing or other agencies), diagnostic services (such as laboratory, ultrasound) and treatments (prescription rights), midwives are able to provide initial responses to problems or needs and can intervene and treat conditions (Fig. 6.2).

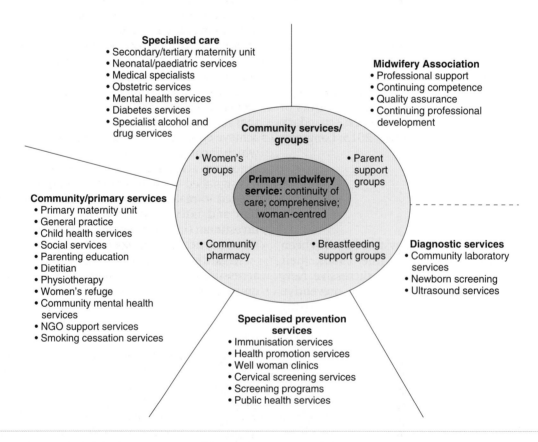

FIGURE 6.2 Primary care as a hub of coordination: networking within the community served and with outside partners
(Adapted from The World Health Report 2008—Primary Health Care (Now More Than Ever). Primary care as a hub of coordination: networking within the community served and with outside partners http://www.int.who.int/whr/2008/en/)

Midwives understand that resolution of health problems should take into account the sociocultural context of the women, their families and communities. In partnership with women and each other, midwives work to empower women and their families towards self-health and self-determination so they can make the best decisions for themselves and also for their families and the wider community. In so doing they utilise public health methodologies.

New Zealand's partnership model of midwifery care is based on the premise that primary healthcare is the cornerstone of maternity services. Combined with the government's overall focus on primary and public health strategies, the model of maternity care has been accepted as the central strategy for improving the health and wellbeing of mothers and babies.

Midwifery, then, is of fundamental importance to the enhancement and maintenance of health. Its ideological framework and holistic agenda provide a platform for community empowerment, potentially ranging along a continuum from individual development through to the collective ability to influence external policy development, legislation and an equitable distribution of resources. Midwives understand that PHC is not merely about moving resources out of the hospitals and into the community; it is also concerned with equity, access, power and politics as well as political activism to ensure that all women have the opportunity to engage in women-centred, holistic services which incorporate body, mind, spirit, land, environment, culture, custom and the social determinants of health, as well as provide accessible, essential, integrated, quality care based upon practical, scientifically sound and socially acceptable methods and technology for all. Best practice maternal health and, of course, midwifery is not just about providing more obstetric services in hospitals; it is more likely achieved through community-based care directly accessed by women and appropriate to their specific needs.

For the vast majority of the world's women, childbearing is a normal, physiological process influenced by culture, family traditions, religion, economics and psychosocial factors. It is a family event that requires a health-oriented approach, even in the presence of co-morbidities. In New Zealand, as in many other countries, midwifery is the PHC workforce whose specific role is to facilitate the transition to parenthood for women and their families regardless of their choice of service provider or place of birth. Australian midwifery is also working to achieve this model of care through the introduction of the endorsed midwife program (Australian College of Midwives (ACM), 2017; Australian Health Practitioner Regulation Agency (AHPRA), 2017; Department of Health (DOH) of Australia, 2017; Nursing and Midwifery Board of Australia (NMBA), 2017). (For further information on the endorsed midwife see Ch. 14.)

The underlying principles of primary healthcare provision apply to maternity services. That is, services should be provided equitably and at the most accessible level of the healthcare system capable of performing them adequately. It is considered internationally that the person best equipped to provide community-based, appropriate technology, and safe and cost-effective care to women during their reproductive lives is the person with midwifery skills who lives in the community alongside the women she attends (WHO, 2004).

Maternal health is not simply a question of providing access to technologically oriented biomedical services. It is a public health issue, for which community interventions that are cost effective, woman focused, appropriate, affordable and sustainable must be implemented. In keeping with primary healthcare's philosophy of self-determination, community-controlled primary healthcare services are initiated, planned and managed by local communities. They aim to deliver high-quality, holistic and culturally appropriate healthcare and have the potential to improve health and wellbeing and reduce delays in seeking and obtaining secondary and tertiary medical services.

Interface between primary and secondary maternity care

A unique aspect of New Zealand's primary healthcare model of maternity care is that primary services are seamlessly integrated with secondary and tertiary services. Secondary maternity care encompasses the provision of comprehensive specialist services, which require referral from PHC, but may or may not require hospitalisation; tertiary maternity care encompasses multidisciplinary care for women and babies with complex needs such as co-morbidities. Women who experience complications during the antenatal, labour, birth and postnatal periods are referred to secondary or tertiary specialist services for either consultation or transfer on a planned or emergency basis. In many cases LMC midwives continue to provide individualised one-to-one midwifery service to women across the various interfaces, collaboratively alongside hospital-based colleagues, including core midwives, ensuring a seamless experience for the woman and her family.

Both New Zealand and Australia have developed mechanisms for linkages between primary, secondary and tertiary maternity services, and these services and referral guidelines are described in the relevant service specifications issued by the Ministry of Health in New Zealand or by Australian State and Federal departments of health (see Ch. 2).

In New Zealand, as in Australia, referral to secondary and tertiary services are guided by the referral guidelines (see Ch. 2). At times, roles and responsibilities can become blurred during the process of referral and consultation, particularly in relation to intrapartum care. In New Zealand LMC midwives follow the woman's journey through the maternity services and provide care in many settings (including within secondary and tertiary hospitals). They may continue to provide care in situations where the woman has secondary care needs in order to provide continuity for the woman. Although midwives are educated to be PHC practitioners, many midwives working as LMCs are also skilled in aspects of secondary care tasks. The provision of care in these circumstances has resourcing implications for both the LMC and hospital services, and can be subject to task shifting from secondary care to primary care services without additional resourcing for LMCs. In Australia a similar situation exists when women negotiate care with an endorsed midwife or other privately practising midwife. Practice is guided by Consultation and Referral guidelines (ACM, 2015) and individual state and hospital policies.

The majority of women give birth within secondary or tertiary hospitals in New Zealand, usually attended by their LMC midwife. This is because the availability of primary maternity (midwife-led) units is limited in many areas, and the disproportionate focus on hospitals and technology which has led to birth being subsumed within hospital care, and a shift away from birth in primary settings (such as home or midwife-led units) to secondary or tertiary hospitals, in spite of a significant body of evidence that well women with uncomplicated pregnancies will have fewer unnecessary interventions if they give birth in primary settings (see Ch. 7).

Due to the closure of so many small primary-level maternity services, Australian maternity services are based largely in secondary and tertiary care hospital facilities or in the primary medical care arena with general practitioners. In 2011 the Commonwealth health ministers recognised that there needed to be a more concerted move towards community and primary healthcare models of maternity care including primary midwifery healthcare (Australian Government DOH, 2011).

Australia legislated changes to the practice of midwives in 2009 with the Health Practitioner Regulation National Law Act (2009), which was designed to promote the provision of community-based primary care through the Eligible Midwife program (now referred to as the Endorsed Midwife program) (ACM, 2017; AHPRA, 2017; NMBA, 2017). Some programs are based on the philosophy and ethos of PHC, but not all.

AUSTRALIA'S NATIONAL PRIMARY HEALTH CARE STRATEGIC FRAMEWORK (2013)

In 2013 Australia introduced the National Primary Health Care Strategic Framework. This was the first national statement, endorsed by the Standing Council on Health, which presented an agreed approach for creating a stronger, more robust PHC system in Australia.

It was developed by the Commonwealth, State and Territory health departments and approved by health ministers, through the Standing Council on Health, in April 2013 under the leadership of the then Federal Labor Minister for Health and Ageing, the Hon. Tania Plibersek. For the first time, it provided a mechanism for coordinated action at the Commonwealth, State and local levels to enable a more harmonised approach in PHC planning and service delivery (Australian Government DOH, 2013).

Inevitably following the change from a Federal Labor government to a Liberal Coalition the following year, many elements of the Framework changed owing to the stronger focus on economic efficiency. Currently Australia places a heavy emphasis on a corporate culture in the healthcare market governed by a logic of cost rather than care and compassion. (For example, the *Medicare local primary healthcare organisations* that had been established in many rural and remote communities and incorporated multidisciplinary practitioners based in local communities were replaced by centralised primary health networks which mainly provide governance for general practitioner services in local health districts.)

The National Primary Healthcare Framework of Australia (2013) outlined a clear vision to achieve a safe, equitable, effective and sustainable health system.

The Framework aims to:
- improve healthcare for all Australians, particularly those who currently experience inequitable health outcomes
- keep people healthy
- prevent illness
- reduce the need for unnecessary hospital presentations
- improve the management of complex and chronic conditions.

The Framework focuses on four strategic outcomes (Australian Government DOH, 2013):
- building a consumer-focused and integrated PHC system
- improving access and reducing inequity
- increasing the focus on health promotion and prevention, screening and early intervention
- improving quality, safety, performance and accountability.

Further work by Javanparast et al. (2022) in evaluating comprehensive primary healthcare (CPHC) in improving population health and health equity in Australia found that regional primary healthcare organisations (RPHCOs) are far from comprehensive and have become more selective over time. The authors include as key criteria for comprehensiveness (1) focus on population health; (2) focus on equity of access and outcomes; (3) community participation and control; (4) integration within the broader health system; (5) intersectoral collaboration; and (6) local responsiveness (Javanparast et al., 2022).

CRITICAL THINKING EXERCISE

Midwifery may view uncomplicated labour and birth a 'primary healthcare' event, whereas the medicalised approach to labour and birth may view it as a 'secondary healthcare' event. How do you define the difference?

Where is the line between primary and secondary care for maternity? Do you think that this line is an arbitrary one or a clear one? What are the advantages of devolving aspects of 'secondary' maternity care to a PHC setting? For women? For midwives? For maternity services?

Where is midwifery most effectively positioned within healthcare systems?

REFLECTIVE CASE STUDY

Midwifery as a primary healthcare service in the context of the COVID-19 pandemic

The New Zealand and Australian governments' response to the COVID-19 pandemic of 'going hard and going early' (swift and decisive stringent lockdowns) meant that very low rates of infection occurred, enabling New Zealand and Australia to subsequently pursue elimination / suppression strategies. These approaches have been lauded internationally as has each government's coordinated national response across a range of health and social services. However, the speed and scope of the lockdown had significant implications for pregnant and birthing women, maternity services and midwives. During the lockdown, for the vast majority of healthcare services, non-acute or routine care could be withdrawn, postponed or provided virtually or by telephone. However, the nature of maternity care required ongoing service delivery throughout the pandemic response. Midwives and maternity services were simply required to continue to provide care in all settings (Bradfield et al., 2021; Crowther, 2021).

In New Zealand a large portion of maternity care is provided in the community by midwives working in a continuity-of-care model. Embedded within primary health are principles enabling rapid adaptation to support the pandemic response. A re-organisation of essential services (including maternity) to minimise all but absolutely necessary in-person contact was required. When contact did occur, social distancing and strict public health measures (such as COVID-19 symptom or risk screening, hand washing, hygiene protocols and use of personal protective equipment (PPE)) were mandatory. The New Zealand College of Midwives developed specific advice for midwives working in the community to guide the frequency and nature of ante- and postnatal contacts using a mixture of telephone and virtual contacts, complemented with minimised in-person contacts for necessary physical assessments. In-person physical assessments were advised to be no longer than 15 minutes in duration with strict social distancing (2 metres apart) to be observed, other than when hands-on physical assessment or care was required (NZCOM, n.d.).

The strong integration between community and hospital maternity services enabled task reallocation in order to meet the public health guidelines. Hospital-based midwives took a greater role in managing in-hospital acute assessments, to avoid community-based midwives having unnecessary contact with hospital. Well-developed professional relationships, strong collegiality and the shared aim of achieving minimal disruption to women's care saw seamless care provision across community and hospital settings, without compromising outcomes for women and their newborns.

In both Australia and New Zealand during the lockdown, women's access to support was strictly limited across the continuum of the childbearing journey, at various key touch points, such as a partner accompanying a woman during a pregnancy ultrasound, to support during labour and birth or assistance and social support postnatally. Midwifery's overarching philosophy of woman-centred partnership care saw a focus on women's choice, safety and social connectivity as paramount throughout this period. For many women and families, midwives were the only healthcare provider whom they had contact with over this period. This comprehensive and holistic way in which midwives practise resulted in them often being a vital source of information and support at a stressful and challenging time for families. This additional burden of care came at a cost to midwives with many reporting increased time required to reassure women, discuss or negotiate changes in care plans and place of birth (NZCOM, n.d.).

In Australia, COVID-19 wreaked havoc with maternity service provision. The ICM, in their survey of professional associations in midwifery throughout the world, found similar themes in all countries (ICM, 2022 in press).

Midwives and maternity services rapidly re-oriented and reorganised care to meet not only the required public health measures to minimise COVID-19 transmission, but also women's changing needs and priorities. The governments' clear messaging, that all unnecessary physical or in-person contact should be avoided, resonated strongly with the public. Many pregnant and birthing women were highly motivated to avoid contact with hospitals unless absolutely required. This meant that more care was provided in community settings, with many women changing birth plans from hospital settings to home or primary maternity units. Many women also chose early discharge from hospital, resulting in more community-based postnatal care by midwives in the early days following birth (ICM, 2022 in press; NZCOM, 2020).

Although midwives responded to changing needs, there were a number of challenges throughout this period. Midwives initially experienced considerable difficulties in accessing sufficient PPE, which created a degree of anxiety and uncertainty as they sought to keep the women in their care, themselves and their families safe. Additional equipment, greater travel requirements and increased access to digital technologies were all costs that midwives were required to meet. Changing care required access to guidance, evidence and information. Many online midwife forums also organically and formally evolved during this period, to provide advice and collegial support to enable the challenges associated with rapid changes in care delivery to be safely met (NZCOM, 2020).

The governments' focus was drawn to the public health response and although the maternity service continued to function well, prioritising and adapting to women's needs, largely due to the adaptable and resilient nature of the midwifery profession, the additional workload and emotional burden on midwives went largely unnoticed, at least initially.

In many countries, maternal and newborn outcomes were compromised during the pandemic as resources were directed to other services and maternity care experienced disruption, resulting in reduced access for women (Chmielewska, 2021). The nature of New Zealand's maternity service, with midwives working within a primary healthcare community-based model, autonomously to their full scope of practice, meant changing needs could be accommodated, thus enabling seamless ongoing access to care for women within a rapid transition and re-orientation of services towards community settings. Midwives literally 'plugged the gaps' for women and their families, where other services withdrew or provided entirely virtual services. Midwives demonstrated a resilient primary healthcare service, which continued to place women's needs in a partnership-oriented model at the centre both in community and hospital settings, in the face of a significant pandemic response (Crowther 2021).

The COVID-19 pandemic has shone a light on the importance of investing in primary healthcare for meeting population health needs. Midwives are essential providers of primary healthcare and can play a major role in this area as well as other levels of the health system: in addition to maternity care, they provide a wide range of clinical interventions and contribute to broader health goals, such as addressing sexual and reproductive rights, promoting self-care interventions empowering women and adolescent girls, and facilitating access to other necessary social and healthcare services.

Conclusion

Primary healthcare is a cornerstone of the health system. It is the hub through which individuals are guided through the system, facilitated by ongoing relationships between clinicians and 'patients' or service users. It offers people the opportunity to participate in decision making about their health and healthcare, and it bridges relationships between personal healthcare and wider population health strategies. It opens opportunities for disease prevention and health promotion, as well as the early detection of disease.

Midwives are PHC practitioners, by the nature of their scope of practice, and because positive outcomes from pregnancy, birth and the postnatal period which are influenced by the interventions that midwives undertake can have a lasting impact and health benefit on maternal and child wellbeing and health. Health systems which enable midwives to practise across their full scope, and work in a PHC capacity in the community providing antenatal, labour and birth and postnatal care, maximise the health gains that can be realised during the childbearing time. Systems which enable continuity of midwifery care will achieve even greater benefits, as the relationship that midwives and women develop through the course of care becomes a platform for effective engagement, empowering women to take ownership over their health and wellbeing.

Review questions

1. What is the difference between public, primary, secondary and tertiary healthcare?
2. List six reasons why midwifery is defined as primary healthcare.
3. Identify four principles of primary healthcare.
4. Describe how midwives can work in partnership with women and their families to improve health literacy of individuals, communities and organisations.

Online resources

Australian College of Midwives: https://www.midwives.org.au.

Australian Government Department of Human Services: https://www.humanservice.gov.au.

Australian Primary Health Care Institute: http://rsph.anu.edu.au/research/centres-departments/australian-primary-health-care-research-institute.

Australian Rural Birthing Index Toolkit: http://ucrh.edu.au/wp-content/uploads/2015/07/ARBI_FINAL_PRINT.pdf.

Midwifery Council of New Zealand: http://www.midwiferycouncil.health.nz.

Ministry of Health (NZ) maternity services: http://www.health.govt.nz/our-work/life-stages/maternity-services.

National Health and Hospital Reform Commission Discussion papers 2009: https://www.google.com.au/?gfe_rd=ctrl&ei=TzcYU63WDMqnN8QeI64GQCg&gws_rd=cr#q=National+Health+and+Hospital+Reform+Commission+Discussion+papers+.

New Zealand College of Midwives: http://www.midwife.org.nz.

New Zealand Health Statistics (formerly NZHIS): http://www.health.govt.nz/nz-health-statistics.

NICE guidelines: https://www.nice.org.uk/guidance/index.jsp?action=byType&type=2&status=3.

References

Australian College of Midwives (ACM). *Endorsed midwives*. 2017. Online: https://www.midwives.org.au/endorsed-midwives.

Australian Government Department of Health (DOH). *National Maternity Services Plan*. 2011. Online: http://www.health.gov.au/internet/main/publishing.nsf/Content/maternityservicesplan.

Australian Government Department of Health (DOH). *National Primary Health Care Strategic Framework*. 2013. Online: http://www.health.gov.au/internet/main/publishing.nsf/Content/6084A04118674329CA257BF0001A349E/$File/NPHCframe.pdf.

Australian Health Practitioner Regulation Agency (AHPRA). *Registration*. 2017. Online: http://www.ahpra.gov.au/Registration.

Australian Institute of Health and Welfare (AIHW). *Primary Health Care in Australia*. Canberra: AIHW. 2016 (Updated 2021). Cat. no. WEB 132. Online: https://www.aihw.gov.au/reports/primary-health-care/primary-health-care-in-australia.

Australian Institute of Health and Welfare (AIHW). *Rural and Remote Health*. Canberra: AIHW. 2020. Online: https://www.aihw.gov.au/reports/australias-health/rural-and-remote-health.

Baum F, Legge DG, Freeman T, et al. The potential for multi-disciplinary primary health care services to take action on the social determinants of health: actions and constraints. *BMC Public Health*. 2013;13:460. Online: http://www.biomedcentral.com/1471-2458/13/460.

Baum F, Freeman T, Sanders D, et al. Comprehensive primary health care under neo-liberalism in Australia. *Soc Sci Med*. 2016;168:43–52.

Blanchet N, Makinen M. *UHC Primary Health Care Self-assessment Tool: Summary Report From Four Country Pilots*. 2016. Online: http://www.jointlearningnetwork.org/resources/uhc-phc-self-assessment-summary-report-from-five-country-pilots.

Boerma T, Eozenou P, Evans D, et al. Monitoring progress towards universal health coverage at country and global levels. *PLoS Med*. 2014;11(9):e1001731.

Bourgeault I, Kuhlman E, Blank RH, et al., eds. *The Palgrave International Handbook of Healthcare Policy and Governance*. Basingstoke, Hants: Palgrave Macmillan; 2015.

Bradfield Z, Wynter K, Hauck Y, et al. Experiences of receiving and providing maternity care during the COVID-19 pandemic in Australia: A five-cohort cross-sectional comparison. *PLoS ONE*. 2021;16(3):e0248488. doi:10.1371/journal.pone.0248488.

Chmielewska B, Barratt I, Townsend R, et al. Effects of the COVID-19 pandemic on maternal and perinatal outcomes: a systematic review and meta-analysis. *Lancet Glob Health*. 2021;9(6):e759-e772. doi:10.1016/ S2214-109X(21)00079-6.

Coreil J, Mull D, eds. *Anthropology and Primary Health Care*. Boulder, CO: Westview Press; 1990:328.

Crowther S, Maude M, Bradford B, et al. When maintaining relationships and social connectivity matter: The case of New Zealand midwives and COVID-19. *Front. Sociol*. 2021; 6:614017. doi:10.3389/fsoc.2021.614017.

Department of Health (DOH) of Australia. *Midwives and Nurse Practitioners*. 2017. Online: http://www.health.gov.au/internet/main/publishing.nsf/Content/midwives-nurse-practitioners.

Dwyer J. *Aboriginal health care and public administration: could a framework of reciprocal accountability reset the relationship?* (PhD thesis). 2016. Online: https://flex.flinders.edu.au/file/aa6f9952-9d1a-470b-9e24-f8368eb87f49/1/Thesis%20Dwyer%202016.pdf.

East CE, Biro MA, Fredericks S, et al. Support during pregnancy for women at increased risk of low birthweight babies. *Cochrane Database Syst Rev*. 2021;4(4):CD000198. doi:10.1002/14651858.CD000198.pub3.

Forrest CB, Starfield B. Entry into primary care and continuity: the effect of access. *Am J Public Health*. 1998;88(9):1330-6.

Gray DJ, Sidaway-Lee K, White E, Thorne A, Evans PH. Continuity of care with doctors—a matter of life and death? A systematic review of continuity of care and mortality. *BMJ Open*. 2018;8(6): e021161.

Haby K, Berg M, Gyllensten H, et al. Mighty Mums—a lifestyle intervention at primary care level reduces gestational weight gain in women with obesity. *BMC Obes*. 2018;5:16.

Health and Disability System Review. *Health and Disability System Review – Final Report – Pūrongo Whakamutunga*. Wellington: HDSR; 2020.

International Confederation of Midwives (ICM). Midwives Speaking Out on COVID-19: The International Confederation of Midwives (ICM) Global Survey. 2022 (in press).

Jatrana S, Crampton P. Primary health care in New Zealand: who has access? *Health Policy (New York)*. 2009;93(1):1–10.

Javanparast S, Baum F, et al. A framework to determine the extent to which regional primary healthcare organisations are comprehensive or selective in their approach. *Int J Health Policy Manag*. 2022;11(4):479–488.

Kildea S, McGhie A, Yu G, et al. Babies born before arrival to hospital and maternity unit closures in Queensland and Australia. *Women Birth*. 2015;28:236–245.

Longman J, Kornelson J, Pilcher J et al. Maternity services for rural and remote Australia: barriers to operationalising national policy. *Health Policy*. 2017;121(11):1161–1168.

Ministry of Health (MOH). *Primary Health Care Strategy*. Wellington: Ministry of Health; 2001. Online: https://www.health.govt.nz/system/files/documents/publications/phcstrat.pdf.

Ministry of Health (MOH). *Better Sooner More Convenient Health Care in the Community*. Wellington: Ministry of Health; 2011a. *Online*. https://www.health.govt.nz/publication/better-sooner-more-convenient-health-care-community.

Ministry of Health (MOH). *Eligibility for Publicly Funded Health Services*. 2011b. Online: https://www.health.govt.nz/new-zealand-health-system/eligibility-publicly-funded-health-services.

Ministry of Health (MOH). *Report on Maternity 2019.* 2021. Online: https://minhealthnz.shinyapps.io/report-on-maternity-web-tool/.

Ministry of Health (MOH). *Achieving Equity.* 2019. Online: https://www.health.govt.nz/about-ministry/what-we-do/work-programme-2019-20/achieving-equity.

Ministry of Health (MOH). *MOH Nationwide Service Framework.* n.d. Online: https://nsfl.health.govt.nz/.

Muldoon L, Hogg W, Levitt M. Primary care (PC) and primary health care (PHC). What is the difference? *Can J Public Health.* 2006;97(5):409–411.

National Aboriginal Community Controlled Health Organisation (NACCHO). *Annual report.* 2009/10. Online: http://www.naccho.org.au/wp-content/uploads/NACCHO-2009-2010-Annual-Report.pdf.

New Zealand College of Midwives (NZCOM). *COVID-19.* n.d. Online: https://www.midwife.org.nz/midwives/covid-19/.

New Zealand College of Midwives (NZCOM) *Midwife Aotearoa New Zealand.* Issue 97, June 2020.

Nove A, Friberg I, de Bernis L, et al. Potential impact of midwives in preventing and reducing maternal and neonatal mortality and stillbirths: a Lives Saved Tool modelling study. *Lancet Global Health.* 2021;9(1): e24-e32.

Nursing and Midwifery Board of Australia (NMBA). *Endorsements.* 2017. Online: http://www.nursingmidwiferyboard.gov.au/Registration-and-Endorsement/Endorsements-Notations.aspx.

Pereira Gray D, Sidaway-Lee K, White E, et al. Improving continuity: the clinical challenge. *InnovAiT.* 2016;9(10):635–45.

SoWMY. *State of the World's Midwifery 2021.* 2021. Online: https://www.unfpa.org/publications/sowmy-2021.

United Nations Population Fund (UNFPA). *The State of the World's Midwifery 2014.* 2014. Online: http://www.unfpa.org/sowmy.

Wilcox CR, Woodward C, Rowe R, et al. Embedding the delivery of antenatal vaccination within routine antenatal care: a key opportunity to improve uptake. *Hum Vaccin Immunother.* 2021;16(5):1221–1224.

Wong Soon HN., Crezee I, Rush E. The role of New Zealand midwives as positive influencers on food literacy with Samoan families: Report on a small Auckland-based study. *J N Z Coll Midwives.* 2021;57:5–11. doi:10.12784/nzcomjnl57.2021.1.5-11.

World Health Organization (WHO). *Universal Health Coverage.* n.d. Online: https://www.who.int/health-topics/universal-health-coverage#tab=tab_1.

World Health Organization (WHO). *Declaration of Alma-Ata, 1978. International Conference on Primary Health Care, USSR, 6–12 September, Alma Ata.* Geneva, Switzerland: WHO European Office; 1978. Online: http://www.euro.who.int/en/publications/policy-documents/declaration-of-alma-ata-1978.

World Health Organization (WHO). *Ottawa Charter for Health Promotion.* Geneva, Switzerland: WHO European Office; 1986.

World Health Organization (WHO). *Pregnancy Safer: The Critical Role of the Skilled Attendant.* Geneva: WHO / ICM / FIGO; 2004. http://www.who.int/maternal_child_adolescent/documents/9241591692/en/. Online.

World Health Organization (WHO). *The World Health Report 2008—Primary Health Care (Now More Than Ever).* 2008. Online: http://www.who.int/whr/2008/en/.

World Health Organization (WHO). Transitions of care. *Technical Series on Safer Primary Care.* Geneva: World Health Organization; 2016.

World Health Organization (WHO). *A Vision for Primary Health Care in the 21st Century. Towards Universal Health Coverage and the Sustainable Development Goals.* Geneva: World Health Organization and the United Nations Children's Fund (UNICEF); 2018 (WHO/HIS/SDS/2018.15). Licence: CC BY-NC-SA 3.0 IGO. Online: https://apps.who.int/iris/bitstream/handle/10665/328065/WHO-HIS-SDS-2018.15-eng.pdf?sequence=1&isAllowed=y.

World Health Organization (WHO). *Universal Health Coverage.* 2021. Online: https://www.who.int/news-room/fact-sheets/detail/universal-health-coverage-(uhc)

World Health Organization (WHO). *Primary Health Care on the Road to Universal Health Coverage: 2019 monitoring report.* 2019. Online: https://www.who.int/publications/i/item/primary-health-care-on-the-road-to-universal-health-coverage-2019-monitoring-report.

Zinsser LA, Stoll K, Wieber F, et al. Changing behaviour in pregnant women: A scoping review. *Midwifery.* 2020;85:102680.

Further reading

Baum F. *The New Public Health.* 3rd ed. Melbourne: Oxford University Press; 2008.

Baum F, Sanders D. Health promotion and primary health care: can they achieve health for all without a return to their earlier, more radical agenda? *Health Promot Int.* 1995;10:149-160. doi:10.1093/heapro/10.2.149.

Baum F, Sanders D. Ottawa 25 years on: a more radical agenda for health equity is still required. *Health Promot Int.* 2011;26 (suppl 2):ii253–ii257. doi:10.1093/heapro/dar078.

Berman G, Paradies Y. Racism, disadvantage and multiculturalism: towards effective anti-racist praxis. *Ethnic Racial Stud.* 2008;33(2):214-232.

Bourdieu P. Forms of capital. In: Richards JC, ed. *Handbook of Theory and Research for the Sociology of Education.* New York: Greenwood Press; 1983:241-258.

Clarke PA. *Aboriginal People and Their Plants.* Dural Delivery Centre, New South Wales: Rosenberg Publishing; 2007.

Coleman JS. Social capital in the creation of human capital. *Am J Sociol.* 1988;94:S95–S120.

Comaroff J. Conflicting paradigms of pregnancy: managing ambiguity in antenatal encounters. In: Davis A, Horobin G, eds. *Medical Encounters: The Experience of Illness and Treatment.* London: Croom Helm; 1977:37-53.

Dahlgren G, Whitehead M. *Policies and Strategies to Promote Social Equity in Health.* Stockholm, Sweden: Institute for Futures Studies (mimeo); 1991.

Kawachi I, Kennedy B. Socioeconomic determinants of health: health and social cohesion: why care about income inequality? *BMJ.* 1997;314:1037.

Lomas J. Social capital and health: implications for public health and epidemiology. *Soc Sci Med.* 1998;47:1181-1188.

Marmot M. The solid facts: the social determinants of health. *Health Promot J Austr.* 1999;9(2):133-139.

Marmot M. *Fair Society, Healthy Lives: The Marmot Review.* London: Marmot Review; 2010.

Marmot M, Wilkinson R, eds. *Social Determinants of Health.* Oxford: Oxford University Press; 2006.

Mehta N. Mind-body dualism: a critique from a health perspective. *Mens Sana Monog.* 2011;9(1):202-209.

Paradies Y, Priest N, Ben J, et al. Racism as a determinant of health: a protocol for conducting a systematic review and meta-analysis. *Syst Rev.* 2013;2:85. Online. http://www.systematicreviewsjournal.com/content/2/1/85.

Putnam RD. Social capital: measurement and consequences. *Can J Policy Res.* 2001;2:41-51.

Reidpath DD. Love thy neighbour it's good for your health: a study of racial homogeneity, mortality and social cohesion in the United States. *Soc Sci Med.* 2003;57:253-261.

Sanders D, Baum F, Benos A, et al. Revitalising primary health care requires an equitable global economic system—now more than ever. *J Epidemiol Community Health.* 2011;65:661-665.

United Nations (UN). *The Millennium Development Goals Report 2008.* 2008. Online: http://www.un.org/millenniumgoals/2008highlevel/pdf/newsroom/mdg%20reports/MDG_Report_2008_ENGLISH.pdf.

United Nations (UN). *The Millennium Development Goals Report 2009.* 2009. Online: http://www.un.org/millenniumgoals/pdf/PR_Global_MDG09_EN.pdf.

United Nations (UN). *The Millennium Development Goals Report 2013.* 2013. Online: http://www.un.org/millenniumgoals/pdf/report-2013/mdg-report-2013-english.pdf.

Wakefield SEL, Poland B. Family, friend or foe? Critical reflections on the relevance and role of social capital in health promotion and community development. *Soc Sci Med.* 2005;60(12):2819-2832.

Walker K. *The Story of Medicine.* New York: Oxford University Press; 1955.

Woolcock M. The place of social capital in understanding social and economic outcomes. *Can J Policy Res.* 2001;2:11-17.

World Health Organization (WHO). *Closing the Gap in a Generation: Health Equity Through Action on the Social Determinants of Health. Final report of the Commission on Social Determinants of Health.* Geneva, Switzerland: WHO; 2008.

World Health Organization (WHO). *Rio Political Declaration on Social Determinants of Health.* Rio de Janeiro, Brazil: World Health Organization; 2011.

CHAPTER 7

Birthplace and birth space

Sally Tracy and Celia Grigg

LEARNING OUTCOMES

Learning outcomes for this chapter are:

1. To explore the safety and impact of the place of birth on women and midwives
2. To explore the risks and benefits of the three locations for place of birth: home, primary maternity unit (PMU) or hospital
3. To describe key factors influencing women's and midwives' decisions around place of birth.

CHAPTER OVERVIEW

This chapter discusses the importance for women, and the role midwives play to encourage, support and facilitate women, to give birth in the most appropriate place for them and their whānau or family. Both 'place' of birth and the 'space' we allocate for giving birth are the major themes of this chapter. The scene is set with a consideration of the concepts of safety, risk and choice, which frame much of the birthplace debate. The chapter reviews where women give birth: whether in secondary or tertiary maternity hospitals; in primary-level midwifery-led maternity units (PMU), either freestanding or alongside a tertiary maternity hospital; or at home. It summarises the current evidence on the clinical outcomes for these settings. It considers what it is about the birth space and its environment that is so important for physiological birth, and women's sense of 'safety' and comfort. It considers why women plan to give birth in different settings including their respective beliefs and values which lead then to make different decisions. Finally, it discusses how midwives can support women to plan to give birth in any of these environments.

KEY TERMS

birth centre
environment

home birth
midwife-led maternity unit

primary maternity unit (PMU)
secondary/tertiary maternity hospital

INTRODUCTION

In the 21st century, birth takes place in the intimate spaces provided in women's homes, in small **birth centres** or primary birth units, and in large hospitals surrounded by an array of technology and personnel. Childbirth is the most common reason for the hospitalisation of women in Australia and Aotearoa New Zealand. However, contemporary maternity services offered in each country differ from each other considerably in context, the system of care they offer and their interface between community and acute facilities. There is worldwide debate surrounding the safety and appropriateness of different birthplaces for well women having uncomplicated pregnancies.

BIRTH MOVES FROM HOME TO HOSPITAL

The turn of the 19th century marked the beginning of the move of childbirth into institutions throughout Britain, Europe, North America, Australia and New Zealand. The history of childbirth in these countries reveals the complex interplay of human and social forces that ultimately dislocated childbearing women from their homes and families, and moved apparent responsibility for childbirth to the medical profession based in hospitals (Graham, 1997). Far from being the rational sequential scientific development that one might expect, such an examination reveals that the systems have been shaped by class and gender, fashion and fallacy, and professional and economic competition (Rowley, 1998).

Place of birth is not easily separated from other aspects of maternity care including caregiver, model of care and the values and beliefs of the society in which it is embedded.

WHAT WAS LOST IN THE MOVE?

Several important things were lost in the move from home to hospital. The first was the opportunity to labour in a familiar **environment**. The second was the close personal and trusting relationship between the woman and her midwife and the continuous support in labour that the midwife provided. The third was the belief in the concept of birth as a social event, a normal, physiological life event. These were, and are still, universal aspects of home-birth provision, and the whole package of care provides clear benefits for women (Walsh, 2004).

The concept of 'environment' is multifaceted and encompasses much more than the geographical location or physical bricks and mortar of the location for birth. It is important to consider that 'environment' also includes the spiritual and emotional space and place in the mind and heart of the woman (Fahy et al., 2008; Simkin & Ancheta, 2001).

In their calls for more home-like environments for birth, more continuity and more choice and involvement in decision making, women may have unknowingly articulated their longing to replicate the idealised birth environment of home. Policy makers have attempted to put back components of the package, and researchers have undertaken numerous studies to explore the safety and impact of differences in location for birth (home, birth centre, primary unit, hospital), type of care provider (medical, midwife, doula), models of care (fragmented versus continuity of care and carer) and philosophies of care (belief in birth as a normal physiological event or only normal in retrospect, and risk embracing or risk averse). However, if the three components of birth at home are an integrated and inseparable package, it becomes apparent that most studies to date have focused on either one or another part of the package. As a consequence, most studies are limited in what they can contribute to our understanding of this complex event.

Current options for birth in Australia include:

- *standard hospital maternity care* at secondary or tertiary level obstetric-led maternity units, where maternity care is offered by a diverse group of practitioners including midwives, obstetricians and GP obstetricians
- *primary level 'alongside hospital' birth centres*, which are next door to labour wards in public hospitals where care is offered by midwives and, in some instances, by private obstetricians
- *primary level (freestanding) midwifery led units* (PMUs) where women book with a named midwife and there is no routine labour involvement of medical staff; these units are geographically separate from any facilities offering onsite obstetric or paediatric services or specialised medical interventions such as epidural analgesia and caesarean sections
- *home birth*, which again differs in Australia and New Zealand. In Australia women and midwives are insured under the public home-birth program, which also differs slightly between states. (Under Medicare, home-birth midwives are not currently insured or indemnified.)

(For further discussion on the funding of these Australian care options see Ch. 2.)

Current options for birth in New Zealand include the following:

- Most women in New Zealand give birth in a secondary or tertiary level obstetric-led hospital, with care provided by lead maternity carers (LMCs) or hospital midwives, and obstetric care as required.
- In many places around the country, you may also have the choice of a birthing centre or small community hospital maternity unit (called a primary maternity unit), with care provided by LMCs, supported by unit midwifery staff. Publicly funded home birth is available throughout the country, where there are LMC midwives offering the option (Box 7.1).

Safety

The primary consideration for women in deciding where to give birth is the safety of themselves and their baby. However, there is ongoing, and sometimes highly politicised,

Box 7.1 New Zealand Ministry of Health advice to women about where to give birth

Women who give birth at home or in a birthing centre or small maternity unit are more likely to have a normal birth than those who give birth in hospital.

You should discuss the place of birth with your midwife or specialist doctor as part of your planning in early pregnancy. Unless you have complications all of these choices are safe.

Giving birth in a birthing centre or small maternity unit, or in hospital

Most women in New Zealand give birth in hospital. In many places around the country, you may also have the choice of a birthing centre or small community hospital maternity unit (called a primary maternity unit). Women giving birth in these smaller units also tend to use less pain relief and have fewer caesarean sections and forceps than those who give birth in hospital. Speak to your midwife (or specialist doctor) about the choices available in your area. You can also see what's available by clicking on your area in the map: https://www.health.govt.nz/your-health/pregnancy-and-kids/services-and-support-during-pregnancy/where-give-birth/find-maternity-facilities-your-area.

If you chose a midwife as your main carer, she will usually be with you during labour and birth. She will have another midwife available to support you and her during and after the birth. They'll work alongside other midwives or doctors if you need additional care. If a specialist doctor is your main carer, they will usually be involved at the time of the birth and you will have a midwife or midwives to care for you during your labour (ask your doctor about this).

Your midwife (or one working on behalf of your specialist doctor) will stay with you for at least 2 hours after the birth.

If you have pregnancy complications or need specialist support, you will be encouraged to give birth in hospital. In some cases, you may need to be under the care of a medical specialist.

Once your baby is born you can stay in hospital for a couple of days and receive care from the hospital-based midwives to assist you to breastfeed your baby and to recover from the birth. Your midwife (or specialist doctor) will visit you every day that you stay in hospital. Your midwife (or one working on behalf of your specialist doctor) will visit within 24 hours of your going home.

(Source: New Zealand Ministry of Health website: https://www.health.govt.nz/your-health/pregnancy-and-kids/services-and-support-during-pregnancy/where-give-birth)

women to give birth, this is not substantiated by current research. There is growing evidence to support **home birth** (Catling-Paull et al., 2013; De Jonge et al., 2009; Hutton et al., 2009; Janssen et al., 2009) and **midwife-led maternity units** as clinically safe for well women (Birthplace in England Collaborative Group, 2011; Davis et al., 2011; Gottvall et al., 2004; Grigg et al., 2017; Grunebaum et al., 2014; Homer et al., 2014; Kruske et al., 2016; Monk et al., 2014; Overgaard et al., 2011; Ryan & Roberts, 2005). It is also necessary to identify other aspects of birthplace which can be as important for childbearing women and their families in their quest for physical safety, such as their psychological, social and cultural safety.

In contemporary Western culture, physical safety is often the only aspect measured. For New Zealand Māori, hauora (health) has been represented as being the four cornerstones of a house—comprising whānau (family), as well as tinana (physical), hinengaro (mental) and wairua (spiritual) safety, with all having equal importance (a model developed by Mason Durie in 1982; see: Ministry of Health (MOH), 2017a). In Australia, maternity services largely reflect modern Western medical values that determine risk and safety. For Aboriginal and Torres Strait Islander women, 'Birth on Country' is a unique and important aspect of safety that until now has never been fully recognised and operationalised. Birth on Country is based on the Aboriginal knowledge of the Dreaming—that health and life are connected as one to the land—and that this link is timeless. In the words of Aboriginal Elder Djapirra Mununggirritj on the importance of Birth on Country to the Yolngu people (AHMAC 2011; Kildea et al., 2013),

> Birth on Country is about all things. Birth on Country brings spiritual meaning to the modern world that we live in now. Birth on Country lies deep and wide … deep … and wide … because it stretches from the ancient to the future, and it is for our generation to continue singing … the identity of the Indigenous people of this world.
>
> (Birthing Yarn—keynote speech given at the National Birthing on Country workshop, Alice Springs, 4th July 2012)

Safety is a relative term for humans in everyday life and cannot be guaranteed generally, or for birth. There are no guarantees of a 'perfect' outcome for the woman or her baby in any setting. Construction of hospitals as the only safe place to give birth misrepresents reality worldwide. However, the large Birthplace in England study identified greater morbidity for women and babies associated with birth in hospital for well women ('low risk' at the start of labour), even accounting for those who transferred to hospital during labour, birth or immediately postpartum (Birthplace in England Collaborative Group, 2011).

The preoccupation with safety can engender alarm, a heightened sensitivity to danger and a sense of personal vulnerability. Much of the anxiety about health is aggravated by a medical technocratic culture that is compelled to identify dangers in order to control them (Crawford

worldwide debate surrounding the safety and appropriateness of different types of birthplaces for women who have uncomplicated pregnancies. While the current thinking is that an obstetric-led hospital is the 'safest' place for all

2004; Moynihan et al., 2002). Women's sense of safety is based on their beliefs and values, not only about birth itself but life in general. A recent Canadian study found women planning to give birth in a freestanding birth centre 'expressed feeling a sense of safety in the birth centre decision-making experience', and that they made that decision 'based on evidence, values and preferences, and experiences' (Wood et al., 2016, p. 17). Women's beliefs and values regarding birth are influenced by a wide range of things, including:

- their personal experiences and those of their family and friends
- the beliefs and values of their partner and sometimes those of their family and friends
- their knowledge-base
- the wider cultural context
- the organisation of maternity care
- local maternity facilities and their reputation
- local 'birth culture', including the local 'risk culture'
- the dominance of obstetrics
- the status and ideology / approach of midwifery
- where most women give birth and what is considered the 'norm' in their community.

Women endeavour to protect the safety of themselves and their baby when making their birthplace plans. This chapter considers safety broadly in order to gain a more comprehensive understanding of the topic and provide evidence to inform all of those concerned with birthplace safety. One of the major influences on women's sense of safety is their belief regarding 'risk'.

REFLECTIVE THINKING EXERCISE

Consider your own thoughts about the safety of birth and different birthplaces. Where would you want to give birth? Who would you feel safe having with you? What would you need there for it to feel safe (services, facilities and environment)?

Risk

The powerful construct of risk is closely linked to the notion of safety and has been extensively written about in relation to birth (Chadwick & Foster, 2014; Coxon et al., 2013; Jordan & Murphy, 2009; McIntyre et al., 2011; Possamai-Inesedy, 2006; Smith et al., 2012; see also Ch. 4).

Risk is a very complex phenomenon and a dominant feature of contemporary Western society. It is an integral and inherent component of pregnancy—and of all life experiences (Enkin, 1994).

Anxiety about pregnancy and childbirth and fears for the safety and wellbeing of themselves and their babies underpin the way many women view childbirth in resource-rich Western society today. Generally, these fears do not stem from a lived experience but from the speculation of risks (Possamai-Inesedy, 2006). In the context of contemporary Western society, women's perception of their risk during pregnancy and birth is out of proportion to their actual risk (Jordan & Murphy, 2009). Yet it seems that as absolute risk of an adverse outcome has decreased over the years, the fear of adverse outcome has increased (Enkin, 1994; Jordan & Murphy, 2009; Possamai-Inesedy, 2006). Arguably it is perception of risk which affects women's behaviours and decision making (Jordan & Murphy, 2009).

Risk relating to childbirth takes many forms. For example, the Australian government policy affecting the closure of rural and remote maternity services and birthplaces leaves women no option other than relocation to give birth in regional centres. This has raised multiple risks including physical and social risks for women—clinical, cultural, emotional, financial—and health-service risks, in addition to legal, financial, political and operational risks (Barclay et al., 2016). The potentially powerful cultural risk experienced by Aboriginal women was reported in a recent study where women stated in their words:

'That link to country is robbed from them—[this is] another form of genocide' (Field Site2).
Another said that 'many women think they stopped birthing here because of land rights. They think their birth certificates say ... so they then can't prove their country [is here]' (Field Site2).

(Barclay et al., 2016, p. 67)

There are ways to effect a change in the all-encompassing and apparently all-consuming context of risk in pregnancy and childbirth. One of the most promising is the method of 'walking' through care in pregnancy and childbirth, prompted by a series of 'decision points' which remind midwives and women to discuss together the need for addressing certain issues as they arise. In New Zealand women and midwives have a booklet to help them navigate their way through the risks that present themselves during pregnancy and labour. The *New Zealand Midwives Handbook for Practice* (NZCOM, 2018) is a comprehensive guide for establishing information sharing and 'partnership' (Guilliland & Pairman, 1995) between women and their caregivers. The handbook is a widely available practical guide written for midwives, women and the general public and aims to set in place a system for the profession and the public to measure both individual midwife practices and midwifery services. The handbook is a practical reminder of the fact that, although women are confronted almost daily with the notion of pregnancy and labour as a risky undertaking, it helps women to map out good reasons for requiring anything that would interfere with the normal birth process, and weigh up the evidence to show that any intervention about to be undertaken will have been well considered from an informed perspective. The prompt for women and midwives to discuss and evaluate together each decision in the context of appropriate and adequate information helps to avoid many unnecessary interventions.

Risk is arguably central to the well-established contrasting models of childbirth (see Table 7.1), which will be called the holistic and technocratic models here, following

Table 7.1 Key features of technocratic and holistic models of childbirth

Technocratic/medical model	Holistic/midwifery/social model
Doctor centred	Woman centred
Obstetrics: experts in pathology	Midwifery: experts in normal physiology
Body–mind dualism; classifying, separating	Holistic; integrating approach
Pregnancy is a medical condition, inherently pathological	Pregnancy is a normal human state, inherently healthy
Birth is only normal in retrospect and requires hospitalisation and medical supervision	Birth is a normal physiological, social and cultural process with environment key
Technology dominant	Technology cautious
Risk selection is not possible, but risk is central	Risk selection is possible and appropriate
Statistical/biological approach	Individual/psychosocial approach
Biomedical focus	Psychosocial focus
Medical knowledge is privileged and exclusionary	Experiential and emotional knowledge valued
Intervention	Observation
Outcome: aims at live, healthy mother and baby	Outcome: aims at live, healthy mother and baby and satisfaction of individual needs of mother/couple

(Sources: Grigg et al., 2014. An interpretation based on Bryers & van Teijlingen (2010), van Teijlingen (2005), Rooks et al. (1989), Davis-Floyd (1992), Jordan (1997))

Davis-Floyd's (1992) terminology. The models identify sets of beliefs which are associated with differing approaches to childbirth (although they may be better represented on a continuum than as two separate and opposing world views) (Davis-Floyd, 1992).

In their chapter outlining the role of midwives and doulas in childbirth Everson and Cheyney (2015) quote from Davis Floyd's description of the two models of childbirth:

The wholistic approach is woman-centred with family as a significant social unit; with woman as active subject; mother and child as one; home as nurturing environment; and bodily, experiential, and emotional knowledge as highly valued. Childbearing is understood as a healthy, normal process best supported by low-tech, high-touch techniques with a midwife as 'skillful guide'.

(Davis-Floyd, pp. 160–1)

Technocratic models, in contrast, are male-centred with social support regarded as unimportant or secondary to primary clinical concerns; with woman as passive object; hospital as 'factory' and babies as 'products'; and technical, scientific knowledge as the only knowledge of value. Childbearing is understood as dysfunctional, even pathological, and best controlled by interventions led by an obstetrician as 'manager/ skilled technician'.

(Davis-Floyd, pp. 160–1)

Research has found women planning to give birth in obstetric-led hospitals hold different sets of beliefs and values on childbirth from those who plan to give birth in midwifery-led contexts (maternity unit or home), which reflect the core tenets of the two models—'technocratic' and 'holistic' respectively. (See Box 7.2.)

It is possible, however, that this dichotomous representation increasingly fails to capture 'the nuances of

Box 7.2 Women describe the difference between technocratic and holistic models of childbirth in a focus group in the NZ EMU study

Technocratic model example

I had a couple of people going 'Oh but it's all just a natural process and it's all good and you should be all fine'; well actually if you look around the world most of the women die in childbirth, that's the riskiest thing women do; I wasn't terribly impressed with that argument.

(TMH planned birth, Fay)

Holistic model example

I think [TMH]—it's a hospital, which if you are sick or if you've had an accident, that's great, that's exactly what you want; but I wasn't sick, I was having a baby—it's a perfectly natural process that millions of women all around the world have managed to do without nice shiny hospitals.

(PMU planned birth, Ivy)

(Source: Grigg et al., 2014, p. 10)

women's experiences or the breadth of contextual influences upon their [birthplace] decisions' (Coxon et al., 2013, p. 3). Davis-Floyd subsequently identified a third 'humanistic' model, which provides a middle ground or stepping stone between the extremes (Davis-Floyd, 2001).

Whichever way women's beliefs are labelled, their perception of the 'risk' of birth and of different birthplaces are complex and influenced by many factors, as are those of midwives'. Canadian obstetrician Andrew Kotaska contends that modern obstetrics is defining ever-smaller increments of perinatal risk, and is becoming dominated by an imperative to avoid any definable risk; which sometimes has the consequence of creating other risks that are often unacknowledged to women and are sometimes greater than those being avoided (Kotaska, 2007). We believe that risk, as it is currently presented by obstetrics, requires reconstruction, which is no easy task given the complexity of childbirth politics and the power of the contemporary Western context (Bryers & van Teijlingen, 2010; Enkin, 1994; Jordan & Murphy, 2009). Reconstruction would require a review of the 'who', 'how', 'when' and 'why' of risk communication. Issues of informed consent, compliance or coercion also need to be addressed, if women are to make informed decisions regarding their planned birthplace (Jordan & Murphy, 2009; Kotaska, 2007; Possamai-Inesedy, 2006).

REFLECTIVE THINKING EXERCISE

What are your own perceptions of risk relating to birthplace, and how would you communicate the 'risks' of different birthplaces to well women?

Choice

'Choice' is an abstract concept that involves the knowledge of the existence of more than one possibility, the ability (both capacity and autonomy) to choose between them, and the act of actually doing so.

Choice is not a simple independent act; rather it is a complex social construct, with numerous interdependent components. It is defined and confined within the existing social context. In the context of pregnancy and childbirth, there are a number of assertions that may be made about the principles, beliefs and values underpinning the ideal of 'choice'.

Firstly, the options available to pregnant women are determined by those with the authority and power to define them. In contemporary Western cultures, it is the medical establishment that largely controls these alternatives.

Secondly, for a choice to be a genuine one the person making it requires access to information and an understanding of all the issues involved. 'Informed Choice' has become enshrined in the law relating to medical care in New Zealand, in the *Health and Disability Services Act, 1993*. The assumption is that if one has information, one has the ability to choose. Unfortunately, information is rarely objective, unbiased and complete, and presented in a form that any reader or listener can fully understand. In many situations information may be packaged by the presenter, in ways which influence the decisions that women and their families make, intentionally or not. Further, some women are unable or unwilling to actively

or meaningfully make informed decisions and accept responsibility for them. Arguably, given all of the above, truly 'informed choice' is an ideal rather than a reality in many situations at the present time.

Thirdly, we know that in maternity care the alternatives are almost never of identifiably equal value. They are often complex and confusingly difficult to analyse, with subtle physiological, psychological or emotional aspects or potential side effects that are difficult to evaluate or quantify. For example, in most Western countries women choosing home birth are seen to be making what is believed by most to be an unsafe and irresponsible choice, despite sound empirical evidence to the contrary.

Fourthly, genuine freedom to choose from a range of real options is rare. In childbirth most choices involve not only the woman as the supposed 'choicemaker', but also caregivers, such as midwives, institutions and the staff that work in them, and the rules and regulations that are inherently choice limiting. All of these 'others' must also support the woman in making any particular choice. For example, women wanting to give birth at home (with a midwife involved) must live in an area where practitioners provide a genuine home-birth service. In Australia, women wanting to have a home birth (and be cared for by a midwife with professional indemnity cover) must satisfy a very strict protocol of risk assessment to become eligible for a publicly funded home-birth. Regardless of how well informed, reasonable or appropriate those women are, they are dependent on others to have any real choice. Thus the philosophical construct of choice is more apparent than real for many childbearing women.

The fallacy of choice can be further illustrated in respect to the concepts of autonomy, power and control—arguably all prerequisites for real choice. Those with the greatest autonomy, power and control determine the choices available for those with the least. Childbearing women are not autonomous agents in the birthing context, regardless of whether they perceive themselves as such. Their ability to determine their own actions is limited in that the options available are predetermined by care providers and policy makers. Despite consumers having rights of autonomy, decision making and complaint (Tracy & Page, 2019), these rights are constrained where they conflict with providers, and they face great pressure to conform to social and institutional norms. Equally, a woman cedes a degree of control to her caregiver when she seeks care (Bryant et al., 2007). The nature of partnership implies a sharing of control. This is not to say that no choices are available, or that women have no autonomy, power or control, or that there are not midwives (and even some doctors) who work hard to share information and support the choices women make. It is the case that the underpinning values and beliefs about the notion of choice are potentially misleading for midwives and childbearing women, who do not know how constructed and constrained their choices are in reality.

In maternity care the notion of choice has also been co-opted and corrupted by obstetrics. Women previously lobbied for birthplace choice when maternity facilities were being centralised into obstetric-led hospitals. They were seeking the choice to give birth somewhere other than a hospital. Subsequently, obstetrics (and some women) adopted the term to support and enable women to 'choose' to give birth in a hospital, or have elective caesarean sections without clinical indication. See Box 7.3.

In order to optimise women's choice in birthplace planning they need access to a supported home-birth service or primary maternity units (PMU), whether freestanding or alongside an obstetric tertiary maternity hospital. PMUs need to be close enough (to women's homes and to the referral hospital) to be a genuine option. The primary units need to have the characteristics and facilities valued by women wanting to use them and be well funded and managed and staffed appropriately, with access to effective transfer arrangements and specialist services, when they are required. However, the provision of the facility alone is not enough. Women also need a midwife, or primary caregiver, who believes in the birth process and women's ability to give birth, in the skills of herself and her colleagues, and supports and attends women who give birth at PMUs or home. Ideally the maternity system needs to be organised to provide well women with continuity of midwifery care for their primary level maternity journey, with the capacity to access specialist facilities and services if they are needed.

> ## Box 7.3 Key features that enable women to 'choose' to give birth in a hospital, or have elective caesarean sections without clinical indication
>
> The features of making a 'choice' about where to give birth, or whether to have a caesarean section, are introduced or packaged to childbearing women with striking similarities. Although the interventions could not be more different, both are:
>
> - presented as an issue of so called 'women's rights' and 'freedom of choice'
> - promoted by medics and some women, both claiming 'feminist' philosophy
> - fairly radical in nature when compared with current practice prior to their introduction
> - promoted as 'fear-reducing' options—hospital birth and the availability of anaesthesia was intended to take away the fear of pain in labour, while elective caesarean section is said to take away all the fears associated with labour
> - presented by clinicians as consumer rather than provider driven
> - debated and contentious in the medical and midwifery fraternity, and by some women, as to the ethics, safety and potential consequences of them both.
>
> (Source: Grigg et al, 2014)

Women need access to information which is balanced, comprehensive and meaningful to them, and to be able to make decisions without coercion from caregivers.

REFLECTIVE THINKING EXERCISE

How would you present information regarding safety, risk and choice to a woman and her partner who are investigating the options open to them? How would you ensure they are in the position to offer 'informed consent'?

Summary

These three complex constructs of safety, risk and choice are central to women's decision making surrounding birth. Currently, it is widely held that obstetrics, espousing the technocratic model, holds the 'authoritative knowledge' on childbirth, has the power to define 'safety' and 'acceptable risk', controls the information women receive and also the 'choices' available to women (Bryers & van Teijlingen, 2010; Davis & Walker, 2013; Edwards & Murphy-Lawless, 2006; Jordan & Murphy, 2009). It is within this context which this chapter discusses birthplace and space.

BIRTHPLACE

Alongside primary maternity units (PMU)

In Australia in 1980, in response to a growing number of home births in Australia, the National Health and Medical Research Council advised maternity units to modify hospital practices and develop a more homelike environment. A small number of birth centres had already been developed in NSW including the birth centre at the Royal Hospital for Women, Sydney. The 1989 Shearman Report on Obstetric Services in New South Wales (NSW Health Department, 1989) made further recommendations along these lines that family-centred birth centres should be developed along with more flexible labour ward practices and accreditation of qualified independent practising midwives. In due course a small number of 'homelike' birth centres were established where women could give birth in a 'less clinical and more homelike atmosphere' (NSW Health, 1989). Alongside the concern that women should be encouraged to give birth in hospital, birth centres were seen as a safer, intermediate option between hospital and home birth, providing a homelike environment with access to medical care if necessary (Griew, cited in Kirkham, 2003). The trend had already begun in the US in the 1970s where many hospitals endeavoured to make their labour rooms 'homelike', although a more accurate term would be 'bedroom-like', since the bed was always the prominent feature. The rooms were decorated and furnished similarly to Western

Table 7.2 Importance of philosophies to alongside birth centres in Australia 1997–2007

Philosophy	Very important	Important	Moderately important	Of little importance	Not important
To provide a non-clinical, homelike environment	11	5	—	—	—
To provide continuity of care, i.e. continuity of philosophy of care	15	1	—	—	—
To provide continuity of carer, i.e. care by a known midwife	9	4	2	1	—
To provide midwifery-led care	16	—	—	—	—
Commitment to normality of pregnancy and birth	16	—	—	—	—
Encourage women's rights and choices	14	2	—	—	—
Encourage family involvement	12	4	—	—	—
Minimal obstetric intervention	14	1	—	1	—
Minimal use of technology	11	2	1	2	—
Minimal pharmacological pain management[a]	9	2	4	—	—

[a]One respondent did not answer this question.
— = zero response.
(Source: Laws et al., 2009)

middle-class bedrooms, with medical equipment concealed from view (Hodnett et al., 2009). The centrality of the hospital bed in a labour room sends a powerful message that the appropriate place in which to labour is the bed (Fannin, 2003). (Midwives who are expert in breech birth attendance have labelled the preoccupation with lying supine on the bed to give birth as a major cause of 'bed dystocia' (Banks, 2014).)

In a study of birth centre characteristics in 2007, a 'commitment to normality of pregnancy and birth' was most commonly reported as the most important philosophy (Laws et al., 2009) (Table 7.2). All birth centres were managed by a midwifery or nursing unit manager, or a clinical nurse specialist, although the models of care within the birth centres varied.

Australia has no nationally agreed definition of a 'birth centre'. The definition that most closely resembles birth centre practice in Australia was proposed in the National Perinatal Epidemiology Unit review of birth centres undertaken in the United Kingdom (Stewart et al., 2005, p. 8. See Box 7.4). The full United Kingdom definition includes both 'freestanding' and 'alongside' birth centres.

However, Australian birth centres are predominantly hospital based. They are most often situated in urban settings alongside a labour ward and integrated wholly within the public hospital structure in terms of funding, staffing and regulation. In most Australian hospitals, the labour ward is situated adjacent to the birth centre so that transfer arrangements involve moving women not more than 50 m from birth centre to labour ward. Although no one single model of birth centre care is used, it is generally agreed that the philosophy of birth centre

Box 7.4   Definition of a birth centre

A birth centre is an institution that offers care to women with a straightforward pregnancy and where midwives take primary professional responsibility for care. During labour and birth, medical services, including obstetric, neonatal and anaesthetic care, are available should they be needed, but they may be on a separate site, or in a separate building, which may involve transfer by car or ambulance.

(Source: Stewart et al., 2005, p. 8)

care includes a homelike, nonclinical environment, autonomous midwifery practice, woman- and family-centered care, and a commitment to and belief in normal, physiological birth.

Over the years the characteristics of birth centres have changed dramatically in Australia. In the decade between 1997 to 2007 there was a decline in the number of birth centres (Laws et al., 2010) with five less birth centres operating in 2007 compared to 1997. Alongside birth centres have also become more conservative over the years in their admission criteria. For example, they are less likely to accept women with a post-dates pregnancy, having a vaginal birth after caesarean section or who are obese. Women may be induced and sometimes receive continuous electronic fetal monitoring in birth centres.

In a national maternity review held in Australia in 2008, submissions received tended to place alongside birth centres in a different light again. They were now seen as a compromise between the medicalised hospital-based system and unfunded, unsupported home birth. Against an overwhelming demand from women for home birth and requests for more midwife-led, non-medicalised options for birth (Dahlen et al., 2010) the Australian government continued to recommend alongside birth centres.

Birthplace in Aotearoa New Zealand

The New Zealand Ministry of Health has developed an interactive map for women to find out what facilities are available to them to give birth:

https://www.health.govt.nz/your-health/pregnancy-and-kids/services-and-support-during-pregnancy/where-give-birth/find-maternity-facilities-your-area

Maternity care in New Zealand is publicly funded, and comprehensive private health insurance cover for pregnancy / childbirth is not available. Most women, supported by their LMC, now give birth in one of the following options. (See Box 7.1)

Birthplace options currently include 18 secondary-level and 6 tertiary-level obstetric-led maternity hospitals, which have midwifery and specialist obstetric, anaesthetic and paediatric services onsite; 54 freestanding primary level midwife-led maternity units offering birthing facilities, which have midwifery services onsite; and funded home birth. In 2014, 87.6% of births occurred in a secondary or tertiary hospital, 9.1% in a freestanding maternity unit and 3.4% were home births (Grigg et al., 2017).

The tertiary hospitals are based in the five largest cities and have more specialised obstetric and neonatal intensive care facilities. Freestanding birth centres are staffed by midwives and have no specialist services onsite. Most of the primary maternity units are situated in rural or semi-rural areas in New Zealand.

Of the women who give birth in New Zealand, Māori women are more likely to give birth in a **primary maternity unit (PMU)** than women of other ethnicities (see Fig. 7.1).

However, researchers from Auckland who studied the choice of place of birth among Pasifika women found that the overwhelming view of the small group of women who participated was that the place to give birth needs to be close to where the family lives and it needs be a place where Pasifika women can feel at home (McAra-Couper et al., 2018).

Hospital birthplace choices are restricted in many areas, with limited numbers of PMUs in most regions, and either a secondary or tertiary hospital available in towns and cities. Planned home birth is a real option. Considerable regional variation is reported with some areas having over 8% home birth rate, and some less than 2%.

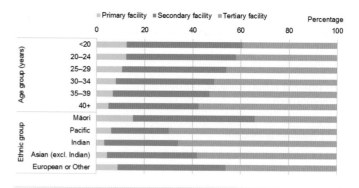

FIGURE 7.1 Distribution of women giving birth at a maternity facility, by type of facility, age group, ethnic group (Source: Extract from NZ Ministry of Health. *Report on Maternity, 2014.* Wellington, NZ: Ministry of Health; 2015:50. ttps://www.health.govt.nz/publication/report-maternity-2014)

Freestanding midwifery-led units in Australia

In Australia the concept of safely giving birth is commonly linked with the immediate onsite availability of specialist medical support. New Zealand, on the other hand, has actively developed and promoted freestanding PMUs over the past decades in an attempt to offer women a real choice for place of birth.

In Australia, market-driven reform agendas, among other things, promoted both the centralisation and privatisation of maternity services. This led to the closure of many smaller maternity units in rural and remote areas of Australia (Monk et al., 2013b). These changes have left a huge gap in the provision of readily accessible maternity care. Paradoxically, it is the 'market' which also underpins the recent innovative developments in maternity care where maternity consumers and professional groups such as nurses and midwives have been supported by the government and able to play a more pronounced role in the formation of maternity policy. As a result, a small number of freestanding PMUs have been developed in urban and regional settings (Monk et al., 2013a); however, they still face the challenge of operating within a culture of childbirth which highly values a medical model of care.

In Australia, birth rates by place of birth are currently (2015) 0.3% home, 1.8% 'birth centres' (both alongside and freestanding PMUs), 97% tertiary maternity hospitals and 0.4% (other) (AIHW, 2017). In contrast, New Zealand currently (2015) has higher rates of planned home birth (3.7%), 9.9% birth rate at freestanding units, and 86.4% in secondary or tertiary hospitals (MOH, 2017b). There has been a marked reduction in the proportion of women giving birth in primary maternity facilities in New Zealand over the last ten years, with one-third fewer women giving birth in these facilities (down from 15.1% in 2006). In Australia, there remain remarkably few PMUs, which face resistance from obstetrics and policy makers, despite efforts by midwifery leaders to increase the primary maternity facilities in both rural and urban areas.

Contributing to the debate about the safety of out-of-hospital settings for childbirth is the perception that caregivers (particularly midwives) in these settings may overemphasise the 'normality' of childbirth and therefore miss or delay recognition of emerging complications. This was the view of Gottvall et al. (2004), who conducted a 10-year retrospective review of the Stockholm Birth Centre, which revealed a trend to higher perinatal mortality in primigravid women. Following scrutiny of each perinatal death by an obstetrician, Gottvall and colleagues (2004) claimed that a potential risk of birth-centre care is the 'philosophy that emphasises a strong belief in the natural process' (p. 77). Hodnett et al. (2005) echoed concerns regarding the emphasis on normal birth and stated that this belief might delay recognition of imminent complications or the ability of the midwife to take averting action. Many of the perinatal deaths in the original Stockholm trial (Waldenstrom et al., 1997) occurred after transfer and were associated with clearly documented suboptimal care in the receiving hospital. Gottvall and colleagues did not comment on this, however.

In contrast, Walsh (2004) refutes any suggestion that birth-centre midwives are over-orientated to normal birth and therefore may delay recognition of complications. Walsh asserts that birth-centre midwives are highly skilled practitioners with an astute awareness of normal labour and that these midwives are particularly diligent in updating their skills in emergency care. Walsh acknowledged that it might very well be the midwife's belief in physiological labour, especially for primigravid women, that enables such women to achieve normal birth in birth centres. In his ethnographic study, Walsh (2006) asserts that very little attention has been paid to organisational dimensions of childbirth care until recently. He claims that freestanding birth centres 'subvert' the processing mentality of modernist organisations such as large maternity hospitals. Birth centres demonstrate greater flexibility in labour care so as to accommodate women's preferences and enhance the autonomy of midwives and women, such that a self-managing and self-regulating ethos flourishes (Walsh, 2006).

Sociologists who have paid particular attention to childbirth also show concern regarding interpretations of safety. Annandale (1988) used both quantitative and qualitative methods to study the structure of birth in a North American birth centre. Her study included 18 months of observation, repeated focus-group interviews and content analysis of 900 women's records over a 5-year period. Obstetricians did not see women unless a risk factor arose; however, Annandale commented that midwives and obstetricians disagreed about what constituted a risk factor. Midwives tended to disagree with the assertion that a post-term induction was high risk, and that intervention was required after 12 hours of ruptured membranes. Annandale found that birth-centre midwives adopted strategies to maintain the 'normal',

such as encouraging women to stay at home until active labour was well established. This strategy reduced the likelihood of transfer to a large hospital for perceived prolonged labour.

Birth outcomes for primary maternity units

In the last five years a substantial body of research has been published on the clinical outcomes of PMUs, almost all of which reported them to have better or similar outcomes for women and babies than hospital births. The existing literature relating to them comes from a range of contexts, with diverse models of maternity care and maternity system organisation, including alongside maternity units and freestanding PMUs. In some settings women receive different models of care dependent on their planned birthplace. For example, women planning to give birth in a PMU may be cared for exclusively by midwives (predominantly offering caseload care), and women planning a hospital birth may receive midwifery and / or obstetric or medical care for some, or all, of their maternity journey. In some contexts PMUs are integrated into the maternity system, while they are considered 'alternative' and outside of standard care provision in others.

There are also a range of study designs utilised in research evaluating PMUs' clinical outcomes and transfers. The majority of the evaluations have used a prospective cohort, retrospective cohort, case study or audit design. While two major RCTs have been undertaken in the context of the opening of a PMU with access to it being dependent on agreement to participate in the study, they were confounded by the two arms receiving different models of care (Rowe et al., 2012; Cheung et al., 2010). RCTs may not be appropriate or possible where women already have ready access to either birthplace type (Hendrix et al., 2009). The main objection to observational studies is their potential for selection bias, which rules out their ability to draw causal inferences (Berger et al., 2012; Yang et al., 2010). Arguably, they are the best design for answering the research questions regarding the identification of differences in clinical outcomes between the different birthplace types, given the complexity of both childbirth and birthplace (Downe, 2010; Enkin, 2012).

The Cochrane review into 'alternative versus conventional settings' (conventional being hospital) for birth only included ten trials, including a total of 11,295 women, relating only to alongside maternity units, with six of them undertaken over 25 years ago (Hodnett et al., 2012).

Recently, research in Australia (Homer et al., 2014; Monk et al., 2014) and New Zealand (Davis et al., 2011; Grigg et al., 2017) has shown the benefit of giving birth in maternity units —both freestanding and alongside delivery wards—when compared to those births that occur in tertiary level maternity hospitals. In both Australia and New Zealand midwifery-led care (Tracy et al., 2005) and robust consultation and referral guidelines (see Ch. 18) are considered to be integral components in determining safe practice.

The 'Birthplace in England' (BE) study is the largest and most comprehensive comparative birthplace research to date (Hollowell et al., 2011). It included 64,538 women, defined as 'low risk': 19,706 planning to give birth in an obstetric unit, 16,710 planning an alongside maternity unit (AMU) birth, 11,282 planning a freestanding maternity unit (FMU) birth and 16,840 planning a home birth. The primary analysis was by intended birthplace at booking. Despite the large study population the rarity of perinatal mortality meant that the study was not powered to detect clinically significant differences in its rate between the different birthplace types. Consequently, a 'composite primary outcome' of perinatal mortality and intrapartum related neonatal morbidities, which ranged in incidence and severity, was used and acknowledged as a study weakness by the collaborative multi-disciplinary research group (Hollowell et al., 2011). The composite outcomes included perinatal mortality (overall incidence 13%) and the intrapartum morbidities of neonatal encephalopathy ('clinical or signs', 46%) meconium aspiration syndrome (30%), brachial plexus injury (8%) and fractured humerus or clavicle (4%). In summary, the research found no significant differences in the (adjusted odds ratio) rate of the primary outcome for women planning a hospital birth, or birth in a freestanding or alongside maternity unit or a home birth (Hollowell et al., 2011). The overall incidence of the composite perinatal outcome was 4.3 per 1000 (inclusive of those with complicating conditions at the start of labour) (Hollowell et al., 2011).

The Birthplace in England study had multiple neonatal and maternal secondary outcomes. A higher rate of neonatal admission was found for the tertiary hospital group, and breastfeeding initiation was less likely to occur for women who planned a tertiary hospital birth (Hollowell et al., 2011). The rates of labour augmentation, analgesia, instrumental vaginal birth and caesarean section, episiotomy and active management of the third stage were all significantly higher in the tertiary hospital group than any of the other settings evaluated (Hollowell et al., 2011). No consistent association was found between birthplace and rates of 3rd and 4th degree perineal tears, blood transfusion or admission to intensive / special care, 'although these adverse outcomes were generally lowest for planned births in freestanding midwifery units' (Hollowell et al., 2011, p. 3).

This comprehensive study is contemporary and set in the British context, making it the dominant reference in the birthplace literature. Following the publication of the Birthplace in England study the evidence base is considered to be strong and robust enough to be incorporated into the latest NICE birthplace guidelines (NICE, 2014), which confirmed the association between maternal morbidity and tertiary hospital birth. (See Box 7.5.)

Home birth

Home birth in New Zealand is encouraged and supported nationally. The New Zealand Ministry of Health has the

---

Box 7.5 Choosing the planned place of birth

The Guideline Group who updated the NICE Guidelines for Intrapartum Care made the following comments in their report. (Clearly the research on which this recommendation was based was undertaken in England—and may not be completely generalisable to either New Zealand or Australia.)

Explain to both multiparous and nulliparous women that they may choose any birth setting (home, freestanding midwifery unit, alongside midwifery unit (alongside an obstetric unit and not requiring ambulance transfer), or obstetric unit) and support them in their choice of setting, wherever that may be:

- *Advise low-risk multiparous women that planning to give birth at home or in a midwifery led unit (freestanding or alongside) is particularly suitable for them because the rate of interventions is lower and the outcome for the baby is no different compared with an obstetric unit. (See Table 6.5.)*

- *Advise low-risk nulliparous women that planning to give birth in a midwifery led unit (freestanding or alongside) is particularly suitable for them because the rate of interventions is lower and the outcome for the baby is no different compared with an obstetric unit. However, if they plan birth at home there is a small increase in the risk of an adverse outcome for the baby. (See Table 6.6.)*

This new recommendation is based on high to very low quality evidence from randomised controlled trials and observational studies and the experience and opinion of the GDG.

(Reproduced from Nunes VD, Gholitabar M, Sims JM, Bewley S. Intrapartum care of healthy women and their babies: summary of updated NICE guidance. On behalf of the NICE Guideline Development Group. *BMJ*. 2014;349:g6886, with permission from BMJ Publishing Group Ltd)

---

following website for women to access and learn more about home birth: https://homebirth.org.nz/

In most other Western countries the topic of home birth generates considerable debate. This is reflected by the differing positions on home birth adopted by professional colleges representing obstetricians and midwives in the UK, USA, Australia, New Zealand and Canada. All appear to rely on the same body of research evidence to arrive at completely different positions (Roome et al., 2016). (See Table 7.3.)

(Note in Table 7.4 that NZCOM does not offer a position statement— possibly because women in New Zealand are free to choose a home birth and are funded to do so, making a 'position statement' redundant.)

Rates of planned home birth vary widely across the developed world, being highest in the Netherlands, at around 30% of all births, in comparison with <1% of births in Australia and the USA, 2% in the UK and 3.3% in New Zealand (Roome et al., 2016).

Table 7.3 Key studies cited by colleges when evaluating safety of home birth

Name of study	Study design	Results for neonatal and perinatal mortality	Colleges that cited this study
Wax et al.[16]	Meta-analysis of 11 cohort studies and one RCT (342,056 planned home births; 207,551 planned hospital births)	Tripling in non-anomalous neonatal mortality (95% CI 1.32–6.25) for home births, no difference in perinatal mortality	RANZCOG, ACOG, ACM, ACNM
De Jonge et al.[1]	Cohort study (321,307 planned home births; 163,261 planned hospital births; 45,120 planned birthing location unknown)	No significant difference	ACM, ACNM, CAM, ACOG
Wiegars et al.[33]	Prospective data analysis of data from midwives ($n=97$) and women at low risk ($n=1836$) from 54 midwifery practices in the Netherlands intending to deliver in hospital ($n=696$) or at home ($n=1140$)	No significant difference	RCOG, ACNM, ACOG, CAM, ACM
Johnson & Daviss[19]	Prospective cohort study of all planned home births ($n=5418$) attended by certified midwives in the USA and Canada in the year 2000	No difference in perinatal mortality when only women at low risk with non-anomalous babies	ACM, ACNM, CAM, ACOG
Janssen et al.[22]	Retrospective cohort analysis of all planned home births attended by a registered midwife from 2000 to 2004 ($n=2889$) and all planned hospital births that would have met eligibility criteria for home births ($n=4752$)	No difference in perinatal mortality across all groups	ACM, ACNM, CAM, ACOG
Hutton & Reitsma[21]	Retrospective cohort of planned home births ($n=6692$) compared with similar women at low risk planning a hospital birth	No difference in perinatal and neonatal mortality	ACNM, CAM, ACM, ACOG
Kennare et al.[34]	Retrospective study using South Australian data on all births and perinatal deaths during the period 1991–2006. Included 1140 home births and 298,860 hospital births	No significant difference in perinatal mortality rate, sevenfold increased risk of intrapartum death, and a 27-fold higher risk of death from intrapartum asphyxia	RANZCOG, CAM, ACOG, ACM

ACM = Australian College of Midwives; ACNM = American College of Nurse-Midwives; CAM = Canadian Association of Midwives; ACOG = American College of Obstetricians; RANZCOG = Royal Australian and New Zealand College of Obstetricians and Gynaecologists; RCT = randomised control trial.
For details of numbered references see original paper.
(Source: Roome et al., 2016)

The most comprehensive home birth clinical outcomes research is from the Dutch context with its integrated and traditionally strong home birth and research culture. Almost all of this research to date has found no differences in maternal or perinatal mortality between home and hospital birth for 'low risk' women (Blix et al., 2012; de Jonge et al., 2009, 2013, 2015; van der Kooy et al., 2017). The only exception is one article reporting a higher perinatal mortality rate for home birth in the Netherlands (Evers et al., 2010). However, de Jonge argues that this later research has not appropriately used the Dutch birth registry data (de Jonge et al., 2017).

Home birth options for women in Australia have become increasingly complex following the changes in regulation, funding and insurance implemented in response to the Maternity Services Review (C of A, 2009). Insurance exemptions, for intrapartum care at home, have been made available to allow midwives to find a possible insurance product to cover the birth component (see AHPRA, 2021). Women who plan to give birth at home find themselves uninsured and having to pay large amounts for their care. There are currently a small number of publicly funded home-birth programs (where women do not need to pay for the care) throughout Australia and acceptance into a program is contingent on women meeting strict, low-risk medical criteria. As a result of the lack of support for home birth in Australia less than 0.3% of Australian births take place at home.

An Australian study of national home-birth outcomes showed that the clinical outcomes for the small number of women who gave birth in publicly funded programs (2005–10) were positive (Catling-Paull et al., 2013). Sassine and colleagues (2021) undertook a national study through social media to explore the characteristics, needs and experiences of women who chose to have a home birth in Australia. They found a concerning number of

Table 7.4 Summary of positions of colleges on home birth

Professional college	Year or date of statement	Position on home births	Details and justifiction
RANZCOG (Australia and New Zealand)	July 2014	Against	Unsafe: tripling in non-anomalous neonatal mortality rate Regional factors
ACM (Australia)	November 2011	For, in women at low risk	Safety, patient autonomy (importance of informed consent and the right of refusal), woman-centred care, importance of birth as a rite of passage
NZCOM (New Zealand)	No statement	No statement	N/A
ACOG (USA)	February 2011 (reaffirmed 2013)	Against, but recognise primacy of autonomy	Lack of RCTs, regional factors (large overseas cohort studies deemed inapplicable to USA health context)
ACNM (USA)	August 2011	For, in women at low risk	Autonomy, more holistic outcomes for mother and family, decreased maternal morbidity, safety, opportunity for students to study normal, undisturbed birth
RCOG and RCM (UK; combined statement)	April 2007 (valid until 2010); both organisations have since welcomed NICE guidelines on place of birth	For, in women at low risk	Lower maternal morbidity, autonomy, psychological and emotional wellbeing, lower intervention rates
SOGC (Canada)	No statement	No statement	N/A
CAM (Canada)	January 2014	For, in women at low risk	Safety (fewer obstetrical interventions with no increase in maternal or neonatal mortality or morbidity), psychological and emotional factors, autonomy

ACM = Australian College of Midwives; ACNM = American College of Nurse-Midwives; CAM = Canadian Association of Midwives; ACOG = American College of Obstetricians; NZCOM = New Zealand College of Midwives; NICE = National Institute for Health and Care Excellence; RANZCOG = Royal Australian and New Zealand College of Obstetricians and Gynaecologists; RCM = Royal College of Midwives; RCT = randomised control trial; SOGC = Society of Obstetricians and Gynaecologists of Canada. (Source: Roome et al., 2016)

women who experienced their hospital birth as traumatic, and reported experiencing a lack of informed consent, and coercion in the hospital setting. Clearly there is a need for Australia to review its standing of planned out-of-hospital birth. Sassine et al. 2021 concluded that there should be better access to midwifery continuity of care, and home-like birth environments and that this could significantly prevent women at higher risk of complications from disengaging with the mainstream maternity system. They said, 'Government support for home birth in the form of Medicare funding would improve access to midwife-attended home birth for many women who currently cannot afford it. A workable solution to the lack of insurance for intrapartum care at home, which includes women with risk factors, is also desperately needed' (Sassine et al., 2021, p. 403).

Although researchers keep adding to the ever-expanding collection of evidence, this research has continued to be steadfastly ignored in Australia for the past thirty years with no apparent good reason for doing so. The most recent Australian research using linked population data published in 2019 examined the clinical outcomes of women with relatively uncomplicated pregnancies

giving birth to a singleton baby between 37 and 41 weeks between 2000 and 2012. The researchers found that in relation to the place of birth, compared with planned hospital births, the odds of normal labour and birth were over twice as high in planned birth centre births (adjusted OR (AOR) 2.72; 99% CI 2.63 to 2.81) and nearly six times as high in planned home births (AOR 5.91; 99% CI 5.15 to 6.78). There were no statistically significant differences in the proportion of intrapartum stillbirths, early or late neonatal deaths between the three planned places of birth (Homer et al., 2019). The Birthplace England Collaboration research reported no difference in the overall adjusted composite perinatal outcome between home, PMUs and tertiary hospitals; it reported poorer composite perinatal outcomes for women having their first baby at home than those giving birth at a freestanding or alongside unit, but better outcomes for women having subsequent babies at home (Hollowell et al., 2011). Tables 7.5 and 7.6 show the outcomes of the Birthplace in England collaboration results according to whether women were having a first baby (Table 7.5) or a second or subsequent birth (Table 7.6). These are different outcomes from the much larger

Table 7.5 Spontaneous vaginal birth, transfer to an obstetric unit, and obstetric interventions according to planned place of birth[a]: low-risk nulliparous women

Outcome	Planned place of birth			
	Home	Freestanding midwifery unit	Alongside midwifery unit	Obstetric unit
Spontaneous vaginal birth	794[b]	813	765	688[b]
Transfer to an obstetric unit	450[b]	363	402	10[c]
Regional analgesia (epidural or spinal)[d]	218[b]	200	240	349[b]
Episiotomy	165[b]	165	216	242[b]
Caesarean birth	80[b]	69	76	121
Instrumental birth (forceps or ventouse)	126[b]	118	159	191[b]
Blood transfusion	12	8	11	16

[a]Figures are instances (n) per 1000 multiparous women giving birth.
[b]Figures from Birthplace in England Collaborative Group (2011) and Blix et al. (2012) (all other figures from Birthplace in England Collaborative Group (2011) only).
[c]Estimated transfer rate from one obstetric unit to a different one owing to lack of capacity or expertise.
[d]The Birthplace in England Collaborative Group (2011) reported spinal or epidural analgesia and Blix et al. (2012) reported epidural analgesia.
(Reproduced from Nunes VD, Gholitabar M, Sims JM, Bewley S. Intrapartum care of healthy women and their babies: summary of updated NICE guidance. On behalf of the NICE Guideline Development Group. *BMJ*. 2014;349:g6886, with permission from BMJ Publishing Group Ltd)

Table 7.6 Spontaneous vaginal birth, transfer to an obstetric unit, and obstetric interventions according to planned place of birth[a]: low-risk multiparous women

Outcome	Planned place of birth			
	Home	Freestanding midwifery unit	Alongside midwifery unit	Obstetric unit
Spontaneous vaginal birth	984[b]	980	967	927[b]
Transfer to an obstetric unit	115[b]	94	125	10[c]
Regional analgesia (epidural or spinal)[d]	28[b]	40	60	121[b]
Episiotomy	15[b]	23	35	56[b]
Caesarean birth	7[b]	8	10	35[b]
Instrumental birth (forceps or ventouse)	9[b]	12	23	38[b]
Blood transfusion	4	4	5	8

[a]Figures are instances (n) per 1000 multiparous women giving birth.
[b]Data from Birthplace in England Collaborative Group (2011) and Blix et al. (2012) (all other data from Birthplace in England Collaborative Group (2011) only).
[c]Estimated transfer rate from an obstetric unit to a different obstetric unit owing to lack of capacity or expertise.
[d]The Birthplace in England Collaborative Group (2011) reported spinal or epidural analgesia and Blix et al. (2012) reported epidural analgesia.[4]
(Reproduced from Nunes VD, Gholitabar M, Sims JM, Bewley S. Intrapartum care of healthy women and their babies: summary of updated NICE guidance. On behalf of the NICE Guideline Development Group. *BMJ*. 2014;349:g6886, with permission from BMJ Publishing Group Ltd)

Dutch studies, and a similar-sized Canadian study, possibly due to factors such as the organisation of the English maternity system and the home birth service in most Trusts, rather than something inherent in women having their first baby.

The USA, with its non-integrated maternity system, also reported higher rates of perinatal mortality than in other contexts and for primiparous women compared with multiparous women giving birth at home (Cheyney et al., 2014). Indeed, Cheyney et al. (2014) propose that 'the lack of integration across birth settings ... contributes to intrapartum mortality due to delays in timely transfer related to fear of reprisal and / or because some women with higher risk pregnancies still choose home birth because there are fewer options that support normal physiologic birth available' (p. 25). Overall, the contemporary research on the clinical outcomes of well (low-risk) women giving birth at home, with registered midwives, in an integrated maternity system with ready access to specialist care if needed, indicates that it is safe, and probably safer than birth in a hospital (See Tables 7.5 and 7.6).

The published studies all strongly support the findings of the comprehensive UK study *Where to be Born?*, which concluded that, given the current state of knowledge, we don't have the evidence to support claims that the safest policy is for all women to give birth in hospital (Macfarlane et al., 2000). Despite the evidence to the contrary, the rhetoric that began over 100 years ago persists, and society still views birth at home (everywhere except the Netherlands and New Zealand) as a poor choice. Indeed, Tew (1995) identified that data had been deliberately misinterpreted in UK studies between 1958 and 1970 to support the claim that 'the family home is the most dangerous place for birth' (p. 29). Tew stated that an impartial observer could clearly see that the perinatal mortality rate was higher in hospitals, yet this fact was distorted in reports of the time. Obstetricians throughout the world used the false interpretation of these statistics to influence the future development of maternity services.

A recent study by McLachlan et al. (2016) in Australia exploring midwives' and doctors' views and experiences of publicly funded home-birthing models found that:

midwife respondents were very supportive of publicly-funded home birth for women with most believing there was consumer demand for the program. Most also believed the program was safe for women and infants. Responding doctors had far more mixed views, with half not supportive of publicly-funded home birth and over one third not convinced of its safety.
(McLachlan et al., 2016, p. 29)

Vedam et al. (2014) found similar differences in professional attitudes towards home birth again divided along disciplinary lines, with midwives more likely to be supportive of planned home birth, and medical staff more likely to view home birth as unsafe.

REFLECTIVE THINKING EXERCISE

Imagine that you are a midwife who cares for women wherever they want to give birth (indeed, this might be a reality for many midwives). Some women want to be at home, others want to be at the small, local birth unit, and still others want to be in the hospital. Ask yourself the following questions.

1. How do I feel about supporting women in each of these locations?
2. Are the feelings different depending on the location?
3. Where do these feelings come from?
4. How do I react when a woman asks me to support her in planning a home birth?
5. How do others react to her decision for a home birth?
6. Why is this so?
7. How inconvenient / uncomfortable / scary is it for me to have to travel to the woman's home? Do I have to support her choice?
8. How inconvenient is it for me to have to travel to the birth centre rather than the hospital?
9. Do we (women and midwives) have any real choices of where to birth in our region?
   a. Is there a need to change anything?
   b. How can I do that?
   c. Who will help me?

Summary

The international evidence published to date is that well women who plan to give birth in a tertiary maternity hospital are more likely to suffer physical problems in the form of peripartum morbidity, such as episiotomy and caesarean section, than those who plan to give birth at home, or in a PMU—whether alongside or freestanding. The notion that the 'interventions' undertaken at the tertiary hospital on well women are either protecting the wellbeing of women or 'saving babies' is not supported by the evidence from comparable contexts. Given the complexity of birth it is difficult to identify causal factors for the increased rate of 'interventions' and their associated morbidities in hospital when compared to home or primary facilities. Arguably, it is not possible to undertake a comprehensive and sufficiently powered randomised study to establish the relative physical safety of home, primary units and tertiary hospital units for well women at 'low risk' of complications. Birthplace research is difficult and complex, with several potential biases and confounding factors. The commonly held anecdotal association of hospitalisation and reduced mortality and morbidity rates has never been supported by evidence. Despite this, the supposition of 'safety' of hospital birth for *all* women remains, arguably as a result of the power of obstetrics and its hold on 'authoritative knowledge' (Goer, 2016). Hospital has become the cultural 'gold standard' by default.

While it is possible that rare and severe incidents might happen at a PMU that might have been prevented or mitigated if the woman was at a tertiary hospital, it is also possible that as many iatrogenic or nosocomial rare and severe incidents happen at a tertiary maternity hospital. Childbearing women and their families are concerned that their 'safety' is optimised and harm minimised; maternity care providers, healthcare funders and planners share these concerns. Even using the narrow outcome measure of physical 'safety' or wellbeing the existing evidence does not support hospitals as safer places for well women to give birth, in the context of professional skilled caregivers, effective referral and transfer systems, and access to specialist facilities and services for those in need of them. Goer (2016) argues that the answer to the question 'Is hospital birth safe for low-risk women?' is 'No'.

THE RETURN OF A FAMILIAR CAREGIVER

The second component of the care package to be lost in the move from home to hospital was the familiar caregiver and the continuous support she provided (Fig. 7.2). This has been addressed through calls for increased continuity of care, which midwives have provided, first in experimental models tested in large randomised controlled trials in Australia (McLachlan et al., 2012; Tracy et al., 2013), and in New Zealand following the changes to the Nurses Act in 1990 leading to midwifery autonomy.

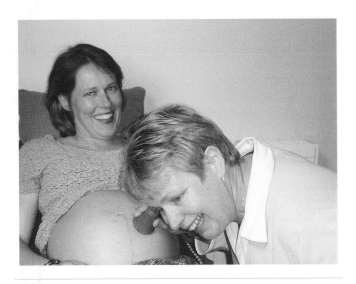

FIGURE 7.2 Auscultation of baby's heart with Pinard stethoscope
(Reproduced with the permission of the New Zealand College of Midwives)

There now exists overwhelming evidence, from nearly 15 randomised controlled trials involving 17,674 women conducted in Australia, Canada, Sweden, Hong Kong, the United Kingdom, Scotland and the United States that midwife-led continuity models of care during childbirth should be the norm, rather than the exception (Sandall et al., 2016). It is clear that any maternity care system that is not founded on this model of care places women at increased risk of interventions such as epidural analgesia and operative birth by forceps, vacuum extraction or caesarean section. Although the short-term effects of such procedures are well documented, it is becoming increasingly apparent that these are all major interventions with potential for unanticipated, adverse, long-term physical and behavioural effects on both mothers and babies. Some effects may be permanent.

The financial costs of the long-term consequences of intervention in childbirth have received less scrutiny, but even the increased costs of the procedures themselves must lead healthcare planners to consider more carefully the models of care to which women are subjected (Roberts et al., 2000; Tracy & Tracy, 2003; Tracy et al., 2013, 2014). These findings cannot be ignored, and many maternity care systems have focused attention on ways and means of increasing opportunities for women to experience continuity of midwifery care with varying degrees of success.

However, although continuous labour support is a form of maternity care that should be available for all women, it is clearly not sufficient in and of itself to promote normal birth. In relation to place of birth, we will consider what it is about continuity of care and continuous labour support that influences outcomes, by exploring the concept of the fear cascade and the physiology of birth (Foureur, 2008; Rowley, 1998). We will also examine the New Zealand maternity care system, which has successfully embraced a model of care that provides continuous labour support for all women. While New Zealand maternity data shows that women still experience relatively high rates of intervention, the rate is notably less than in other Western countries, including Australia (see Ch. 3) (Ministry of Health, 2017b).

WHAT IS A 'NORMAL BIRTH'?

Continuous labour support aims to decrease intervention in childbirth and thereby increase the numbers of women who experience 'normal' birth. Much debate has arisen around the concept of 'normal' birth, and for the purposes of this chapter it is defined as follows: labour occurs at term, is spontaneous in onset, and there is no requirement for augmentation or analgesia; the birth occurs spontaneously, vaginally, and the mother and baby are healthy. Some authors have estimated that, in the 21st century, less than one-third of women in 'developed' countries will be enabled to give birth as nature intended (Sandall, 2004). Many women are fearful of the process and shocked by their experiences. Rates of intervention vary between and within countries, between different locations for birth (hospital, birth centre and home), and between different models of maternity care in the same settings (public and private, fragmented care and continuity of care) (see Table 7.7).

Very few trials and even fewer national data collection systems report birth outcomes in terms of the numbers of women who experience normal birth. Therefore the extent (or disappearance) of normal birth has been unintentionally hidden from our gaze until very recently.

'Continuity of care' versus 'continuous labour support'

Continuity of care describes the actual provision of care by the same caregiver or small group of caregivers throughout pregnancy, during labour and birth, and in the postnatal period. This model usually implies, but may not always include, continuous one-to-one support throughout labour. Continuous labour support describes the process of one-to-one supportive care from a companion throughout labour (Homer et al., 2008). It is apparent from at least one systematic review that continuous labour support provided by a non-hospital caregiver is more effective at reducing interventions than support provided by members of the hospital staff (Hodnett et al., 2005). This raises interesting questions as to why the impact of continuous labour support differs depending on the type of caregiver. Hodnett & colleagues (2005) propose that the difference results from the ability of non-hospital caregivers to give greater attention to the mother's needs, since such companions are not distracted by the diverse responsibilities of hospital employees and organisational issues such as shift changes and staff shortages. We propose that this explanation is too simplistic. If the proposal of Hodnett et al. (2005) were valid,

Table 7.7 Birth outcomes for low-risk first-time mothers who received caseload midwifery care at a major tertiary teaching hospital (RHW) in Sydney, 2014[a]

Outcome	Midwifery group practice		Routine (all other public models)		Private obstetric care	
	$n = 482$	(95% CI)	$n = 647$	(95% CI)	$n = 250$	(95% CI)
Spontaneous onset	58.5	(54.1–62.9)	32.0	(28.4–35.6)	28.0	(22.4–33.6)
C/S for singleton births	15.4	(12.1–18.6)	19.5	(16.4–22.5)	17.6	(12.9–22.3)
Elective C/S	1.6	(0.5–2.8)	5.3	(3.5–6.9)	17.2	(12.5–21.9)
Instrumental	24.5	(20.6–28.3)	27.0	(23.6–30.5)	34.4	(28.5–40.3)
Vaginal birth	58.5	(54.1–62.9)	48.2	(44.3–52.1)	30.8	(25.1–36.5)

[a]Rates per 100 women.
CI = confidence interval; C/S = caesarean section; RHW = Royal Hospital for Women, Sydney.
(Source: Tracy et al., 2014)

we could expect to find low rates of intervention in maternity care systems where both continuity of care and continuous one-to-one support throughout labour from non-hospital caregivers was the norm.

REFLECTIVE THINKING EXERCISE

Consider the factors that contribute to intervention intrapartum. Is there research evidence to support these interventions? How can midwives who provide continuity of care reduce the rate of interventions that occur in their practice? How can midwives who provide only intrapartum care reduce the interventions for the women they care for?

CRITICAL THINKING EXERCISE

1. Summarise the findings of research evidence in relation to place of birth to enable you to share this information with clients.

2. Compile a list of conditions (maternal and fetal) that warrant intrapartum care in a secondary / tertiary hospital.

3. Compile a guideline that shows which women could be suitable for home birth or birth-centre (primary unit) birth.

4. Review research evidence in relation to prolonged pregnancy and induction of labour. Reflect on induction of labour statistics and whether induction is congruent with research evidence.

5. Review the research evidence in relation to electronic fetal monitoring including admission cardiotocograph. Is electronic fetal monitoring used judiciously in your setting?

6. Apply critical thinking as to how midwives can enhance their own belief about physiological birth and convey this belief to the women in their care.

BIRTH SPACE

In a typical hospital labour ward the bed is the central piece of furniture and in spite of its pastel colours the implication is that the woman will use the bed to give birth. Within this birth space there is usually a chair, a cupboard, a television and sometimes a crib. These create a domestic setting. Behind the bed, hidden by curtains or movable panels, or in a storage space next to the room, is the traditionally necessary technological equipment to meet the needs of medical intervention if the need should arise. The organisation of the entire setting is a function of the patterns of movement that occur during medical intervention (Lepori, 1994; see Box 7.6).

Healthcare design has mostly focused on functional service delivery, though there is increasing evidence pointing to the role of hospital design on healthcare outcomes (Ulrich et al., 2008). Aspects of design that have been found to impact outcomes in hospital settings include: natural light and sunshine, design features that limit noise, soft floor furnishings and windows exposing views of natural landscapes. These aspects have a particular impact on the levels of stress and anxiety experienced not only by patients within these settings but also by staff. We have described how labour and birth involve a complex interplay of hormonal, emotional and physiological factors and it is easy to see how environments that increase stress, anxiety and fear can change a labouring woman's neurohormonal constitution. The environment can also direct a woman's activity in labour, thereby impacting on the physiology of labour and birth at the biomechanical level. A birth environment that features a bed and offers little other space or support for an active labour encourages a passive birth. Labour progress in this situation may not be optimised because the woman is not benefiting from the pressure that the fetal head exerts on the cervix when the woman is in an upright position or from the widening of the pelvic diameters that can be achieved when the woman is able to squat, for example, in the second stage of labour. Fig. 7.3 shows the range of body postures the ideal birth space supports.

Box 7.6   Extracts from Italian architect Bianca Lepori on spatial requirements for an active birth

Spatial requirements that support active participation of women in the birth

A place designed for childbirth should nowadays guarantee the security offered by technology without denying freedom of expression to the woman …

… From the woman's point of view it seems that in order to improve birth environments it is not necessary to return to a home atmosphere, but rather to create a freer atmosphere … women tend to individuate territory in a protected empty space, sheltered by low furnishings where they solidly work with gravity, their feet firmly on the floor, while hanging, kneeling, holding themselves in order for the pelvic floor to relax and allow birth to take place.

If left to their own choice women identify a centered territory that is not programmed, not defined by external authorities, seldom pre-arranged, always spontaneously determined during delivery and birth as a focus of action and concentration …the natural path is a spiral leading toward the centre of a woman's concentration and ability to and therefore towards her own control and choice.[1]

Women who can give birth naturally do not need particular colours, nor beautiful furniture that reminds them of their homes: they need a space in which to express themselves, in which to wait; they need the space-time to let it happen. The only thing they really need is not to be forced into a particular position. Even pain dissolves with movement; pain killers are a consequence of stillness.[2]

(Lepori, 1994, pp. 83–4)

(Sources:
[1]Bianca Lepori (1994). Freedom of movement in birth places. *Children's Environments;* 11(2):81–7
[2]Bianca Lepori (1992). *La Nascita e i Suoi Luoghi.* Como, Italy: RED Edizioni.)

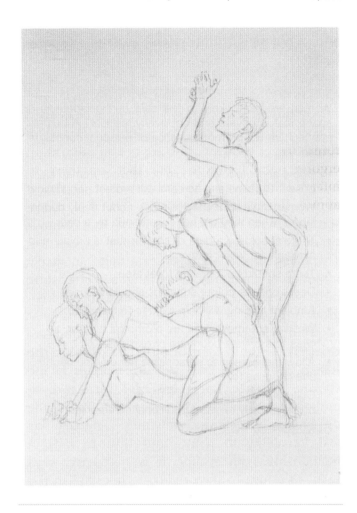

FIGURE 7.3 Range of body postures to be supported
(Source: Bianca Lepori, 1994, Freedom of movement in birth places)

What is the ideal environment for maximising the potential for normal birth? Many would argue that home is the ideal environment, though, given that most women plan to give birth in hospital settings, it is important that we give some serious consideration to the design of hospital or primary maternity facilities.

Drawing on published research and interviews with expert midwives, researchers Foureur et al. (2010a) have developed a tool to measure the optimality of birth environments: the Birth Unit Design Spatial Evaluation Tool. Four domains are canvassed in the tool: characteristics affecting the fear cascade, facility characteristics, the aesthetic aspects of the unit, and the essential support elements for women and families. Factors included in the fear cascade include the conspicuousness of medical equipment and the degree to which a domestic rather than a medical ambiance prevails. Facility characteristics include things like access to a bath and other props that support an active labour and birth. Aesthetics include the colours, textures, views and artwork, and support elements include access to food and drinks, and hospitality for her supporters. The authors hypothesise that there is a relationship between birth unit design and a safe and satisfying birth experience (Foureur et al., 2010b). When a woman feels physically and emotionally comfortable in an aesthetically pleasing environment, when the environment works to promote relaxation rather than anxiety, when she is invited to be active and when she knows that her supporters are accommodated, the opportunity for normal birth is maximised (Box 7.7). The delicate interplay of hormones and biomechanics responsible for labour and birth has been described as a 'dance'; they must work in concert rather than against one another to bring about normal labour and birth, and environment is just one of the factors that mediate this 'dance' (Walsh, 2007, p. 34).

Box 7.7   Characteristics of a space in which women feel safe and relaxed during labour and birth

Women are most likely to feel safe during labour in a space that is private and not overly 'clinical'. A homely atmosphere will promote a sense of personal control. In particular:

- Doors and windows should not leave a woman exposed. Curtains and screens will protect her privacy.
- Women are encouraged to move about freely during labour when they are not constrained by a bed.
- There should be a bath or shower that is private and available for water immersion.
- There should be a private toilet area.
- Deep, opaque colour schemes should be used.
- Ambient lighting will help women to feel calm.
- Walking and movement are promoted by easy access to a private courtyard or gardens.
- Allow the woman to personalise her environment if she chooses to.
- Culturally safe birth spaces are important for supporting locally relevant traditional ceremonies.

(Based on Jenkinson et al., 2014)

It is not only women who are impacted by the environment. In a study by Davis and Walker (2010) caseload midwives in New Zealand reported that the hospital environment also engendered fear in them. One midwife commented, 'I think there is more fear, it's sort of sucked into the walls or something' (p. 386). For another midwife, it was the predominance of medical equipment that focused her attention on risk:

The big resuscitation tray for the baby … It's all aimed at when things go wrong and even though you try … it reinforces that things can go wrong, doesn't it. And it does for the woman, for her family and for me … You're just … aware that, it sort of, I don't know, it introduces fear in the midwife and the woman.

When comparing their practice in different environments, midwives reported that they practised differently in the hospital setting. They had a lower threshold for referral to medical practitioners in this environment and were less likely to feel comfortable with situations that would not have concerned them at home or in a birth centre or PMU (for example, a labour that slows for a period of time). We will explore the impact of environment on midwives further in the next section of this chapter.

Focusing on the childbearing woman again, continuity of care is another strategy that aims to facilitate normal birth by addressing the fear cascade. Continuous one-to-one support in labour provides an opportunity to ensure that labour is undisturbed and the fear cascade is not initiated (Buckley, 2003).

The influence of the birth room on the promotion of a normal physiological childbirth

In a study exploring midwives experiences of how the birthing room affects them in their work to promote a normal physiological birth, Andrén et al. (2021) found that birth rooms reflect four opposing constituents. Table 7.8 sets out the components of the birth space that contribute to this phenomenon of either promoting a pathogenic-oriented care approach or one that protects the mother from disturbing elements both inside and outside the room. (See also Fig. 7.4.)

Three basic needs for the mother and her new baby

In his chapter relating to birth territory, Michel Odent begins by outlining the physiological context within which birth occurs. In balancing the antagonism between adrenaline and oxytocin, a labouring woman needs to feel secure, without feeling observed, in a warm enough place, and to be protected against any sort of neocortical stimulation (language, light, lack of privacy, being aware of possible danger) (Odent, 2008, p. 131) (Box 7.8).

Research has shown that the environment can have a very important role to play in preventing the inhibitory effects of neocortical activity on the process of giving birth. Ideally the neocortex remains unstimulated so that the hypothalamus and the pituitary gland can release their hormones that facilitate labour. For example, it is known that mammals do not release oxytocin in the presence of high levels of adrenaline.

Odent (2008) proposes three basic necessities that should be incorporated into birth spaces to protect women from neocortical activity in a bid to promote an ideal hormonal balance during labour and birth.

1. *Language and silence*: Communicating with the labouring woman stimulates her brain to respond. Therefore, remaining silent and unobtrusive, asking only necessary questions and keeping a low profile help the woman to remain in a state of deep hormonal balance.
2. *Bright lights*: Brain activity (neocortical stimulation) can be enhanced by visual stimulation. Keeping the light low will allow the woman to position herself spontaneously for labour and prevent overactive responses that keep her from being 'connected' to her labouring body.
3. *Feeling observed and the need for privacy*: Arousal occurs when a woman feels she is being observed. This explains the mammalian behaviour to find a private secluded place to give birth.
   See Fig. 7.5.

Table 7.8 How the birth room affects midwives' work to promote a normal physiological birth

Room constituents	Salutogenic-oriented maternity care emphasises that women are continuously moving between the two endpoints dis-ease and ease/health.	Pathogenic-oriented maternity care classifies women as 'healthy or not' (at a certain level of risk).
CONSTITUENT	PRIVATE room	PUBLIC room
	• Monitor progress in room	• CTG monitors on public display in the office
	• Door closed	• Door open
	• Bathtub (in room)	• Bathtub (elsewhere)
	• No risk of being seen/heard through a window	• Observe what is going on outside the window
CONSTITUENT	HOME-LIKE room	HOSPITAL-LIKE room
	• Lighting can be dimmed, creates cosy, calm, and enclosing atmosphere	• Fluorescent lamps in the ceiling giving a strong light
	• Earthy wall colours/plants	• White sterile walls
	• Bed is covered with pretty duvet covers to make it more inviting	• Bed with a sheet and a plastic protective mat
	• Promotes nesting and taking possession of the room	• Medical equipment on view indicates that giving birth is a risky event
CONSTITUENT	Room PROMOTING ACTIVITY	Room PROMOTING PASSIVITY
	• Sufficient floorspace to move around with visible options for movement such as balls, walking trays, yoga mats, or a large bathtub inside the room	• Bed is the main feature and midwives work around it • Medical equipment, such as the CTG device, the nitrous oxide tubes, drip stands and infusion pumps, are placed around the head end of the bed
CONSTITUENT	Room promoting the midwife's PRESENCE	Room promoting the midwife's ABSENCE
	• Room provides space for the midwife to 'be'	• Midwives can read CTG graph sitting in the coffee room
	• Care arranged for one midwife per mother giving birth	• Alarm systems ring and disturb the midwives indicating others' needs in the wider labour ward
	• Midwives work allows them to give a continuous presence	• Fragmented workload with more than one woman to care for

Source: Derived from research published by Andrén et al. (2021)

REFLECTIVE THINKING EXERCISE

Take a careful look at the birth spaces in your local unit and ask yourself the following questions.

1. Can women labour undisturbed in this environment?
2. How can I ensure that no one disturbs the woman unnecessarily?
3. Am I disturbing her by talking too much?
4. Is there a sign on the door asking people to knock and wait for a reply if they want to come in?
5. Do unknown staff members walk in unannounced?
6. Are there locks on the door?
7. Can we hear the woman next door giving birth?
8. How private is the space?
9. Who 'owns' the space when a woman is in labour and giving birth there?
10. Is the woman free to move around—to sit, stand, walk, squat, lean, lie down?
11. Are there en suite facilities for her to shower or use a bath during labour or birth?
12. Where is the bed located and what kind of bed is it?
13. Is there a space for her family support people?
14. How welcoming is it for them?
15. Is food and drink available?
    a. Is there a need to change anything?
    b. How can I do that?
    c. Who will help me?

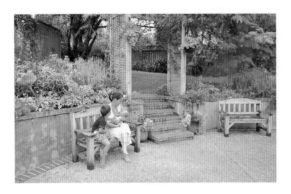

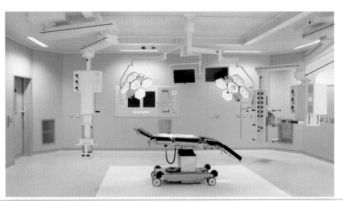

FIGURE 7.4 Courtyard garden at the Helensville Birth Centre, NZ, providing a private, calming, natural environment.
(Source: Helensville Birthing Centre. Helensville Birthing Centre. http://www.helensvillebc.co.nz/)

Box 7.8   Environmental factors that disturb the balance between adrenaline and oxytocin in labour

Oxytocin is a small peptide consisting of only nine amino acids and is produced in neurons in two nuclei within the hypothalamus—the paraventricular nucleus and the supraoptic nucleus. Some of the neurons project to the posterior pituitary, from where oxytocin is released into the circulation to exert its well-known contractile effects on uterine muscles during labour and on myoepithelial cells during breastfeeding.

Human beings are different from other mammals where childbirth is concerned, because they have developed to an extreme degree the part of the brain called the neocortex—the brain of the intellect. An involuntary process such as birth can be inhibited by the thinking brain. A labouring woman needs to be protected against neocortical stimulation. A silent midwife is important because language is the main stimulant of the neocortex. When we feel observed we have a tendency to observe ourselves, thus stimulating the neocortex.

In spite of medical science accepting that natural oxytocin is needed to initiate and maintain labour, the birth systems in the developed world do not help it to flow. Oxytocin requires a dark, quiet, non-threatening environment to flow, but birth units tend to be brightly lit and noisy with unknown people coming in and out of a room, often trying to intervene.

The main lesson of modern physiology is that parturition is an involuntary process related to the activity of archaic brain structures. One cannot help an involuntary process, but certain situations can inhibit it. This leads to the realisation that labouring women do not need direct, active help. They mostly need protection against any factor that might increase the level of adrenaline or stimulate the neocortex.

(Source: Michel Odent (2004) Knitting midwives for drugless childbirth? *Midwifery Today*. pp. 21–2; www.midwiferytoday.com)

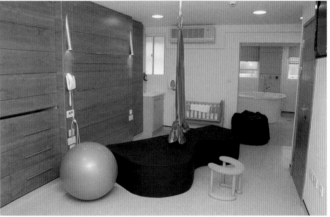

FIGURE 7.5 Comparing a space for observation and intervention (top) with a space for private birth (below)
(Sources: (above) iStockphoto/baranozdemir; (below) iStockphoto/thelinke)

BELIEF IN BIRTH AS A NORMAL PHYSIOLOGICAL PROCESS

Not only is the birth environment an important factor impacting on childbearing women, it also exerts a powerful force on midwives. A study conducted by Marion Hunter in New Zealand provides important insights into the power of the place of birth to influence the midwife's belief in birth as a normal physiological process (Hunter, 2000, 2003). In a series of in-depth interviews conducted with caseload midwives who cared for women in both large (secondary/tertiary) and small (primary) maternity facilities, Hunter discovered that the midwives overwhelmingly preferred to provide labour care in small maternity units, where they felt they were more able to attend to women, as opposed to attending to machines, and where they had developed additional midwifery skills. They described this as practising 'real midwifery'. In the small unit, the midwives felt truly autonomous, able to take time to let labour unfold rather than rush a woman along as if on a conveyor belt, able to give the woman time to settle into her labour before intruding with a vaginal examination (VE) to assess progress, and more able to tolerate the woman making noise without fear that they would be regarded as a less-than-competent midwife. Importantly, the midwives revealed how the additional responsibility of being alone in the small unit caused them to reflect carefully on their skills and ability to manage any challenge, keeping them alert and watchful. Despite the additional responsibility and feeling that they would 'carry the can' if anything went wrong, they were unshaken in their belief in the normal process of birth and had the confidence to enable the process to occur with minimal intervention. Hunter (2003) proposed that the following skills are necessary for midwives who practise in PMUs:

- the confidence to provide intrapartum care in a low-technology setting
- being comfortable with using embodied knowledge and skills to assess a woman and her baby, as opposed to using technology
- being able to let labour 'be' and not interfere unnecessarily
- the confidence to avert or manage problems that might arise
- the confidence to trust the process of labour and be flexible with respect to time
- being willing to employ other options to manage pain, without access to epidurals
- being solely responsible for outcomes without access to onsite specialist assistance
- being a midwife who enjoys practising 'real midwifery'.

'Real midwifery' was articulated by one of the participants, named Elizabeth, as follows (Hunter, 2003, p. 241):

> At [the small maternity unit] it's like real midwifery in a way, because you're not interfering ... When you are using the synto and the epidural, a lot of it's taken away from the woman and, in a lot of respects, probably taken away from you a little bit as well.
>
> ...I think with real midwifery, a lot of it is not doing, in a way letting it happen, being there, but you're still there and you still want to make sure that things are happening as they should ... And I think real midwifery can be not being that overpowering person there.

Midwives in PMUs need to have a belief in normal birth and the skills to be unobtrusive while still ensuring that labour is progressing normally. Women also need to believe that they are able to labour and give birth in a primary facility (Lundgren, 2005). Antenatal visits and childbirth education classes held at primary units foster women's confidence and enhance their commitment to labouring in a primary facility. In the study by Hunter (2000, 2003), the midwives endeavoured to influence women with regard to place of birth, as evidenced by the following words from one of the participants:

> With first-time mums when they come to me, we talk about who has actually influenced them into thinking they need to be at a large hospital. We talk about the statistics that show women are actually safer in a smaller hospital, and a good percentage of them will end up coming to the smaller hospital.
>
> (Rosemary, in Hunter, 2000 [unpublished thesis])

Rosemary could be referring to a number of studies, including a landmark study undertaken by Rosenblatt and colleagues (1985), which showed that New Zealand women had good outcomes in primary facilities and that such facilities had an important place within a population that is dispersed throughout urban and remote rural areas. Tracy et al. (2006) reinforced findings of positive outcomes in smaller units for primiparous and multiparous women in Australia. Data from over 330,000 low-risk women was analysed in relation to outcomes after the establishment of labour. The findings revealed that adverse outcomes were not associated with birth centres and hospitals with low numbers of birth per annum.

RESEARCH ACTIVITY

Access a map of the region where you reside and plot the location of birthing units, secondary and tertiary hospitals. Find out the home-birth statistics for your region. If you reside and practise in an urban area, compare your region with a remote region within your country. Compare the midwifery skills required by midwives working in tertiary hospitals to those skills required by midwives practising in remote rural regions.

Being confident to provide intrapartum care in a low-technology setting

Most of the participants interviewed in Hunter's study (2000, 2003) stated that they were proficient with the technology in the large hospital. Yet they preferred practising in primary units, where there is low use of technology. Participant Elizabeth emphasised this point:

> The technology has got its place. I can go from having a woman on a Syntocinon® infusion and an epidural pump, to the next day, at the small unit, and the woman is squatting in the corner, or whatever, and it is totally different.
>
> (Hunter, 2000 [unpublished thesis])

For the midwife, being hands-off and just being there for the woman is often more challenging than being constantly busy attending to equipment and machines.

Being confident to avert or manage problems that might arise, and being solely responsible for outcomes without access to onsite specialist assistance

Situations arise in the course of midwifery practice where the midwife must promptly avert or manage problems. Midwives carry the memories of emergency occasions with them in their subconscious or conscious minds. Some memories are of positive outcomes, whereas other memories represent the trauma thrust upon the woman and the midwife. It is important that practice is not coloured by a problem focus. However, our memory tends to occlude the numerous occasions when we have driven our cars without incident, yet we vividly recall the one time that we had an accident. Midwives admitted that the responsibility for outcomes was greater when they practised intrapartum care in freestanding PMUs. It could take hours before the woman was transferred via ambulance to the large hospital and assessed by a specialist obstetrician. In the interlude, it is the midwife who assesses the emergency situation, provides interim care and organises the urgent transfer to the large hospital.

Midwives stressed the need to be aware and alert, and to react in a timely manner in order to provide intrapartum care safely within primary units. A midwife in a primary unit has to know what to do immediately—there are no doctors to respond to an emergency bell.

The following participant gives an example of responding to an emergency situation:

> I had a postpartum haemorrhage the other night of 1000 mL in the small unit. I gave intramuscular syntometrine and intravenous Syntocinon® and I ended up putting up a drip. I knew the placenta was complete and knew the uterus wasn't contracting well. Her pulse didn't accelerate, her blood pressure never wavered, the blood had clotted; so she was able to stay there. So you just do what you would do. You don't wait and see.
>
> (Mary, in Hunter, 2000 [unpublished thesis])

Mary's assessment skills are evident in the scenario above. She had checked the placenta thoroughly and thus ruled out retained products. The woman had been administered two oxytocic drugs—intravenous Syntocinon® ensures rapid uterine contractility and intramuscular syntometrine is used to obtain a longer-acting contraction of the uterus. Mary then inserted an intravenous line to administer fluids and to provide access for an ongoing Syntocinon® infusion. She did not waste precious minutes trying to insert the intravenous line initially. A tourniquet can be applied to give immediate intravenous access for a slow bolus of Syntocinon® 5 IU administration. The woman's pulse did not accelerate and, hence, Mary was reassured that the woman was not becoming hypovolaemic and shocked.

⚲ CLINICAL POINT

Options re: place of birth

When undertaking a birth plan with Shay, I revisited that she was happy to birth in a primary unit. I explained that studies have shown good outcomes for low-risk women in primary units and home birth. Shay had read adverse publicity about primary units in the media recently, including statements from the Royal Australian and New Zealand College of Obstetricians and Gynaecologists (RANZCOG, 2017) stating that birth was not as safe in primary units. I asked Shay if she felt frightened by this publicity and if this might affect her ability to labour

within the primary unit. She responded with her opinion: 'To have an obstetrician present at every birth would be like having a vet present every time a cow calved.' She said that would be 'ridiculous'. She commented that women needed to help themselves in order to labour well by changing positions and walking around. Shay's belief in physiological birth reinforced my belief and helped to cement working in partnership. Several weeks later, Shay had a beautiful water birth and was matter-of-fact about her ability to birth physiologically as if this was an everyday occurrence.

REFLECTIVE THINKING EXERCISE

Think about the hospital labour ward with which you are most familiar and imagine that you are greeting a woman in early labour who has never been there before. Ask yourself the following questions.

1. What makes this place familiar to me—is it the smell when I walk in the door? Do I even notice it anymore? I wonder what it smells like to this woman—safe and comforting, or antiseptic and scary?

2. I wonder what it sounds like to her. Is it noisy right now? What kinds of noises are there—clanking sounds of metal on metal and harsh surfaces, lots of voices, telephones and beeping machinery?

3. What does it look like—bright lights, busy people, paperwork on the desk, equipment lining the corridor, signs on the wall, businesslike, efficient? Is this comforting to her? I wonder how her family (who are with her) feels right now.

4. What do I see when we walk into her room together? I wonder what she sees first and what impression it has on her and how she feels.

Remember, 'environment' encompasses all five senses—sight, hearing, touch, taste and smell—and each of these senses has an impact on the mind and heart, and therefore the physiology of childbirth.

a. Is there a need to change anything?

b. How can I do that?

c. Who will help me?

WHAT INFLUENCES PLACE OF BIRTH DECISIONS?

It is unclear the extent to which the different beliefs and values held by midwives and/or women influence the clinical outcomes in respective birth environments.

Transfer

Transfer has the potential to impact on the physical and / or emotional wellbeing of those involved and on social perception of home and primary units as safe birthplaces. Recent New Zealand and Australian research has reported the reasons and timing of antenatal, labour and postnatal transfers from primary units, the time frames involved in transfers and the outcomes for those who transferred (Grigg et al., 2015; Kruske et al., 2015).

All of the research identifies one or more themes of control (which can involve participation in decision making); communication—including support, information and relationships (with midwives where there is continuity); and, in some contexts without continuity of care, experience of loss (Cheyne et al., 2012; Fox et al., 2018; Grigg et al., 2015; Overgaard et al., 2012; Patterson et al., 2015; Rowe et al., 2012).

There is also some literature reporting midwives' (or caregivers') views or experience of transfer from rural maternity units (Cheyne et al., 2012; Patterson et al., 2015) and alongside maternity units (Deery, 2010; Kuliukas et al., 2016) and home (Fox et al., 2018). A range of themes are reported, including: 'making the mind shift', 'sitting on the boundary', 'timing the transfer', 'community interest', 'the midwife's internal conversation', 'feeling out of place' and 'the midwives' need for debrief'. The 'us and them' dynamic was identified as influential for both home-birth midwives and hospital staff (midwives and obstetricians) (Fox et al., 2018).

Why, how and when women decide where to plan to give birth

How and when do women decide where to plan to give birth, and who influences that decision? Birthplace decision making occurs in, and is strongly influenced by, the social, cultural and political context within which women and their families live.

The New Zealand Evaluating Maternity Units (EMU) research project recruited well women planning to give birth in either an obstetric-led tertiary level hospital or a freestanding midwifery-led primary level maternity unit (Grigg et al., 2014). In a survey (six weeks postpartum) women were asked about the extent to which certain people and factors influenced their birthplace decision making (571 women responded—81% response rate). The women were asked first where they planned to give birth and why in open-ended questions. They were then asked to rate how much various people influenced them ('a lot', 'some', 'a bit' or 'none') in a closed 'Likert scale' question. Both groups of women perceived themselves as the main decision maker (Fig. 7.6), with their partners being the next most influential, followed by their midwives (all women had their own LMC midwife providing continuity of care).

Interestingly, almost 40% of the women planning a tertiary hospital birth rated their midwife as having no influence on their birthplace decision (Fig. 7.7). Midwives were significantly (<0.001) more influential for women planning a PMU birth (Grigg et al., 2014, p. 8).

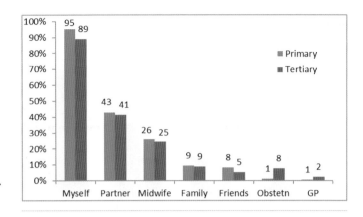

FIGURE 7.6 People who had 'a lot' of influence on women's birthplace decision
(Source: Grigg et al., 2014)

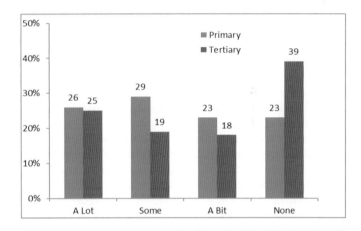

FIGURE 7.7 Influence of 'my midwife' on birthplace decision
(Source: Grigg et al., 2014)

In contexts where women genuinely have birthplace choices, their decision making appears to reflect their worldview and personal beliefs, which are strongly influenced by the sociopolitical and cultural context in which they live. Patterson et al. (2015) found women's birthplace planning 'was a complex decision ... influenced by their personal, social and cultural history'. Grigg et al. (2014) found that different views and beliefs about childbirth were illustrated by the divergent rationales given by the two groups of women. The tertiary hospital women actively and almost exclusively chose it for its specialist services / facilities. The availability of pain relief and avoidance of intrapartum transfer was only occasionally mentioned. In contrast, the PMU women often gave several reasons, with closeness to home, ease of access, avoidance of early postnatal transfer, the atmosphere or feel of the unit most frequently mentioned (Fig. 7.8). Avoidance of 'unnecessary intervention' was also important for some (Grigg et al., 2014).

The focus on influential people and factors in birthplace decision making might obscure the power of women's beliefs and values, which are often deeply held. The wider

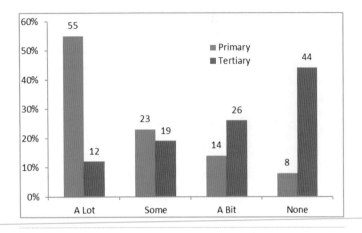

FIGURE 7.8 Influence of 'atmosphere or feel of unit' (Source: Grigg et al., 2014)

sociocultural context is also influential; it includes the organisation of maternity care, the local maternity facilities and their reputation, the local 'birth' and 'risk' cultures, the dominance of obstetrics, the status and ideology of local midwifery, and what is considered the 'norm' in their community (Bryers & van Teijlingen, 2010; Davis-Floyd, 1994; Edwards & Murphy-Lawless, 2006; Kirkham, 2003; Noseworthy et al., 2013).

Research seeking to identify enabling factors or underlying belief systems which drive women's decision making has more commonly studied women intending to give birth at home than in primary units (Catling et al., 2014; Murray-Davis et al., 2014). This has recently been explored for women planning a home birth in Australia (Catling et al., 2014) and a PMU or tertiary hospital birth in New Zealand (Grigg et al., 2015). Both studies found safety to be paramount and 'confidence' to be a prominent theme, with women planning birth at home or a PMU. Grigg et al. (2015) identified 'confidence' as the overarching concept influencing the five core themes: process, self, midwife, system and place. Amongst women who decided to give birth in a PMU, confidence is needed with respect to:

1. process—the process of birth
2. self—their ability to give birth
3. midwife—their midwife
4. system—the health system, for transfer and access to specialist facilities / staff
5. place—the intended birthplace itself.

Women who planned a primary unit birth expressed greater levels of confidence in most of the five core themes above than those who planned a tertiary hospital birth (Grigg et al., 2014).

Birth process

Women who believe that pregnancy is a normal physiological event are more likely to have confidence in the birth process. Holding this belief is a core tenet of the 'holistic' model of birth. The NZ EMU study found the women who planned hospital births did so almost exclusively for its specialist services/facilities—95% of tertiary hospital survey respondents (Grigg et al., 2014). This rationale appeared to express a strong lack of confidence in the birth process, with many women using terms such as 'if anything goes wrong', 'just in case'; and 'if needed' (Grigg et al., 2014).

Self

Earlier work by Davis-Floyd (1992) identified women in her study with a holistic viewpoint as having greater faith in the ability of their own bodies to give birth than in technology's capacity to protect them from harm.

Midwife

Almost all of the NZ EMU study participants (in both groups) expressed confidence in their midwife (Grigg et al., 2014). The context of this study is one of full (relational) continuity of care regardless of planned or eventual birthplace, which may have influenced the confidence the participants expressed in their midwife. In a context without continuity of care, British research found that women did not have confidence in midwives' skills (Lavender & Chapple, 2005). In a broader context for birth planned outside tertiary level hospitals, recent Australian research found women planning a publicly funded home birth had confidence in their midwives (Catling-Paull et al., 2011). Canadian research also found women planning either hospital or home birth with midwifery care had confidence in their midwives (Murray-Davis et al., 2014).

System

Like recent Australian research into publicly funded home birth (Catling-Paull et al., 2011), the NZ EMU study found the PMU group had confidence in the maternity system and the availability of appropriate resources and believed that transfer could occur in an acceptable, safe and timely manner, should it be required (Grigg et al., 2014). In contrast, the tertiary hospital group did not express confidence in the transfer system, believing that transfer from a (freestanding) primary unit might take too long, be unpleasant and potentially unsafe. The organisation of the maternity system and its impact on the efficacy and efficiency of referral, collaboration and transfer can influence women's experience of and confidence in it, although it is rarely studied (Skinner & Foureur, 2010).

Place

Confidence in a primary unit as a safe place to give birth is based on the understanding that a safe birth does not necessarily require hospitalisation and medical supervision. The NZ EMU study results identified several things the women value in a PMU when accounting for their birthplace decision (Grigg et al., 2014). For example, its 'low tech' or 'un-hospital-like' environment, closeness to home, calm, quiet, comfortable, 'small', relaxed environment, with water / pool for labour and birth, where staff (midwives) on duty have both time and skills to care for and support them. The significance of the environment for birth has been well documented previously

(Fahy et al., 2008; Hammond et al., 2013; Havill, 2012). The reputation of a unit in a community has also been identified as influential in women's birthplace decisions (Barber et al., 2006; Patterson, 2009). In order for women to plan to give birth in a PMU women need access to this type of facility, whether freestanding or alongside a tertiary obstetric hospital. The facility needs to be close enough to both women's homes and to the tertiary hospital to be a genuine option. The units need to have the characteristics and facilities valued by women wanting to use them, and be well funded and managed and staffed appropriately, with access to effective transfer arrangements and specialist services, when they are required.

Building confidence in order to enable women to plan to give birth away from a hospital environment is a complex and difficult process. Confidence is based on beliefs. Beliefs can be deeply held and value laden and are influenced by a range of personal, social, cultural and political factors. It is well understood that beliefs regarding birth are strongly context-bound and most powerfully influenced by the complex contrasts of safety, choice and risk (Bryers & van Teijlingen, 2010; Coxon et al., 2013; Edwards & Murphy-Lawless, 2006).

Midwives' skills

Kirkham (2003) argues that the birth centre is the place where 'the complex skills underpinning normal birth can be developed, nurtured and learned' (p. 12). Whether the birth centre needs to be freestanding or whether these same skills can be nurtured in a birth centre that is part of a hospital remains to be seen. The Birthplace in England study suggests that geographical distance or separation from an obstetric unit has a protective effect on normal birth since freestanding birth centres had better outcomes than alongside birth centres (Birthplace in England Collaborative Group, 2011). Birth centres may offer the greatest opportunity for both women and midwives to rediscover a profound belief in the inherently normal physiological process of birth. As with birth at home, birth centres are founded on a belief in the normality of birth, which appears to be the most influential aspect of the birth environment to consider.

Global strategies to centralise childbirth into large tertiary centres on the grounds of safety pose a serious threat not only to home birth and birth centres but also to rural communities, which are faced with the loss of PMUs as locations for birth. The challenge facing maternity services today in countries like Australia and New Zealand is how to preserve primary-level birth facilities. A population-based Australian study of all women who gave birth from 1999 to 2001 showed that, for low-risk women, small maternity units were not associated with higher rates of perinatal mortality, regardless of parity (Tracy et al., 2006). In New Zealand, a mixed-methods study by Patterson et al. (2011) highlights the importance of maternity services to rural communities. Patterson and colleagues found that midwives erred on the side of caution and were proficient in accounting for distance as well as geographical and climate-related challenges that might impact on transfer to higher-level units. In a survey receiving responses from two-thirds of all rural maternity units in New Zealand, they also found that 83% of women beginning labour in a rural maternity unit gave birth there. Half of all in-labour transfers were for slow labour progress, a situation that is rarely acute in nature. This evidence is important and should be reassuring to rural women and service providers.

Our current maternity care context is dominated by biomedical discourses focusing on childbirth as risk. Within this context, birth environments other than the obstetric hospital are constructed as unsafe, despite overwhelming evidence to the contrary. Obstetric intervention in childbirth is increasing and physiological birth is becoming less common. Midwifery skills, the art of 'real midwifery', is at risk because midwives are pressed more and more to practise to obstetric rather than midwifery norms. This is particularly the situation in obstetric settings. This is a perplexing situation because high-level evidence demonstrates the superiority of midwifery-led care in helping women to achieve a safe, satisfying physiological childbirth experience, yet midwives are pressed to adopt the practices of a profession who cannot demonstrate a record of such achievement.

Conclusion

The three components of women's care that were lost when the place of birth changed from home to hospital were the familiar environment, the close personal and trusting relationship with a midwife who provided continuous care throughout labour, and a strong belief in the normal physiology of birth. All three components of the care 'package' function together to keep birth normal. The environment for birth not only includes the geographical space where the event will unfold, but is influenced by less-visible but no-less-powerful forces that include relationships with midwives and the beliefs, knowledge and skills they bring to practising real midwifery. The challenge for all midwives is to consider these three elements in their own practice location (see Box 7.9).

Box 7.9   YouTube: A new space for birth?

In her paper titled 'YouTube: A new space for birth?', Robyn Longhurst concludes:

… that although youTube has the potential to open up new windows on birth, this potential is not yet being realized. youTube does not overcome or render insignificant material expressions of power, instead it typically privileges US experiences of birth, reiterates discourses of 'good' mothering and censors particular (mainly vaginal) representation …

Currently, youTube does not pluralise understandings of birth. This does not mean that viewers will simply succumb to birthing as it is represented online but rather they will variously reject, embrace or selectively accommodate these images. The way people construct and view videos of birth is mediated through gender differences and also through differences in sexuality, class, ethnicity, age, and culture …The politics that surround birth in 'real' space are reflected and reinforced in cyberspace.

(Extract from 'YouTube: A new space for birth?' by Robyn Longhurst, 2009)

In 2007, Laura Shanley sent a letter to staff at YouTube titled 'Censorship on YouTube'.

Many wonderful childbirth videos have been deleted by youTube supposedly because they violate your obscenity policies. Homebirth and natural childbirth videos are specifically being targeted, yet many are far less graphic than hospital birth videos which show close up images of vaginas being cut by doctors (episiotomies) and other interventions. Perhaps when birth is presented as a medical event it is viewed as acceptable but when it is presented as a natural, loving act between a woman, her baby and her partner it is viewed as sexual and therefore obscene.

Shanley makes an interesting point. She received a message from the YouTube team in response to her letter explaining that her video 'An unassisted childbirth' after being 'flagged' by members of the YouTube 'community' and reviewed by YouTube staff, had been removed owing to its 'inappropriate nature'.

Review questions

1. What does the theoretical model known as the fear cascade contribute to our understanding of how the place of birth affects birth outcomes?
2. What role(s) does oxytocin play in birth outcomes?
3. What were the reasons for women moving from home to hospital to give birth at the turn of the 20th century?
4. Why do different accounts of childbirth explain these events differently?
5. How similar are the childbirth histories of women and midwives in New Zealand and Australia?
6. What three things were lost when women moved from home to hospital for birth?
7. What are the potential consequences of intervention in childbirth?
8. How many women choose home birth in Australia or New Zealand?
9. Do midwives and other providers enable 'choice' for women regarding place of birth?
10. What midwifery skills are needed in order to provide care to women either at home or in primary maternity settings?

Acknowledgements

We wish to acknowledge the major contribution made by the previous authors, Deborah Davis and Marion Hunter.

References

AHPRA. 'Ministers extend professional indemnity insurance exemption for privately practising midwives'. 2021. Online: https://www.nursingmidwiferyboard.gov.au/News/2021-12-22-Ministers-extend-insurance-exemption-for-privately-practising-midwives.aspx

Australian Health Ministers Advisory Council (AHMAC). *National Maternity Services Plan, 2011*. Canberra: Australian Health Ministers Advisory Council, Commonwealth of Australia; 2011.

Andrén A, Begley C, Dahlberg H, et al. The birthing room and its influence on the promotion of a normal physiological childbirth: a qualitative interview study with midwives in Sweden, *Int J of Qual Studies Health Wellbeing*. 2021;16:1

Annandale E. How midwives accomplish natural birth: managing risk and balancing expectations. *Soc Probl*. 1988;32(2):95–110.

Australian Institute of Health and Welfare (AIHW). *Australia's Mothers and Babies*. Canberra: AIHW; 2017

Banks M. *The obstetric bed: resistance in action, 2014*. Online: http://www.birthspirit.co.nz/

Barber T, Rogers J, Marsh S. The birth place choices project: phase one. *B J Midwifery*. 2006;14(10):609–13.

Barclay L, Kornelsen J, Longman J, Robin S et al. Reconceptualising risk: Perceptions of risk in rural and remote maternity service planning. *Midwifery*. 2016;38: 63–70.

Berger M, Dreyer N, Anderson F, et al. Prospective observational studies to assess comparative effectiveness: The ISPOR good research practices task force report. *Value in Health*. 2012;15: 217–30.

Birthplace in England Collaborative Group. Perinatal and maternal outcomes by planned place of birth for healthy women with low risk pregnancies: The Birthplace in England national prospective cohort study. *Br Med J*. 2011;116:1177–1184.

Blix E, Huitfeldt AS, Oian P, et al. Outcomes of planned home births and planned hospital births in low-risk women in Norway between 1990 and 2007: a retrospective cohort study. *Sex Reprod Healthcare*. 2012; 3:147–53.

Bryant J, Porter M, Tracy SK, et al. Caesarean birth: consumption, safety, order, and good mothering. *Soc Sci Med*. 2007;65: 1192–1201.

Bryers M H, van Teijlingen E. Risk, theory, social and medical models: a critical analysis of the concept of risk in maternity care. *Midwifery*. 2010;26(5):488–96.

Buckley S. Undisturbed birth: nature's blueprint for ease and ecstasy. *J Perinat Psychol Health*. 2003;17(4):261–288.

Catling-Paull C, Coddington R, Foureur M, Homer C. Publicly funded homebirth in Australia: a review of maternal and neonatal outcomes over 6 years. *Medical Journal of Australia*. 2013; 198: 616–620.

Catling-Paull C, Dahlen H, Homer CSE. Multiparous women's confidence to have a publicly-funded homebirth: a qualitative study. *Women Birth*. 2011;24:122–128.

Catling-Paull C, Dahlen H, Homer CS. The influences on women who choose publicly-funded home birth in Oz. *Midwifery*. 2014;30:892–898.

Chadwick, RJ, Foster D. Negotiating risky bodies: Childbirth and constructions of risk. *Health, Risk & Society*. 2014; 16(1), 68–83.

Cheung N, Mander R, Wang X, et al. Clinical outcomes of the first midwife-led normal birth unit in China: a retrospective cohort study. *Midwifery*. 2010;27:582–7.

Cheyne H, Dalgleish L, Tucker J, et al. Risk assessment and decision making about in-labour transfer from rural maternity care: a social judgment and signal detection analysis. *BMC Medical Informatics and Decision Making*. 2012;12(122):13. Epub 31 October 2012.

Cheyney M, Bovbjerg M, Everson C, et al. Outcomes of care for 16,924 planned home births in the United States: The Midwives Alliance of North America Statistics Project, 2004 to 2009. *J Midwifery Womens Health*. 2014;59(1):17–27.

Commonwealth of Australia (C of A). *Improving Maternity Services in Australia: The Report of the Maternity Services Review*. Canberra: Commonwealth of Australia; 2009. http://www.health.gov.au/internet/main/publishing.nsf/Content/maternityservicesreview-report.

Coxon K, Sandall J, Fulop N. To what extent are women free to choose where to give birth? How discourses of risk, blame and responsibility influence birth place decisions. *Health Risk Soc*. 2013;16(1):1–17. doi:10.1080/13698575.2013.859231.

Crawford R. Risk ritual and the management of control and anxiety in medical culture. *Health*. 2004;8(4):505–528

Davis D, Walker K. Case-loading midwifery in New Zealand: making space for childbirth. *Midwifery*. 2010;26(6):603–608.

Davis D, Baddock S, Pairman S, et al. Planned place of birth in New Zealand: does it affect mode of birth and intervention rates among low-risk women? *Birth*. 2011;38(2):111–119.

Davis D, Walker K. Towards an 'optics of power': technologies of surveillance and discipline and case-loading midwifery practice in New Zealand. *Gend Place Cult*. 2013;20:597–612.

Davis-Floyd R. *Birth as an American Rite of Passage*. Berkeley: University of California Press, 1992.

Davis-Floyd R. The technocratic body: American childbirth as cultural expression. *Soc Sci Med*. 1994;38(8):1125–1140.

Davis-Floyd R. The technocratic, humanistic, and holistic paradigms of childbirth. *Int J Gynaecol Obstet*. 2001;75 (supp 1): S5–S23.

Deery R. Transfers from midwife led to obstetric led care: some insights from midwives. *Essentially MIDIRS*. 2010;1(3):17–22.

de Jonge A, van der Goes B, Ravelli A, et al. Perinatal mortality and morbidity in a nationwide cohort of 529,688 low-risk planned home and hospital births. *Br J Obstet Gynaecol*. 2009; 116:1177–1184.

de Jonge A, Mesman JA, Manniën, et al. Severe adverse maternal outcomes among low risk women with planned home versus hospital births in the Netherlands: nationwide cohort study. *BMJ*. 2013;346:f3263.

de Jonge A, Geerts CC, van der Goes BY, et al. Perinatal mortality and morbidity up to 28 days after birth among 743 070 low-risk planned home and hospital births: a cohort study based on three merged national perinatal databases. *BJOG*. 2015; 122(5):720–8.

de Jonge A, Wouters M, Klinkert J, et al. Pitfalls in the use of register-based data for comparing adverse maternal and perinatal outcomes in different birth settings. *BJOG*. 2017;124(10): 1477–1480.

Downe S. Beyond evidence-based medicine: complexity and stories of maternity care. *J Eval Clin Pract*. 2010;16:232–7.

Edwards NP, Murphy-Lawless J. The instability of risk: women's perspectives on risk and safety in birth. In: Symon A, eds. *Risk and Choice in Maternity Care: An International Perspective*. Philadelphia: Churchill Livingstone Elsevier; 2006:35–49.

Enkin M. Risk in pregnancy: the reality, the perception, and the concept. *Birth*. 1994;21(3):131–134.

Evers AC, Brouwers HA, Hukkelhoven CW, et al. Perinatal mortality and severe morbidity in low and high risk term pregnancies in the Netherlands: prospective cohort study. *BMJ*. 2010;341: c5639.

Everson C, Cheyney M. Between two worlds: doula care, liminality, and the power of mandorla spaces in doulas and intimate labour: boundaries, bodies, and birth. In: Casteneda AN, Johnson Searcy J, eds., Bradford, Ontario: Demeter Press; 2015.

Fahy K, Foureur M, Hastie C. *Birth Territory and Midwifery Guardianship*. Oxford: Elsevier; 2008.

Fannin M. 2003 Domesticating birth in the hospital: "Family-centered" birth and the emergence of homelike birthing rooms. *Antipode*. 2003;35(3):513–535.

Foureur M. Creating birth space to enable undisturbed birth. In: Fahy K, Foureur M, Hastie C, eds. *Birth Territory and Midwifery Guardianship*. Oxford: Elsevier; 2008:57–78.

Foureur M, Leap N, Davis D, et al. Developing the birth unit design spatial evaluation tool (budset) in Australia: a qualitative study. *HERD*. 2010a;3(4):43–57.

Foureur M, Davis D, Fenwick J, et al. The relationship between birth unit design and safe, satisfying birth: developing a hypothetical model. *Midwifery*. 2010b;26(5):520–525.

Fox D, Sheehan A, Homer C. Birthplace in Australia: processes and interactions during the intrapartum transfer of women from planned homebirth to hospital. *Midwifery*. 2018 Feb; 57:18–25.

Goer H. Duelling Statistics: Is out-of-hospital birth safe? *The Journal of Perinatal Education*. 2016; 25(2): 75–79.

Gottvall K, Grunewald C, Waldenstrom U. Safety of birth centre care: perinatal mortality over a 10 year period. *Br J Obstet Gynaecol*. 2004;111:71–78.

Graham I. *Episiotomy: Challenging Obstetric Intervention*. London: Blackwell Science; 1997.

Griew K. Birth centre midwifery down under. In: Kirkham M, ed. *Birth Centres. A Social Model for Maternity Care*. London: Elsevier, 2003, 209–222.

Grigg C, Tracy S, Daellenbach R, et al. An exploration of influences on women's birthplace decision-making in New Zealand: a mixed methods prospective cohort within the Evaluating Maternity Units study. *BMC Pregnancy and Childbirth*. 2014; 14(210):14.

Grigg C, Tracy S, Schmied V, et al. Women's experiences of transfer from primary maternity unit to tertiary hospital in New Zealand: part of the prospective cohort Evaluating Maternity Units study. *BMC Pregnancy and Childbirth*. 2015;15(339):1–12. Epub 18 December 2015.

Grigg C, Tracy SK, Tracy MB, et al. Evaluating Maternity Units: a prospective cohort study of freestanding midwifery–led primary maternity units in New Zealand – clinical outcomes. *BMJ Open*. 2017; 7(8):e16288.

Grunebaum A, McCullough L, Sapra K, et al. Early and total neonatal mortality in relation to birth setting in the United States, 2006–2009. *Am J Obstet Gynecol*. 2014;211(390):e1–7.

Guilliland K, Pairman S. *The midwifery partnership: a model for practice. Department of Nursing and Midwifery Monograph Series 95/1*. Victoria University of Wellington, New Zealand: 1995.

Hammond A, Foureur M, et al. Space, place and the midwife: exploring the relationship between the birth environment, neurobiology and midwifery practice. *Women Birth*. 26(4) (2013), pp. 277–281.

Hendrix M, Van Horck M, Moreta D, et al. Why women do not accept randomisation for place of birth: feasibility of a RCT in the Netherlands. *BJOG*. 2009;116:537–44.

Hodnett ED, Downe S, Edwards N, et al. Homelike versus conventional institutional settings for birth. *Cochrane Database Syst Rev*. 2005;(1):Art. No.: CD000012, doi:10.1002/14651858. CD000012.pub2.

Hodnett E, Stremler R, Edwards N, et al. 2009. Re-conceptualising the hospital labor room: the PLACE (Pregnant and Laboring in an Ambient Clinical Environment) pilot trial. *Birth*. 36,159–166.

Hodnett ED, Downe S, Walsh D. Alternative versus conventional institutional settings for birth. *Cochrane Database Syst Rev*. 2012; (8):Art. No.: CD000012. doi:10.1002/14651858.CD000012.pub4.

Hollowell J, Puddicombe D, Rowe R, et al. *The Birthplace national prospective cohort study: perinatal and maternal outcomes by planned place of birth: final report Part 4. Birthplace in England research programme*. NIHR Service Delivery and Organisation programme; 2011. Online: https://www.npeu.ox.ac.uk/birthplace.

Homer CSE, Cheah SL, Rossiter C, et al. Maternal and perinatal outcomes by planned place of birth in Australia 2000–2012: a linked population data study. *BMJ Open*. 2019;9.

Homer C, Brodie P, Leap N. *Midwifery Continuity of Care: a Practical Guide*. Sydney: Elsevier; 2008.

Homer C, Thornton C, Scarf V, et al. Birthplace in New South Wales, Australia: an analysis of perinatal outcomes using routinely collected data. *BMC Pregnancy and Childbirth*. 2014;14(206):1–12. Epub 14 June 2014.

Hunter M. *Autonomy, Clinical Freedom and Responsibility: the Paradoxes of Providing Intrapartum Midwifery Care in a Small Maternity Unit As Compared with a Large Obstetric Hospital (MA thesis)*. Palmerston North, New Zealand: Massey University; 2000.

Hunter M. Autonomy, clinical freedom and responsibility. In: Kirkham M, ed. *Birth Centres: a Social Model for Maternity Care*. London: Elsevier Science; 2003:239–249.

Hutton EK, Reitsma AH, Kaufman K: Outcomes associated with planned home and planned hospital births in low-risk women attended by midwives in Ontario, Canada, 2003–2006: A retrospective cohort study. *Birth*. 2009, 36:180–189.

Janssen P, Saxell L, Page L, et al. Outcomes of planned home birth with registered midwife versus planned hospital birth with midwife or physician. *Can Med Assoc J*. 2009;181:6–7. doi:10.1503/cmaj.081869.

Jenkinson B, Josey N, Kruske S. *Birthspace: An Evidence-based Guide to Birth Environment Design*. Brisbane: Queensland Centre for Mothers and Babies, The University of Queensland; 2014. Online: https://espace.library.uq.edu.au/view/UQ:339451/UQ339451_fulltext.pdf.

Jordan B. Authoritative knowledge and its construction. In: Davis-Floyd R, Sargent C, eds. *Childbirth and Authoritative Knowledge*. Berkley, CA: University of California Press; 1997: 55–79.

Jordan R, Murphy P. Risk assessment and risk distortion: finding the balance. *J Midwifery Womens Health*. 2009;54:191–200.

Kildea S, Magick Dennis F, et al. *Birthing on Country Workshop Report, Alice Springs, 4th July*. Brisbane: Australian Health Minister's Advisory Council, 2013.

Kirkham M. Birth Centres: *A Social Model for Maternity Care*. London: Elsevier Science; 2003.

Kotaska A. Combating coercion: breech birth, parturient choice, and the evolution of evidence-based medicine. *Birth*. 2007; 34:176–180.

Kruske S, Schultz T, Eales S, et al. A retrospective, descriptive study of maternal and neonatal transfers, and clinical outcomes of a primary maternity unit in rural Queensland, 2009–2011. *Women Birth*. 2015;28:30–39.

Kruske S, Kildea S, Jenkinson B, et al. Primary Maternity Units in rural and remote Australia: results of a national survey. *Midwifery*. 2016; 40:1–9.

Kuliukas L, Lewis L, Hauck Y, et al. Midwives' experiences of transfer in labour from a Western Australian birth centre to a tertiary maternity hospital. *Women and Birth*. 2016; 29:18–23.

Lavender T, Chapple J. How women choose where to give birth. *The practising midwife*. 2005;8(7):10–5.

Laws P, Lim C, Tracy SK, et al. Characteristics and practices of birth centres in Australia. *Australian and New Zealand Journal of Obstetrics and Gynaecology*. 2009;49:290–5.

Laws P, Lim C, Tracy SK, et al. Changes to booking, transfer criteria and procedures in birth centres in Australia from 1997 to 2007: a national survey PSANZ. *Journal of Paediatrics and Child Health*. 2010;46(Suppl. 1):57–96.

Lepori B. Freedom of movement in birth places. *Children's Environments*. 1994;11(2):81–87. Online: http://www.colorado.edu/journals/cye/11_2/11_2article1.pdf.

Lundgren I. Swedish women's experience of childbirth 2 years after birth. *Midwifery*. 2005;21(4):346–354.

Macfarlane A, McCandlish R, Campbell R. There is no evidence that hospital is the safest place to give birth. *Br Med J*. 2000;320:798.

McAra-Couper J, Farry A, Marsters N, et al. Pasifika women's choice of birthplace. *New Zealand College of Midwives Journal*. 2018(54).

McIntyre M, Chapman Y, Francis K. Hidden costs associated with the universal application of risk management in maternity care. *Aust Health Rev*. 2011;35:211–215.

McLachlan HL, Forster DA, Davey MA, et al. Effects of continuity of care by a primary midwife (caseload midwifery) on caesarean section rates in women of low obstetric risk: the COSMOS randomised controlled trial. *BJOG*. 2012;119(12):1483–1492.

McLachlan H, McKay H, Powell R, Small R, Davey MA, Cullinane F, Newton M, Forster D. Publicly-funded home birth in Victoria, Australia: Exploring the views and experiences of midwives and doctors. *Midwifery*. 2016;35:24–30.

Ministry of Health (MOH). *Māori health models – Te Whare Tapa Whā*. Wellington, NZ: Ministry of Health; 2017a. Online: https://www.health.govt.nz/our-work/populations/maori-health/maori-health-models/maori-health-models-te-whare-tapa-wha.

Ministry of Health. *Report on Maternity 2015*. Wellington: Ministry of Health; 2017b. https://www.health.govt.nz/system/files/documents/publications/report-on-maternity-2015-updated_12122017.pdf

142

Monk AR , Tracy S, Foureur M, et al. Australian primary maternity units: past, present and future. *Women Birth*. 2013a;26(3): 213–8.

Monk AR, Tracy SK, Foureur M, et al. Evaluating midwifery units (EMU): lessons from the pilot study. *Midwifery*. 2013b;29(8): 845–51.

Monk A, Tracy M, Foureur M, et al. Evaluating Midwifery Units (EMU): a prospective cohort study of freestanding midwifery units in New South Wales, Australia. *BMJ Open*. 2014;4(e006252):12.

Moynihan R, Heath I, Henry D, Selling sickness: the pharmaceutical industry and disease mongering. *BMJ*. 2002; 324:886–91.

Murray-Davis B, McDonald H, Rietsma A, et al. Deciding on home or hospital birth: Results of the Ontario choice of birthplace survey. *Midwifery*. 2014;30(7):869–76.

National Institute for Health and Care Excellence (NICE). *Intrapartum care for healthy women and babies: clinical guideline*. 2014 (updated 2017). Online: nice.org.uk/guidance/cg190 https://www.nice.org.uk/guidance/cg190/resources/intrapartum-care-for-healthy-women-and-babies-pdf-35109866447557.

Noseworthy DA, Phibbs SR, Benn CA. Towards a relational model of decision-making in midwifery care. *Midwifery*. 2013 Jul;29(7):e42–8.

NSW Health Department. *Final report of the ministerial task force on obstetric services in NSW: The Shearman Report*. Sydney: NSW Department of Health; 1989.

NZCOM. *Midwives Handbook for Practice New Zealand College of Midwives, org?* New Zealand, 2018.

Odent M. Birth Territory: The besieged territory of the Obstetrician. In: Fahy K, Foureur M, Hastie C, eds. *Birth Territory and Midwifery Guardianship*. Oxford: Elsevier; 2008:131.

Overgaard C, Moller A, Fenger-Gron M, et al. Freestanding midwifery unit versus obstetric unit: a matched cohort study of outcomes in low-risk women. *BMJ Open*. 2011;2(e000262):12.

Overgaard C, Fenger-Gron M, J S. The impact of birthplace on women's birth experiences and perceptions of care. *Soc Sci Med*. 2012;74:973–81.

Patterson J. *A time of travelling hopefully: a mixed methods study of decision making by women and midwives about maternity transfers in rural Aotearoa, New Zealand*. [Unpublished PhD thesis]. http://researcharchive.vuw.ac.nz/handle/10063/1028: Victoria Univeristy of Wellington; 2009.

Patterson JA, Foureur M, Skinner JP. Patterns of transfer in labour and birth in rural New Zealand. *Rural Remote Health*. 2011;11:1710. Online: http://www.rrh.org.au. accessed Dec 9th 2021.

Patterson J, Skinner J, Foureur M. Midwives 'decision making about transfers for 'slow' labour in rural New Zealand. *Midwifery*. 2015;31:606–12.

Possamai-Inesedy A. Confining risk: choice and responsibility in childbirth in a risk society. *Health Sociol Rev*. 2006;15: 406–414.

Roberts CL, Tracy S, Peat B. Rates for obstetric intervention among private and public patients in Australia: population-based descriptive study. *BMJ*. 2000;321:137–141.

Rooks J, Weatherby N, Ernst E, et al. Outcomes of care in birth centres: the national birth centre study. *N Engl J Med*. 1989; 321(26):1804–1811.

Roome S, Hartz D, Tracy S, et al. Why such differing stances? A review of position statements on home birth from professional colleges. *BJOG*. 2016;123(3):376–82.

Rosenblatt RA, Reinken J, Shoemack P. *Regionalisation of Obstetric and Perinatal Care in New Zealand: A Health Service Analysis*. Wellington: Unpublished report for the New Zealand government; 1985.

Rowe R, Kurinczuk J, Locock L, et al. Women's experience of transfer from midwifery unit to hospital obstetric unit during labour: a qualitative interview study. *BMC Pregnancy Childbirth*. 2012;12(129):1–15. Epub 15 November 2012.

Rowley MJ. *Evaluation of Team Midwifery Care in Pregnancy and Childbirth: a Randomised Controlled Trial (PhD thesis)*. Newcastle NSW: University of Newcastle; 1998.

Royal Australian and New Zealand College of Obstetricians and Gynaecologists (RANZCOG). *Home births*. 2017. Online: https://ranzcog.edu.au/RANZCOG_SITE/media/RANZCOG-MEDIA/Women%27s%20Health/Statement%20and%20guidelines/Clinical-Obstetrics/Home-Births-(C-Obs-2)-Review-July-17.pdf?ext=.pdf

Ryan M, Roberts C. A retrospective cohort study comparing the clinical outcomes of a birth centre and labour ward in the same hospital. *Aust J Midwifery*. 2005;18(2):17–21.

Sandall J. Normal birth: a public health issue. *Pract Midwife*. 2004; 7(1):4–5.

Sandall J, Soltani H, Gates S, et al. Midwife-led continuity models versus other models of care for childbearing women. *Cochrane Database of Systematic Rev*. 2016(4):CD004667, doi:10.1002/14651858.

Sassine H , Burns E, Ormsby S, et al. Why do women choose homebirth in Australia? A national survey. *Women and Birth*. 2021;34:396–404.

Simkin P, Ancheta R. *The Labor Progress Handbook*. Oxford: Blackwell Science; 2001.

Skinner J, Foureur M. Consultation, referral, and collaboration between midwives and obstetricians: lessons from New Zealand. *J Midwifery Womens Health*. 2010;55(1):28–37.

Smith V, Devane D, Murphy-Lawless J. Risk in maternity care: a concept analysis. *Int J Childbirth*. 2012;2:126–135.

Stewart M, McCandlish R, Henderson J, et al. *Report of a Structured Review of Birth Centre Outcomes*. Oxford: National Perinatal Epidemiology Unit, 2005.

Tew M. Safer Childbirth? *A Critical History of Maternity Care*. 2nd ed. London: Chapman & Hall; 1995.

Tracy SK, Tracy MB. Costing the cascade: estimating the cost of increased obstetric intervention in childbirth using population data. *Br J Obstet Gynaecol*. 2003;110 (8):295–300.

Tracy SK, Hartz D, Nicholl M, et al. An integrated service network in maternity: the implementation of a free standing midwifery led unit. *Australian Health Review*. 2005;29(3):332–339.

Tracy SK, Dahlen H, Wang A, et al. Does size matter? A population-based study of birth in lower volume maternity hospitals for low-risk women. *Br J Obstet Gynaecol*. 2006;113(1):86–97.

Tracy SK, Hartz DL, Tracy MB, et al. Caseload midwifery care versus standard maternity care for women of any risk. 2013; M1723–32.

Tracy SK, Welsh A, Hall B, et al. Caseload midwifery compared to standard or private obstetric care for first time mothers in a public teaching hospital in Australia: a cross sectional study of cost and birth outcomes. *BMC Pregnancy Childbirth*. 2014;14:46.

Tracy SK, Page L. Notions of choice and continuity in promoting normal birth. In Downe S and Byrom S, eds. *Squaring the Circle: researching normal childbirth in a technological world Pinter and Martin*, London.

Ulrich R, Zimring C, Xuemei Z, et al. Evidence-based healthcare design. *HERD*. 2008;7(3):61–125.

van der Kooy J, Birnie E, Denktas S, et al. Planned home compared with planned hospital births: mode of delivery and Perinatal mortality rates, an observational study. *BMC Pregnancy Childbirth*. 2017;17(1):177.

van Teijlingen E. A critical analysis of the medical model as used in the study of pregnancy and childbirth. *Sociol Res Online*. 2005;10(2):doi:10.5153/sro.1034. Online: http://www.socresonline.org.uk/10/2/teijlingen.html.

Vedam S, Stoll K, Schummers L, et al. The Canadian birth place study: examining maternity care provider attitudes and interprofessional conflict around planned home birth. *BMC Pregnancy Childbirth*. 2014:(October) 28;14:353. doi: 10.1186/1471-2393-14-353.

Waldenstrom U, Nilsson C, Winbladh B. The Stockholm birth centre trial: maternal and infant outcomes. *Br J Obstet Gynaecol.* 1997;104:410–418.

Walsh D. Birth centres unsafe for primigravidae. *Br J Midwifery.* 2004;12(4):206.

Walsh D. Subverting the assembly line: childbirth in a freestanding birth centre. *Soc Sci Med.* 2006;62:1330–1340.

Walsh D. *Evidence-Based Care for Normal Labour and Birth: a Guide for Midwives.* London: Routledge; 2007.

Wood et al. 2016 Choosing out of hospital birth centre: exploring women's decision-making experiences. *Midwifery.* 2016; 39:12–19.

Yang W, Zilov A, Soewondo P, et al. Observational studies: going beyond the boundaries of randomised controlled trials. 2010. 2010;88s:s3–s9.

CHAPTER 8

Ways of looking at evidence and measurement

Sally K Tracy

LEARNING OUTCOMES

Learning outcomes for this chapter are:

1. To explore the dimensions of research in midwifery
2. To introduce some of the common terms used in research, in both qualitative and quantitative methods
3. To understand the basis for evidence-based midwifery
4. To identify some of the tensions in the evidence-based movement.

CHAPTER OVERVIEW

The purpose of this chapter is to explore some of the dimensions of research in midwifery. It is intended to be used as an introductory tool for understanding the basics of evidence-based practice.

KEY TERMS

case–control study
cohort study
confidence interval
cross-sectional study

evidence-based midwifery
experimental method
intervention study
level of evidence

qualitative research
quasi-experimental method
randomised controlled trial (RCT)
systematic review

INTRODUCTION

Some ways of knowing have traditionally occupied spaces at the edge of the dominant vision—the same kinds of spaces as are filled by the lives and experiences of the socially marginalised, including women. Thus, neither methods nor methodology can be understood except in the context of gendered social relations. Understanding this involves a mapping of how gender, women, nature and knowledge have been constructed both inside and outside all forms of science.

(Oakley, 2000, p. 4)

Research is a process of gathering facts and exploring relationships. The end result is a body of knowledge that can be used to guide midwifery practice and provide the basis for further exploration of ideas. As you travel along research paths you will become very familiar with two terms: quantitative and qualitative methodologies.

In the *quantitative* school of thought, the researcher identifies and measures facts that are considered to be objective. On the other hand, a *qualitative* researcher may be concerned with explaining or understanding how people view their world.

These two schools are based on the following underlying methods:

- In quantitative research it is believed that the theory and hypothesis should be developed before the research is undertaken. This is known as *deductive method*. It follows the thinking of Karl Popper (1979) that scientific knowledge is gained through the development of ideas and the attempt to refute them with empirical research. The dominant philosophy underlying quantitative scientific method is *positivism*. Positivism assumes that phenomena are measurable using the deductive principles of the scientific method—that is, the investigator starts with a theory and a hypothesis that is tested by the data (deduction).
- On the other hand, the qualitative school of thought holds that research should precede theory and not be limited to a passive role of verifying and testing theory; rather, it should help to shape the development of theory (Bowling, 2014) by the process of *induction*.

Both these strategies are used to develop the knowledge of midwifery.

Whichever method we use to try to find answers to a certain problem or situation, there are certain things that help us measure how successful the research is in answering our question. Two important concepts found in all reliable research are known as *reliability* (the repeatability of the research) and *validity* (the extent to which the tools or instruments used in the research actually measure what they set out to measure). (For further information on these concepts see Ch. 22 of this book, also Borbasi et al., 2016.)

For all research, regardless of the method, a basic formula sets out the cycle of events that occur in a research process (Fig. 8.1).

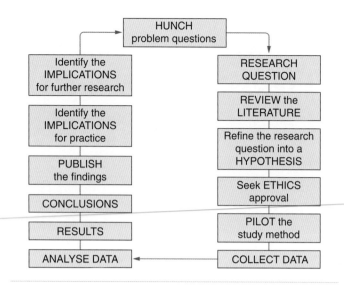

FIGURE 8.1 The research cycle

QUALITATIVE RESEARCH METHODS

Qualitative research contributes to the understanding of social aspects of health issues through direct observation of the nuances of social behaviour (Green & Britten, 1998; Pope & Mays, 2013). Qualitative research is useful to investigate practitioners' and people's attitudes, beliefs and preferences, and the whole question of how evidence is turned into practice. The value of qualitative methods lies in their ability to pursue systematically the kinds of research questions that are not easily answerable by experimental methods. Rigorously conducted qualitative research is based on explicit sampling strategies, systematic analysis of data and a commitment to examining counter-explanations. Ideally, methods should be transparent, allowing the reader to assess the validity and the extent to which the results might be applicable to their own clinical practice. Qualitative research does not usually produce numerical rates and measures (Corbin & Strauss, 2014; Green & Britten, 1998). Researchers who use qualitative methods seek a different truth (Greenhalgh, 2014). They aim to make sense of, or interpret, phenomena using a holistic perspective that preserves the complexities of human behaviour (Black, 1994). The research often provides us with a picture of 'behind the scenes', how people are feeling, or what other forces are at work that may not be discovered in a quantitative investigation of facts. Nevertheless, in developing practice and policy, qualitative research has yet to emerge fully from the shadow of its powerful quantitative 'other': the **randomised controlled trial (RCT)** (Porter, 2010).

An example of how research can identify what is happening 'behind the scenes' is described in the following case study, which describes a quantitative and a qualitative study exploring the same phenomena. The 'behind the scenes' behaviour that affected the introduction of evidence-based leaflets into maternity hospitals in the United Kingdom was recorded by Stapleton et al. (2002) when they undertook a qualitative study alongside an RCT by O'Cathain et al. (2002). In the experimental study, the researchers concluded that, in everyday practice, evidence-based leaflets were not effective in promoting informed choice for women using maternity services (O'Cathain et al., 2002). The qualitative study (Stapleton et al., 2002) mounted alongside this RCT provided a rich insight into what was happening with the information leaflets, and found that the way in which the leaflets were disseminated affected promotion of informed choice in maternity care. The qualitative study provided the evidence for 'behind the scenes' bullying and coercive behaviours that had become a normal way of doing things in these maternity units. The culture into which the leaflets were introduced supported existing normative patterns of care and this ensured informed compliance rather than informed choice (Stapleton et al., 2002).

Overview of qualitative methods

As a midwife you will be intimately involved in finding the answers to many questions through research evidence. However, the scope of this chapter permits only a very brief overview of some of the terms and methods you will encounter. The following summary of some of the qualitative research methods used in scientific research will give you a very brief introduction to the terminology and concepts used in qualitative research.

Phenomenology

Phenomenology is a method of constructing the meaning of (a phenomenon from) someone's experience—for example, their 'lived experience'. The researcher not only explores what people experience but also how it is that they experience what they experience! For example, a midwife might utilise phenomenology if she wanted to study the unique experiences of midwives working in a group practice in Aotearoa New Zealand:
- Data are gathered through in-depth interviews.
- The sample is drawn only from those who have experienced the phenomenon.
- The analysis is derived from interview transcripts. The participants' 'voices' are examined line by line, to identify key statements that describe participants' experiences and to identify common themes that illustrate the researcher's interpretation of the phenomenon.

(See Grigg et al., 2015.)

Ethnography

Ethnography is used by the researcher to construct the meaning of culture—that is, the researcher tries to understand the insider's 'emic' view of the world. The researcher enters an unknown world and tries to make sense of it from the insider's point of view. For example, a midwife may choose ethnography to 'explore the nature of interactions between midwives and breastfeeding women within postnatal wards of a large tertiary hospital in Australia':
- Data are gathered through participant observation and interviews, and the researcher interprets the cultural patterns observed during these interactions.
- The sample is taken from people in a cultural group who are living in the phenomenon. These are known as the key informants and/or the general informants. The key informants are those with special knowledge who are prepared to teach the researcher.
- The analysis is undertaken on field notes (sometimes video) and observations, and meaning is sought from cultural symbols in the informants' language.

(See Harte et al., 2016.)

Narrative

Narrative inquiry is a research methodology encompassing a number of approaches such as autobiography, biography, cultural, life history, oral history and life stories. For example, narrative research allows us to learn about women by listening to their stories. The narrative provides information that does not pertain simply or directly to the unfolding events. The same sequence of events told by another person to another audience might be presented differently without being any less 'true'. First, it has a finite and longitudinal time sequence—that is, it has a beginning, a series of unfolding events and (we anticipate) an ending. Secondly, it presupposes both a narrator and a listener, whose different viewpoints affect how the story is told. Thirdly, the narrative is concerned with individuals—rather than simply reporting what they do or what is done to them, it concerns how those individuals feel and how people feel about them.

Narratives help to set a person-centred agenda and challenge received wisdom, and they may generate new hypotheses. Narratives offer a method for addressing existential qualities such as inner hurt, despair, hope, grief and moral pain, which frequently accompany, and may even constitute, people's illnesses and wellbeing (Greenhalgh, 2016; Greenhalgh & Hurwitz, 1999; Lindsay & Schwind, 2016):
- Data are gathered by collecting the respondent's story.
- The sample is a convenience sample.
- The analysis of the narrative is an interpretive act—that is, interpretation (the discernment of meaning) is central to the analysis of narratives. Actual transcripts are presented in the results of narrative research.

(See Fraser & MacDougall, 2017.)

Historical research

Historical research is mainly narrative rather than numerical. Much conventional scholarship continues to focus on the search for a single, knowable, verifiable past (Swanson & Holton, 2005):
- The data consist of a systematic compilation of information regarding people, events and occurrences in the past.
- The sample tries to identify all data sources (e.g. docu-

ments, radio, interview or television transcripts, film, paintings and sculpture).

- The analysis involves the validity of external criticism; reliability delineates data sources by internal criticism. The reader 'hears' the narrator's 'voice' and 'sees' the actions in the story with the eyes of an 'internal' or 'external' focaliser, who may or may not be identical to the narrator (Norkus, 2004).

Grounded theory

Grounded theory focuses on human behaviour and perceptions and the factors that influence them. Through an inductive approach it facilitates the development of theories, which emerge from the data in a manner that means most hypotheses and concepts not only come from the data, but also are systematically worked out in relation to the data during the course of research (Corbin & Strauss, 2014). Grounded theory is particularly useful when little is known about the area of interest. It aims to find underlying social forces that shape human behaviour. For example, a researcher might want to explore how 'novice midwives incorporate a woman-focused philosophy into their practice in a "high-risk" maternity unit':

- Data are derived from interviews and skilled observations of individuals interacting in a social setting.
- The sample is purposive—the researcher deliberately samples a particular group or setting of people who are experiencing the circumstance.
- During analysis, the researcher's task is to sift and decode the data to make sense of the situation, events and interactions observed. Often this analytical process starts during the data collection phase. Variants of content analysis involve an iterative process of developing categories from the transcripts or field notes, testing them against hypotheses and refining them (Corbin & Strauss, 2014; Hall et al., 2011; Pope et al., 2000).

For an example of interpreting qualitative data in midwifery, see Jyai Allen's work on the "endorphic" response in midwifery (Allen et al., 2017).

Other methods

Other qualitative research methods include:
- *documents*—study of documentary accounts of events, such as meetings
- *passive observation*—systematic watching of behaviour and talk in naturally occurring settings
- *participant observation*—observation in which the researcher also occupies a role or part in the setting, in addition to observing
- *in-depth interview*—face-to-face conversation for the purpose of exploring issues or topics in detail; it does not use preset questions, but rather is shaped by a defined set of topics
- *focus groups*—a method of group interview that explicitly includes and uses the group interaction to generate data (Greenhalgh, 2014).

Reading and critiquing qualitative research: questions to ask

Mays & Pope (2000) suggest the following questions to ask of qualitative studies:
- Has the study contributed to our knowledge?
- Was the research question clear?
- Would a different method have been more appropriate? Was the design appropriate for the question?
- Is the context adequately described?
- Was the sampling strategy clearly described and justified?
- How was the fieldwork undertaken? Was it described in detail? Could the evidence (e.g. fieldwork notes, interview transcripts, recordings, documentary analysis, etc.) be inspected independently by others; if relevant, could the process of transcription be independently inspected?
- Were the procedures for data analysis clearly described and theoretically justified? Did they relate to the original research questions? How were themes and concepts identified from the data? Was the analysis repeated by more than one researcher to ensure reliability?
- Was there an audit trail, so that another researcher could repeat each stage of the research?
- Was enough of the original evidence presented systematically in the written account to satisfy the sceptical reader of the relationship between the interpretation and the evidence? (For example, were quotations numbered and sources given?)

CRITICAL THINKING EXERCISE

Search the literature for a study that uses each of the above methodologies, and compare the written studies to see what questions are asked and how these are answered (Boxes 8.1, 8.2 and 8.3). Could the same question be answered by each of the different methodologies?

For an interactive experience of looking at methodologies and analysis of qualitative research go to: https://methods.sagepub.com/methods-map

Evidence-based practice

Sackett et al. (1996, 2000; Box 8.4) identified five steps in putting evidence into practice:
1. Fit what you want to know into a question that can be answered.
2. Go looking for the best research to answer it.

Box 8.1 What is a Boolean operator?

Boolean operators connect your search words together to either narrow or broaden your set of results.

The three basic Boolean operators are: 'and', 'or' and 'not'.

Box 8.2 How to search for a research paper

How to search for a paper on Medline or the Cochrane Library:

To look for an article you know exists, search by text words (in title, abstract, or both) or use field suffixes for author, title, institution, journal and publication year.

For a maximally sensitive search on a subject, search under both MESH headings (exploded) and text words (title and abstract), then combine the two by using the Boolean operator 'or'.

For a focused (specific) search on a clear-cut topic, perform two or more sensitive searches as in step 2, and combine them by using the Boolean operator 'and'.

To find articles that are likely to be of high methodological quality, insert an evidence-based quality filter for therapeutic interventions, aetiology, diagnostic procedures or epidemiology, and/or use maximally sensitive search strategies for randomised trials, systematic reviews and meta-analyses.

Refine your search as you go—for example, to exclude irrelevant material, use the Boolean operator 'not'.

Use subheadings only when this is the only practicable way of limiting your search, as manual indexers are fallible and misclassifications are common.

When limiting a large set, browse through the last 50 or so abstracts yourself rather than expecting the software to pick the best half dozen.

(Source: Greenhalgh, 2014)

Box 8.3 Definitions

Some common terms used in research:

- *Case studies*—focus on one or a limited number of settings; used to explore contemporary phenomena, especially where complex interrelated issues are involved. Can be exploratory, explanatory or descriptive, or a combination of these.

- *Consensus methods*—include Delphi and nominal group techniques and consensus development conferences. They provide a way of synthesising information and dealing with conflicting evidence, with the aim of determining the extent of agreement within a selected group.

- *Constant comparison*—iterative method of content analysis where each category is searched for in the entire data set and all instances are compared until no new categories can be identified.

- *Content analysis*—systematic examination of text (field notes) by identifying and grouping themes and coding, classifying and developing categories.

- *Epistemology*—theory of knowledge; scientific study which deals with the nature and validity of knowledge.

- *Field notes*—collective term for records of observation, talk, interview transcripts or documentary sources. Typically includes a field diary, which provides a record of the chronological events and development of research as well as the researcher's own reactions to, feelings about and opinions of the research process.

- *Hawthorne effect*—impact of the researcher on the research subjects or setting, notably in changing their behaviour.

- *Naturalistic research*—non-experimental research in naturally occurring settings.

- *Purposive or systematic sampling*—deliberate choice of respondents, subjects or settings, as opposed to statistical sampling, concerned with the representativeness of a sample in relation to a total population. Theoretical sampling links this to previously developed hypotheses or theories.

- *Reliability*—extent to which a measurement yields the same answer each time it is used.

- *Social anthropology*—social scientific study of peoples, cultures and societies; particularly associated with the study of traditional cultures.

- *Triangulation*—use of three or more different research methods in combination; principally used as a check of validity.

- *Validity*—extent to which a measurement truly reflects the phenomenon under scrutiny.

(Source: Pope & Mays, 2006)

3. Critically estimate the research for how close it is to the truth and whether it could be clinically useful.
4. Try to use the suggestions in practice.
5. Reflect on, or evaluate, what happens.

In *The New Midwifery*, Professor Lesley Page describes evidence in terms of 'a process of involving women in making decisions about their care and of finding and weighing up information to help make those decisions' (Page & McCandlish, 2006, p. 360). The five steps to **evidence-based midwifery** (Box 8.5) were adapted by Professor Page from the original work in this area undertaken by Sackett et al. in 1996.

In step 3, seeking and assessing evidence, the original authors added that it is important to decide how *valid* something is. In other words, how close to the truth is it? It is also important to find out how *useful* it is—that is,

Box 8.4 Evidence-based practice

The aim of evidence-based practice, to quote Professor David Sackett, is 'the conscientious, explicit and judicious use of current best evidence in making decisions about the care of individual patients ... the integration of individual clinical expertise with the best available external clinical evidence from systematic research' (Cooke & Sackett, 1996, p. 535). In other words, it is the combination of clinical judgment and clinical practical experience with information we gather to help us learn.

Box 8.5 Page's five steps to evidence-based midwifery

1. Find out what is important to the woman and her family.
2. Use information from the clinical examination.
3. Seek and assess evidence to inform decisions.
4. Talk it through.
5. Reflect on outcomes, feelings and consequences.

(Source: 3Page & McCandlish, 2006)

Box 8.6 The PICO method (with the addition of T for time)

PICO is a way of breaking a question into its components:

P Population or Patients

I Intervention or Indication

C Comparison group or Control

O Outcome.

Additionally:

T Time describes the duration for your data collection.

C C refers to the context in which the identified studies were undertaken.

how applicable to practice is the evidence? One thing to remember is that evidence-based midwifery should never be a 'cookbook' approach to what we do. The evidence that we bring to practice from the literature or from research informs practice in conjunction with a woman's individual preference for a clinical decision (Cooke & Sackett, 1996; Page & McCandlish, 2006).

One of the ways of checking whether a research paper addresses the area of inquiry you are interested in is to see whether the question the research seeks to answer applies to your area of interest. To do this, we divide the question into its components to make sure it is relevant. This is known as the PICO method (Box 8.6); the mnemonic PICO helps to remember each component. For example:

- Does it involve a P*opulation* of interest, or does the population closely resemble the one you want to understand?
- Is the I*ntervention* or treatment relevant for your area of interest?
- Is the C*omparison* group appropriate?
- Is the O*utcome* one that you are interested in?

(You may sometimes see a 'T' on the end of PICO—researchers may specify the time the studies were undertaken; and similarly you may sometimes see 'C' on the end of PICO—this refers to the context in which the identified studies were undertaken.)

Appendix 8.1 at the end of this chapter lists questions to ask in evaluating a clinical guideline.

When assessing qualitative research, however, the PICO method may not be so easy to interpret and the following table is an innovative new method showing how to interpret the PICO method when assessing qualitative research—reproduced here from a paper by Cooke et al. (2012) 'Beyond PICO: the SPIDER tool for qualitative evidence synthesis' (Fig. 8.2).

Evidence-based everything

Evidence-based obstetric care ... had its origins in the early 1970s ... this was a shift away from opinion-based obstetrics, which up until then had been the dominant paradigm.

(King, 2005, p. 3)

The foundation and primary focus of evidence-based care is within the specialty of medical epidemiology, to ensure the practice of effective medicine, in which the benefits to an individual patient or population outweigh any associated harm to that same patient or population (Gray, 2009, p. 11). The underlying belief is that meaning can be discerned from population patterns and that a relationship exists between mathematics and material reality. The epidemiologist's focus of study is the whole population, in which outcomes are described in averages and percentages, rates and risks. Then the science of chance is applied in the form of a statistical framework that gives the reader an indication of the measurement error or the uncertainty with which the result is believed to be true. This is better known as the '**confidence interval**' (Jolley, 1993). Epidemiology seeks to provide answers through the analysis of accumulated results of hundreds or thousands of comparable cases in population samples. The language of mathematics is used to describe the findings in terms of 'probability' and 'risk'. Such answers, arrived at through studying population samples in randomised trials and cohort studies, cannot be mechanistically applied to the individual, however: 'In large research trials the individual participant's unique and multidimensional experience is expressed as (say) a single dot on a scatter plot to which we apply mathematical tools to produce a story about the sample as a whole' (Greenhalgh, 1999, p. 324). In other words, the answers that we gain from doing research at a population level tell us about the general population in averages and frequency measures;

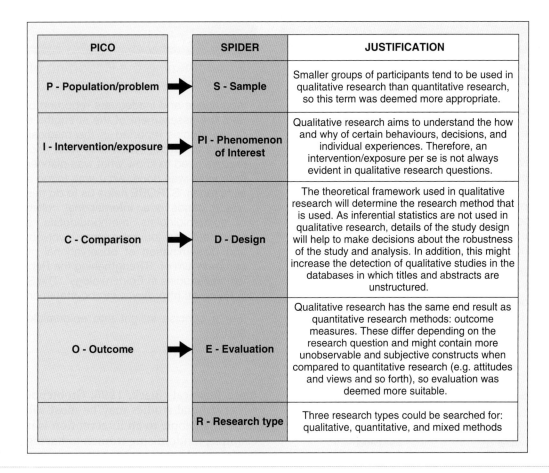

PICO	SPIDER	JUSTIFICATION
P - Population/problem	S - Sample	Smaller groups of participants tend to be used in qualitative research than quantitative research, so this term was deemed more appropriate.
I - Intervention/exposure	PI - Phenomenon of Interest	Qualitative research aims to understand the how and why of certain behaviours, decisions, and individual experiences. Therefore, an intervention/exposure per se is not always evident in qualitative research questions.
C - Comparison	D - Design	The theoretical framework used in qualitative research will determine the research method that is used. As inferential statistics are not used in qualitative research, details of the study design will help to make decisions about the robustness of the study and analysis. In addition, this might increase the detection of qualitative studies in the databases in which titles and abstracts are unstructured.
O - Outcome	E - Evaluation	Qualitative research has the same end result as quantitative research methods: outcome measures. These differ depending on the research question and might contain more unobservable and subjective constructs when compared to quantitative research (e.g. attitudes and views and so forth), so evaluation was deemed more suitable.
	R - Research type	Three research types could be searched for: qualitative, quantitative, and mixed methods

FIGURE 8.2 Beyond PICO the SPIDER tool for qualitative evidence synthesis
(Source: Cooke et al., 2012)

they do not tell us the story of the individuals who took part. In asking 'What works?' we are suggesting that research will show us how to do things the best way. The danger here is that we may unwittingly focus on very narrow 'evaluative' studies—that is, studies that demonstrate the effectiveness of an intervention, such as the RCT, when in fact information from a whole range of types of studies answering a variety of questions may be more useful. (See the story of the information leaflets earlier in this chapter.) In reality we practise within a complex and mostly unpredictable reality in which learning from trial and error may be an important way to make progress (Churruca et al., 2019).

At the turn of the 20th century, epidemiological research began to explicitly incorporate social science perspectives related to health data that could inform public policy. One of the first substantial prospective epidemiological analyses to be undertaken was a study of the socioeconomic and nutritional determinants of infant mortality in the United States in 1912, by Julia Lathrop (Krieger, 2000). As sociologist Ann Oakley pointed out, the history of experimentation and social interventions are 'conveniently overlooked by those who contend that randomised controlled trials have no place in evaluating social interventions. It shows clearly that prospective experimental studies with random

allocation to generate one or more control groups is perfectly possible in social settings' (Oakley, 1998, p. 1240). The usefulness of the population-based results of an RCT depends on the translation of the concepts and measures used to describe groups of people into a language that can inform the decisions of an individual (Steiner, 1999).

The RCT is currently considered to be the orthodox and 'gold standard' scientific experimental method for evaluating new treatments. The ethical basis for entering patients in RCTs, however, is currently under debate (Box 8.7). Some doctors espouse the uncertainty principle whereby randomisation to treatment is acceptable when an individual doctor is genuinely unsure which treatment is best for a patient. Others believe that clinical equipoise, reflecting collective professional uncertainty over treatment, is the soundest ethical criterion (Webster et al., 2016). The scientific principles that are applied to the design and conduct of primary research, such as the RCT, are also applied to secondary research, such as the systematic review (Chalmers et al., 1992). Indeed, many regard epidemiology as 'an arcane quantitative science penetrable only by mathematicians' (Grimes & Schulz, 2002, p. 58). However, it must be pointed out that 'statistics is at most complementary to the breadth

Box 8.7 Research ethics

The ethical principle governing research is that respondents should not be harmed as a result of participating in research, and that they should always be asked for their informed consent to participate.

This principle is widely agreed among researchers. Participants should be asked to give their consent in writing after they have had written information about the aims, risks, discomforts, benefits, procedures, questionnaires and the way confidentiality and anonymity will be preserved. Hospitals and universities have ethics committees to oversee the operations of research projects from an ethical and scientific standpoint often referred to HREC (Human Research Ethics Committee).

Before you undertake any research you must undertake to satisfy the ethics committee at the hospital or university where you work by submitting an ethics application for approval before any research begins.

Box 8.8 What is STROBE?

STrengthening the Reporting of OBservational studies in Epidemiology

Incomplete and inadequate reporting of research hampers the assessment of the strengths and weaknesses of the studies reported in the medical, midwifery and nursing literature. When they read and review studies, readers need to know what was planned (and what was not), what was done, what was found and what the results mean. STROBE helps us to do this in a systematic way. It stands for an international, collaborative initiative of epidemiologists, methodologists, statisticians, researchers and journal editors involved in the conduct and dissemination of observational studies, with the common aim of 'STrengthening the Reporting of OBservational studies in Epidemiology'. The STROBE website is found at: http://www.strobe-statement.org/

(For a concise insight into epidemiology see Saracci (2010).)

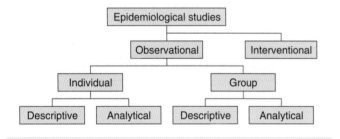

FIGURE 8.3 Types of epidemiological studies

and judgment' of the knowledge gained from epidemiological research (Jolley, 1993, p. 28).

Fig. 8.3 outlines the kinds of studies you will encounter in the scientific literature, both medical and midwifery, that are based on the epidemiological method. In order to find where the 'best evidence' is to support our practice we are encouraged to give research studies a ranking from the highest level, or the 'gold standard', to the lowest level of research evidence. These rankings are made explicitly on the ranking of research methods from the most reliable to the least reliable. This 'evidence hierarchy' provides an initial screening test as to whether data from research studies are derived from methods that are more likely or less likely to guide readers towards truthful conclusions (Grootendorst et al., 2010; Gupta, 2003). (Further discussion on this topic, and current debates, definitions and controversies, can be found on the Centre for Evidence-Based Medicine website at http://www.cebm.net/.)

Experimental trials are limited when the study size is too small to detect rare or infrequent adverse outcomes, or when the outcome of interest is long term and the trial would need to continue for an improbable length of time. In all these cases, observational studies may be considered

more practical (Black, 1996; Grootendorst et al., 2010). Observational studies may be most valuable where randomising people to an intervention is inappropriate—for example, randomising women to having water birth or to having an elective caesarean section is inappropriate and also disregards the 'effect that choice itself has on therapeutic outcome' (McPherson, 1994, p. 7) (Box 8.8).

There is no doubt that there are limitations of empiricism as a value-neutral truth, and as the only structure for analysing our decision making. As one physician put it, 'Evidence-based decision models may be very powerful—but are like computer generated symphonies in the style of Mozart—correct but lifeless' (Saunders, 2000, p. 22). From the sociologist's viewpoint, the implementation of RCTs in real-life settings causes some hazards, such as low participation and high attrition rates, problems with informed consent, unanticipated side effects of the intervention, and possible problematic relations between research and policy. Ann Oakley, a sociologist well known for her research on housework and on childbirth asks, 'What may a society obsessed with quantification have lost in terms of the value of more intimate knowledge, intuition, emotions and all the other qualities that (we) soft social scientists are renowned for going on about?' (Oakley, 1998, p. 1242).

The **experimental method** allows the investigator to have control over the population group she or he is studying, by deciding which groups will be exposed to a factor under study and which groups will become the control group. This method involves manipulating one variable to determine whether changes in one variable cause changes in another variable. A feature of the experimental method is that the investigator can randomly allocate a subject to the experimental or the control group (Schneider & Lilienfeld, 2015).

It may consist of questionnaires, biophysical measures, structured observations and clinical trials.

In the sample, the subjects may be randomly allocated to the experimental or the control group.

Analysis includes inferential statistics provided in tables, which give the significance of findings in terms of a probability (*p*) value, or the confidence intervals.

CRITICAL THINKING EXERCISE

Apply the PICO (T and / or C) formula to the M@NGO and COSMOS trials (McLachlan et al., 2012; Tracy et al., 2013)

Quasi-experimental method is similar to the above, but there may be no control or randomisation. Non-experimental methods are used to gather data to describe events as they occur. These may consist of surveys, for example. The data are analysed and presented using descriptive statistics such as frequency distributions and histograms. Relationships and associations may be inferred, but not cause and effect. These methods will be covered in more detail later in this chapter.

THE RANDOMISED CONTROLLED TRIAL

A randomised controlled trial (RCT) is an experiment in which two or more interventions, including a control intervention or no intervention, are compared by being randomly allocated to participants (CONSORT Group, 2010, 2017). RCTs are often referred to as 'clinical trials'. In an RCT or clinical trial, each participant is randomised to either receive or not receive the intervention. A clinical trial must have at least one prospectively assigned *concurrent* control or comparison group (Moher et al., 2012; Schulz et al., 2010).

The rationale for conducting an RCT is to compare the outcomes of treatment given to different groups of people, while at the same time preventing the effect of systematic 'bias' on the results. The application of randomisation is the logical way to control bias in assessing the effects of certain treatments (Chalmers, 1989). The idea is not to worry about the characteristics of the patients, but to be sure that the division of the patients into two groups is done by some method independent of human choice—that is, by the use of random numbers (Cochrane in Black et al., 1984, p. 115) (Box 8.9).

In controlling the selection bias, the aim is to be able to distinguish the effect of a certain treatment on a group of people that is separate from and not affected by the individual characteristics of that group of people. In the RCT, the logical application of controlling bias is to allocate the people who will be part of the trial by randomising them to either the treatment or the control group (Fig. 8.4).

Box 8.9 CONSORT

Have you seen this word when reading about randomised controlled trials? It stands for: **CON**solidated **S**tandards **O**f **R**eporting **T**rials. You can find out more at: http://www.consort-statement.org/.

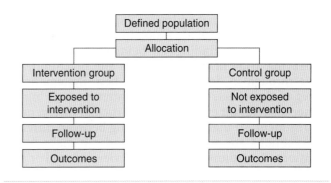

FIGURE 8.4 Allocation of a treatment group and a control group in an intervention study (including the randomised controlled trial)

The term 'random' does not mean the same as haphazard, but has a precise technical meaning. By random allocation we mean that each person has an equal chance, of being given each treatment, but the treatment to be given cannot be predicted. If there are two treatments, the simplest method of random allocation gives each patient an equal chance of getting either treatment; it is equivalent to tossing a coin. In practice, most people use either a table of random numbers or a random-number generator on a computer. This is simple randomisation. Possible modifications include block randomisation, to ensure closely similar numbers of patients in each group, and stratified randomisation, to keep the groups balanced for certain prognostic patient characteristics (Altman & Bland, 1999; CONSORT Group, 2010). There are points to consider here in midwifery, however. When data are derived exclusively from RCTs or meta-analysis, the results give us a clear idea of the efficacy of the intervention for an 'average' randomised patient (Box 8.10).

Box 8.10 The 'average' patient

One immediate problem in using the results of RCTs is that the conclusions refer to an 'average patient' who fulfilled the criteria for admission. When transferred to clinical medicine from an origin in agricultural research, randomised trials were not intended to answer questions about the treatment of individual patients. The trials have almost always been used to offer an average value for efficacy in groups of patients receiving the compared therapies.

(Source: Feinstein & Horwitz, 1997, p. 534)

Randomised controls offer 'the protection of the public from potentially damaging uncontrolled experimentation and a more rational knowledge about the benefits to be derived from professional interventions' (Oakley, 1998, p. 1242).

THE SYSTEMATIC REVIEW

A **systematic review** is a concise summary of the best available evidence that addresses a sharply defined clinical question (Sackett et al., 2000). In a world where more and more research findings are being published, there is a dizzying array of information for the practitioner to wade through in deciding what is best. Systematic reviews of the effects of healthcare attempt to bring together the relevant evidence on a particular intervention or treatment, so that people choosing between different interventions are more informed and can make better decisions. Regardless of whether a review is broad or narrow, the reviewer tries to identify as many of the eligible studies as possible, so that these can be included as fully as possible in the review.

If appropriate, the reviewer might conduct a meta-analysis, in which the results of different trials are statistically combined to provide a more precise estimate of the average difference between the effects of the interventions being compared. In all systematic reviews, the evidence being brought together for a particular intervention needs to be as free from bias and as reliable as possible. This is why most reviews of the effects of interventions rely exclusively on randomised trials. The process of bringing together the evidence also needs to minimise bias, and be rigorous and robust. The ultimate aim of any systematic review of randomised trials should be to ensure that relevant data on all randomised participants from all relevant trials are included (McKenzie et al., 2016; Shamseer et al., 2015).

The value of systematic reviews depends greatly on the availability and quality of the results of primary research: 'Knowledge development must be cumulative in the sense that related knowledge generated from separate research studies is integrated into a more comprehensive understanding of the topic at hand' (Kirkevold, 1997, p. 977).

One of the key parts of any review is to consider how similar or different the available primary studies are and what impact any differences have on the studies' results. Between-study differences or *heterogeneity* in results can result from chance, from errors in calculating accuracy indices, or from true heterogeneity—that is, from differences in design, conduct, participants, tests and reference tests.

The steps required to undertake a systematic review are as follows:

1. The problems to be addressed are specified in the form of well-structured questions.
2. The inclusion and exclusion criteria, which will be used to determine whether a study will be included in the search, are defined.
3. Literature searches are conducted to identify potentially relevant studies that shed light on the questions.
4. The quality of the selected studies is assessed.
5. The evidence concerning study characteristics and results is summarised, differences between studies are explored and, when feasible and appropriate, meta-analysis is undertaken to help in collating results.
6. Inferences and recommendations for practice are generated from interpretation and exploration of clinical relevance of the findings (Khan, 2005; Machi & McEvoy, 2016).

A systematic review of the literature allows for estimations of the effects of healthcare interventions by identifying the individual, clinical and contextual factors that influence the effectiveness of that care. Overall conclusions are drawn from many studies that are believed to address the same or similar research hypotheses. An overview provides a broader look at the subject in question, as it is based on a number of studies in different settings and includes a variety of participants. Overviews are also useful in identifying the uncertainties and gaps in the research. Meta-analysis uses statistical techniques to combine and summarise results of multiple studies that may or may not be contained within a systematic review. It can provide more precise estimates of the effects of healthcare by combining more data than those derived from individual studies (Shamseer et al., 2015). The benefits of meta-analysis include a consolidated and quantitative review of a large and often complex, and sometimes conflicting, body of literature (Haidich, 2010). The systematic review differs from meta-analysis in that it does not necessarily statistically combine the results of studies that are critically reviewed.

Specific characteristics of a systematic review include:

- formal criteria on which studies are eligible for inclusion—this is done in order to avoid selection bias regarding inclusion or exclusion of studies
- a clear set of objectives with an explicit, reproducible methodology
- a systematic search that attempts to identify all studies meeting the eligibility criteria
- assessment of the validity of findings—expression of the statistical uncertainties inherent in each study by appropriate use of the confidence interval
- in the interpretation of results, taking into account the limitation of some studies in inferring causality (Higgins & Green, 2011; Shamseer et al., 2015).

The systematic review is an important tool, for a number of reasons. Progress in midwifery care is achieved through research that refines, extends or refutes prior theoretical concepts to build onto that system of scientific knowledge. Knowledge that is cumulative can then be integrated into one systematic review in order to achieve a more comprehensive understanding (Chalmers et al., 1992; Kirkevold, 1997). The value of systematic review has been demonstrated by the success of systematic review providers such as the Cochrane database. Research must be accessible to clinicians and consumers if research-based practice is to become a reality, and the Cochrane database is one way for midwives to find systematic reviews without having to trawl through the internet (see: https://www.cochrane.org/search/site/cochrane/reviews).

META-ANALYSIS

The *Cochrane Handbook for Systematic Reviews of Interventions* (Higgins & Green, 2011) quotes the following reasons for considering a meta-analysis:

1. *To increase power*—power is the chance of detecting a real, statistically significant effect, if it exists. Many individual studies are too small to detect small effects, but when several are combined there is a higher chance of detecting an effect.
2. *To improve precision*—the estimation of a treatment effect can be improved when it is based on more information.
3. *To answer questions not posed by the individual studies*—primary studies often involve a specific type of patient and explicitly defined interventions. A selection of studies in which these characteristics differ can allow investigation of the consistency of effect and, if relevant, allow reasons for differences in effect estimates to be investigated.
4. *To settle controversies arising from apparently conflicting studies or to generate new hypotheses*—statistical analysis of findings allows the degree of conflict to be formally assessed, and reasons for different results to be explored and quantified.

Warning: Of course, the use of statistical methods does not guarantee that the results of a systematic review are valid, any more than it does for a primary study. Moreover, like any tool, statistical methods can be misused. Meta-analyses of poor-quality studies may be seriously misleading. If bias is present in each (or some) of the individual studies, meta-analysis will simply compound the errors, and produce a 'wrong' result that may be interpreted as having more credibility (Higgins & Green, 2011, section 9.1.4).

The methods used for meta-analysis generally follow these basic principles:

Meta-analysis is typically a two-stage process. In the first stage, a summary statistic is calculated for each study. For controlled trials, these values describe the treatment effects observed in each individual trial. For example, the summary statistic may be a risk ratio if the data are dichotomous or a difference between means if the data are continuous.

In the second stage, a summary (pooled) treatment effect estimate is calculated as a weighted average of the treatment effects estimated in the individual studies (Higgins & Green, 2011, section 9.4.2).

You will no doubt be familiar with the Cochrane Library graphs illustrating the probability of an outcome between two groups who have been treated differently (the treatment group and the control group). When deciding what this shows—that is, the treatment effects—the questions to ask are:

1. What is the direction of effect?
2. What is the size of effect?
3. Is the effect consistent across studies?
4. What is the strength of evidence for the effect?

See if you can work out the answers to these questions when exploring Fig. 8.5. This figure demonstrates the outcome in terms of having to manually remove the placenta between a group of women (treatment group) who were given IM Syntometrine as the oxytocic of choice and comparing this outcome with the group of women (control group) who had been randomly allocated *not* to receive this treatment. Remember: the line that passes down the middle of the graph is called the 'line of no effect' (Box 8.11). (This will be explained more fully later in the chapter.) To go back to our four questions:

1. *Answer:* the effect is very minimally on the positive side (the right-hand side) of 1. This tells us that the treatment had a mildly positive effect—that is, having an active management of the third stage of labour was

Review: Active versus expectant management in the third stage of labour
Comparison: Active vs expectant management (all women)
Outcome: Manual removal of placenta

Study	Treatment n/N	Control n/N	Relative Risk (Fixed) 95% CI	Weight %	Relative Risk (Fixed) 95% CI
Abu Dhabi 1997	3/827	9/821		19.9	0.33 [0.09, 1.22]
Brighton 1993	1/103	0/90		1.2	2.63 [0.11, 63.64]
Bristol 1988	16/846	22/849		48.4	0.73 [0.39, 1.38]
Dublin 1990	19/705	1/724		2.2	19.51 [2.62, 145.36]
Hinchingbrooke 1998	15/748	13/764		28.3	1.18 [0.56, 2.46]
Total	3229	3248		100.0	1.21 [0.82, 1.78]

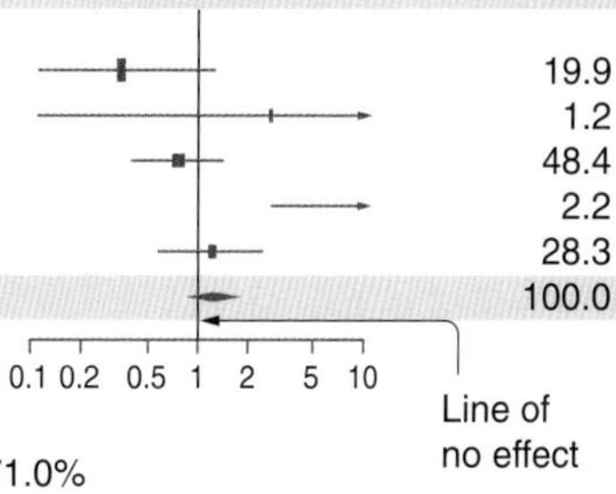

0.1 0.2 0.5 1 2 5 10

Line of no effect

Total events: 54 (Treatment), 45 (Control)
Test for heterogeneity chi-square = 13.80 df = 4 p = 0.008 T^2 = 71.0%
Test for overall effect Z = 0.95 p = 0.3

FIGURE 8.5 Example of a systematic review and meta-analysis
(Based on Begley et al., 2015)

Box 8.11   Reading a Cochrane table

See Fig. 8.5 for an example of a Cochrane table.

The 'forest plot' is the diamond at the bottom. It depicts the pooled odds ratios.

The horizontal lines correspond with each trial included and show the difference between groups—best single; the width of the line demonstrates the 95% confidence interval of this estimate.

The black line down the middle of the picture is known as the 'line of no effect'.

If the confidence interval (the horizontal lines) crosses the line of no effect (the vertical line), this means either that there is no significant difference between the interventions, or that the sample size was too small for us to be confident of where the true result lies.

The various individual studies give point estimates of the relative risks, and the confidence intervals are so wide on some studies that they go off the page. This is depicted as an arrow.

The tiny diamond below all the horizontal lines represents the pooled data from the trials, with a new, much narrower confidence interval.

If the diamond overlaps the line of no effect, we can say there is probably little difference between the two interventions in terms of the primary end point (defined at the top of the graph).

Heterogeneity can involve some serious statistics. However, the question to ask is whether there is greater variation between the results of the trials than would be conceivable through chance.

You need to think how you would interpret these results in practice.

associated with having to have a manual removal of the placenta. This is called the *direction* of the effect.

2. *Answer:* the size of the effect is very small as well, because we can see that the confidence intervals of four of the studies and the pooled result all cross the line of no effect.
3. *Answer:* no, the effect is not consistent across all studies.
4. *Answer:* the confidence interval crosses 1, or the line of no effect, and therefore the strength of the evidence is not strong. The outcome may have occurred due to *chance*.

The different types of review are summarised in Box 8.12.

SYNTHESISING RESEARCH

Gathering research, getting rid of rubbish and summarising the best of what remains captures the essence of the science of systematic review. Nevertheless, although the need to synthesise research evidence has been recognised for well over two centuries, it was not until the 20th century that researchers began to develop explicit methods for this form of research.

IMPLEMENTATION SCIENCE OR KNOWLEDGE TRANSLATION

One of the biggest challenges in health is being able to move from the position of knowing the evidence to being able to apply it in practice (Box 8.13). The term 'knowledge translation' (KT) has gained traction in addressing the challenges in translating research to knowledge in order to start closing the 'know-do' gap (WHO, 2006). Knowledge

Box 8.12   Types of reviews currently in use for gathering evidence

- **Systematic review:** aims to review evidence on a clearly formulated question that uses systematic and explicit methods to identify, select and critically appraise relevant primary research, and to extract and analyse data from the studies that are included in the review. The methods used must be reproducible and transparent. (See the **P**referred Reporting Items for Systematic Reviews and Meta-Analyses (PRISMA) statement at http://www.prisma-statement.org/documents/PRISMA-P-checklist.pdf.)

  - The review question is identified.

  - A comprehensive search is made to find all the relevant studies.

  - Explicit criteria is used to either include or exclude the studies.

  - The studies must be critically appraised for quality.

  - Explicit methods are used to extract or synthesise the study findings.

- (Some systematic reviews may go further to synthesis the statistical outcomes into a meta-analysis.)

  Strengths: identifies all available research that is relevant to a particular review question and by using a known formula they can easily be replicated / updated.

  Weaknesses: uses a necessarily narrowly defined review question and therefore can only provide specific answers to specific questions.

(See also Page et al., 2021.)

- **Critical review:** aims to demonstrate that the writer has extensively researched the literature and critically evaluated its quality. It is more than a description, however; it typically manifests in a hypothesis or a model, not an answer.

  Strengths: provides an opportunity to 'take stock' and evaluate what is of value from the previous body of work.

Box 8.12 Types of reviews currently in use for gathering evidence—cont'd

Weaknesses: the emphasis is on the conceptual contribution of each item of included literature, not on formal quality assessment.

- **Literature review:** describes 'published materials which provide an examination of recent or current literature'. Generally, a literature review involves some process for identifying materials for potential inclusion—whether or not requiring a formal literature search—for selecting included materials, for synthesising them in textual, tabular or graphical form and for making some analysis of their contribution or value.

  Strengths: identifies what has been accomplished previously, allowing for consolidation, for building on previous work, for summation, for avoiding duplication and for identifying omissions or gaps.

  Weaknesses: lacks an explicit intent to maximise scope or analyse data collected. Authors may select only literature that supports their worldview, lending undue credence to a preferred hypothesis.

- **Mapping review/systematic map:** aims to map out and categorise existing literature on a particular topic, identifying gaps in research literature from which to commission further reviews and/or primary research.

  Strengths: can show whether the total population of studies is sufficiently similar for a coherent synthesis. This type of review may characterise studies in other ways such as according to theoretical perspective, population group or the setting within which studies were undertaken.

  Weaknesses: mapping reviews are necessarily time constrained and lack the synthesis and analysis of more-considered approaches. They do not usually include a quality assessment process, characterising studies only on the basis of study design.

- **Meta-analysis:** is 'a technique that statistically combines the results of quantitative studies to provide a more precise effect of the results'. Most importantly, it requires that the same measure or outcome be measured in the same way at the same time intervals.

  Strengths: from its early origins in the social sciences, meta-analysis has grown in popularity, primarily because of the facility to take individual studies, not in themselves sufficient to impact on practice, and to assimilate them into a composite evidence base.

Small or inconclusive studies lacking in statistical significance can nevertheless make a contribution to the larger picture.

  Weaknesses: critics of meta-analysis argue the inappropriateness of combining 'apples and oranges', i.e. studies that are not sufficiently similar. One essential fact remains—a meta-analysis cannot be better than its included studies allow.

- **Narrative review:** see Literature review, above.

- **Mixed studies review/mixed methods review:** refers to any combination of methods where at least one of the components is a literature (usually systematic) review. In bringing together outcome studies with studies that describe the actual processes that were used, these reviews attempt to bring the 'what works' of the former together with the 'how and why does it work' of the latter to start to address the more complex issue of 'what works under which circumstances'.

  Strengths: capitalises on the corresponding weaknesses of the 'what works' effectiveness of a systematic review and alternative, more-theory-driven approaches.

  Weaknesses: may compound the methodological challenges of appraising and synthesising both quantitative and qualitative research with the added difficulty of integrating the results.

- **Overview:** is a generic term used for 'any summary of the [medical] literature'.

  Strengths: provides a broad summation of a topic area for those coming to a subject for the first time.

  Weaknesses: frequently used as a non-discriminant word for reviews of varying rigour and quality.

- **Qualitative systematic review/qualitative evidence synthesis:** is a method for integrating or comparing the findings from qualitative studies.

  Strengths: complements research evidence obtained through epidemiological research from a user-reported or practitioner-observed perspective. It can be used to explore a point of view from those in the service and those experiencing the service.

  Weaknesses: there is a debate centring on whether the dominant model for qualitative evidence synthesis is the classic systematic review method, or whether it is more appropriate to adapt and adopt concepts from primary qualitative research (e.g. grounded theory, theoretical saturation, purposive sampling, etc.).

(Based on Grant MJ, Booth A. A typology of reviews: an analysis of 14 review types and associated methodologies. *Health Information and Libraries Journal.* 2009;l26:91–108. doi:10.1111/ j.1471-1842.2009.00848.x, with permission of John Wiley & Sons)

translation can be defined as 'ensuring that stakeholders are aware of and use research evidence to inform their health and healthcare decision-making'; this definition recognises that there are a wide range of stakeholders or target audiences for knowledge translation, including policy makers, professionals (practitioners), consumers (i.e. patients, family members and informal carers), researchers and industry (Grimshaw et al., 2012, p. 2).

There is a plethora of interventions and policies aimed at changing practice habits of midwives and obstetricians, but little evidence exists on the most effective interventions to change professional practice in line with emerging

<table>
<tr><td>

Box 8.13 Embedded implementation design

This is a practice-based research method that relies heavily on connecting with communities within which the research is planned. The research involves 'knowledgeable researchers' (ideally those who live and work within, or are embedded in) the service where changes are being designed working with the academic researchers to facilitate change. In this way the researcher builds the capacity for change and implementation through consultation and partnership at the outset with the women who would benefit from the changes proposed. This method shifts the power from the 'researcher' on one hand and 'the researched' on the other into a working partnership promoting change.

(Braithwaite, 2017; Braithwaite et al., 2018; Churruca et al., 2019; Greenhalgh et al., 2016)

</td></tr>
</table>

research. Chauhan et al. (2017) in an overview of available reviews found that behaviour change interventions, including interactive and multifaceted continuous education, training with audit and feedback, enabling patients through advanced information technology-based systems, and collaborative team-based interventions, can effectively modify healthcare professionals' practice and patient outcomes. Interestingly the researchers concluded that financial incentives did not influence long-term practice change.

In Australia, midwives in Victoria have used normalisation process theory (NPT) to provide a framework to consider issues of implementation, embedding, continuation and sustainability of the caseload midwifery model. Researchers have embedded an element of implementation science in trying to understand the factors that impact on the introduction, sustainability and growth of these models. The researchers found that the normalisation process model provided a framework within the COSMOS trial to examine some issues prospectively, through both the evaluation research design (relating to the implementation of the model of care into practice) and the analysis of findings (Forster et al., 2011).

CRITICAL THINKING EXERCISE

Find the COSMOS, WAVE and ECO studies from Victoria, Australia, and determine how implementation science was used to translate research into practice. (See Forster et al. (2011) and the work from the COSMOS trial (McLachlan et al., 2012).)

For further information on knowledge transfer see the following two Canadian websites:
Rx for Change: https://www.cadth.ca/rx-change
Health Systems Evidence: https://www.healthsystemsevidence.org.

COMPLEX INTERVENTIONS, HEALTHCARE POLICY AND REALIST REVIEW

Researching complex interventions is an area that is attracting increasing interest in healthcare. In bringing to the fore the perspective of managers and decision makers, and in recognising the messy, non-linear nature of decision making, realist review is one way to overcome the constraints of evidence-based decisions in healthcare policy and management (Box 8.14).

In the four-stage approach outlined by Pawson et al. (2005), the process begins with the decision makers and reviewers negotiating the reasons for the review and how it will be used. The next step is to search for and review the evidence, followed by continuous contact and negotiation between decision makers and reviewers. Finally, there is a bringing together of the results of the review and synthesis to enable decision makers to reach a deeper understanding of the intervention they are considering and its likely impact. It follows from this view that research syntheses used to inform policy and management decisions are less about converging on answers and recommendations than about using evidence to illuminate choices and to explore the consequences of alternative courses of action.

THE HIERARCHY OF EVIDENCE

You may see guidelines written with a **'level of evidence'** ranking beside the advice given (Table 8.1). These rankings or levels are given to the research evidence to help decision makers gauge the strength of the evidence for a particular course of treatment or action. Most studies are ranked according to whether they have controlled for the possibility of bias and whether they have a strong scientific study design. It will not surprise you to note that the systematic review—which is a collection of RCTs attempting to answer the same question—is top of the list.

(For more information on the levels of evidence hierarchy see the Oxford Levels of Evidence Working Group at the Oxford Centre for Evidence-based Medicine; the 2016 levels of evidence are at: https://www.cebm.net/2016/05/ocebm-levels-of-evidence/.

CRITICAL THINKING EXERCISE

What are the differences between the following:

- bad science based on poor evidence?
- inadequate science based on insufficient evidence?
- no science based purely on dogma?

(Source: Sharpe, 2000, p. 29)

Box 8.14 Realist review for researching complex systems

According to Pawson et al. (2005, p. 25): 'Complex service interventions can be conceptualised as dynamic complex systems thrust amidst complex systems, relentlessly subject to negotiation, resistance, adaptation, leak and borrow, bloom and fade, and so on'.

In evaluating complex systems the researcher takes an approach to reviewing and synthesising research evidence that is believed to be well suited to the study of complex social interventions.

Realist review is a relatively new strategy for synthesising research that has an explanatory rather than judgmental focus. It seeks to unpack the mechanism of how complex programs work (or why they fail) in particular contexts and settings.

Realist review is not a method or formula, but rather a logic of enquiry that is inherently pluralist and flexible, embracing both qualitative and quantitative, formative and summative, prospective and retrospective, and so on. It seeks not to judge but to explain, and is driven by the question 'What works for whom in what circumstances and in what respects?' Under realism, the basic evaluative question—'What works?'—changes to 'What is it about this program that works for whom in what circumstances?'

Realist review learns from (rather than controls for) real-world phenomena such as diversity, change, idiosyncrasy, adaptation, cross-contamination and program failure. It engages stakeholders systematically—as fallible experts whose insider understanding needs to be documented, formalised and tested, and provides a principled steer away from failed one-size-fits-all ways of responding to problems.

Realist review differs from an experimental randomised trial, for example. In the latter the experimental propositions that are being tested relate to whether the treatment (and the treatment alone) is effective. As well as random allocation of participants, safeguards such as the use of placebos and double blinding are utilised to protect this causal inference. The idea is to remove any shred of human intentionality from the investigation. Realist review using active programs, by contrast, only works through the stakeholders' reasoning and knowledge of that reasoning as integral to understanding its outcomes. Broadly speaking, we should expect that, in tracking the successes and failures of interventions, reviewers will find at least part of the explanation in terms of the reasoning and personal choices of different actors and participants.

By taking program theory as its unit of analysis, realist review has the potential to maximise learning across policy, disciplinary and organisational boundaries.

Table 8.1 NHMRC evidence hierarchy: designations of 'levels of evidence' according to type of research question

Level	Intervention[1]	Diagnostic accuracy[2]	Prognosis	Aetiology[3]	Screening intervention
I[4]	A systematic review of level II studies	A systematic review of level II studies	A systematic review of level II studies	A systematic review of level II studies	A systematic review of level II studies
II	A randomised controlled trial	A study of test accuracy with: an independent, blinded comparison with a valid reference standard,[5] among consecutive persons with a defined clinical presentation[6]	A prospective cohort study[7]	A prospective cohort study	A randomised controlled trial
III-1	A pseudorandomised controlled trial (i.e. alternate allocation or some other method)	A study of test accuracy with an independent, blinded comparison with a valid reference standard,[5] among non-consecutive persons with a defined clinical presentation[6]	All or none[8]	All or none[8]	A pseudorandomised controlled trial (i.e. alternate allocation or some other method)

Continued

Table 8.1 NHMRC evidence hierarchy: designations of 'levels of evidence' according to type of research question—cont'd

Level	Intervention[1]	Diagnostic accuracy[2]	Prognosis	Aetiology[3]	Screening intervention
III-2	A comparative study with concurrent controls: • Non-randomised, experimental trial[9] • Cohort study • Case–control study • Interrupted time series with a control group	A comparison with reference standard that does not meet the criteria required for level II and III-1 evidence	Analysis of prognostic factors amongst persons in a single arm of a randomised controlled trial	A retrospective cohort study	A comparative study with concurrent controls: • Non-randomised, experimental trial • Cohort study • Case–control study
III-3	A comparative study without concurrent controls: • Historical control study • Two or more single-arm study[10] • Interrupted time series without a parallel control group	Diagnostic case–control study[6]	A retrospective cohort study	A case–control study	A comparative study without concurrent controls: • Historical control study • Two or more single-arm study
IV	Case series with either post-test or pretest/post-test outcomes	Study of diagnostic yield (no reference standard)[11]	Case series, or cohort study of persons at different stages of disease	A cross-sectional study or case series	Case series

(Sources and explanatory notes 1–11 can be found at: http://sydney.edu.au/medicine/21st-century/presentations/2013/NHMRC-hierarchy-of-evidence.pdf; Merlin T, Weston A, Tooher R. Extending an evidence hierarchy to include topics other than treatment: revising the Australian 'levels of evidence'. *BMC Med Res Methodol*. 2009;9:34. doi: 10.1186/1471-2288-9-34; © Merlin et al; licensee BioMed Central Ltd, 2009)

Box 8.15, the story of Semmelweis, gives an example of evidence versus dogma.

REFLECTIVE THINKING EXERCISE

What do you think of the hierarchical system for ranking evidence?

To recap, the results of RCTs are considered to be evidence of the highest grade, whereas observational studies are viewed as having less validity because they reportedly overestimate treatment effects:

[Studies are] classified according to grades of evidence on the basis of the research design, using internal validity (that is, the correctness of the results) as the criterion for hierarchical ranking. The highest grade is reserved for research involving properly randomised controlled trials, and the lowest grade is applied to descriptive studies (such as case series) and expert opinion. Observational studies, both cohort studies and case–control studies, fall at intermediate levels. Although the quality of studies is sometimes evaluated within each grade, each category is considered methodologically superior to those below it. This hierarchical approach to study design has been promoted widely in individual reports, meta-analyses, consensus statements, and educational materials for clinicians.

(Concato et al., 2000, p. 1887)

Culpepper & Gilbert (1999) point out that, because the evidence hierarchy privileges certain types of data and certain types of research methodologies, phenomena not easily amenable to investigation by these privileged methods may be neglected or presumed less worthy of inquiry than those interventions best suited to the preferred methods.

INTERVENTION STUDIES

The RCT is an example of an **intervention study**. In such a study, we do not just observe exposures and outcomes in a population. We actively allocate an exposure (or intervention) to one of the study groups; the group that does not receive the intervention acts as a control group. We then follow the groups over a period of time. We compare the frequency of the outcome in the experimental group—those receiving the intervention—with the frequency of the outcome in the group not allocated the intervention. See, for example, the RCTs into continuity of midwifery care conducted by Flint et al. (1989), Homer et al. (2001); McLachlan et al. (2012); Rowley et al. (1995) and Tracy et al. (2013).

Box 8.15   Semmelweis

The story of Semmelweis is well known. In 1848 he published his findings that the rate of fatal postpartum sepsis was 12% for obstetricians attending women in childbirth after having performed an autopsy and not washing their hands, compared with 3% for those attended by midwives who did not perform autopsies. The medical fraternity totally and unequivocally rejected his probability-based evidence. He was denounced and driven from his job, his country, and perhaps his mind, dying in a mental institution at the age of 47 (Goodman, 1999).

Before accountability was determined by 'best evidence', the collective medical tradition in these years was to leave the job of clinical evaluation to the individual. The American Medical Association (AMA) code of ethics (1847) contended that character was as important a qualification as knowledge:

> ... character must be the foundation upon which ethical action is to be built. Proper conduct among men and affairs must be left to the man, his tact, his judgment, his education and his experience.

(Sharpe, 2000, p. 30)

The AMA at the turn of the century further counselled discretion and silence with regard to the practice of colleagues. No ethical alarm bells rang, then, when Charles Meigs, chairman of midwifery at Jefferson Medical College in Philadelphia, in 1859 (11 years following the disclosure by Semmelweis) stated:

> I have practiced midwifery for many long years; I have attended some thousands of women in labour ... passed through repeated epidemics of childbed fever, both in town and in hospital ... After all this experience however, I do not, upon careful reflection and self-examination, find the least reason to suppose I have ever conveyed the disease from place to place in any single instance ... a gentleman's hands are clean.

(Sharpe, 2000, p. 30)

COHORT
1 Follow the cohort over time.
2 Classify into those who are exposed and those who are not exposed.
3 Record those who have the outcome and those who do not have the outcome.

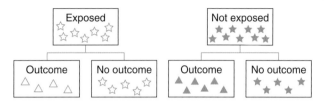

FIGURE 8.6 Cohort studies

CASE CONTROL STUDY
1 Identify the individuals with the outcome of interest (cases).
2 Identify a group who do not have the outcome (controls).
3 Assess difference between the two groups in the past exposure.

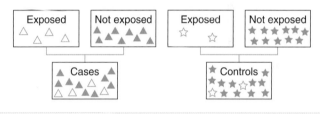

FIGURE 8.7 Case–control studies

slow and expensive to carry out. They are also inefficient in investigating rare outcomes—that is why we do case–control studies where we select all cases with a rare outcome and match them for variables of interest.

Cohort studies

In a **cohort study** (Fig. 8.6) we:
1. select a study population or cohort of people who do not initially have the outcome of interest
2. classify the members of the cohort according to whether or not they have been *exposed* to the potential risk factor
3. follow the entire cohort over time and compare the incidence of the *outcome(s)* in the exposed individuals with the incidence in those not exposed.

Cohort studies are particularly useful for rare exposures and in situations where we are interested in studying more than one outcome. However, they are generally

Case–control studies

In a **case–control study** (Fig. 8.7) we:
1. identify individual cases of the *outcome* of interest
2. identify a representative group of individuals who do not have the outcome; these individuals act as controls
3. compare cases and controls to assess whether there were any differences in their past exposure to one or more possible risk factors.

Cross-sectional studies

In a **cross-sectional study**, we measure the frequency of a particular exposure(s) and/or outcome(s) in a defined population *at a particular time*. Cross-sectional studies can be either descriptive or analytical.
- In a descriptive cross-sectional study, we simply describe the frequency of the exposure(s) or outcome(s) in a defined population.

161

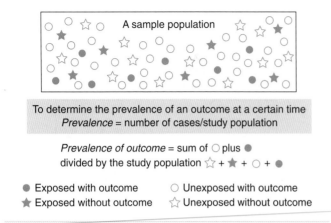

FIGURE 8.8 Analytical cross-sectional study design

- In an analytical cross-sectional study (Fig. 8.8), we:
  - simultaneously collect information on both the *outcome* of interest and the *exposure* to the potential risk factor(s)
  - then *compare* the frequency of the outcome in the people exposed to each risk factor with the frequency in those not exposed.

The *prevalence* is the proportion of persons in a defined population that have the outcome under study at a specific point in time. It equals the number of cases divided by the total number of people in the study population at a given time. The *incidence* of an outcome refers to the number of new cases with the outcome in a population in a defined time period.

Ecological studies

Ecological studies compare the exposure status and outcome status of *groups* rather than individuals. An ecological study thus looks for an association between an exposure and an outcome at the group level. In other words, we look to see whether the outcome is more frequent in groups where the exposure is more frequent. For each group, the exposures and outcomes are measured for the group as a whole. So, it is not possible to link the exposure of any particular individual to his or her outcome.

BIAS IN RESEARCH STUDIES

Bias refers to any errors in the design or conduct of a study that result in a conclusion that is different from the truth. It is particularly important that potential sources of bias are identified at the stage of study design (Fig. 8.9, Box 8.16) because you cannot usually adjust or make allowance for bias at the analysis stage. To put it very simply, if you study the wrong people, or get the wrong data from them, no amount of analysis will make it right. So, bias can ruin a study irretrievably.

The subject of bias is hotly debated in the evidence-based movement. Technical bias, publication bias and source-of-funding bias are all potential sources of systematic bias that affect the total pool of evidence and skew it in favour of experimental and commercially profitable interventions (Song et al., 2010):

- *Technical bias* favours research that we know how to do, and therefore is towards phenomena that we know how to investigate. Technical bias creates a systematic bias that influences what kinds of data are created.
- *Publication bias* refers to the differential publication by medical journals of positive and/or statistically significant results (Song et al., 2010). The purpose of this practice is to make the medical literature more interesting by publishing studies where new interventions are shown to be effective. However, through publication bias, clinicians may be exposed to a group of studies that misleadingly suggests the superiority of new interventions. Furthermore, publication bias, like technical bias, can ultimately lead to the neglect of

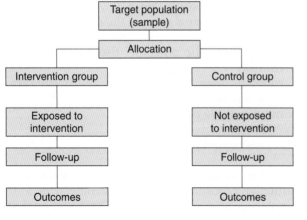

Potential sources of bias and where it may occur:

Selection bias
There may be systematic differences in the comparison groups
Solution: randomise

Performance bias
There may be systematic differences in the care apart from that being evaluated

Attrition bias
There may be systematic differences in the withdrawals from the trial
Solution: account for all the subjects

Detection bias
There may be systematic differences in the outcome assessment
Solution: 'blinding' of participants and/or observers

FIGURE 8.9 Potential sources of bias
(Based on sources of bias in trials of healthcare interventions in Higgins & Green *Cochrane Handbook for Systematic Reviews of Interventions*, Ch. 8, Section 8.5, 2011)

Box 8.16 Types of bias

Definitions of *interpretation* biases:

- *confirmation bias*—evaluating evidence that supports one's preconceptions differently from evidence that challenges these convictions
- *rescue bias*—discounting data by finding selective faults in the experiment
- *auxiliary hypothesis bias*—introducing ad hoc modifications to imply that an unanticipated finding would have been otherwise had the experimental conditions been different
- *mechanism bias*—being less sceptical when underlying science furnishes credibility for the data
- *'time will tell' bias*—when different scientists need different amounts of confirmatory evidence
- *orientation bias*—the possibility that the hypothesis itself introduces prejudices and errors and becomes a determinant of experimental outcomes.

(Source: Reproduced from Kaptchuk TJ. Effect of interpretive bias on research evidence. *BMJ*. 2003;326(7404):1453–1455. doi: 10.1136/bmj.326.7404.1453, with permission from *BMJ* Publishing Group Ltd)

certain types of phenomena. Because getting published counts significantly in researchers' career advancement, researchers may choose to study a restricted group of topics that are most likely to yield publishable results—that is, topics that do not fall in the 'grey zones' of clinical practice (practices whose usefulness is uncertain or for which older research data have been equivocal) (Naylor, 1995). Together, these scientific and social constructionist arguments undermine the assumption in evidence-based medicine (EBM) that EBM-preferred data are a representative body of data most likely to lead to truthful conclusions about the medical interventions they represent (Greenhalgh et al., 2014; Gupta, 2003).

- *Source-of-funding bias:* another area for ethical concern is the effect that EBM has on the authority and power of doctors vis-à-vis other groups. EBM prioritises certain types of clinical research and thus increases the pressure for this research to be *conducted and funded*. This results in several particular outcomes. Research-funding decisions are made in the context of competing priorities, so that decisions to fund clinical research are also decisions not to fund other things. As the majority of evidence-based research is conducted by physicians, EBM becomes a way of entrenching medical authority in determining to what degree research will be funded, what questions will be researched and by whom, and thus which results will be given priority in clinical decision making. This occurs at the expense of those who might wish to contribute to setting the research agenda and to determining what research should be funded (Gupta, 2003, p. 118).

CONFIDENCE INTERVAL

The confidence interval (CI) does as the name suggests—it allows us to feel confident (or not!) that we can apply the results we have found in our sample to the whole population. Another way of saying this is that we can *infer* the results from research to the population at large if certain situations exist (such as when we are dealing with a 'normal distribution' and are able to take a 'random sample' from the same population we are studying). Let's say we calculate from a sample of 100 healthy pregnant women that the mean weight (the average number of kilograms) they will gain during pregnancy will be 12 kg. Let's say this will be a close approximation to the average weight gained. If we were then to repeat this experiment 100 times over, with randomly selected women from the same population, we would be able to say with more certainty that the result we got (say it is 12 kg) is the average weight we would expect healthy pregnant women to gain in pregnancy. Of course you can see that this is a large undertaking—this is where the confidence interval comes in. Using fairly complicated statistics, we can calculate the 95% confidence interval for the average weight gain in healthy women in pregnancy. Then we can say (without having to physically repeat the experiment 100 times) that if we repeated the experiment 100 times we could be sure that, 95% of the time, the mean weight gain would be somewhere around 12 kg. The two numbers on either side of the confidence interval tell us where the true value lies in the population. Going back to our example, we might record our finding in the following way:

average weight gained in pregnancy
=12.0 kg (95% CI 10.5–14.2)

(Our sample was randomly selected from a population of healthy pregnant women in Sydney in 2005.)

This tells us that in our study the average was 12 kg, and we can infer that, 95 out of 100 times, the true value in the population will be somewhere between 10.5 and 14.2 kg. (The statistics have saved us from having to do the study 100 times and record all the weights!) Another way of saying this is that, once we construct a confidence interval, we have a range of values that we can be confident includes the true value of the mean. You will meet confidence intervals when you read any good-quality research papers.

(This is an introductory guide to help you understand the very basics about confidence intervals. I have recommended further reading at the end of this chapter.)

ODDS RATIO

One of the ways in which we can understand how an exposure or an intervention is associated with the outcome we are interested in observing is to calculate the odds ratio (OR) (Fig. 8.10). The odds ratio could be loosely described as the probability of an event happening in two groups. If the odds of an event are greater than one, then the event is said to be *more likely to occur*. Conversely, if

Review: Continuity of caregivers for care during pregnancy and childbirth
Comparison: Continuity of caregivers during pregnancy and childbirth
Outcome: Not feeling well-prepared for child care

Study	Treatment n/N	Control n/N	Peto Odds Ratio 95% CI	Weight %	Peto Odds Ratio 95% CI
Flint 1989	399/503	434/498		100.0	0.57 [0.41, 0.80]
Total (95% CI)	399/503	434/498		100.0	0.57 [0.41, 0.80]

0.1 0.2   1   5 10

Test for heterogeneity chi-square = 0.00 df = 0
Test for overall effect = −3.31 p = 0.0009

FIGURE 8.10 Odds ratio for association between continuity of care during pregnancy and not feeling well prepared for child care (Based on Hodnett, 2000)

Review: Active versus expectant management in the third stage of labour
Comparison: Active vs expectant management (all women)
Outcome: Maternal dissatisfaction with third stage management

Study	Treatment n/N	Control n/N	Relative Risk (Fixed) 95% CI	Weight %	Relative Risk (Fixed) 95% CI
Hinchingbrooke 1998	27/748	46/718		100.0	0.56 [0.35,0.90]
Total	748	718		100.0	0.56 [0.35,0.90]

0.1 0.2 0.5 1   2   5 10

Total events: 27 (Treatment), 46 (Control)
Test for heterogeneity: not applicable
Test for overall effect: Z = 242 p = 0.02

FIGURE 8.11 Relative risk for association between active versus expectant management, and maternal dissatisfaction (Based on Begley et al., 2015)

Review: Continuity of caregivers for care during pregnancy and childbirth
Comparison: Continuity of caregivers during pregnancy and childbirth
Outcome: Not feeling well prepared for labour

Study	Treatment n/N	Control n/N	Peto Odds Ratio 95% CI	Weight %	Peto Odds Ratio 95% CI
Flint 1989	359/503	396/498		100.0	0.64 [0.48, 0.86]
Total (95% CI)	359/503	396/498		100.0	0.64 [0.48, 0.86]

0.1 0.2   1   5 10

Test for heterogeneity chi-square = 0.00 df = 0
Test for overall effect = −2.99 p = 0.003

FIGURE 8.12 Odds ratio for association between continuity of care during pregnancy and not feeling well prepared for labour (Based on Hodnett, 2000)

the odds ratio is less than one, then the event is *less likely to occur*. This is a very simplistic description of a very complex statistical measure.

You are most likely to come across odds ratios in reading the Cochrane graphs in systematic reviews, so I will illustrate how to read the odds ratio using a Cochrane graph.

The graph in Fig. 8.10 illustrates the odds of continuity of care during pregnancy and childbirth on the likelihood of not feeling well prepared for childcare. As you can see, the odds ratio is 0.57, which is less than 1, and therefore we can deduce that continuity of care is less likely to be associated with *not* feeling well prepared for child care.

Another example of the odds (in this case the risk ratio) being less than 1 is shown in Fig. 8.11. (A slightly confusing issue arises here, where the authors have used the measure 'relative risk' rather than an odds ratio. For

Review: Active versus expectant management in the third stage of labour
Comparison: Active vs expectant management (all women)
Outcome: Vomiting between delivery of baby and discharge from labour ward

Study	Treatment n/N	Control n/N	Relative Risk (Fixed) 95% CI	Weight %	Relative Risk (Fixed) 95% CI
Bristol 1988	102/846	55/849		74.8	1.86 [1.36, 2.55]
Dublin 1990	10/86	2/114		2.3	6.63 [1.49, 29.47]
Hinchingbrooke 1998	47/748	17/764		22.9	2.82 [1.64, 4.87]
Total	1680	1727		100.0	2.19 [1.68, 2.86]

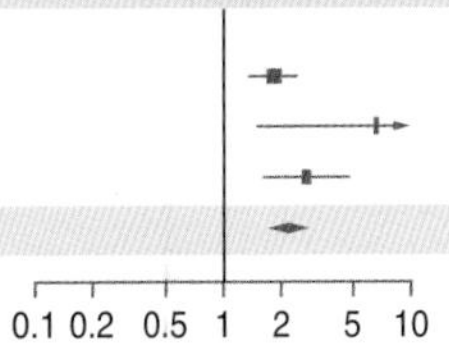

0.1 0.2 0.5 1 2 5 10

Total events: 159 (Treatment), 74 (Control)
Test for heterogeneity chi-square = 3.99 df = 2 p = 0.14 I^2= 49.8%
Test for overall effect: Z = 5.80 p < 0.00001

FIGURE 8.13 Odds ratio for association between active or expectant management and vomiting
(Based on Begley et al., 2015)

our purposes, at this stage of critical analysis they are interchangeable. At an advanced level of statistics, the meanings are slightly different.)

Let's turn to Fig. 8.12. Can you say in your own words what it is telling us?

Now for an example of the odds being greater than 1: Fig. 8.13 tells us that when comparing active versus expectant management of the third stage of labour when women in the treatment group were given IM Syntometrine as the oxytocic of choice, and comparing this outcome with the group of women (control group) who had been randomly allocated *not* to receive this treatment, there is a greater likelihood of vomiting between delivery of the baby and discharge from the labour ward. The pooled risk ratio is 2.19, with a 95% confidence interval of 1.68–2.86. This tells us that the women who were given an oxytocic in the third stage of labour had a greater likelihood of vomiting after birth than those who did not receive the treatment.

An alternative approach to outcome evaluation is that of 'optimality' (Box 8.17).

In summary, this has been a whistle-stop introduction to odds and risk ratios. You are advised to look at the Further reading list at the end of the chapter for more information.

One of the ways in which we can discern whether the results of research are going to be useful to us in clinical practice is to consider the relationship between the odds ratios, the line of no effect and another measure called the line of equivalence (which will not be explained here). For further reference and discussion regarding the relationship between the odds ratio and the line of no effect, please see Alderson (2004).

LIKELIHOOD RATIO

A likelihood ratio is the percentage of ill people with a given test result divided by the percentage of well individuals with the same result. Ideally, abnormal test results should be much more typical in ill individuals than in those who are well (high likelihood ratio), and normal test results should be more frequent in well people than in sick people (low likelihood ratio). Likelihood ratios near unity have little effect on decision making; in contrast, high or low ratios can greatly shift the clinician's estimate of the probability of disease (Grimes & Schulz, 2005).

Box 8.17   Optimality

The concept of 'optimality' offers an alternative approach to evaluating the outcomes of clinical care. Optimality looks for the desired best possible outcome, rather than the occurrence of undesired adverse (and rare) events. In essence, it replaces the focus on risk and adverse outcomes with a focus on measuring the frequency of 'optimal' (good, desired) outcomes.

Optimality is different from the concept of 'normality'. 'Normal' is frequently defined in healthcare as the absence of abnormalities or adverse events. However, definitions of what is normal must be based on decisions about what constitutes the broad range of normal. The Dutch authors Wiegers et al. (1996) who originally used the 'optimality' approach for measuring patient care stressed that the index is not a static one, but rather requires close evaluation of its internal validity as it applies to different practice situations. The tool must be adapted to accommodate different or changed insights into maternity care.

(Sources: Murphy & Fullerton, 2001; Wiegers et al., 1996)

Conclusion

Turning the phrase 'evidence-based' into 'evidence-informed' was the subject of debate in the UK in 2000; through use of the word 'informed' we are more likely to be mindful of the process of midwifery knowledge that midwives understand to originate from the way women themselves understand their bodies and the process of giving birth. Professor Lesley Page, in 'The backlash against evidence-based care', contends that 'evidence-based' does not necessarily mean practice based on a positivist, reductionist knowledge generated solely from within the scientific medical paradigm (Page, 1996). Others, such as Professor Mavis Kirkham, claim that through research we can question the status quo, that research is also the means with which we can move from being 'expert, professional and oppressed' to an alliance with women giving birth (Kirkham, 2010).

A strategic relationship between women and midwives can challenge both the economically driven imperative for research and the legislation and control of accepted practice, and in doing so it may promote the care of previously excluded groups of women. Midwives have the opportunity to show leadership in undertaking research that is relevant to women and makes judicious use of precious research funds. To quote from Dr Mary Stewart's research, 'the technocratic paradigm has become authoritative and highly valued, whereas a more holistic model, incorporating concepts of intuition and shared knowledge, has less credence' (Stewart, 2001, p. 281).

There is no doubt that evidence-based healthcare in its broadest meaning has the potential to better the lives of all women in childbirth, simply because it claims to be based in 'science' as opposed to 'authority'. It is a powerful tool with which to question the authority of obstetric practice and intervention. It is also the means with which we offer accountable and responsible care to women through informed decision making. The RCT is currently regarded as a highly effective methodology for investigating the introduction of new technologies and treatments before they become introduced routinely. What a pity, then, that the introduction of epidurals and other highly interventionist technology was never evaluated by any rigorous, or for that matter even second-rate, scientific investigation before its wholesale incorporation into routine practice. In the arena of 'evidence-based everything' the RCT is an immensely valuable tool, but there is room for other methodologies and there is also room for improvement (Box 8.18). The RCT is a relatively new and evolving method of seeking truth in maternity care that has helped to change the lives of midwives and women so far. As Chalmers noted, 'the greatest potential for improving research may lie in greater public involvement. Partly because of perverse incentives to pursue particular research projects researchers often seem to design trials to address questions that are of no interest to patients' (Chalmers, 1989, p. 1168).

Box 8.18   Let's have socially equitable comparisons (SECs)

As well as being vigilant in ensuring that research is ethical and meaningful to those who are researched, the use of appropriate language is something that cannot be underestimated. Ann Oakley wrote:

> Over a few commiserative drinks one evening a clinical colleague and I decided that if randomized controlled trials were renamed socially equitable comparison tests social scientists might like them better. It does not exactly run off the tongue, I know, but then neither does randomized controlled trial. Are there any takers out there?

(Oakley, 1998, p. 1241)

Count me in! Renaming the things 'socially equitable comparisons' (SECs) would locate the research language in a place much closer to the language of birth if we were to suggest having SECs rather than undertaking an RCT!

Review questions
---

1. What are the essential elements of a well-designed epidemiological study?

2. Name one intervention used in midwifery care that has not been researched. How would you research its effectiveness?

3. List five interventions you routinely use in your practice. Is there any published evidence to support these interventions? If so, what level of evidence (in the hierarchy of evidence) are they?

4. Using an example from practice, describe the steps you would take in applying the five steps of evidence-based practice.

5. Find an example of two areas of practice where the research underlying the practice is based on trials with a large crossover rate. How can you justify using this evidence?

6. If a study is analysed using an 'intention-to-treat' methodology, would you be more likely to believe the results of this trial than a population-based descriptive study? Why? What bias is likely to be evident?

7. Are randomised controlled trials meant to answer questions about the care of an individual woman? Why, or why not?

8. Name some 'grey zones' of clinical practice where there is no evidence or very little evidence to support your actions.

9. What is the goal of qualitative research? Is it useful? Give an example of qualitative research that has influenced your practice.

10. How can qualitative methods complement quantitative ones?

Online resources

Agency for Healthcare Research and Quality (US): http://www.ahrq.gov/.

Australian Clinical Practice Guidelines: http://www.clinicalguidelines.gov.au/.

CASP (Critical Appraisal Skills Programme; making sense of evidence): http://www.casp-uk.net/.

Centre for Evidence Based Medicine: http://www.cebm.net/.

Cochrane Library: http://www.cochrane.org.

CONSORT Group. Extensions of the CONSORT Statement; 2017: http://www.consort-statement.org/extensions.

Evidence for Policy and Practice Information and Coordinating Centre (EPPI Centre), Social Science Research Unit, Institute of Education, London EPPI Centre: http://eppi.ioe.ac.uk/cms/.

Government guidelines: http://www.guideline.Gov.

MIDIRS Midwifery Digest UK: https://www.midirs.org/.

STrengthening the Reporting of OBservational Studies in Epidemiology: http://www.strobe-statement.org/.

References

Alderson P. Absence of evidence is not evidence of absence. *BMJ.* 2004;328(7438):476–477. doi:10.1136/bmj.328.7438.476.

Altman DG, Bland JM. Statistics notes. Treatment allocation in controlled trials: why randomise? *BMJ.* 1999;318(7192):1209.

Begley CM, Gyte GM, Devane D, et al. Active versus expectant management for women in the third stage of labour. *Cochrane Database Syst Rev.* 2015;(3):CD007412, doi:10.1002/14651858.CD007412.pub4.

Black N. Why we need qualitative research. *J Epidemiol Community Health.* 1994;5:425–426.

Black N. Why we need observational studies to evaluate the effectiveness of health care. *BMJ.* 1996;312(7040):1215–1218.

Black N, Boswell D, Gray A, et al. *Health and Disease: A Reader.* Milton Keynes, UK: Open University Press; 1984.

Borbasi S, Jackson D, eds. *Navigating the Maze of Research: Enhancing Nursing and Midwifery Practice.* 4th ed. Sydney: Mosby Australia/Elsevier; 2016.

Bowling A. *Research Methods in Health: Investigating Health and Health Services.* 4th ed. Maidenhead, UK: McGraw-Hill Education; 2014.

Braithwaite J. *Complexity Science in Healthcare: A White Paper.* Sydney: Macquarie University; 2017.

Braithwaite J, Churruca K, Long J, et al. When complexity science meets implementation science: a theoretical and empirical analysis of systems change. *BMC Med.* 2018;16(1):63.

Chalmers I. Evaluating the effects of care during pregnancy and childbirth. In: Chalmers I, Enkin M, Keirse MJNC, eds. *Effective Care in Pregnancy and Childbirth: Childbirth.* Oxford: Oxford University Press; 1989:1168.

Chalmers I, Dickersin K, Chalmers TC. Getting to grips with Archie Cochrane's agenda. *BMJ.* 1992;305(6857):786–788.

Churruca, K., et al. The time has come: Embedded implementation research for health care improvement. *J Eval Clin Pract.* 2019;25(3): 373-380

Chauhan BF, Jeyaraman M, Mann AS, et al. Behavior change interventions and policies influencing primary healthcare professionals' practice—an overview of reviews. *Implement Sci.* 2017;12:3. doi:10.1186/s13012-016-0538-8.

Concato J, Shah N, Horwitz RI. Randomized, controlled trials, observational studies, and the hierarchy of research designs. *N Engl J Med.* 2000;342(25):1887–1892. doi:10.1056/nejm200006223422507.

CONSORT Group. CONSORT 2010; 2010. Online: www.consort-statement.org/consort-2010.

CONSORT Group. *Extensions of the CONSORT Statement*; 2017. Online: www.consort-statement.org/extensions.

Cooke A, Smith D, Booth A. Beyond PICO: the SPIDER tool for qualitative evidence synthesis. *Qual Health Res.* 2012;22(10):1435–1443. doi:10.1177/1049732312452938.

Cooke IE, Sackett DL. Evidence-based obstetrics and gynaecology. *Baillière's Clin Obstet Gynaecol.* 1996;10(4):535–549. doi:10.1016/S0950-3552(96)80003-4.

Corbin J, Strauss A. *Basics of Qualitative Research: Techniques and Procedures for Developing Grounded Theory.* 4th ed. Los Angeles: SAGE Publications; 2014.

Culpepper L, Gilbert TT. Evidence and ethics. *Lancet.* 1999;353(9155):829–831. doi:10.1016/s0140-6736(98)09101-6.

Feinstein AR, Horwitz RI. Problems in the "evidence" of "evidence-based medicine". *Am J Med.* 1997;103(6):529–535.

Flint C, Poulengeris P, Grant A. The 'Know Your Midwife' scheme—a randomised trial of continuity of care by a team of midwives. *Midwifery.* 1989;5(1):11–16.

Forster D, Newton M, McLachlan HL, et al. Exploring implementation and sustainability of models of care: can theory help? *BMC Public Health.* 2011;11(suppl 5):S8.

Fraser H, MacDougall C. Doing narrative feminist research: intersections and challenges. *Qual Soc Work.* 2017;16(2):240–254.

Goodman SN. Probability at the bedside: the knowing of chances or the chances of knowing? *Ann Intern Med.* 1999;130(7):604–606.

Grant MJ, Booth A. A typology of reviews: an analysis of 14 review types and associated methodologies. *Health Info Libr J.* 2009;26(2):91–108. doi:10.1111/j.1471-1842.2009.00848.x.

Gray JAM. *Evidence-based Healthcare and Public Health: How to Make Decisions About Health Services and Public Health.* 3rd ed. New York: Churchill Livingstone/Elsevier; 2009.

Green J, Britten N. Qualitative research and evidence-based medicine. *BMJ.* 1998;316(7139):1230–1232.

Greenhalgh T. Narrative based medicine: narrative based medicine in an evidence based world. *BMJ.* 1999;318(7179):323–325.

Greenhalgh T. *How to Read a Paper: The Basics of Evidence-based Medicine.* 5th ed. Chichester, UK: Wiley; 2014.

Greenhalgh T. *Cultural Contexts of Health: The Use of Narrative Research in the Health Sector.* Copenhagen: World Health Organization; 2016.

Greenhalgh T, Howick J, Maskrey N. Evidence based medicine: a movement in crisis? *BMJ.* 2014;348:g3725. doi:10.1136/bmj.g3725.

Greenhalgh T, Hurwitz B. Narrative based medicine: why study narrative? *BMJ.* 1999;318(7175):48–50.

Greenhalgh T, Jackson C, Shaw S, et al. Achieving *Research Impact Through Co-creation in Community-Based Health Services: Literature Review and Case Study.* Milbank Q. 2016;94(2):392–429.

Grigg C, Daellenbach R, Kensington M, et al. Women's birthplace decision-making, the role of confidence: part of the Evaluating Maternity Units study, New Zealand. *Midwifery.* 2015;31(6):597–605.

Grimes DA, Schulz KF. An overview of clinical research: the lay of the land. *Lancet.* 2002;359(9300):57–61. doi:10.1016/s0140-6736(02)07283-5.

Grimes DA, Schulz KF. Refining clinical diagnosis with likelihood ratios. *Lancet.* 2005;365(9469):1500–1505. doi:10.1016/s0140-6736(05)66422-7.

Grimshaw JM, Eccles MP, Lavis JN, et al. Knowledge translation of research findings. *Implement Sci.* 2012;7:50.

Grootendorst DC, Jager KJ, Zoccali C, et al. Observational studies are complementary to randomized controlled trials. *Nephron Clin Pract.* 2010;114(3):c173–c177. doi:10.1159/000262299.

Gupta M. A critical appraisal of evidence-based medicine: some ethical considerations. *J Eval Clin Pract.* 2003;9(2):111–121.

Haidich AB. Meta-analysis in medical research. *Hippokratia*. 2010; 14(suppl 1):29–37.

Hall WA, Tomkinson J, Klein MC. Canadian care providers' and pregnant women's approaches to managing birth: minimizing risk while maximizing integrity. *Qual Health Res*. 2011;22(5): 575–586.

Harte JD, Sheehan A, Stewart SC. Childbirth supporters' experiences in a built hospital birth environment exploring inhibiting and facilitating factors in negotiating the supporter role. *HERD*. 2016;9(3):135–161. doi:10.1177/1937586715622006.

Higgins JPT, Green S. *Cochrane Handbook for Systematic Reviews of Interventions*. Version 5.1.0. London: Cochrane Collaboration; 2011.

Hodnett ED. Continuity of caregivers for care during pregnancy and childbirth. *Cochrane Database Syst Rev*. 2000;(2):CD000062, doi:10.1002/14651858.cd000062.

Homer CS, Davis GK, Brodie PM, et al. Collaboration in maternity care: a randomised controlled trial comparing community-based continuity of care with standard hospital care. *BJOG*. 2001;108(1):16–22.

Jolley D. The glitter of the table. *Lancet*. 1993;342(8862):27–29.

Kaptchuk TJ. Effect of interpretive bias on research evidence. *BMJ*. 2003;326(7404):1453–1455. doi:10.1136/bmj.326. 7404.1453.

Khan KS. Systematic reviews of diagnostic tests: a guide to methods and application. *Best Pract Res Clin Obstet Gynaecol*. 2005;19(1):37–46. doi:10.1016/j.bpobgyn.2004.10.012.

King JF. A short history of evidence-based obstetric care. *Best Pract Res Clin Obstet Gynaecol*. 2005;19(1):3–14. doi:10.1016/ j.bpobgyn.2004.09.003.

Kirkevold M. Integrative nursing research—an important strategy to further the development of nursing science and nursing practice. *J Adv Nurs*. 1997;25(5):977–984.

Kirkham M. *The Midwife–Mother Relationship*. 2nd ed. London: Macmillan Education; 2010.

Krieger N. Epidemiology and social sciences: towards a critical reengagement in the 21st century. *Epidemiol Rev*. 2000;22(1): 155–163.

Lindsay GM, Schwind JK. Narrative inquiry: experience matters. *Can J Nurs Res*. 2016;48(1):14–20. doi:10.1177/0844562116652230.

Machi LA, McEvoy BT. *The Literature Review: Six Steps to Success*. Los Angeles: SAGE; 2016.

McKenzie JE, Beller EM, Forbes AB. Introduction to systematic reviews and meta-analysis. *Respirology*. 2016;21(4):626–637. doi:10.1111/resp.12783.

McLachlan H, Forster D, Davey M, et al. Effects of continuity of care by a primary midwife (caseload midwifery) on caesarean section rates in women of low obstetric risk: the COSMOS randomised controlled trial. *BJOG*. 2012; 19(12):1483–1492.

McPherson K. The Cochrane Lecture. The best and the enemy of the good: randomised controlled trials, uncertainty, and assessing the role of patient choice in medical decision making. *J Epidemiol Community Health*. 1994;48(1):6–15.

Mays N, Pope C. Qualitative research in health care. Assessing quality in qualitative research. *BMJ*. 2000;320(7226):50–52.

Merlin T, Weston A, Tooher R. Extending an evidence hierarchy to include topics other than treatment: revising the Australian 'levels of evidence'. *BMC Med Res Methodol*. 2009;9:34. doi:10.1186/1471-2288-9-34.

Moher D, Hopewell S, Schulz KF, et al. CONSORT 2010 explanation and elaboration: updated guidelines for reporting parallel group randomised trials. *Int J Surg*. 2012;10(1):28–55. doi:10.1016/j.ijsu.2011.10.001.

Murphy PA, Fullerton JT. Measuring outcomes of midwifery care: *development of an instrument to assess optimality. J Midwifery Womens Health*. 2001;46(5):274–284.

Naylor CD. Grey zones of clinical practice: some limits to evidence-based medicine. *Lancet*. 1995;345(8953):840–842.

Norkus Z. Historical narratives as pictures: on elective affinities between verbal and pictorial representations. *JNT*. 2004;34(2): 173–206.

O'Cathain A, Walters SJ, Nicholl JP, et al. Use of evidence-based leaflets to promote informed choice in maternity care: randomised controlled trial in everyday practice. *BMJ*. 2002; 324(7338):643.

Oakley A. Experimentation and social interventions: a forgotten but important history. *BMJ*. 1998;317(7167):1239–1242.

Oakley A. *Experiments in Knowing: Gender and Method in the Social Sciences*. Cambridge: Polity Press; 2000.

Oxford Centre for Evidence-Based Medicine (OCEBM) Working Group. *The Oxford; 2016 Levels of Evidence*. Oxford: OCEBM; 2016. Online: https://www.cebm.net/2016/05/ocebm-levels-of-evidence/.

Page L. The backlash against evidence-based care. *Birth*. 1996; 23(4):191–192.

Page LA, McCandlish R. *The New Midwifery: Science and Sensitivity in Practice*. 2nd ed. Edinburgh: Churchill Livingstone; 2006.

Page MJ, McKenzie JE, Moher D, et al. The PRISMA 2020 statement: an updated guideline for reporting systematic reviews *BMJ*. 2021;372:n71. doi:10.1136/bmj.n71.

Pawson R, Greenhalgh T, Harvey G, et al. Realist review—a new method of systematic review designed for complex policy interventions. *J Health Serv Res Policy*. 2005;10(suppl 1):21–34. doi:10.1258/1355819054308530.

Pope C, Mays N. *Qualitative Research in Health Care*. 3rd ed. Oxford: Blackwell; 2006.

Popper KR. *Objective Knowledge: An Evolutionary Approach*. 2nd ed. Oxford: Clarendon Press; 1979.

Porter S. The role of qualitative research in evidence-based policy and practice. *J Res Nurs*. 2010;15(6):495–496. doi:10.1177/ 1744987110383102.

Rowley MJ, Hensley MJ, Brinsmead MW, et al. Continuity of care by a midwife team versus routine care during pregnancy and birth: a randomised trial. *Med J Aust*. 1995;163(6):289–293.

Sackett DL, Rosenberg WM, Gray JA, et al. Evidence based medicine: what it is and what it isn't. *BMJ*. 1996;312(7023):71–72.

Sackett DL, Straus SE, Richardson WSR, et al. *Evidence-based Medicine: How to Practice and Teach EBM*. 2nd ed. Edinburgh: Churchill Livingstone; 2000.

Saracci R. *Epidemiology: A Very Short Introduction*. Oxford: OUP; 2010.

Saunders J. The practice of clinical medicine as an art and as a science. *Med Humanit*. 2000;26(1):18–22.

Schneider D, Lilienfeld DE. *Lilienfeld's Foundations of Epidemiology*. New York: Oxford University Press; 2015.

Schulz KF, Altman DG, Moher D. CONSORT 2010 statement: updated guidelines for reporting parallel group randomised trials. *PLoS Med*. 2010;7(3):e1000251. doi:10.1371/journal. pmed.1000251.

Shamseer L, Moher D, Clarke M, et al. Preferred reporting items for systematic review and meta-analysis protocols (PRISMA-P) 2015: elaboration and explanation. *BMJ*. 2015;350:g7647. doi:10.1136/bmj.g7647.

Sharpe VA. Behind closed doors: accountability and responsibility in patient care. *J Med Philos*. 2000;25(1):28–47. doi:10.1076/0360-5310(200002)25:1;1-V;FT028.

Song F, Parekh S, Hooper L, et al. Dissemination and publication of research findings: an updated review of related biases. *Health Technol Assess*. 2010;14(8):iii, ix–xi, 1–193. doi:10. 3310/hta14080.

Stapleton H, Kirkham M, Thomas G. Qualitative study of evidence based leaflets in maternity care. *BMJ*. 2002; 324(7338):639.

Steiner JF. Talking about treatment: the language of populations and the language of individuals. *Ann Intern Med.* 1999;130(7):618–622.

Stewart M. Whose evidence counts? An exploration of health professionals' perceptions of evidence-based practice, focusing on the maternity services. *Midwifery.* 2001;17(4):279–288. doi:10.1054/midw.2001.0286.

Swanson RA, Holton EF. *Research in Organizations: Foundations and Methods in Inquiry.* Oakland, CA: Berrett-Koehler; 2005.

Tracy SK, Hartz DL, Tracy MB, et al. Caseload midwifery care versus standard maternity care for women of any risk: M@NGO, a randomised controlled trial. *Lancet.* 2013;382(9906):1723–1732.

Webster F, Weijer C, Todd L, et al. The ethics of future trials: qualitative analysis of physicians' decision making. *Trials.* 2016;17:12. doi:10.1186/s13063-015-1137-8.

Wiegers TA, Keirse MJ, Berghs GA, et al. An approach to measuring quality of midwifery care. *J Clin Epidemiol.* 1996;49(3):319–325.

World Health Organization (WHO). *Bridging the "Know-Do" Gap.* Geneva, Switzerland: WHO Press; 2006.

Further reading

Altman DG. *Practical Statistics for Medical Research.* London: Chapman Hall; 1991.

Berkman L, Kawachi I. *Social Epidemiology.* Oxford: Oxford University Press; 2000.

Bowling A. *Research Methods in Health: Investigating Health and Health Services.* Buckingham, UK: Open University Press; 2002.

Clarke M. Individual patient data meta-analyses. *Best Pract Res Clin Obstet Gynaecol.* 2005;19(1):47-55.

Cochrane AL. *Effectiveness and Efficiency: Random Reflections on Health Services.* London: Nuffield Provincial Hospitals Trust; 1972.

Coggon D, Rose G, Barker DJP. *Epidemiology for the Uninitiated.* London: BMJ Books; 2003.

CONSORT Group. *Extensions of the CONSORT Statement;* 2017. Online: http://www.consort-statement.org/extensions.

Darlington Y, Scott D. *Qualitative Research in Practice: Stories From the Field.* Buckingham, UK: Open University Press; 2002.

Douglas E, Liamputtong P. *Qualitative Research Methods.* Melbourne: Oxford University Press; 2005.

Doyle L. Sex and gender: the challenge for epidemiologists. *Int J Health Sci.* 2003;33(3):569-579.

Duley L. Evidence and practice: the magnesium sulphate story. *Best Pract Res Clin Obstet Gynaecol.* 2005;19(1):57-74.

Egger M, Smith GD, Altman DG. *Systematic Reviews in Healthcare: Meta-Analysis in Context.* London: BMJ Publishing; 2001.

Enkin M. For and against: clinical equipoise and not the uncertainty principle is the moral underpinning of the randomised controlled trial. *BMJ.* 2000;321:756-758.

Gordis L. *Epidemiology.* Philadelphia: WB Saunders; 1996.

Greenhalgh T. *How to Read a Paper: The Basics of Evidence-Based Medicine.* 4th ed. London: BMJ Books; 2014.

Greenhalgh T, Hurwitz B. *Narrative-Based Medicine: Dialogue and Discourse in Clinical Practice.* London: BMJ Books; 1998.

Greenhalgh T, Robert G, Macfarlane F, et al. Storylines of research: a meta-narrative perspective on systematic review. *Soc Sci Med.* 2005;61(2):417-430.

Grimes DA, Shulz KF. Refining clinical diagnosis with likelihood ratios. *Lancet.* 2005;365(9469):1500-1505.

Holloway I, ed. *Qualitative Research in Health Care.* Maidenhead, UK: Open University Press; 2005.

Kranzler G, Moursund J. *Statistics for the Terrified.* 2nd ed. New Jersey: Prentice Hall; 1999.

Lomas J. Research and evidence-based decision making. *Aust N Z J Public Health.* 1997;21(5):439-440.

Mays N, Pope C. *Qualitative Research in Healthcare.* 2nd ed. London: BMJ Books; 1999.

MIDIRS Midwifery Digest UK. Online: https://www.midirs.org/.

Oakley A. *Experiments in Knowing: Gender and Method in the Social Sciences.* Cambridge: Polity Press; 2000.

Page L, McCandlish R. *The New Midwifery: Science and Sensitivity in Practice.* 2nd ed. London: Churchill Livingstone; 2006.

Sackett DL, Straus SE, Richardson WS, et al. *Evidence-Based Medicine: How to Practice and Teach EBM.* 2nd ed. Edinburgh: Churchill Livingstone; 2000.

Sacks HS, Berrier J, Reitman D, et al. Meta-analyses of randomized controlled trials. *N Engl J Med.* 1987;316(8):450-455.

Saracci R. *Epidemiology: A Very Short Introduction.* Oxford UK: OUP; 2010.

Vernon B, Tracy S, Reibel T. Compliance, coercion and power have huge effect in maternity services. *BMJ.* 2002;325:43.

Weijer C, Shapiro SH, Cranley Glass K. For and against: clinical equipoise and not the uncertainty principle is the moral underpinning of the randomised controlled trial. *BMJ.* 2000;321(7263):756-758.

World Health Organization (WHO). *Bridging the "Know-Do" Gap.* Geneva, Switzerland: WHO Press; 2006.

Appendix 8.1 Evaluating a clinical guideline

Who developed the guideline?

- Are the members of the guideline development team identified?
- Are all clinical perspectives represented?
- Are all cultural perspectives represented (e.g. African-American, Pacific Islander)?
- Is patient input or participation documented?
- Are the sponsors of the guideline identified?
- Are there potential conflicts of interest?
- Why did they develop the guideline?
- Is there a clear statement of the guideline objective?
- Is the gap between current practice and outcomes and the recommended practice and outcomes clearly stated?
- Is the guideline development process described? (If so, what process was used?)
  - Explicit evidence based (includes projections of healthcare outcomes for a defined population)
  - Evidence based
  - Consensus process
  - Process of development not described
- What is the strength of the evidence?
- Is there a description of the strategy used to obtain information from the medical literature?
- Is there a description of the strategy used to critically appraise and synthesise the evidence?
- Is the evidence presented in terms of absolute differences in outcome (as compared with relative differences)?
- Are the major recommendations of the guideline based on high-quality evidence?

Does the guideline possess the attributes of a good guideline?

- Are the patients that the guideline applies to clearly described and are exceptions stated?
- Is the guideline clear and brief?
- Does it provide genuine clinical guidance?
- Is it flexible (does it allow for clinical judgment)?
- Can the change in care be measured?
- Can it be implemented in your care delivery system?
- Is the information the guideline is based on current?
- Has the guideline been successfully piloted or implemented?

(For further reading see: *A Guide to the Development, Evaluation and Implementation of Clinical Practice Guidelines*. Online: https://www.nhmrc.gov.au/guidelines/publications/cp30.)
(Sources: Flodgren G, Hall AM, Goulding L, et al. Tools developed and disseminated by guideline producers to promote the uptake of their guidelines. *Cochrane Database Syst Rev*. 2016;8:CD010669. doi: 10.1002/14651858.CD010669.pub2; New Zealand Guidelines Group and Group Health Cooperative of Puget Sound, http://www.nzgg.org.nz.)

The woman

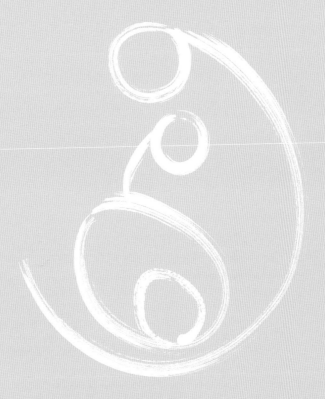

CHAPTER 9

Social and environmental determinants of health

Claire MacDonald and Lesley Dixon

LEARNING OUTCOMES

Learning outcomes for this chapter are:

1. To investigate the relationship between health and the social determinants of health
2. To explore how interrelationships between social, cultural, environmental, economic and genetic factors contribute to health disparities among women and between genders
3. To identify the importance of the social determinants of health for midwives and women during childbirth
4. To explore the theories and pathways of causation from the social determinants to health outcomes
5. To identify key actions that can be taken on the social determinants of health to reduce health inequities and improve health outcomes.

CHAPTER OVERVIEW

This chapter will identify the environmental context and social conditions in which people live. It discusses the complex interrelationship between social factors such as income and education on women's health and the pathways by which these social determinants exert their influence and operate over time and across generations. It provides an outline of the theories that suggest causative pathways between the social determinants and health outcomes and identifies some of the actions that, if taken, have the potential to reduce inequity and improve health outcomes.

KEY TERMS

environmental determinants of health
equality
equity
inequality

inequity
population health
poverty
social determinants of health

social justice
wealth

INTRODUCTION

Whilst midwives seek to optimise health at an individual and whānau/family level when working with women and their families, it is important to also consider how women's health is influenced by their place within society—this includes their culture, social relationships, social engagement, expectations, opportunities and challenges. This chapter reviews how the prevailing political theory, context and resulting government policies along with social position, culture and social context have the potential to influence women's health at both an individual and a population level.

Social determinants of health (SDH) is a term that has gained prominence in recent years and outlines a concept which identifies that political, societal and environmental factors affect the health of individuals within populations. A life-course approach underpins the SDH with an understanding that factors which influence health outcomes accrue over years and even over generations. Founded on the ethical principles of equity and social justice, the SDH concept identifies that health inequities are a result of the unequal distribution of power, prestige and resources among groups within society. Furthermore, health inequities are unjust because they are avoidable yet not avoided (Commission on the Social Determinants of Health (CSDH), 2007). When looking at the health of a population amongst countries with similar levels of income, studies have consistently found that those countries with lower income inequality have better population health (as measured by life expectancy and other indicators) compared with countries with greater income inequality (Detollenaere et al., 2018; Dewan et al., 2019; Diderichsen et al., 2012; Picket & Wilkinson, 2015). We therefore have an opportunity to improve health outcomes for all members of society by taking actions that reduce inequalities.

In 2005 the World Health Organization (WHO) set up the Commission on Social Determinants of Health, chaired by Professor Sir Michael Marmot, to collate global evidence about SDH. The Commission's subsequent report identifies how the distribution of income, wealth, influence and power at the societal level affects health outcomes at the individual level (CSDH, 2008). This report has been influential globally in focusing the discussion on actions to address unequal access to the SDH and thus reduce inequity as a means of improving population health. Environmental health links closely with SDH, the environment being an important part of the global/macro-level influences on population health.

(See Box 9.1 for definitions of terms.)

SOCIETY AND THE SOCIAL DETERMINANTS OF HEALTH

For midwives, an understanding of the SDH comprises two interwoven concepts: firstly, the social, structural and political conditions in which people are 'born, grow, live, work, and age' (CSDH, 2008, p. 1) influence their health behaviours and outcomes; and secondly, there is social

---

Box 9.1 Definitions

Health and wellbeing

'Health is a state of complete physical, mental and social well-being and not merely the absence of disease or infirmity' (WHO, 1948). This definition, which conceptualises health as more than simply the absence of disease, has endured as the guiding tenet of WHO policy, and underpins discussions of health in this chapter. Its implications extend beyond the health service, which exists primarily to treat illness and injury. Prevention is the key because in many cases by the time illness manifests it is too late to return to a full state of health according to this definition.

Determinants

The use of the term 'determinants' does not imply a deterministic relationship between the determinants and health outcomes; nor does it imply the absence of free will about 'life choices'. Instead, determinants refer to macrosocial influences that affect health, such as poverty, that prove very difficult for individuals to alter.

(Thorogood, 2015, p. 62)

Individual versus population health

The discussion in this chapter considers health and its determinants from a population perspective, not from an individual perspective. This means that rates of outcomes in the population change according to certain exposures, but this does not mean that individuals within those populations necessarily experience the outcomes in question.

Equity/equality

The words 'equality' and 'inequality' are often used interchangeably with 'equity' and 'inequity'. However, Baum (2015) and others make the important distinction that equality pertains to 'sameness' whereas equity refers to 'fairness'. Thus, some inequalities are simply differences, whereas those differences that are unjust and preventable are called inequities.

---

patterning of health and illness where exposures to the SDH, and thus health outcomes, are inequitably distributed across population and income groups. This is known as the social gradient of health. Understanding and acting on the SDH fits into the social model of health, which recognises that people come into pregnancy from all sectors of society, and that health and disease are a product of multiple, intersecting determinants.

Baum (2015) identifies a number of focal points for health inequities including socioeconomic status (SES) and employment, gender, ethnicity and indigeneity, and location (rural/urban). Many of the differences in health outcomes according to gender and ethnicity are underpinned by SES. Women are more likely to be in low-paid or part-time work than men. Pākehā and Australian

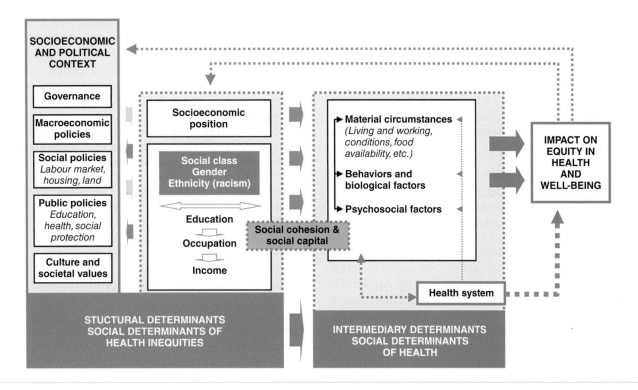

FIGURE 9.1 Commission on Social Determinants of Health final conceptual framework
(Source: WHO, 2010, p. 6)

Europeans are overrepresented at the privileged end of the social gradient in wealth and income, whereas indigenous Māori, Aboriginal and Torres Strait Islanders as well as former refugees are overrepresented in the lowest income brackets, the former as a result of ongoing colonial processes and the latter as a result of displacement and forced migration. However, SES does not explain the entire differential in health outcomes for these groups.

The CSDH conceptual framework was developed to support an improved understanding of how the SDH can influence the health of the individual (Fig. 9.1).

The framework identifies the structural mechanisms (socioeconomic and political context along with social position) that cause, influence or generate social stratification and define individual socioeconomic position. These occur at the global/macro and community/mesa level and have an influence at the micro/individual and family level on material circumstances, behaviours and psychosocial factors. The following section explains the aspects of this conceptual framework and how these influences work together to support or undermine health and wellbeing at each of these levels.

The bigger picture (global/macro level)

Governance and policy

When health is considered as a social phenomenon it becomes clear that how the health of a population is promoted and managed is an inherently political activity (Baum, 2015). For many governments the health agenda and health policy have focused on ensuring access to and provision of medical services for its population. Depending on the country, healthcare is subsidised nationally from taxation or individually through health insurance. However, health (rather than the treatment of illness) as defined by the WHO is linked to broader social policy and requires action within several different sectors such as housing, education and employment (WHO, 2010). The extent to which health is prioritised, the model of health that is privileged and the level of intersectoral action for health that can be achieved is influenced by the prevailing political ideology, global pressures and historical, social and cultural norms in each country.

In order to understand the philosophy which underpins government policy it is necessary to consider the historical economic philosophies that have been the drivers of the modern political agenda and policies.

Aotearoa New Zealand and Australia are known as liberal democratic societies. Political parties subscribe to divergent ideologies which are part of a spectrum underpinned by capitalism. In simple terms, economic policy at the right of the spectrum, sometimes known as libertarian democracy, is underpinned by a belief that the free market will meet most of society's needs with a smaller place for government in providing services. The role of government is seen as facilitating the market to grow the economy with minimal regulation. Individual responsibility is central and health is often seen as a product of healthcare provision as per the biomedical model and good personal health decisions. To the left of the spectrum, social democratic parties believe in a larger role for government to regulate the market in order that those who lack economic power have adequate resources to meet their needs. Individual responsibility is important but is seen as being socially constructed, thus efforts to improve the conditions in which people make decisions are central. Social security is inherently linked with health and healthcare (Baum, 2015).

The changing face of politics and economics

New Zealand was an early adopter of two major changes to health and social policy that spread internationally. The first began in 1938 following the Great Depression, when Michael Joseph Savage's Labour government sought to enact a world-first, taxation-funded public health system as part of a suite of social security measures through the Social Security Act (SSA) (*Social Security Act 1938*). The architects of the 1938 health service innovations recognised that health is inextricably linked with social security—in other words, ensuring adequate income so that nobody suffers from circumstances not of their creation. Similar policies were implemented in Australia and the rest of the industrialised world as part of the postwar consensus in the 1950s and 1960s. A strong focus on specific disease eradication or reduction, together with the creation of the welfare state and other policies which sought to minimise poverty rates, resulted in major health and life expectancy gains. High levels of employment were achieved through Keynesian economic policies which promoted job creation, and through government borrowing and spending, in order to increase the purchasing power of individuals and thus create economic growth (Baum, 2015).

The economic crises of the 1970s and rising unemployment provided an opportunity for the second of these major economic transitions to be implemented, this time to a neoclassical economic paradigm, often known as neoliberalism (Boston, 1999). During the 1980s, structural adjustment policies were adopted and known as Rogernomics in New Zealand, Reaganism in the USA and Thatcherism in the UK. Australia implemented these changes somewhat more gradually, maintaining social policies together with some significant neoliberal changes until the Howard Coalition government brought a commitment to this agenda over its 1996–2007 terms (Baum, 2015). The central aims were to promote economic growth by decreasing public spending, reducing the role of the public sector, debt repayment and deregulation of the market, along with privatisation and trade liberalisation (CSDH, 2008).

In the decade from 1984, manufacturing declined and moved offshore resulting in high inflation, high interest rates and a surge in unemployment in New Zealand (Kelsey, 2015). Welfare provisions were decreased and there was a move from a social-citizenship model of welfare towards a needs-based model. This was implemented in the New Zealand in the 1991 Budget, which dropped benefits below the minimum wage (Stephens, 1999), a

measure that was embedded by subsequent administrations (Boston, 2013). Chenoweth (2008) describes a gradual dismantling of the welfare state in Australia from the late 1980s onwards, beginning with people who were long-term unemployed and disregarding the social and structural problems that contributed to individuals' circumstances.

Reforms in both countries included a reduction in government assistance and services accompanied by a flattening of the tax rates including cuts for the rich and increases for the poor (Chenoweth, 2008; Easton, 2008). These policies effectively ensured wealth was 'redistribut[ed]' towards the better-off' (Dalziel, 1999, p. 60). The effects disproportionately affected the poor and increased inequality between social groups, with worse impacts for Māori and Polynesian people in Aotearoa (Stephens, 1999).

Mass Māori urbanisation had begun during the Depression and World War II as Māori moved to cities for work (Rei, 1993) predominantly in the manual and blue-collar sector, which was hardest hit by the decline in manufacturing. Howard-Wagner's (2017) analysis of the effect of neoliberalism on Australian Aboriginal and Torres Strait Islander people identifies that, from 1996, government policy focused on assimilating Indigenous Australians into the mainstream economy through 'an individualistic framework of individual rights' (p. 1340). Living on remote homelands without employment in the mainstream economy was deemed by the federal Minister for Indigenous Affairs in 2005 as 'unviable' and a 'lifestyle choice', and she instead encouraged urbanisation for employment and service access. Howard-Wagner (2017) argues that these neoliberal government policies have been paternalistic, and 'represent a deeply invasive and insidious racial project and a form of contemporary colonialism' (p. 1346).

Trade agreements and transnational corporations

The 1990s saw a global shift in trade liberalisation and investment through international agreements underpinned by the liberal economic policies of the World Bank and International Monetary Fund (Baum, 2015). The dramatic increase in the size, wealth and power of transnational corporations (TNCs) resulted in their control of 80% of the world's trade by 2013 (United Nations Conference on Trade and Development, 2013). A 2017 analysis of the annual revenues of governments and corporations indicates that of the top 100, only 29 are countries while 71 are corporations (Babic et al., 2017). Such market domination has enabled TNCs to exert control over national governmental policy to favour their interests (Wade, 2013). This has disempowered workers, unions and unemployed people by influencing labour policy and, in some countries, decreased workplace safety (Benach et al., 2007). Kelsey (2015) describes how governments have subsequently entered into free trade agreements that prioritise the rights of corporations over those of citizens. The provisions of trade and investment liberalisation agreements can limit governments in their abilities to legislate strongly for public health (Labonte & Sanger, 2006a, 2006b) or for policies directed towards reducing poverty related to inequality.

Culture, societal norms and values

These dramatic shifts in political and economic philosophy and direction occurred in response to the underlying social concerns that created fertile conditions for change. Broadly speaking, the development of the welfare state and the egalitarian focus of social policy occurred in the wake of the Great Depression and fitted with the sense of community and collectivism engendered by living through two world wars. Subsequently, as Curtis (2002) argues, the sociopolitical ferment of the rights movements during the 1960s and 1970s, which resulted in socially progressive change on many other levels, also heralded the transition from collectivism to individualism. Together with the oil shocks and economic crisis of the 1970s, the rise of individualism provided the conditions for neoliberalism to be introduced and subsequently to be entrenched as the guiding value in the population. With its emphasis on individual responsibility for success or failure, the focus is diverted away from the *conditions that enable* self-determination. Inequality in social status and health is thus constructed as the result of individual endeavour or failure instead of the result of the organisation of policy and society.

The belief that those at the lower end of the social gradient of health are responsible for their own poverty and ill health is known as *victim blaming*, and is a result of individualism in society and policy. Those at the most deprived end of the gradient are systematically disadvantaged and then blamed for their disadvantage, while those at the privileged end of the gradient are systematically advantaged and take credit for their own success. In other words, disempowerment results from ignoring the causes and only focusing on the symptoms of poverty. Empowerment therefore becomes possible when root causes are addressed.

Individualism and collectivism both have positive and negative characteristics. Individualism is associated with both victim-blaming and isolation but also autonomy and agency, while collectivism is associated with stability and access to help but also paternalism. The challenge for government and health policy is in finding the right balance. Policies that are too heavily weighted towards collectivism can negate the right of the individual to make their own choices. Policies that subscribe uniquely to an individualistic philosophy result in a lack of attention to the circumstances of people's lives, which are created by social and economic policy and which create the context of their decision making.

Midwifery itself regained its status as an autonomous profession in New Zealand in 1990 through the assertion of individual rights (Guilliland & Pairman, 2010), which fitted within the emergent neoliberal paradigm of the then Labour government (Davies, 2017). For a more detailed discussion of the ethical and philosophical foundations of politics as relevant to the SDH, see Baum (2015).

Cultural norms and values differ between populations and groups within countries. Although generalisations can be problematic, broadly speaking Pākehā / Australian European norms are more individualistic whereas indigenous Māori and Aboriginal social structure and rights concepts are more collective (Grimes et al., 2015; Miller, 2018), as are those of some other ethnic groups. This is relevant for health in a number of ways, particularly because the culture of the dominant group is often seen as the norm for a whole country and is privileged by governments, who reflect it through a greater proportion of voters.

Social, cultural, economic and political change

Social change refers to the influence of human interactions and culture shifts on institutions and politics and often involves social movements working outside political systems to protest the status quo and bring about change. A social movement generally consists of a network of people who organise formal or informal interactions to bring about or impede social, political, economic or cultural change. There are several different types of social movement—such as reform movements (e.g abortion rights), revolutionary movements (political change) and reactionary movements.

Social movements seek to shift power imbalances and challenge injustice through multiple means, such as organised political campaigns, protest, direct action and civil disobedience. Social movements engage in agenda setting to influence thinking and aspects of culture, which often has the deepest impact within democratic societies.

Historically, social movements have created important change, for example, women's suffrage, the anti-nuclear movement and civil rights, the movement against apartheid, the Indigenous land-rights movement in Australia, the Māori protest movement women's rights including access to legal and safe abortion, LGBTIQ+ rights, and many others. With the introduction of the internet, social movements have been able to reach wider, often global audiences, which has increased their potential reach and scale (Boxes 9.2, 9.3 and 9.4).

Community (mesa level)

Societal organisation and power structures create social stratification, assigning social positions and status (Diderichsen et al., 2012). This results in differential exposures to health-damaging conditions and different consequences of ill health according to social position (and ability to access healthcare). Social position is influenced by education, occupation, income, gender and ethnicity. Lower socioeconomic position is associated with poorer education, fewer amenities, increased risk of

177

Box 9.2   The #MeToo movement

The #MeToo (also Me Too) movement was started as a way of helping sexual abuse survivors be heard and understood. It has broken the silence surrounding sexual abuse and sexual harassment and become an international protest which has raised awareness of the prevalence and pernicious impact of sexual violence. The movement was started by Tarana Burke in 2006 who used the phrase Me Too among women of colour who had been sexually abused. Following widespread allegations of sexual abuse against an American film producer in 2017, the hashtag was adopted and spread virally internationally, with the expression translated into different languages. The movement has helped to empower women and it calls on men to stand against behaviour that objectifies women. It now works to support marginalised people and communities to identify and prevent sexual violence.

Box 9.3   The #BlackLivesMatter movement

The Black Lives Matter movement was founded in 2013 in response to the police killings of people of colour in the USA. The aim of the movement is to 'eradicate white supremacy and build local power to intervene in violence inflicted on Black communities by the state and vigilantes' (Black Lives Matter, n.d.). In 2020, the death of George Floyd at the hands of the police in Minneapolis, Minnesota caused demonstrations across America and around the world. The #BlackLivesMatter movement is now a member-led global network of more than 40 chapters. The movement shines a spotlight on racism and racial inequality as a continued, widespread problem and has been adopted by indigenous and minority ethnic groups in Aotearoa and Australia to highlight and fight against discrimination (Black Lives Matter, 2018).

Box 9.4   The climate movement

The climate movement is a collective of non-government organisations that individually and collectively engage in activities to protest the environmental destruction being caused by a reliance on fossil fuels. The aim of the movement is to identify environmental issues and compel government action to reduce the impact of global warming and the risk it brings of social and ecological collapse. The climate movement advocates for the reduction of carbon emissions and the transition to carbon-neutral policies. Many of the organisations use nonviolent civil disobedience as a means of identifying issues and compelling action (e.g., Extinction Rebellion) whilst others provide information, education and advocacy to put pressure on local and national politicians to support climate solutions (e.g., The Climate Reality Project).

Events such as Earth Day, Zero Hour and School Strike 4 Climate have seen widespread strikes, marches and other actions involving millions of people globally. The movement's continued activities have resulted in governments increasingly recognising climate change as an international emergency that requires collective global political and economic action to resolve.

unemployment and job insecurity, poorer working conditions and increased risk of unsafe neighbourhoods—all of which have an impact on family life and health.

Gender and ethnicity are relevant to health because of how they influence social position through privilege and discrimination.

Gender and sexual diversity

Gender involves 'culture-bound conventions, roles and behaviours that shape relations between and among women and men and boys and girls' (WHO, 2010, p. 33). Furthermore, 'Lesbian, gay, bisexual, transgender, queer, and intersex (LGBTQI) individuals face high rates of physical and mental health issues and reduced access to medical and social services' (WHO, 2016, n.p.). Within

society there is often structural and systematic discrimination in access to power, prestige and resources which is a result of gender discrimination. Gender divisions are not always visible but result in a lack of opportunity, status and control over resources, all of which increase exposure to poorer health. There are a number of examples throughout this chapter of how gender intersects with other social determinants of health to affect health outcomes for people in pregnancy and birth.

In her investigation of the United Nations System of National Accounts, Waring (1988) drew attention to the fact that women's work in production and reproduction was almost entirely unvalued, as was the notion of a healthy environment. Conversely, any activity that resulted in the circulation of money and economic growth, including war and oil spills, was considered economically valuable owing to its contribution to gross national product. More than three decades later, the paradigm of economic growth continues to impact on the value of women's work and contribution to society. This manifests in a number of ways, including persistent wage inequality between men and women in spite of legislation requiring equal pay for equal work (Australian Trade Union Archives, 1973–1988; *Equal Pay Act 1972*), and the 'motherhood penalty'—the pay gap between parents and non-parents of both sexes (Statistics New Zealand & Ministry for Women, 2017). Feminism is a political and social movement which seeks to ensure equal opportunities for women in education and employment and establish equal political, personal and social rights for women.

Intersectional feminism acknowledges the diverse and multiple social identities that people may have, which can overlap and compound experiences of privilege and discrimination (UN Women, 2020). The term was coined by law professor Kimberlé Crenshaw in 1989 to bring to light the experiences and realities of women of colour, which had not been as visible or acknowledged in the feminist movement until that point. WHO (2021, n.p.) refers to *intersectionality* thus:

> *Gender is hierarchical and produces inequalities that intersect with other social and economic inequalities. Gender-based discrimination intersects with other factors of discrimination, such as ethnicity, socioeconomic status, disability, age, geographic location, gender identity and sexual orientation, among others.*

Reproductive justice is an organising and theoretical framework for intersectional feminist activism which has evolved as a movement over the last three decades to acknowledge the importance of, and advocate for, access to the means to fully exercise reproductive rights. By applying intersectionality to reproductive politics (Ross, 2017), reproductive justice recognises that sexual and reproductive health and the ability to exercise agency are shaped and constrained by social positioning (Morison & Herbert, 2018). This framework has been used by a number of indigenous women's groups in Australia and internationally to regain self-determination in health and primary healthcare provision (Dudgeon & Bray, 2020). Closely aligned with all of these concepts is cultural safety, a framework developed in Aotearoa (Ramsden, 2015) which involves a process of self-reflection about a midwife's own culture, identity and world view. It seeks to lay the foundation for delivering safe care to women, wāhine and gender-diverse pregnant people according to who they are, which includes understanding and equalising power in the relationship. For more information, see Chapter 17 for a discussion on cultural safety and gender-inclusive midwifery care.

See Box 9.2.

Racism

Although life expectancy has been increasing in New Zealand and Australia, there continue to be inequitable health outcomes related to ethnicity. Average life expectancy is 84.5 years for 'European or other' New Zealand women, but 77.1 for Māori women and 79.0 years for Pasifika women (Stats NZ, 2021). In Australia, life expectancy for Aboriginal and Torres Strait Islander women is 75.6 compared with 83.4 for non-indigenous women (Australian Institute of Health and Welfare (AIHW), 2021a). When considering maternal and perinatal health, ethnic disparities are clear—with Māori, Pasifika and Aboriginal women and babies experiencing disproportionately high levels of perinatal mortality (AIHW, 2021b; Perinatal and Maternal Mortality Review Committee, 2021); and infant hospitalisations (Lawton et al., 2016) compared with other ethnic groups. The authors of this last study point out that ethnicity itself is not a risk, rather that differential exposures to risk factors occur because of the inequitable distribution of resources by ethnic group.

Ethnicity manifests itself in adverse health outcomes through the mechanism of racism at individual, institutional and systemic levels across time. Racism is recognised as a SDH in itself, and thus an important public health issue (Moewaka et al., 2014). White privilege and racism towards non-Europeans underpin the inequitable distribution of health outcomes between ethnic groups in Aotearoa and Australia. Racism and racial discrimination are described by Becares & Atatoa-Carr (2016, p. 1) as 'systemic oppression existent in social institutions [which] ensures that both socioeconomic disadvantage and its detrimental effect on health are continuously transmitted throughout generations'.

Colonisation set the foundations for inequitable access to resources and thus poorer health outcomes for indigenous Māori and Aboriginal people compared with the settlers, which have been built on and compounded to the present day. Durie (1999) points to disparities in Māori health across the spectrum of social indicators that have arisen due to the multiple, damaging effects of colonisation. Land alienation, loss of cultural identity and racism all need to be addressed for Māori and Aboriginal people to achieve health and participation in society at all levels. As Durie (1999, p. 3) states:

> *entrapment in lifestyles which lead to poor health and risk taking, is so closely intertwined with poverty traps and deculturation that macro-solutions become as important, if not more important, than targeted interventions at individual or community levels.*

The ongoing longitudinal study 'Growing up in New Zealand' (Becares & Atatoa-Carr, 2016) found strong associations between lifetime experiences of ethnically motivated interpersonal attacks and unfair treatment on pre- and postnatal mental health for Māori, Pasifika and Asian women, noting a dose-dependent and cumulative effect. Women who had experienced racist treatment by a health professional were 66% more likely to suffer from postnatal depression compared with women who did not report these experiences. Discrimination in other sectors including employment and housing also affected women's mental health. The authors conclude that racial discrimination has a severe, direct effect on maternal mental health, which can then affect the child and family, and needs to be addressed.

A more detailed discussion on Aboriginal health is provided in Chapter 1 and on Māori health in Chapter 11. See also Box 9.3.

Education

Education level follows the social gradient, is related to early childhood development and is independently associated with health outcomes, cognition in old age and life expectancy (Marmot, 2015). Education level influences income via the jobs one has access to and the likelihood of unemployment, thus impacting on health (Marmot, 2015).

As an example of how both privilege and poverty can be transferred between generations, Hart & Risley (2003) measured how many words were addressed to children in their first 3 years by their parents. The researchers calculated that children of professional parents had 30 million more words addressed to them than did children of parents living with socioeconomic hardship (20,000 more words per day). At age 3 years, children living in wealthier families had a broader vocabulary and added new words faster than children of families in hardship. This gap persisted and widened, with measurable differences at 9–10 years old in vocabulary and reading comprehension that followed the patterns set down in the first 3 years. This uneven playing field promotes opportunities for wealthier children as they grow and reduces them for poorer children.

Work

Work affects health in several ways. It may be health enhancing by providing a secure, good income, high status, job satisfaction and social interaction. Conversely, work can have a negative impact on health when it is poorly paid, low status, stressful, insecure, isolating, undignified or affects circadian rhythms (night work). Employment law and employment conditions influence the work environment. Laws that support precarious work such as short-term, temporary or zero-hours contracts are deleterious to the physical health and mental health of the individual (CSDH, 2008). The health impact for workers in the 'gig economy' that has emerged with the development of digital platforms that provide low-cost, on-demand services (such as ride-share apps) is an area of concern and research investigation (Bajwa et al., 2018; Freni-Sterrantino & Salerno, 2021). Low-status work is also associated with increased exposures to health hazards, while higher-status work often involves daytime work, regular hours and permanent contracts, which minimise uncertainty and support improved health.

Income, wealth and poverty

As an indicator of socioeconomic position, income provides the most direct measure of material resources for individuals and families. It has a dose–response association with health, where health improves as income rises along the social gradient. It also has a cumulative effect over the life course but can change most on a short-term basis owing to the vagaries of employment/unemployment (dependent on occupation). There are various components of income which involve not just wages but also dividends, child and other dependent support, and pension (superannuation) payments.

Income is often limited for parents following the birth of a baby. This is due to the reduced ability of both parents to work and/or pay for childcare, resulting in a reduced income. In New Zealand and Australia, median family income varies according to ethnicity and family type (two parents compared with single-parent families), with the median income for non-indigenous population groups significantly higher than indigenous populations (AIHW, 2019; Perry, 2019a).

Rashbrooke (2016) points out that 'Income is what people need to get through the present, while wealth allows them to plan for the future'. **Wealth** or 'net worth' takes into account assets, savings and investments. In Australia and Aotearoa wealth is accrued to a far greater degree by those of European descent than Aboriginal, Māori, or Pasifika people (Oxfam Australia, 2019; Stats NZ, 2018). This is due in large part to white privilege and the intergenerational transmission of wealth that dates back to the confiscation of Māori and Aboriginal land into Pākehā and Australian European ownership during colonisation. In Australia between 1887 and 1970, strict laws and policies gave control of contracts between indigenous people and employers to a 'protector' or 'administrator'. Collusion, fraud and non-payment of wages by these white authorities was common, as was the forced labour of Aboriginal people. This is known as a period of 'stolen wages' and resulted in an inquiry by the Australian Human Rights Commission (Human Rights and Equal Opportunity Commission, 2006), class-action lawsuits and repayments (Grant Thornton, 2020). The influence of colonisation is ongoing through the dominance of Pākehā/Australian European culture, governance, education and concepts of individual property ownership, enabling privileged access to resources and employment, which in turn facilitates wealth accrual (Consedine, 2005). Wealth contributes to health by increasing access to good nutrition, housing, education and healthcare and also by providing a buffer for unexpected expenses that would otherwise be highly stressful.

Poverty intersects with multiple other determinants but the definition is dependent on context. Absolute poverty, also called physical or extreme poverty, relates to survival and the ability to consistently source the necessities of life, namely food, shelter and clothing. This is more commonly discussed in the context of resource-poor countries, while analysis in developed countries centres on relative poverty or social deprivation, where inequality is the central focus (Bourguignon, 1999). In this context poverty is often defined by a threshold measure of living in a household with an income less than 60% of the median income after housing expenses are taken into account. Poverty has several synonyms in the literature, including socioeconomic deprivation, hardship, material disadvantage (Baum, 2015), 'lack of economic resources' (Statistics New Zealand & Ministry of Pacific Affairs, 2011) and, of particular relevance to this discussion, 'having income less than that needed for a healthy life' (Marmot, 2015, p. 184). Both absolute and relative poverty have negative impacts on health.

The impact of material deprivation on health is starkly illustrated by the differences in health and life expectancy between resource-rich and resource-poor countries. However, large disparities are also evident in Australasia, particularly between indigenous and settler groups, and so-called 'diseases of poverty', which exist in higher levels in Australia and New Zealand than many industrialised countries. For example, acute rheumatic fever is associated with poverty and household crowding. Together, Māori and Pasifika people in New Zealand and Indigenous Australians have the highest documented rates of this infection in the world, at 12–124 times higher levels than among European/other New Zealanders (Bennett et al., 2021) and Australians respectively (Katzenellenbogen et al., 2020).

The Human Development Index is a metric which includes health, education and standard of living as benchmark measurements. In 2014, out of 187 countries, Australia and New Zealand ranked favourably at 8th and 14th respectively (United Nations Development Programme (UNDP), 2020). However, Marmot (2016) points out the enormous disparity experienced by indigenous people: 'If Australian Aborigines were considered as a separate country, they would rank 122'. Without adequate income, those in poverty experience worse health, shorter lives, and longer periods of disability at the end of life compared with those with higher incomes (Marmot, 2015).

Individual or micro level

Material circumstances

Material circumstances are directly related to available income and include living and household costs, travel and commuting costs and access to healthcare. Housing is a fixed cost paid for by all households. Government policies and legislation which have promoted housing property as an investment commodity and reduced the availability of social housing provision have led to increasingly unaffordable housing in Australasia (Howden-Chapman, 2015). Since the global financial crisis in 2008, house prices have steadily increased, and further escalated since 2020 during the COVID-19 pandemic (Greenaway-McGrevy & Phillips, 2021; KPMG Economics' 2021), with both supply and affordability being considered in 'crisis' (Maalsen et al., 2020; McArthur, 2020; Wetzstein, 2021) as more people are priced out of the market. Housing debt and household indebtedness have reached new record highs despite government efforts to address the situation (Barber et al., 2021). In addition, rents appear to be increasing at a faster rate than wage increases.

Poorer households are much more likely to spend more than 30% of their after-tax income on accommodation (the level at which the Ministry of Social Development (MSD) defines housing affordability) (MSD, 2016) and housing accounted for more than half of income expenditure for 40% of quintile 1 (most deprived) households in 2017–18 (Perry, 2019b). Health-based housing legislation was announced in 2017 and passed in 2019 in Aotearoa; the healthy homes standards include minimum requirements for rental homes in heating, insulation, drainage, draft-stopping, ventilation and moisture ingress (Tenancy Services, 2021). Australian rental accommodation standards are variable across states and fall short of the New Zealand standards (Australian Housing and Urban Research Institute, 2018). High rent reduces disposable income for other basic necessities such as heating and clothing to mitigate excess cold and damp in poor-quality housing, which results in excess winter hospitalisations (Howden-Chapman, 2015). Security of tenure is compromised in state housing and the private rental market (Howden-Chapman, 2015), and is independently associated with mental and physical health status (Macintyre et al., 2000). High rental costs also result in household crowding, which affects Pasifika, Māori and Indigenous Australians more than Pākehā or European Australians (AIHW, 2020; Baker et al., 2013; Stats NZ, 2020). Several close-contact infectious diseases are attributable to household crowding, which may be rendered more severe through the other effects of poverty, including inadequate nutrition, heating and reduced access to healthcare (Baker et al., 2013).

In Australia, Aboriginal people are systematically disadvantaged in relation to housing, with high rates of homelessness and inadequate housing including lack of bathroom facilities and electricity or gas (Baum, 2015).

Psychosocial

Psychosocial circumstances relate to social relationships, supports, stressors and coping strategies. According to the New Zealand Health Survey (Ministry of Health (MOH), 2020a), both psychological distress and diagnosed mental health conditions have increased for most groups over time, are strongly correlated with social deprivation, affect more women of reproductive age (15–44) than men, and more Māori and Pasifika women than other ethnicities. A major contributor is the stress associated with the anxiety of trying to meet daily living expenses with inadequate income. In controlled experiments in the USA and India, Mani et al. (2013) found that financial stress for those in poverty resulted in a reduction in cognitive functioning, equivalent to a 13-point drop in IQ or the loss of a whole night's sleep. When the financial stress was relieved, cognitive function returned to normal. This relationship was not seen for higher income controls. Financial stress is associated with increased rates of negative health behaviours including smoking and drinking alcohol. Gregg et al. (2005) found that when those in financial hardship were provided with more money through child benefits and tax credits designed to benefit the poorest, they spent less on alcohol and cigarettes, which were coping strategies that were no longer needed once the stress of making ends meet was gone.

Behaviours and biological factors include nutrition, physical activity and social hazards (tobacco, alcohol and drug addictions) along with an individual's biological/genetic factors. There is now an improved understanding of the 'critical periods' in which exposure can have a lifelong effect on the structure and functions of organs, tissues and body systems and the biological programming of the child. The burgeoning field of epigenetics is investigating how physical, nutritional and emotional exposures from conception through to early childhood have the potential to influence lifelong health.

181

Adequate income and time are required for the purchase and preparation of nutritious food, which can become a discretionary item after fixed expenses (rent, electricity and phone) are paid. In New Zealand, fruit and vegetable consumption, as a proxy for good nutrition, is lower in deprived areas than in less-deprived areas (MOH, 2020a). Food insecurity is more prevalent among groups experiencing socioeconomic disadvantage and living in remote rural areas, including Indigenous Australians, due to the history of colonisation and successive government policies that disadvantage this population (Bowden, 2020; Davy, 2016).

CLINICAL POINT

Using an SDH lens it becomes clear that obesity is the result of inequality as poverty creates an obesogenic pathway with fewer healthy choices available. Parker & Pausé (2018) found that women felt stigmatised during antenatal care, suggesting a victim-blaming culture which misses valuable opportunities for empowerment in the midwifery partnership. Midwives need to consider carefully how they discuss healthy eating and weight gain during pregnancy to ensure they work in partnership.

Health problems can cause a reduction in quality of life for women before childbearing, and become comorbidities during pregnancy, resulting in an inequitable distribution of maternal morbidity and mortality along the social gradient (PMMRC, 2021).

Breastfeeding rates are positively correlated with SES, meaning that the health benefits of breastfeeding are enjoyed more by well-resourced women and their babies than those living with hardship (AIHW, 2020; MOH, 2020b), while the cost burden of infant formula is increased. Factors influencing breastfeeding are maternal education, support from family and access to supportive healthcare providers (McIntyre et al., 2001).

CRITICAL THINKING EXERCISE

Interventions based on behavioural messaging are ineffective at a population level when the circumstances in which people make decisions (the structural factors) are not addressed (Baum & Fisher, 2014). Using the CSDH conceptual framework (see Fig. 9.1), consider how each factor contributes to inequities in obesity rates.

Obesity is highly visible. How might the social stigma caused by the rhetoric of individual responsibility and victim-blaming contribute to health?

HEALTHCARE SYSTEM

Australia and New Zealand have publicly funded health systems to support access to healthcare for all (see Ch. 2) but also a mix of public and private systems for delivering healthcare. In Australia the government funds a health insurance scheme called Medicare, which administers the publicly funded universal healthcare system. In New Zealand all accidents are covered by the Accident Compensation Corporation (ACC) and hospital care is provided free of charge through District Health Boards (which includes emergency care). However, primary community care from general practitioners, whilst subsidised, also requires some co-payments. Both of these systems are designed to support **access** to healthcare for their populations.

Women of childbearing age (15–44), especially in the most deprived areas, have the highest unmet need for primary healthcare, at far greater levels than men. The New Zealand Health Survey (MOH, 2020a) found that cost and/or lack of transport were the main reasons women (especially younger women) either did not visit their GP or have prescriptions filled. Maternity care is free of charge in Australasia and improves health outcomes through screening, education, support and intervention where there is clinical need; however, there is lower engagement for women of lower SES. Where complications arise, therefore, they are more likely to be picked up later on when the opportunities for prevention have become much more limited, and when consequences may be more severe (PMMRC, 2021).

ENVIRONMENTAL DETERMINANTS OF HEALTH

The environmental factors influencing health can be considered from the individual (proximal) to the global (distal). Health-harming exposures at home or at work (e.g. cold, damp homes, lead paint, asbestos, carbon monoxide from traffic, air pollution, noise pollution and industrial chemicals) fit into the rubric of environmental health, and influence population and individual health. They intersect with other SDH through differential exposure along the social gradient. This can also be seen at an urban planning level where wealthier suburbs have better infrastructure and urban design (green spaces that promote physical activity, better roads and amenities including easy access to healthier food outlets) than poorer suburbs. At a global level, changes in the hydrological cycle through climate change increase water scarcity through changing patterns of drought and flooding (UN Water, 2014), which affects the crops on which populations rely for survival. Famine and displacement cause major mortality and morbidity. The technology that has enabled the increase in the earth's carrying capacity for human beings has also altered the equilibrium on which planetary health relies. Our current resource use is not equitably allocated between rich and poor countries and cannot be sustained for future generations (Hassan et al., 2005; McMichael, 1999a; Meadows et al., 2004; Wackernagel et al., 2002). See Box 9.4.

HOW DO THE SOCIAL DETERMINANTS OF HEALTH INFLUENCE OUTCOMES?

It is generally accepted that health outcomes are linked and correlate with the SDH and that there is a social gradient of health. However, whether there is a causal pathway from environmental and societal factors to disease has been debated, often along ideological lines. Critics have accused social epidemiology of being 'casual about causality' (Harper & Strumpf, 2012, p. 796) owing to its production of mostly descriptive rather than interventional studies. A better understanding of the causal pathway is important if effective interventions are to be found and funded. Pickett & Wilkinson (2015) examined the epidemiological evidence for this relationship in their causal review. There are three main theoretical approaches that attempt to explain how the SDH influence health; these are psychosocial approaches, social production of disease and ecosocial theory.

1. Psychosocial factors

The primary emphasis of this theory is on the psychosocial factors that arise owing to living in an unequal society. This theory argues that social inequality causes increased stress, which in itself leads to poor health. A growing body of research has produced evidence to explain how social status contributes to health via the physiological response to acute and chronic stress which is caused by low social status (Marmot, 2015). *Allostasis* is the necessary process by which the body responds to stressful events by activating 'neural, neuroendocrine and neuroendocrine–immune mechanisms' (McEwen, 1998, p. 33) in order to maintain homeostasis. *Allostatic load* is the term used to describe the 'wear and tear' on the body due to frequent or chronic exposure to stress, and it increases the long-term risk of disease. In their synthesis of the evidence, Braveman & Gottlieb (2014, p. 24) explain:

> *Examples include observations that stress can induce pro-inflammatory responses, including production of IL-6100 and C-reactive protein, and that lower income and educational achievement contribute to higher blood pressure and unfavorable cholesterol profiles. Physiological regulatory systems thought to be affected by social and environmental stressors have included the hypothalamic–pituitary–adrenal axis; sympathetic (autonomic) nervous system; and immune/inflammatory, cardiovascular, and metabolic systems.*

Other research links altered neuroendocrine patterns to compromised health with perceptions and experience of social status (Wilkinson & Pickett, 2010). The theory suggests that for people living in what are perceived as lower social positions there is the constant comparison to others in higher status social positions. This comparison can produce feelings of shame, inadequacy and worthlessness, which can result in chronic stress and undermine health (WHO, 2010).

Critiques of this approach argue that the focus on stress and stressed people results in less attention on who and what generates the psychosocial challenges and supports and how resource distribution is shaped by social/political and economic policies (Krieger, 2001). In addition, this approach fails to incorporate how changes over time have impacted on health.

2. Social production of disease/political economy of health framework

This theoretical approach argues that the association between income inequality and health is due to structural causes of inequalities and not just the individual's perceptions of their social status (Krieger, 2001). The economic processes and decisions that shape the available public services are central concerns so that income inequality is one of a cluster of material conditions that affect health. This approach identifies power structures within political processes and ideologies that shape economic and social policy and resource distribution. This in turn shapes what other infrastructure and systems are available to the individual—such as education, transport, environment, housing and food affordability—and which therefore affect the individual's health.

3. Ecosocial theory

This approach integrates social and biological factors and was introduced by Krieger (2001) and further developed by others (McMichael, 1999b; Susser & Susser, 1996) to include wider social and environmental changes. It argues that there is a need to identify and explore the biological mechanisms concomitantly with social organisation and ecology as ways of understanding health. The more we know about biology and our biological responses the better we understand how these are influenced by the way society is organised and the environment we live in, which in turn supports more exploration of these effects on biology.

McMichael's (1999b) environmental health work expands on this theory and is closely connected to the SDH. Since the 1960s we have begun to recognise the far-reaching human health consequences of our environmental exploitation (Frumkin, 2010) as environmental degradation is now threatening our species. Humanity evolved within ecosystems and our health relies on their continuance. The transition from hazards-based environmental health theory to one of 'habitat thinking' is a move from separation to integration, from being 'apart from' to being 'a part of' nature (Myers & Kent, 2005, p. 291). Habitat thinking was and is inherent in many indigenous knowledge systems. We must see ourselves as part of the whole rather than separate from it, which leads to a reconceptualisation of the necessary solutions to focus on ecosystem health. This shift in understanding has been integrated

183

into public health, initially by scholars and subsequently in global policy such as the UN Sustainable Development Goals (UNDP, 2017).

SOCIAL COHESION AND SOCIAL CAPITAL

Most societies, regardless of country, are stratified to some degree with members differentiated into particular groups (Øyen, 2002). Being a member of a group can open some privileges and rights or reduce access to those privileges/rights. The poor or socially deprived often suffer social exclusion, especially if they do not conform to societal norms and values as defined by the dominant group.

Larsen (2013, p. 2) defines social cohesion as 'the belief held by citizens of a given nation-state that they share a moral community, which enables them to trust each other'. Social cohesion is built on integration, and considered the 'glue' or bonds that keep societies together. A society that is socially cohesive is considered to be one that works towards the inclusion and wellbeing of all members of that society to create a sense of belonging and trust. The aim of social inclusion is that all members of society have equal power within that society.

Social capital comprises the resources and benefits that occur when members of society work and cooperate together towards a common aim. It can involve economic, cultural and social networks and is associated with trust, reciprocity and cooperation (Øyen, 2002). Social capital is a very necessary safety net for people who cannot rely on privileged access to resources, such that members of a group provide physical, emotional and resource support to each other (Øyen, 2002). Integrating society to reduce stratification and increase social cohesion and the ability to work together can improve social capital for that society. It requires the strengthening of individual capacity and the capacity of the community to identify, resolve and improve the quality of the lives of everyone in that community/society (De Oliveira, 2002). This can be done through cooperation and partnerships which support trust and reciprocity; it needs to be fostered by government agencies and organisations amongst communities.

Social capital features prominently in Māori health promotion, which aims to transition from an experience of social exclusion caused by low SES and disconnection from te ao Māori, to the health-enhancing state of social inclusion (Shaw et al., 2006). This is most likely to be achieved through increased economic participation in society/Te Oranga and facilitated access to te reo and mātauranga Māori, culture and wāhi Māori, economic resources as guaranteed in Te Tiriti o Waitangi (1840) (see Box 9.5), social resources and an expectation of a normalised experience of 'being Māori' in society (Durie, 1999).

Box 9.5 Te Tiriti and the social determinants of health

Te Tiriti o Waitangi (1840), the founding document of the nation of New Zealand, provides for equity in Article Three (see Appendix 11.2). The 1984 Hui Whakaoranga formally recognised a Māori understanding of health including spirituality, culture and Māori identity (Durie, 1998). Since then, several advances have been made in Māori health policy and provision, with a strong focus on Māori autonomy, aiming to enact the provision of Te Tiriti o Waitangi for Tino Rangatiratanga (self-determination) in health (Durie, 2009). Māori health promotion models have been developed, including Te Pae Mahutonga (Durie, 1999). Addressing the social determinants of health including poverty is central to this model.

The Waitangi Tribunal has been hearing Kaupapa (thematic) inquiries including claims relating to the Crown's failure to uphold Te Tiriti in relation to health and Mana Wāhine (Waitangi Tribunal, 2021). The findings are becoming influential in the struggle to change the health sector and government policy to meet the needs of Tangata Whenua, where the Crown has been abrogating its responsibilities.

REFLECTIVE CASE STUDY

In Brazil, the Comunidade Solidária was a government-led program aimed at encouraging parents' involvement with school life and mobilising people to take care of their own health. This program included 'top down' and 'bottom up' approaches which were complementary and mutually reinforcing. The results indicated increased solidarity within the community, improved individual and community confidence and skills along with increased trust in the government. This program identified that skills, expertise, organisational capability and networks need to be considered as resources and can be used to improve and increase social capital (De Oliveira, 2002).

ACTIONS ON SDH

The CSDH builds on the work of previous WHO publications, in particular the Ottawa Charter, which provided a multifaceted, intersectoral intervention framework for health promotion, recognising that several fundamental conditions are required for health, namely 'peace, shelter, education, food, income, a stable ecosystem, sustainable resources, social justice and equity' (WHO, 1986, *Ottawa Charter for Health Promotion*, p. 1). By setting up the CSDH, the WHO demonstrated global leadership and guidance on how to reduce inequity and support improved global health in the contemporary context.

Five shared political factors are considered important to improved **population health** (CSDH, 2008, p. 33):

1. A commitment to health as a social goal
2. A social welfare orientation/philosophy
3. Community participation in decision-making processes (that are relevant to health)
4. Universal access and healthcare for all social groups
5. Intersector linkages of government departments to promote health.

When these factors are achieved, in both wealthy and low-income countries, there have been improved health outcomes and reduced health inequities. The high level of population health in Nordic countries is attributed to a long-term commitment to 'universalist policies based on equality of rights to benefits and services, full employment, gender equity and low levels of social exclusion' (CSDH, 2008, p. 33). Cuba, Costa Rica, China, Sri Lanka and Kerala in India have achieved equal or better population health (as measured by life expectancy) than the USA despite spending less per capita on healthcare (Organization for Economic Cooperation and Development (OECD), 2014), illustrating that a high national income is not necessary when these principles are followed.

The WHO (2010) set out a conceptual framework for action that can reduce inequity and improve health through the SDH (Fig. 9.2). This diagram identifies the need for action to occur at all levels, with context-specific strategies which work on the structural determinants and seek to integrate different sectors (governmental and environmental) and which also work to improve the participation and empowerment of all within society. For this to occur, health needs to be prioritised as a central, rather than competing, factor in government policy across the spectrum from the health service to economic and social policy sectors. Health justice is achieved by 'good policy for health' rather than just 'good health policy' (Sen, 2009, p. viii).

Multisector action on the SDH is challenging in the global neoliberal context, as discussed in the section on macro-level determinants. Hunter et al. (2010) describe a process of 'lifestyle drift', where governments begin the policy-making process with a commitment to addressing SDH, but ultimately move 'downstream' to interventions directed at individual behavioural change, which Baum & Fisher (2014) argue is ineffective in the context of poverty. This is, of course, a logical and appealing avenue for governments that are operating in an individualised, neoliberal climate, because of the difficulty in moving against supranational power structures such as trade agreements and TNCs (Baum & Fisher, 2014). Examples of lifestyle drift include dietary guidelines (still current in 2022) to reduce obesity in Australia, which overtly place responsibility on

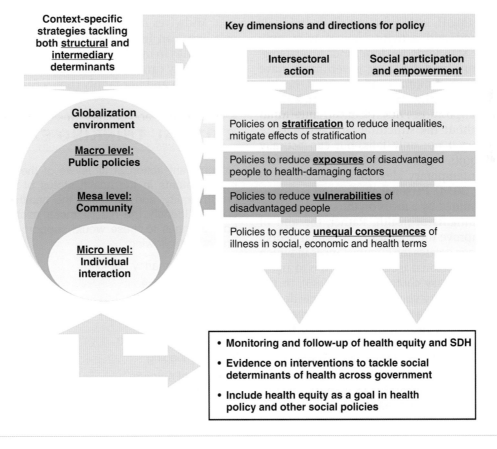

FIGURE 9.2 Framework for tackling SDH inequities
(Source: WHO, 2010, p. 8)

Box 9.6 Midwifery practice points

Midwives work at the nexus of individualised care and population health, and see women living in a variety of different circumstances. Exposures and outcome measurements relating to the social and environmental determinants of health are population based, not individual. They are relevant for midwives in practice for a number of reasons.

- Health, social and economic policy forms the context within which midwives provide care to women.
- Political ideology and international agreements influence the way governments respond to health and resource pressures.
- Focusing on behavioural change without considering the structural changes necessary to improve the circumstances for everyone in society is ineffective at a population level and can do more harm than good. This is because those who are well resourced are

more likely to take up recommendations whereas those who are poorly resourced are less able to do so. A healthy lifestyle is far easier to achieve when women and families are well resourced than when resources are limited.

- Individualism is central to the dominant culture in New Zealand and Australia. This enables a high level of autonomy in decision making by some groups, but also creates a victim-blaming culture.
- Midwives can support women to make behavioural changes for health but need to understand that women and families are also influenced by their circumstances, which in turn are influenced by social and economic policy and cultural norms.
- Social stigma for obesity and smoking can increase stress and is counterproductive to the empowerment that facilitates healthy decision making.

the individual: 'the rising incidence of obesity and type 2 diabetes in our population is evidence of the need for Australians to improve their health by making better dietary decisions' (National Health and Medical Research Council, 2013, p. 3). Similarly, the New Zealand Childhood Obesity Plan (MOH, 2015), focuses on individuals making healthy food and activity choices with only voluntary industry standards for food and advertising. Subsequent additions under a new government have continued a focus on voluntary adoption of health-enhancing policies, rather than regulation (MOH, 2020c).

Health policy that promotes behavioural change at an individual level without the structural changes that are necessary to support it not only fails, but can actually increase health inequities and stigmatises those who 'fail' to conform to a contemporary ideal of 'health' (Baum & Fisher, 2014; Parker, 2014). Personal agency and responsibility are not undermined by a focus on the social and environmental determinants of health. Rather, the aim of policy change to improve the conditions in which people live, work, play and age creates the circumstances in which everyone can exercise personal agency. The aim is to 'make the healthy choice, the easy choice' (WHO, 1986). In the context of food and activity choices, action is needed to move from an obesogenic to a salutogenic *environment*.

Midwifery is a primary healthcare service that brings healthcare into the community and provides individualised care to women within their family/whānau as they identify, recognising their context for health and health behaviours. Antenatal care is an essential health service and an important determinant of health (WHO &

World Bank, 2017), but cannot alone mitigate the health problems caused by lack of access to the wider SDH. Health messaging by midwives is part of antenatal care, and with an individualised relationship the messages can be delivered in a way that is relevant to the woman's context. Midwives need to recognise that pressures on women's lives can influence the level of ease or difficulty a woman has in making behavioural change, whilst government policy can either enhance or decrease the health of the woman and her family (Box 9.6).

CRITICAL THINKING EXERCISE

Government action at all levels of the SDH is needed for improvements in the health status of the population and health equity, and to 'make the healthy choice, the easy choice'. Identify the macro/mesa/micro-level factors and how changes to these would support improved health for one of the following:

- Early pregnancy booking
- Antenatal care
- Housing insulation schemes
- Parenting education
- Smoking reduction
- Safe sleeping
- Optimal nutrition
- Parental leave.

Conclusion

This chapter began with the WHO's 1948 holistic definition of health as a state of complete wellbeing, not just the absence of disease, and an acknowledgement that the majority of the health service exists to treat, rather than prevent, health problems. Studying the social and environmental determinants of health allows us to see the 'big picture', to understand that population health is a product of the structure of society and its social systems. Just as individuals develop their identity through their upbringing, family norms, schooling, socioeconomic status and cultural context, so too are health behaviours and health exposures influenced by these proximal factors. The circumstances of life in which children are born, grow, live, work and age are created by the distal factors comprising national and international governance and government policy across all sectors including macroeconomic policy, social security, education, labour and housing. In turn, the policy direction of any given government or international body is underpinned by political ideology. A study of the SDH is, therefore, a study of power.

The social patterning of health outcomes along the social gradient of health illustrates how resources are inequitably distributed in society. That differential health outcomes occur according to ethnicity, particularly indigeneity, is a reflection not of innate differences but rather of how society has historically and politically been structured to privilege some groups and discriminate against others. Colonisation, as an ongoing process, has resulted in unequal access to wealth, power and ultimately health.

By moving our understanding from 'downstream' to 'upstream' factors, the multifactorial and interconnected influences on health outcomes are revealed. Chronic stress appears to be a central pathway from the SDH to health outcomes. The three main theoretical approaches underpinning the SDH identify the impact of stress on biological systems, how social status creates chronic stress, how social organisation and power structures create social stratification and how our place as part of an ecosystem affects population health.

Effective action on the SDH to improve population health and reduce health inequities involves multisectoral approaches at macro, mesa and micro levels, which requires that health is a central value in policy making.

As midwives, it is important to understand how women's, babies' and families' health is influenced by the wider political context, through government policies and societal values and beliefs, which in turn shape the living environment of individuals. These policies also create the context of midwives' work both through employment and contractual arrangements as well as mandating public health messaging to pregnant women/people in their diversity. Poverty and discrimination are fundamentally disempowering and strongly affect women's ability to prioritise health-related decisions. The goal of action on the SDH is to improve the circumstances in which people live and make decisions, in order to facilitate autonomy, empowerment and integration, and ultimately promote the wellbeing of parents and their babies through generations.

Review questions

1. What does the term 'social determinants of health' mean?
2. How is a focus on the SDH different from the traditional 'causes' of health outcomes such as hypertension, body weight and smoking?
3. At what level of the conceptual framework of the SDH is action likely to have the biggest effect on population health outcomes? Why?
4. What are some of the challenges to action on the SDH?
5. Why is it relevant for midwives to understand the SDH?

Online resources

Australian Bureau of Statistics: http://www.abs.gov.au.
Australian Institute of Health and Welfare (AIHW) reports: Mothers & babies: https://www.aihw.gov.au/reports-data/population-groups/mothers-babies/reports.
Ministry of Health (NZ). Report on Maternity Series: https://www.health.govt.nz/nz-health-statistics/health-statistics-and-data-sets/report-maternity-series.
Perinatal and Maternal Mortality Review Committee reports: https://www.hqsc.govt.nz/our-programmes/mrc/pmmrc/.
Stats NZ: https://www.stats.govt.nz/.

References

Australian Housing and Urban Research Institute (AHURI). *When it comes to rental property standards, what can Australia learn from New Zealand? New Zealand rental property standards go further in protecting tenants health and safety (AHURI Brief).* Melbourne: AHURI; 2018. Online: https://www.ahuri.edu.au/research/ahuri-briefs/when-it-comes-to-rental-property-standards-what-can-australia-learn-from-new-zealand.
Australian Institute of Health and Welfare. *Indigenous income and finance.* Canberra: AIHW. 2019; Sept. Online: https://www.aihw.gov.au/reports/australias-welfare/indigenous-income-and-finance.

Australian Institute of Health and Welfare. *Australia's children. Cat. no. CWS 69*. Canberra: AIHW; 2020. Online: https://www.aihw.gov.au/reports/children-youth/australias-children/contents/executive-summary.

Australian Institute of Health and Welfare (AIHW). *Deaths in Australia*. 2021. Online: https://www.aihw.gov.au/reports/life-expectancy-death/deaths/contents/life-expectancy.

Australian Institute of Health and Welfare (AIHW). *Stillbirths and neonatal deaths in Australia 2017 and 2018*. Perinatal statistics series no. 38. Cat. no. PER 115; 2021b. Canberra: AIHW. Online: https://www.aihw.gov.au/reports/mothers-babies/stillbirths-and-neonatal-deaths-in-australia-2017/summary.

Australian Trade Union Archives. *Australian Conciliation and Arbitration Commission; 1973–1988*. Online: http://www.atua.org.au/biogs/ALE1402b.htm.

Babic M, Fichtner J, Heemskerk E. States versus corporations: rethinking the power of business in international politics. *The International Spectator*. 2017;52(4):20–43. doi:10.1080/03932729.2017.1389151.

Baker M, McDonald A, Zhang J, et al. *Infectious Diseases Attributable to Household Crowding in New Zealand: A Systematic Review and Burden of Disease Estimate*. 2013. Online: http://www.healthyhousing.org.nz/wp-content/uploads/2010/01/HH-Crowding-ID-Burden-25-May-2013.pdf.

Bajwa U, Gastaldo D, Di Ruggiero E, et al. The health of workers in the global gig economy. *Global Health*. 2018;14(124). doi:10.1186/s12992-018-0444-8

Barber P, Tanielu R, Ika A. *State of the Nation 2021 Report*. Auckland: The Salvation Army Social Policy and Parliamentary Unit; 2021. Online: https://www.salvationarmy.org.nz/research-policy/social-policy-parliamentary-unit/latest-report.

Baum F. *The New Public Health*. 4th ed. Melbourne: Oxford University Press; 2015.

Baum F, Fisher M. Why behavioural health promotion endures despite its failure to reduce health inequities. *Sociol Health Illn*. 2014;36(2):213–225. doi:10.1111/1467-9566.12112.

Becares L, Atatoa-Carr P. The association between maternal and partner experienced racial discrimination and prenatal perceived stress, prenatal and postnatal depression: findings from the growing up in New Zealand cohort study. *Int J Equity Health*. 2016;15(1):155. doi:10.1186/s12939-016-0443-4.

Benach J, Muntaner C, Santana V. *Employment Conditions and Health Inequalities. Final Report to the WHO Commission on Social Determinants of Health*. 2007. Online: http://www.who.int/social_determinants/resources/articles/emconet_who_report.pdf.

Bennett J, Zhang J, Leung W, et al. Rising ethnic inequalities in acute rheumatic fever and rheumatic heart disease, New Zealand, 2000–2018. *Emerg Infect Dis*. 2021 Jan;27(1):36–46. doi:10.3201/eid2701.191791

Boston J. New Zealand's welfare state in transition. In: Boston J, Dalziel P, St John S, eds. *Redesigning the Welfare State in New Zealand*. Auckland: Oxford University Press; 1999:3–19.

Boston J. Child poverty in New Zealand: why it matters and how it can be reduced. Paper presented at the Children in Crisis Conference, Waikato University, 2013.

Bourgignon F. *Inclusion, Justice, and Poverty Reduction: Absolute Poverty, Relative Deprivation and Social Exclusion*. 1999. Online: http://www.gdsnet.org/BourgignonRelativeDeprivation.pdf.

Bowden, M. Understanding food insecurity in Australia: CFCA Paper No. 55. Southbank, VIC: Australian Institute of Family Studies. Online: https://aifs.gov.au/cfca/publications/understanding-food-insecurity-australia.

Braveman P, Gottlieb L. The social determinants of health: it's time to consider the causes of the causes. *Public Health Rep*. 2014;129(suppl 2):19–31.

Chenoweth, L. Redefining welfare: Australian social policy and practice. *Asian Social Work Policy Rev*. 2(1), 53–60. doi:10.1111/j.1753-1411.2008.00009.x.

Commission on Social Determinants of Health (CSDH). *Achieving Health Equity: From Root Causes to Fair Outcomes: Commission on Social Determinants of Health Interim Statement*. Geneva: World Health Organization; 2007.

Commission on Social Determinants of Health (CSDH). *Closing the Gap in a Generation: Health Equity Through Action on the Social Determinants of Health*. Geneva: World Health Organization; 2008.

Consedine R. White privilege: the hidden benefits. In: Consedine R, Consedine J, eds. *Healing our History: The Challenge of the Treaty of Waitangi*. Auckland: Oxford University Press; 2005:60–74.

Curtis A. *The century of the self (radio program)*. UK: BBC 4; 2002.

Dalziel P. Macroeconomic constraints. In: Boston J, Dalziel P, St John S, eds. *Redesigning the Welfare State in New Zealand*. Auckland: Oxford University Press; 1999:60–74.

Davies L. Midwifery: A Model of Sustainable Healthcare Practice? (Doctoral thesis). Christchurch: University of Canterbury; 2017.

Davy D. Australia's efforts to improve food security for Aboriginal and Torres Strait Islander peoples. *Health Hum Rights*. 2016;18(2):209–218.

De Oliveira M. Citizen participation and social capital formation. In: UNESCO, eds. *Social Capital and Poverty Reduction: Which Role for the Civil Society Organizations and the State?* Paris: UNESCO; 2002:15–19.

Detollenaere J, Desmarest A, Boeckxstaens P, et al. The link between income inequality and health in Europe, adding strength dimensions of primary care to the equation. *Soc Sci Med*. 2018;201:103–110. doi:10.1016/j.socscimed.2018.01.041.

Dewan P, Rørth R, Jhund P, et al. Income inequality and outcomes in heart failure. *JACC: Heart Failure*. 2019;7(4):336–346. doi:doi:10.1016/j.jchf.2018.11.005.

Diderichsen F, Andersen I, Manual C, et al. Health inequality – determinants and policies. *Scand J Public Health*. 2012;40(8 suppl):12–105.: https://doi.org/10.1177/1403494812457734.

Dudgeon P. Bray A. Reproductive justice and culturally safe approaches to sexual and reproductive health for indigenous women and girls. In Ussher J, Chrisler J, Perz J, eds. *Routledge International Handbook of Women's Sexual and Reproductive Health*. Taylor & Francis. Abingdon: Routledge, Taylor & Francis Group; 2020:542–555.

Durie M. *Whaiora: Māori Health Development*. Auckland: Oxford University Press; 1998.

Durie M. Te Pae Mahutonga: a model for Māori health promotion. *Health Promotion Forum N Z Newsl*. 1999;49:2–5.

Durie M. *Pae Ora: Māori health horizons (lecture transcript)*. 2009. Online: https://www.health.govt.nz/our-work/populations/maori-health/he-korowai-oranga/pae-ora-healthy-futures.

Easton B. Does poverty affect health? In: Dew K, Matheson A, eds. *Understanding Health Inequalities in Aotearoa New Zealand*. Dunedin: Otago University Press; 2008:97–106.

Freni-Sterrantino A, Salerno V. A plea for the need to investigate the health effects of gig-economy. *Front Public Health*. 2021;9:638767. doi:10.3389/fpubh.2021.638767.

Frumkin H. Introduction. In: Frumkin H, eds. *Environmental Health: From Global to Local*. 2nd ed. Hoboken: Wiley; 2010:XXIX–LVII.

Grant Thornton. *Stolen Wages Settlement*. 2021. Online: https://www.stolenwages.com.au/.

Greenaway-McGrevy R. Phillips P. House prices and affordability. *N Z Econ Pap*. 2021;55(1):1–6. doi: 10.1080/00779954.2021.1878328.

Gregg P, Waldfogel J, Washbrook E. *Expenditure Patterns Post-Welfare Reform in the UK: Are Low-income Families Starting to*

Catch up? 2005. Online: http://eprints.lse.ac.uk/6259/1/Expenditure_Patterns_Post-Welfare_Reform_in_the_UK__Are_low-income_families_starting_to_catch_up.pdf.

Grimes A, MacCulloch R, McKay F. *Indigenous Beliefs in a Just World: New Zealand Māori and other Ethnicities Compared.* 2015. Online: http://www.motu.org.nz/wpapers/15_14.pdf.

Guilliland K, Pairman S. *Women's Business: The Story of the New Zealand College of Midwives 1986–2010.* Christchurch, NZ: New Zealand College of Midwives; 2010.

Harper S, Strumpf EC. Social epidemiology: questionable answers and answerable questions. *Epidemiology.* 2012;23(6):795–798. doi:10.1097/EDE.0b013e31826d078d.

Hart B, Risley T. The early catastrophe: the 30 million word gap by age 3. *Am Educ.* 2003;Spring:4–9.

Hassan R, Scholes R, Asch N, et al. Ecosystems and their services around the year 2000. In: Hassan R, Scholes R, Ash N, eds. *Ecosystems and Human Well-being: Current State and Trends.* Vol. 1. Washington: Island Press; 2005:1–23.

Howard-Wagner, D. Governance of indigenous policy in the neo-liberal age: indigenous disadvantage and the intersecting of paternalism and neo-liberalism as a racial project. *Ethn Racial Stud.* 2017;41(7), 1332–1351. doi:10.1080/01419870.2017.1287415.

Howden-Chapman P. *Home Truths: Confronting New Zealand's Housing Crisis.* Wellington: Bridget Williams Books; 2015.

Human Rights and Equal Opportunity Commission. *Inquiry into Stolen Wages. Submission of the Human Rights and Equal Opportunity Commission to the Senate Legal and Constitutional References Committee.* 2006. Online: https://humanrights.gov.au/our-work/legal/inquiry-stolen-wages.

Hunter D, Popay J, Tannahill C, et al. Getting to grips with health inequalities at last? *BMJ.* 2010;340(7742):323–324. doi:10.1136/bmj.c783.

Katzenellenbogen J, Bond-Smith D, et al. Contemporary incidence and prevalence of rheumatic fever and rheumatic heart disease in australia using linked data: the case for policy change. *American Heart Assoc.* 2020;9:e016851. doi:10.1161/JAHA.120.016851.

Kelsey J. *The FIRE Economy: New Zealand's Reckoning.* Wellington: Bridget Williams; 2015.

KPMG Economics. *The Impact of Covid-19 on Australia's Residential Property Market: KPMG Economics report.* Australia: KPMG; 2021.

Krieger N. Theories for social epidemiology in the 21st century: an ecosocial perspective. *Int J Epidemiol.* 2001;30(4):668–677.

Labonte R, Sanger M. Glossary of the World Trade Organisation and public health: part 1. *J Epidemiol Community Health.* 2006a;60(9):738–744.

Labonte R, Sanger M. Glossary of the World Trade Organisation and public health: part 1. *J Epidemiol Community Health.* 2006b;60(8):655–661.

Larsen CA. *The Rise and Fall of Social Cohesion: The Construction and De-construction of Social Trust in the US, UK, Sweden and Denmark.* Oxford: Oxford University Press; 2013.

Lawton B, Stanley J, Filoche S, et al. Exploring the maternal and infant continuum—ethnic disparities in infant hospital admissions for respiratory disease. *Aust N Z J Public Health.* 2016;40(5):430–435. doi:10.1111/1753-6405.12505.

Maalsen S, Rogers D, Ross L. Rent and crisis: Old housing problems require a new state of exception in Australia. *Dialogues Hum Geogr.* 2020;10(2):225–229.

McArthur J. *Somewhere to live: Exploring solutions to the housing affordability crisis in Aotearoa New Zealand.* Auckland: The Helen Clark Foundation; 2020.

McEwen B. Stress, adaptation and disease. Allostasis and allostatic load. *Ann N Y Acad Sci.* 1998;840:33–44.

McIntyre E, Hiller J, Turnbull D. Attitudes towards infant feeding among adults in a low socioeconomic community: what social support is there for breastfeeding? *Breastfeed Rev.* 2001;9(1):13–24.

Macintyre S, Hiscock R, Kearns A. Housing tenure and health inequalities: a three-dimensional perspective on people, homes and neighbourhoods. In: Graham H, eds. *Understanding Health Inequalities.* Buckingham: Open University Press; 2000:129–142.

McMichael A. Hazard to habitat: rethinking environment and health. *Epidemiology.* 1999a;10(4):460–464.

McMichael A. Prisoners of the proximate. Loosening the constraints on epidemiology in an age of change. *Am J Epidemiol.* 1999b;149(10):887–897.

Mani A, Mullainathan S, Shafir E, et al. Poverty impedes cognitive function. *Science.* 2013;341:976–980.

Marmot M. *The Health Gap: The Challenge of an Unequal World.* London: Bloomsbury; 2015.

Marmot M. *Social justice and health: making a difference (lecture transcript).* 2016. Online: http://www.abc.net.au/radionational/programs/boyerlectures/social-justice-and-health-making-a-difference/7804552.

Meadows D, Randers J, Meadows D. *Overshoot. Limits to Growth: The 30-year Update.* White River Junction, VT: Chelsea Green; 2004.

Miller K. Balancing individualism and collectivism in an Australian Aboriginal context. In: McIntyre-Mills J, Romm N, Corcoran-Nantes Y, eds. *Balancing Individualism and Collectivism: Social and Environmental Justice.* Champaign, IL: Springer; 2018:199–209.

Ministry of Health. *Annual Update of Key Results 2019/20: New Zealand Health Survey.* 2020a. Online: https://www.health.govt.nz/publication/annual-update-key-results-2019-20-new-zealand-health-survey.

Ministry of Health (MOH). *Childhood Obesity Plan.* 2015. Online: http://www.health.govt.nz/our-work/diseases-and-conditions/obesity/childhood-obesity-plan.

Ministry of Health. *Report on Maternity 2018 web tool.* 2020b. Wellington: Ministry of Health. Online: https://www.health.govt.nz/publication/report-maternity-web-tool.

Ministry of Health. *Obesity.* 2020c. Online: https://www.health.govt.nz/our-work/diseases-and-conditions/obesity.

Ministry of Social Development (MSD). *The Social Report 2016: Te pūrongo oranga tangata.* 2016. Online: http://socialreport.msd.govt.nz/documents/2016/msd-the-social-report-2016.pdf.

Moewaka Barnes M, Borell B, McCreanor T. Theorising the structural dynamics of ethnic privilege in Aotearoa. Unpacking 'this breeze at my back'. *IJCIS.* 2014;7(1):1–14.

Morison T, Herbert S. Rethinking 'risk' in sexual and reproductive health policy: the value of the reproductive justice framework. *Sex Res Social Policy.* 2018;16(4):434–445.

Myers N, Kent J. *The New Atlas of Planet Management.* Berkeley: University of California Press; 2005.

National Health and Medical Research Council. *Australian Dietary Guidelines.* 2013. Canberra: National Health and Medical Research Council. Online: https://www.nhmrc.gov.au/adg.

Organization for Economic Cooperation and Development (OECD). Life expectancy. In: Indicators OS, eds. *Society at a Glance 2014.* Paris: OECD; 2014.

Oxfam Australia. *The Inequality that Divides Us: Australian Inequality Fact Sheet.* 2019. Online: https://www.oxfam.org.au/wp-content/uploads/2019/03/2019-Davos-factsheet.pdf.

Øyen E. Social capital formation: a poverty reducing strategy? (paper presented at the UN Summit +5, UNESCO/MOST and CROP/ISSC). In: (n.a.) *Social Capital and Poverty Reduction.* Paris: UNESCO; 2002:9–12. Online: http://unesdoc.unesco.org/images/0013/001325/132556e.pdf.

Parker G. Mothers at large: responsibilizing the pregnant self for the "obesity epidemic". *Fat Stud.* 2014;3(2):101–118. doi:10.1080/21604851.2014.889491.

Parker G, Pausé C. Pregnant with possibility: negotiating fat maternal subjectivity in the "war on obesity". *Fat Stud.* 2018;7(2):124–134. doi:10.1080/21604851.2017.1372990.

Perinatal and Maternal Mortality Review Committee. *Fourteenth Annual Report of the Perinatal and Maternal Mortality Review Committee | Te Pūrongo ā-Tau Tekau mā Whā o te Komiti Arotake Mate Pēpi, Mate Whaea Hoki.* Wellington:Health Quality and Safety Commission; 2021. Online: https://www.hqsc.govt.nz/our-programmes/mrc/pmmrc/publications-and-resources/publication/4210/.

Perry B. *Household incomes in New Zealand: Trends in indicators of inequality and hardship 1982 to 2018.* 2019a. Wellington: Ministry of Social Development. Online: https://www.msd.govt.nz/about-msd-and-our-work/publications-resources/monitoring/household-incomes/index.html.

Perry B. *The material wellbeing of NZ households: Overview and Key Findings.* 2019b. Wellington: Ministry of Social Development. Online: https://www.msd.govt.nz/about-msd-and-our-work/publications-resources/monitoring/household-incomes/index.html.

Pickett KE, Wilkinson RG. Income inequality and health: a causal review. *Soc Sci Med.* 2015;128:316–326. doi:10.1016/j.socscimed.2014.12.031.

Rashbrooke M. *Understanding Inequality.* 2016. Online: http://www.inequality.org.nz/understand/.

Rei T. Te Rōpū Wāhine Māori Toko i te Ora, Māori Women's Welfare League 1951. In: Else A, eds. *Women Together: A History of Women's Organisations in New Zealand, Ngā Rōpū Wāhine o te Motu.* Wellington: Daphne Brasell Associates Press & Historical Branch, Department of Internal Affairs; 1993:34–38.

Ramsden I. 'Towards cultural safety'. In Wepa D, ed. *Cultural Safety in Aotearoa New Zealand.* 2nd ed. Melbourne: Cambridge University Press; 2015:5–25.

Ross, L. Reproductive Justice as intersectional feminist activism. *Souls.* 2017;19(3):286–314.

Sen A. Foreword. In: Ruger JP, eds. *Health and Social Justice.* Oxford: Oxford University Press; 2009:vi–ix.

Shaw M, Dorling D, Davey Smith G. Poverty, social exclusion and minorities. In: Marmot M, Wilkinson R, eds. *Social Determinants of Health.* Oxford: Oxford University Press; 2006:211–239.

Statistics New Zealand (Stats NZ), Ministry of Pacific Affairs. *Health and Pacific Peoples in New Zealand.* 2011. Online: http://archive.stats.govt.nz/browse_for_stats/people_and_communities/pacific_peoples/pacific-progress-health.aspx.

Statistics New Zealand (Stats NZ), *Ministry for Women. Effect of Motherhood on Pay—Summary of Results: June 2016 Quarter.* 2017. Online: http://archive.stats.govt.nz/browse_for_stats/income-and-work/Income/motherhood-penalty-summary.aspx.

Stats NZ. *Household net worth statistics: Year ended June 2018.* 2018. Online: https://www.stats.govt.nz/information-releases/household-net-worth-statistics-year-ended-june-2018.

Stats NZ. *Almost 1 in 9 people live in a crowded house.* Wellington: Stats NZ; 2020. Online: https://www.stats.govt.nz/news/almost-1-in-9-people-live-in-a-crowded-house.

Stats NZ. *National and subnational period life tables: 2017–2019.* 2021. Online: https://www.stats.govt.nz/information-releases/national-and-subnational-period-life-tables-2017-2019.

Stephens R. Poverty, family finances and social security. In: Boston J, Dalziel P, St John S, eds. *Redesigning the Welfate State in New Zealand.* Auckland: Oxford University Press; 1999: 238–259.

Susser M, Susser E. Choosing a future for epidemiology ii. From black box to Chinese boxes and eco-epidemiology. *Am J Public Health.* 1996;86(5):674–677.

Tenancy Services. *About the healthy homes standards.* Wellington: Ministry of Business, Innovation and Employment; 2021. Online: https://www.tenancy.govt.nz/healthy-homes/about-the-healthy-homes-standards/.

Te Tiriti o Waitangi; 1840. Online: http://www.treatyofwaitangi.maori.nz/.

Thorogood C. Models of health. In: Pairman S, Pincombe J, Thorogood C, et al., eds. *Midwifery: Preparation for Practice.* 3rd ed. Sydney: Elsevier; 2015:56–71.

United Nations Conference on Trade and Development. *World Investment Report 2013.* 2013. Online: http://unctad.org/en/PublicationsLibrary/wir2013_en.pdf.

United Nations Development Programme (UNDP). *Sustainable Development Goals.* 2017. Online: http://www.undp.org/content/undp/en/home/sustainable-development-goals.html.

United Nations Development Programme (UNDP). *Human Development Index Ranking. Human Development Report 2020.* Online: http://hdr.undp.org/en/content/latest-human-development-index-ranking.

UN Water. *A Post-2015 Global Goal for Water: Synthesis of Key Findings and Recommendations From UN-Water.* 2014. Online: http://www.un.org/waterforlifedecade/pdf/27_01_2014_un-water_paper_on_a_post2015_global_goal_for_water.pdf.

UN Women. *Intersectional feminism: what it means and why it matters right now.* 1 July 2020. Online: https://www.unwomen.org/en/news/stories/2020/6/explainer-intersectional-feminism-what-it-means-and-why-it-matters.

Wackernagel M, Schulz NB, Deumling D, et al. Tracking the ecological overshoot of the human economy. *Proc Natl Acad Sci USA.* 2002;99(14):9266–9271. doi:10.1073/pnas.142033699.

Wade M. Inequality and the West. In: Rashbrooke M, eds. *Inequality: A New Zealand Crisis.* Wellington: Bridget Williams; 2013:39–52.

Waitangi Tribunal. *Kaupapa Inquiries.* 2021. Online: https://waitangitribunal.govt.nz/inquiries/kaupapa-inquiries/.

Waring M. *Counting for Nothing: What Men Value and What Women are Worth.* Wellington: Allen & Unwin; 1988.

Wetzstein, S. Assessing post-GFC housing affordability interventions: a qualitative exploration across five international cities. 2021;21(1):70–102. doi: 10.1080/19491247.2019.1662639.

Wilkinson R, Pickett K. *The Spirit Level: Why Equality is Better for Everyone.* London: Penguin; 2010.

World Health Organization (WHO). Preamble to the Constitution of the WHO (paper presented at the International Health Conference, New York, 1948). Online: http://www.who.int/about/mission/en/.

World Health Organization (WHO). *Ottawa Charter For Health Promotion.* Geneva: World Health Organization; 1986.

World Health Organisation (WHO). Solar O, Irwin A. A Conceptual Framework for Action on the Social Determinants of Health. Social Determinants of Health Discussion paper 2 (Policy and Practice). Geneva: World Health Organisation; 2010.

World Health Organization (WHO). *Gender, Equity and Human Rights: Health and Sexual Diversity.* 2016. Online: http://www.who.int/gender-equity-rights/news/health-sexual-diversity/en/.

World Health Organization (WHO). *Gender and Health.* 2021. Online: https://www.who.int/health-topics/gender.

World Health Organization & World Bank. *Tracking Universal Health Coverage: 2017 Global Monitoring Report.* 2017. Online: http://documents.worldbank.org/curated/en/640121513095868125/pdf/122029-WP-REVISED-PUBLIC.pdf.

Statutes

Equal Pay Act; 1972. Public Act No. 118 (NZ).

Social Security Act; 1938. § 2GEO. VI, 7 Stat. 62–146 (NZ).

Further reading

Baum F. *The New Public Health*. 4th ed. Melbourne: Oxford University Press; 2015.

Commission on Social Determinants of Health (CSDH). *Closing the Gap in a Generation: Health Equity Through Action on the Social Determinants of Health*. 2008. Geneva: World Health Organization.

Grimes A, MacCulloch R, McKay F. *Indigenous Beliefs in a Just World: New Zealand Māori and Other Ethnicities Compared*. 2015. Online: http://www.motu.org.nz/wpapers/15_14.pdf.

Kazancigil A, Øyen E, Fournier F, et al. *Social Capital and Poverty Reduction: Which Role for the Civil Society Organizations and the State?* 2002. Online: http://unesdoc.unesco.org/images/0013/001325/132556e.pdf.

Marmot M. *The Health Gap: The Challenge of an Unequal World*. London: Bloomsbury; 2015.

Miller K. Balancing individualism and collectivism in an Australian Aboriginal context. In: McIntyre-Mills J, Romm N, Corcoran-Nantes Y, eds. *Balancing Individualism and Collectivism: Social and Environmental Justice*. Champaign, IL: Springer; 2018:199–209.

Rashbrooke M. *Inequality: A New Zealand Crisis*. Wellington: Bridget Williams; 2013.

World Health Organization (WHO). *A Conceptual Framework for Action on the Social Determinants of Health*. 2010. Online: http://www.who.int/social_determinants/publications/9789241500852/en/.

World Health Organization (WHO). *Gender, Equity and Human Rights: Health and Sexual Diversity*. 2016. Online: http://www.who.int/gender-equity-rights/news/health-sexual-diversity/en/.

Wilkinson R, Pickett K. *The Spirit Level: Why Equality is Better for Everyone*. London: Penguin; 2010.

CHAPTER 10

Midwives working with Aboriginal and Torres Strait Islander women

Donna Hartz and Juanita Sherwood

LEARNING OUTCOMES

Learning outcomes for this chapter are:

1. To identify considerations unique to Aboriginal and Torres Strait Islander Australians
2. To appreciate the complexity of health status in Aboriginal and Torres Strait Islander peoples and to recognise the heterogeneity of indigenous Australians
3. To identify the impact that colonisation continues to have on the health and wellbeing of Aboriginal and Torres Strait Islander peoples
4. To explore the concept of 'birthing on country'
5. To recognise individual, professional and institutional racism in maternity care and its health implications
6. To identify strategies for midwives to work respectfully and effectively in partnership with Aboriginal and Torres Strait Islander women and their respective community-controlled health services.

CHAPTER OVERVIEW

Author Donna Hartz is an Aboriginal midwife with over 30 years' experience working in maternity service reform in Australia, in particular continuity of midwifery care models. Her recent work has been on the evaluation of urban Aboriginal models of midwifery care and the promotion and development of education pathways for Aboriginal people into midwifery training. Juanita Sherwood shares her views as an Aboriginal woman and nurse who has worked in the area of Aboriginal health, Aboriginal child and family health education, and research in urban, rural and remote communities throughout Australia, also for over 20 years. Previous chapter foundation authors Sue Kildea and Sue Kruske, both non-indigenous midwives, brought over 20 years' experience of working in remote Aboriginal communities and experience working in rural and urban areas in the area of Aboriginal Maternal and Infant Health. All current and past authors are leaders in the national initiative of Birth on Country program aimed at addressing maternal and infant health outcomes and social disparities by rekindling traditional birth knowledge and community-led birth services within the Aboriginal and Torres Strait communities irrespective of location.

The chapter provides an overview of the specific challenges facing Aboriginal and Torres Strait Islander childbearing women in Australia. It explores the inequalities between the health status of our first Australians and non-Aboriginal people, and the reasons for these. It also explores maternity and midwifery services, and highlights factors that midwives need to consider in improving their midwifery services to Aboriginal and Torres Strait Islander women.

KEY TERMS

Aboriginal and Torres Strait Islander peoples
Birthing on Country
colonisation
connection to country
cultural competence and cultural safety
ethnocentrism
indigenous peoples
respect
white privilege

INTRODUCTION

In Australia, British colonisation has had profound effects on the health and wellbeing of **Aboriginal and Torres Strait Islander peoples** resulting in disparities in the life expectancy, burden of disease and social determinants of health compared with the non-Aboriginal population (Jackson Pulver et al., 2010). Colonisation for Aboriginal people has been marked by genocide, dispossession of lands, systemic incarceration and removal of children (Human Rights and Equal Opportunity Commission, 1997). This has resulted in persistent intergenerational grief and loss that has been compounded by government policy and societal ignorance around the effects of colonisation in fragmenting Aboriginal and Torres Strait Islander cultural and traditional mores and laws (Jackson Pulver et al., 2010).

Midwives have a pivotal role to play in supporting Aboriginal and Torres Strait Islander women and families to heal and also in providing and guiding them into the safest environment for them to grow their families and promote better health outcomes. To work effectively with Aboriginal and Torres Strait Islander Australians, midwives require an understanding of some of the key factors that influence the health and wellbeing of communities and how these can affect access to healthcare services. This chapter will provide an overview of these factors and will outline some of the principles and practices known to make a difference to services and outcomes. Most importantly, midwives need to be able to work comfortably and effectively across cultures. We will provide some insight into this complex area and have included some strategies that should assist such interactions. Stories from the field will be used to highlight some of the key points.

ABORIGINAL AND TORRES STRAIT ISLANDER HEALTH IN AUSTRALIA

In 2020 there were 22,016 Aboriginal and Torres Strait Islander births registered, an increase of 91 babies from 2019. This represents 7.5% of all births registered in 2020 (Australian Bureau of Statistics (ABS), 2021). The majority (79%) live in cities and non-remote regional areas, with about one-third of all indigenous[a] Australians living in major cities (35%). A further 22% lives in inner regional areas, 22% in outer regional areas, 8% in remote areas and 14% very remote areas (Australian Institute of Health and Welfare (AIHW), 2017a). These demographics present additional challenges in healthcare service delivery to the last of these groups.

The significant differences in health status for Aboriginal and Torres Strait Islander Australians, when compared with non-indigenous Australians, is well documented and reflected in the different population pyramid shown in Fig. 10.1. Comparisons with other indigenous populations also show that Australia's indigenous population have a worse life expectancy than other indigenous populations in comparable colonised countries (AIHW, 2011).

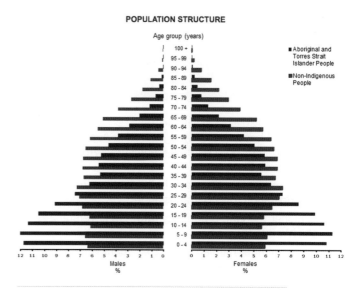

FIGURE 10.1 Population pyramid for Aboriginal and non-Aboriginal populations
(Source: Australian Bureau of Statistics (2017a) Aboriginal and Torres Strait Islander Population 2016, Cat: 2071.0)

Closing the gap

In 2005, the Social Justice Commissioner, Tom Calma, argued for governments to make a commitment to accepting a human rights approach to the health inequality of Aboriginal Australians. Taking a human rights approach to the inequalities in Australia was increasingly being advocated. In 2007, non-government organisations launched the 'Close the Gap' campaign that was ultimately supported by all Australian governments. This campaign aimed to close key gaps in outcomes in areas of health, education and employment between indigenous and non-indigenous Australians. Six targets were selected as essential elements in closing the gap and a number of strategic areas for action were identified, with key indicators for improving maternal and infant health including: improved antenatal care provision, alcohol and smoking reduction in pregnancy, reducing the rate of low-birth-weight babies, reducing the rate of teenage pregnancy and birth, and addressing the causes of maternal mortality and early childhood hospitalisations (Steering Committee for the Review of Government Service Provision (SCRGSP), 2009). However, in 2021 the majority of targets have not been met and the Australian government is now revisiting the initiative and has made a commitment through Closing the Gap 2021 (Department of Prime Minister and Cabinet, 2020).

Maternal and infant health

Improvements in some maternal health indicators is evident, such as the rates of smoking in pregnancy, teenage pregnancy, low birth weight and antenatal attendance; however, there remain disparate outcomes for Aboriginal and Torres Strait Islander mothers and babies (see Box 10.1). When compared with non-indigenous Australians, these

Box 10.1 Comparative maternal and babies demographics and health statistics for Aboriginal and Torres Strait Islander Australians[a]

Maternal demographics

- 6% of all births (18,560) registered in Australia where one or both parents identified as Aboriginal and Torres Strait Islander.
- 4.3% of women who gave birth identified as Aboriginal or Torres Strait Islander.
- A higher teenage pregnancy rate—15% versus 2% (AIHW, 2017b).
- Were younger median age—25.5 years versus 31.2 years (all mothers).
- Have more babies—with total fertility rates per woman of 2.12 versus 1.7 (all women) (ABS, 2017b).

Health statistics

- While more Aboriginal and Torres Strait Islander women attend for care in the first trimester—57% versus 63%—they still have one less antenatal visit.
- There is also a higher incidence of co-morbidities:
  - smoking 45% versus 12% (these rates are improving)
  - obesity 33% versus 20%
  - pre-existing diabetes 13% versus 9%
  - gestational diabetes 3.8% versus 1.1%
  - chronic hypertension 1.9% versus 0.9%
  - gestational hypertension 4.5% versus 3.9% (AIHW, 2017a).

Babies statistics

- In 2015 the perinatal mortality rate was around 12 per 1000 births compared with 8 per 1000 births.
- Major contributors to mortality were pre-term birth (25% versus 13%) and congenital abnormalities (32% versus 18%).
- Higher pre-term birth rates (14% versus 8%).
- Improving but still higher rate of low birth weights (11.9% versus 6.2%) (AIHW, 2017a).

[a]Versus non-indigenous Australians.

women experience more complications in pregnancy and birth including gestational diabetes, hypertension, lower-birth-weight babies and death of babies. They have a higher fertility rate, tend to have babies at a younger age and generally do not present for antenatal care so early compared with the mainstream average. It is important to appreciate that the way Aboriginal and Torres Strait Islander people view health and wellbeing is different to the way Western healthcare providers understand health and expect Aboriginal Australians to behave. Statistics such as those presented in this chapter need to be explored in the light of a problematic history between Indigenous and non-indigenous Australians that is played out clearly in the inequity of health status between them. The statistics are of concern and require redress, but not by further problematising or blaming indigenous Australians (ABS, 2021; AIHW, 2017b). Some overarching and comparative statistics are shown in Box 10.1. The figures show improved perinatal mortality rates (Fig. 10.2) but little change in low-birth-weight babies over time (Fig. 10.3).

WHY THE DIFFERENCE IN HEALTH OUTCOMES?

Colonisation

Colonisation is a critical determinant of **indigenous peoples'** health worldwide and a key causal agent of the heavy burden of disease, poor socioeconomic status, severe disadvantage and the maintenance of political controlling regimes that highlight the discrepancies between Aboriginal peoples' morbidity and eventual mortality and that of the rest of the Australian population (Czyzewski, 2011; Sherwood, 2010). This picture is related to a history of colonisation, genocide, oppression, social exclusion, Western-informed healthcare, loss of land and people, sustained institutionalised racism and the devaluing of Aboriginal knowledge, law, languages and culture (Briscoe, 2003; Ermine et al., 2004; Kunitz, 1996; Toussaint, 2003; Trudgen, 2000; Wilkinson & Marmot, 1998). It is the fundamental discrepancies of health status that allow for comparative descriptions such as resource-poor countries' health status in a resource-rich nation (Bartlett, 1998; Bhatia & Anderson, 1995). Aboriginal health today must be considered in the light of historical and political circumstances that shaped, engineered and ignored the very basic needs of Aboriginal and Torres Strait Islander Australians.

It is estimated that Aboriginal people have lived in Australia for 40,000 to 60,000 years (Kleinert & Neale, 2000), with some evidence to suggest that they may have been here for 120,000 years (Broome, 2002). Aboriginal people, however, consider the time to be 'forever'—as Galarrwuy Yunupingu said, 'Our ancestors have been here since the beginning of time' (1997, p. 1). The population was considered to range between 500,000 and 1,000,000 prior to European arrival, but by the 1920s it had been reduced to approximately 60,000 (Broome, 2002).

The history of the past 220 years provides a vital context of which many health professionals are not aware. It is essential knowledge, however, for understanding why and how colonisation was such a brutal and devastating experience for Aboriginal people. With colonisation came new diseases, loss of culture and difficulties in maintaining the hunter–gatherer lifestyle. Many epidemic and endemic diseases were unknown before colonisation (Callaghan, 2001).

At first contact, Aboriginal people were observed to be a healthy population. Archaeological evidence suggests that morbidity was related mainly to injury and wear and tear,

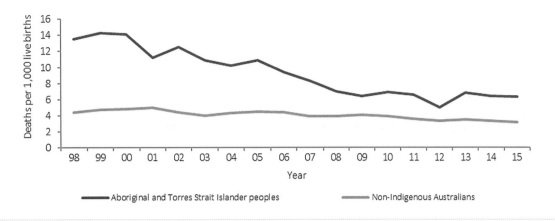

FIGURE 10.2 Infant mortality rates per 1000 live births, by indigenous status (NSW, Qld, WA, SA and the NT), 1998 to 2015
(Source: ABS and AIHW analysis of National Mortality Database in Department of Prime Minister and Cabinet, 2017; https://www.pmc.gov.au/sites/default/files/publications/Aboriginal_and_Torres_Strait_Islander_HPF_2014%20-%20edited%2016%20June2015.pdf)

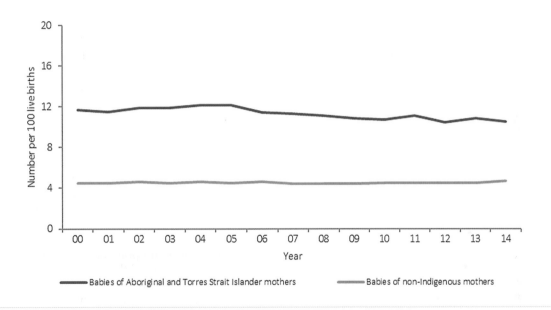

FIGURE 10.3 Low birth weight per 100 liveborn singleton babies, by indigenous status of mother (NSW, Vic, Qld, WA, SA and NT), 2000 to 2014
(Source: ABS and AIHW analysis of National Mortality Database in Department of Prime Minister and Cabinet, 2017; https://www.pmc.gov.au/sites/default/files/publications/Aboriginal_and_Torres_Strait_Islander_HPF_2014%20-%20edited%2016%20June2015.pdf)

rather than non-communicable diseases (Saggers & Gray, 1991). Diet, exercise and lifestyles linked to the traditional culture and lifestyle ensured general wellbeing on all levels. The injuries caused by invasion and encroachment of land by the new settlers led to loss of land, nutrition, trade, cultural practices and autonomy of action (Reid & Lupton, 1991). Settlement occurred over 100 years, commencing in New South Wales (NSW) in the 1780s and completing in the Northern Territory (NT) in the 1880s. This process was resisted by Aboriginal tribal groups and was met with frontier warfare and, later, settler reprisals—now acknowledged as massacres (Connor, 2003).

Survivors were incarcerated onto reserves, islands and missions for 'protection'. The policy of 'protection' spanned from 1883 to 1937 and was orchestrated to regulate, manage and control Aboriginal people. It is this policy that fundamentally entrenched many of the determinants that affect Aboriginal health today, and occurred through the enforcement of sedentary lifestyles, extremely poor and overcrowded housing, and appalling diets that were rationed to families (Reid & Lupton, 1991). These conditions spelt the beginning of the so-called lifestyle (chronic/non-communicable) diseases among the Aboriginal population, as well as contributing to malnutrition that led to widespread infant and child mortality (Kidd, 2000). Government underfunding in the areas of health and housing infrastructure was also established during this era (Kidd, 2000).

Under various state and Commonwealth Protection Acts, the authority was given to remove Aboriginal children

195

from their families. The initial premise for removal was the aim of educating and civilising the children. They were removed from loving families and placed in institutions where they were poorly fed and trained as apprentices to work for non-Aboriginal peoples (Haebich, 1988). These children are now known as the 'Stolen Generation' (Human Rights and Equal Opportunity Commission (HREOC), 1997), and their trauma was officially recognised only recently with an apology in 2008 from the Prime Minister to all Aboriginal people and the Stolen Generation for their 'profound grief, suffering and loss'.

Many men and women sought employment outside of their respective encampments to subsidise family rations. Wages for Aboriginal people up until the 1970s were less than those paid to non-Aboriginal people, although the work was the same. In most cases wages were directed to either local or state 'Protectors', entrenching a lifestyle of poverty. These wages were utilised by the government for the building of mainstream infrastructure, leading to the claim of 'stolen wages' (Kidd, 2000).

Policies of assimilation (1950s–60s) and integration (1967–72) encouraged Aboriginal people to adopt European ways and abandon their culture (Johnston, 1991). This was difficult, as they had effectively been denied the privileges and rights other Australians had enjoyed for generations. Aboriginal and Torres Strait Islander peoples continued to have poor access to healthcare services, education, clean drinking water and suitable housing or employment opportunities.

> An important premise of this [assimilation] policy was that prejudice towards Aborigines was insoluble, and that only by breeding out Aboriginality could these people expect to be treated as equals.
>
> (Rowley 1970, p. 343, cited in Saggers & Gray, 1991, p. 388)

By 1969, Australian states (except for Queensland) had removed most of the restrictions that were placed on Aboriginal people, granting them full citizenship rights and, in 1962, the opportunity to vote (Broome, 2002).

The 1967 referendum enabled constitutional revision to include Aboriginal peoples in the census and gave the Commonwealth greater authority in the area of law making for Aboriginal and Torres Strait Islander Australians (Prentis, 2009). Thus Aboriginal and Torres Strait Islander health became a funded agenda, and both the Department of Aboriginal Affairs and the self-determination policy were established in 1972. However, this policy was seriously undermined by the Federal Liberal Party while John Howard, who commenced in 1996, was at the helm. During his terms there was continued underfunding in the area of Aboriginal and Torres Strait Islander health and primary care services.

The battle for equal rights and removal of inequalities continues today, as years of systemic discrimination and racism have led to a 'multi-causal cycle of poverty', which was reinforced by a lack of self-determination and of access to education, employment, housing and basic healthcare services (Broome, 2002). On 15 June 2007 the NT government

released the publication *Little Children are Sacred: The Report of a Board of Inquiry Into the Protection of Aboriginal Children From Sexual Abuse* (Wild & Anderson, 2007). The inquiry, chaired by Rex Wild and Patricia Anderson, was established in August 2006 and investigated ways to protect children from sexual abuse and neglect. The report made 97 recommendations regarding alcohol restrictions, the provision of healthcare and many other issues relating to child abuse and neglect in regional Aboriginal communities. The report concluded that sexual abuse of children in Aboriginal communities in the NT had reached crisis levels, demanding that it be designated an issue of urgent national significance by both the Australian and NT governments (Wild & Anderson, 2007). In response the government prepared the NT National Emergency Response (also referred to as 'The Intervention') which was a controversial package of changes to legislation that was identified by the United Nations as being racially discriminatory, along with changes to welfare provision, law enforcement, land tenure and other measures, introduced in 2007. The NT National Emergency Response was replaced in 2011 by the Stronger Futures legislation. This too is a controversial policy directive that has support from the Australian parliament and some Aboriginal leaders but has also been criticised by many Aboriginal leaders and national and international organisations including Amnesty International, Concerned Citizens of Australia and many of the major Christian Church denominations. There has been much written about these most recent changes, with one website providing many links: http://concerne-daustralians.com.au/. An example of some of the concerns that have been expressed is provided in Box 10.2.

Connection to country

Apart from the universal value of land as an economic base and a place to live, for indigenous peoples the land is the foundation of social unity and of cultural identity and the source of spiritual sustenance (Durie, 2003). When people are dispossessed of their cultural, spiritual, social and economic base their cultural, spiritual, social and economic wellbeing will suffer—for generations. Therefore, the present circumstances faced by Aboriginal peoples are inextricably linked to their past.

> Aboriginal concept of health is holistic, encompassing mental health and physical, cultural and spiritual health. Land is central to wellbeing. This holistic concept does not merely refer to the 'whole body' but in fact is steeped in the harmonised interrelations which constitute cultural wellbeing. These inter-relating factors can be categorised largely as spiritual, environmental, ideological, political, social, economic, mental and physical. Crucially it must be understood that when the harmony of these inter-relations is disrupted, Aboriginal ill-health will persist.
>
> (Swan & Raphael, 1995, p. 13)

Aboriginal people consider they were created through the life-force of their Dreaming ancestors, along with their respective lands, flora and fauna. All indigenous persons,

Box 10.2

Letter printed on 16 May 2013 sent to the Chief Minister in the NT from Reverend Dr Djiniyini Gondarra, spokesperson for the Yolngu people:

The majority of our people live in the Third world conditions, with poverty, unemployment and disadvantage a part of everyday life. The struggle of families to raise their children properly comes from this lack of stability, not from a lack of responsibility. Like everyone else in the world, we love our children deeply and want the best for them. We need support to do this. Not for our children to be taken away from us … Since the Intervention started in 2007, we've seen family support services almost disappear, whilst more and more of our children are being taken away by child protection services … you claim that only one child has been taken away and given up for adoption in the last 10 years. But the fact is, about 60 children are being taken away every month in the NT by child protection services. Children are being taken away from us at numbers not seen since the Stolen Generations … Our families live in fear. If our babies do not put on weight, child protection officers come in force to take them away. We already live under such heavy control, with no respect or support given to us. This law will paralyse our people … Help us give our children the standard of life they deserve, instead of destroying our families … The dysfunction in our communities is caused by decades of neglect, and is now further exacerbated by the disempowering policies of the federal and NT governments. As people with dignity, we also want to improve the lives of our people, especially the children who represent our future. But we need your help to do this, not your punishment and more pain for our people. …

(Gondarra, 2013. https://www.smh.com.au/national/elder-slams-nt-forced-adoption-plan-20130520-2jw5t.html; © Rev Dr Djiniyini Gondarra OAM)

regardless of their nation, have as a result of this creation a metaphysical and geographical relationship with all of the living and non-living beings of their respective Dreaming creators (Hume, 2002). Deborah Bird Rose writes:

By Dreaming Law no country is dominated by another. Autonomy, the right to be self-governing without reference to a higher social authority, informs the reflexivity of person/group/country. Within their own country, mature adults expect not to be dominated by others. This is where they are needed and wanted, and this is where they have the indisputable right to be.

(Bird Rose, 2000, p. 121)

This statement represents Indigenous people's worldviews (i.e. their ways of knowing, being and doing), and is distinctly different to the Western worldview.

For Aboriginal peoples, country is much more than a place. Rock, tree, river, hill, animal, human—all were formed of the same substance, by the ancestors who continue to live in land, water and sky. Country is filled with relations speaking language and following Law, no matter whether the shape of that relation is human, rock, crow or wattle. Country is loved, needed and cared for; and country loves, needs and cares for her peoples in turn. Country is family, culture, identity; country is self (Kwaymullina, 2005). The connection that Aboriginal people have to land or country, through their spiritual and physical ancestry, is transgenerational, experiential and significant. Land is the lifegiver to all peoples in the world and provides for all needs. Aboriginal people have long respected and reciprocated this relationship and have historically endeavoured to maintain their union through law, ceremony, cultural practice and protocols.

The Aboriginal people of Australia are owned by the land. The connection starts at birth and remains until each member is laid back within the earth to again become part of her. To lose connection to country is to cause ill-health. As Bill Neidjie, Aboriginal Elder, explains,

Yes, this country, your country, my country … I love im.
I don't want to lose country, somebody take im.
Make you worry.
If somebody take im your country, you'n'me both get sick.
Because feeling … this country where you brought up
And just like you'n'me mother.
Somebody else doing it wrong … you'n'me feel im.
Anybody, anyone … you'n'me feel

(Neidjie, 1989)

A distressful inappropriate birthing experience can also cause ill-health. Rawlings (1998) explains that the birthing experience cannot act as a true rite of passage when a woman is not surrounded by those who care for her cultural and spiritual needs, even if her physical needs are being met. This point could be argued for all women. Rawlings (1998) provides the example of the Ngaanyatjarra[b] women who grieve for the way the placenta is handled when women birth in hospitals. The quote below illustrates a similar belief stated by a Yolngu[c] woman:

smoking will close up and heal the soreness of childbirth … it should be available in hospital … the placenta should not be burnt as the mother might then get a sickness in the womb, it is alright to freeze it till it can be buried by the families at home.
(East Arnhem Aboriginal Health Worker (Kildea, 1999))

Some Aboriginal women believe that when babies and mothers return from the regional centres, they return in a weak state and need cultural ceremonies such as the 'smoking ceremony' to be performed to make them strong again (Carter et al., 1987). Failing to observe the relevant rituals and laws during pregnancy and birth presents a grave risk to the health of both the mother and baby and the long-term health of her people. For Aboriginal women, separated from their land, language, culture and families during the birth of their children, removal to the regional hospital represents an at times unacceptable risk (Roberts, 2001). Some Aboriginal women identify giving birth in the hospital as the cause of infant mortality. As a result of not being welcomed properly into the world, and the appropriate ceremonies not being performed, the baby's weakened spirit gets sick (Mills & Roberts, 1997).

REFLECTIVE THINKING EXERCISE

Some Aboriginal women in remote areas are frightened of being taken off country and away from family and hence attempt to hide from the healthcare staff when they are pregnant because they do not want to be flown out for birth. Women who are flown out for birth can be separated from family for up to 6 weeks; staying on their own in a strange environment, they are at risk of getting depressed and not eating well, further exacerbating the risk of a small-for-dates baby.

How would you respond to this situation? What sort of strategies could you employ to encourage the women to access antenatal care?

A MIDWIFE'S STORY

Alex Godsen, Visiting Community Midwife, Palm Island

One of the things I like most about working with Aboriginal families is their pragmatic approach to birthing. There is an inherent belief that it's normal and the thought of it becoming a medical event is alien and frightening. On Palm Island, we offer only antenatal care, so women have to go to Townsville and await the birth of their baby—a policy that the women often question verbally and with their feet. Noby was one Aboriginal woman I worked with, and at 38 weeks gestation, I organised for her to fly to Townsville. She went, but she wasn't happy. She told her partner that she was going back to Palm Island and that she'd have her baby when Alex was there on Tuesday. And she did! I arrived on Tuesday morning and she was in good labour, and about an hour later a baby girl was born on country. Being born on country is very important to Aboriginal families.

Social determinants of health

There is indisputable evidence that a person's social and economic circumstances will strongly affect their health, with those further down the social ladder suffering higher rates of serious illness and premature death (Australian Indigenous HealthInfoNet, 2017; World Health Organization (WHO), 2018; see also Ch. 9). Aboriginal and Torres Strait Islander families have significantly lower education status, incomes, home ownership and employment rates, compared with non-indigenous Australians (United Nations General Assembly, 2017). Their national imprisonment rates are also 13 times higher, still increasing since 2000 and the gap is widening, with Indigenous women representing 34% of the female prison population (Price Waterhouse Cooper, 2017), with the majority of these women of childbearing age. Prison policy expert Eileen Baldry, of the University of NSW, said the increase should be cause for alarm. She stated 'Aboriginal women often lacked the social support afforded to the general population, while being at higher risk of domestic violence, mental or cognitive impairments, homelessness and poverty. ... It has continued despite warnings that there should be other ways to deal with this, largely through providing support for these women' (Browne, 2012).

Although Indigenous disadvantage is well documented, almost half of Australian people believe that Aboriginal and Torres Strait Islander peoples are *not disadvantaged* (Reconciliation Australia, 2021). It is important that these beliefs be explored, as they support the underlying racism in Australian society. The lack of recognition creates disharmony within society and is acted out in ways that further marginalise and discriminate against Aboriginal and Torres Strait Islander Australians.

There are strong links between education, income and health, but it is also known that social and psychological circumstances that cause stress, and a lack of control over one's circumstances in life, are detrimental to health (Wilkinson & Marmot, 1998). It has been argued that unfavourable social conditions and ineffective self-management are greater determinants of health in disadvantaged populations than is a lack of access to medical care (Pincus et al., 1998). These concepts are not new to Aboriginal Australians, who have always seen health in a broader context than that which is solely related to disease.

THE ABORIGINAL AND TORRES STRAIT ISLANDER DEFINITION OF HEALTH

The Aboriginal and Torres Strait Islander definition of health does not relate to physical health alone but rather encompasses a holistic approach including the social, emotional, spiritual and cultural wellbeing of an individual, together with community capacity and governance (National Aboriginal and Torres Strait Islander Health Council (NATSIHC), 2000). Thus, health programs must address all of these issues if they are to provide a service that is appropriate to Aboriginal peoples. Comprehensive primary healthcare has been identified as the most appropriate model of care for Aboriginal Australians (NATSIHC, 2000). Primary healthcare includes (culturally) appropriate, accessible healthcare with community participation in the planning, organisation, operation and control of the healthcare service (WHO, 1978).

Equity

There is misunderstanding and a lack of awareness among non-indigenous communities about Aboriginal and Torres Strait islander peoples, their health and healthcare. Education is at the heart of change in this situation, and midwives can play a role in this in society. A basic principle of equity is that health expenditure should reflect the relative needs of the population. Current estimates indicate that while there is an increase in funding this does not translate equitably, with an expenditure rate of 1.38 times greater than for non-indigenous Australians but a rate of 2.3 times the burden of disease and illness for Aboriginal Australians (Department of Prime Minister and Cabinet, 2020). Compounding this is the fact that Aboriginal and Torres Strait Islander Australians have significantly poorer access to healthcare services; it is probable that this is not the only cause of their poor health statistics.

REFLECTIVE THINKING EXERCISE

What can you do in your workplace to make services more accessible to Aboriginal and Torres Strait Islander women? What strategies would you use as an individual working in the system? What could you do as a collective, working with your peers?

Access

Community-controlled healthcare services were established in the early 1970s in response to Aboriginal and Torres Strait Islanders' appalling health status, and lack of access to culturally safe and affordable health service provision. The major philosophies underpinning these services are *self-determination* and *primary healthcare*. The 1978 Alma-Ata Declaration has provided a foundation that has been very useful in developing these services; however, it must be noted that many of the services had a strong commitment to self-determination that predated the signing of the Alma-Ata (WHO, 1978). Community-controlled healthcare services have had an impact far beyond their own organisations. They have played an advocacy role in relation to Aboriginal and Torres Strait Islander issues, attempting to ensure that conditions and concerns were noted and addressed by appropriate bodies, particularly in the area of health.

Australia's size and geography present added challenges for people living in rural and remote areas, as does the tropical north where weather will cut off road access for 6 months of the year. We have seen the closure of many small maternity units over the last 10–15 years, which has resulted in more women having to travel long distances to access services. The reasons for closures include workforce shortages and maldistribution, loss of doctors with obstetric and anaesthetic skills, lack of access to onsite caesarean section, concerns about safety,

indemnity issues and perceived higher costs (ACRRM & RDAQ, 2004; Hirst, 2005). The impact this has on families is significant, with considerable Australian data now supporting birth for 'low-risk' women in primary units attended by skilled attendants with appropriate referral mechanisms (Kruske et al., 2015; Monk et al., 2014).

A MIDWIFE'S STORY
Sarah Ireland, Remote Area Nurse Midwife, Wadeye

I have worked as a midwife in remote Aboriginal communities looking after women and their families. In this work you have the true capacity to make a positive and empowering influence in a woman's life, the future of her baby and, with that, the community as a whole. For me it has meant the chance to really experience continuity of care, but I wish I could offer women more choice about giving birth in the community. Working with Aboriginal women means every day I have to be: reflective; creative; humorous; humble; hopeful; inspiring; and also gentle. I have learned so much from my Aboriginal mentors and feel professionally satisfied when we work alongside each other. It's not always easy work, but it's the sort of unforgettable real stuff that I will remember and look back on with fondness when I am a very old, grey-haired woman!

What constitutes 'safe birthing services' is strongly contested, with many Aboriginal and Torres Strait Islander women seeing birth as a normal life event—one where family, the land and culture are all significant factors (Kildea, 2006). Being removed from these during birth is seen by some women to be the cause of the poorer health outcomes. There have long been requests from women, and many government-sponsored report recommendations, stating that birthing in remote communities should be trialled (Kildea, 2006). Yet a lack of political will, opposition from the medical profession and a generalised fear of birthing in remote areas seem to prevent this from occurring. This is despite the excellent outcomes that are occurring in remote Inuit communities many hours away from surgical services (Van Wagner et al., 2012).

BIRTHING ON COUNTRY

In recognising the challenges faced of both access to, and acceptability of, maternity services, the Australian Governments prioritised improvements in maternity services for Aboriginal and Torres Strait Islander families and services, in particular in rural and remote areas. These initiatives relate directly to developing and supporting an Aboriginal and Torres Strait Islander maternity care workforce and developing and expanding culturally safe maternity care for Aboriginal and Torres Strait Islander people. ('Cultural safety' is the preferred term of the Congress of Aboriginal and Torres Strait Islander Nurses and Midwives (CATSI-NaM, 2017, 2018)). A key priority is to establish **Birthing on Country** programs (Kildea et al., 2016).

The term 'Birthing on Country' was conceptualised at a national workshop in 2012 with Aboriginal and Torres Strait Islander Community Elders and a wide range of stakeholders. Ms Djapirri Mununggirritj, a Yolgnu elder from north-eastern Arnhem Land, articulated the meaning of Birthing on Country to be understood:

> ... as a metaphor for the best start in life for Aboriginal and Torres Strait Islander babies and their families because it provides an integrated, holistic and culturally appropriate model of care; not only bio-physical outcomes ... it's much, much broader than just the labour and delivery ... (it) deals with socio-cultural and spiritual risk that is not dealt with in the current systems. It is important that the Birthing on Country project move from being aspirational to actual. The Birthing on Country agenda relates to system-wide reform and is perceived as an important opportunity in 'closing the gap' between Indigenous and non-Indigenous health and quality of life outcomes.
>
> (ACM, CATSINaM & CRANAplus, 2016, p. 8)

Since this workshop the Birthing on Country Model and Evaluation Framework has been developed and endorsed by the Australian Government. The key elements of Birthing on Country are listed in Box 10.3.

Collectively, the Australian College of Midwives (ACM), CATSINaM and CRANAplus have developed a position statement progressing the Birth on Country agenda (see: https://www.birthingoncountry.com/resources). Real progress is being made with this agenda, which is reflected by the government-funded and research support for two programs. In urban Brisbane, Queensland, a partnership program with the local Aboriginal community, the Mater Mothers Hospital and university researchers is under way—'Birthing in our Community: Improving the Maternal Infant Health Care for Aboriginal and Torres Strait Islander Women and Families'. This program offers a fully integrated service for expectant mothers and their families to help them enjoy the best experience possible, as well as support their health and welfare during this exciting time with a Midwifery Group Practice, continuity-of-care model for all Aboriginal and Torres Strait Islander mothers planning to birth at the Mater Mothers' Hospital from early pregnancy through to around 6 weeks post-birth.

A national Birth on Country project is also under way; titled 'Building on Our Strengths (BOOSt): Developing and Evaluating Birthing on Country Primary Maternity Units', it is informed by the highest-quality midwifery and maternity service evidence and Aboriginal knowledge, and is community controlled. This project is facilitating the redesign of health services to provide 24/7 continuity of midwifery care and birthing in an Aboriginal birth centre. Aboriginal leadership and a team with expertise in Aboriginal health and research will translate what works in other settings, and other countries, into practice here in Australia (see: http://www.habs.uq.edu.

Box 10.3 Birthing on Country key elements

Description of the key elements of the Birthing on Country service model (Kildea et al., 2016)

- **Aboriginal governance:** in each site maintained through a *Steering Committee* with strong, and at least 51%, representation from Aboriginal people and/or organisations. A key consideration is acknowledging and responding to the local diversity within Aboriginal communities.

- **Continuity of midwifery carer:** within a Midwifery Group Practice model networked to a regional or higher-level service, offering 24/7 care from a named midwife from first presentation in pregnancy until handover to child health services at 6 weeks postnatal.

- **A standalone birth unit (primary maternity unit)** that incorporates traditional practice; recognises the connection with land and country; incorporates a holistic definition of health; values both indigenous and non-indigenous ways of knowing, learning and risk assessment; and incorporates culturally safe service delivery developed by, or with, Aboriginal people. Care will be provided for all women, and those with no identified risk factors offered local birth. Women with risk factors will be carefully monitored and offered more support and continuity than is currently provided.

- **Cultural capability framework including cultural and clinical supervision model:** framework is under development. A supervision model is currently being piloted in the Brisbane site where an Aboriginal psychiatrist and a psychologist provide monthly supervision of staff.

- **Aboriginal health workers and student midwife development:** we are building on the evidence base of how to create supportive career pathways with Aboriginal workers embedded in the team with cadetships also available to support student midwifery training.

- **Cultural strengthening and revival program** that improves family functioning and parental self-esteem, and has the opportunity of reducing family violence, through recognising intergenerational trauma and building resilience, incorporating therapeutic healing and strengthening cultural connection (to be developed).

au/article/2017/10/million-dollar-boost-groundbreaking-maternity-program). The Birthing on Country project by the Australian College of Midwives is integral to the research programs and is providing considerable leadership in the promotion of the understanding of Birthing on Country and also significant funding towards the BOOSt project.

MAKING A DIFFERENCE
Working in partnership

Working in partnership is a key principle of midwifery care and a recurrent theme presented throughout this textbook (see Ch. 17). Partnership with an individual woman will result in unique care based on her unique needs. This is important for all women but particularly for Aboriginal and Torres Strait Islander women, who have huge diversity in their values and beliefs but are often stereotyped as a homogeneous group. This also enables the underpinning of the cultural, social, historical and environmental influences of health and wellbeing from the community's perspective. In an area as complex as Aboriginal and Torres Strait Islander peoples' health, the prevailing view often fails to recognise the multiple layers of complexity that influence health and wellbeing.

Working in partnership requires midwives to transfer the focus of professional attention away from 'problems', 'deficits' and 'weaknesses' and towards the strengths or power of the woman and her community. This in turn assists the midwife towards developing a collaborative and equal partnership with women, focusing on building individual, family and community assets. By focusing on the woman's strengths, midwives are more likely to increase the woman's capacity and self-esteem, and her likelihood to respond to interventions (Darbyshire & Jackson, 2004).

Working in partnership with women does not deny the expertise of the midwife; it merely identifies the complementary expertise of the woman (Davis et al., 2002). This partnership is particularly important when working with marginalised groups, such as Aboriginal peoples, who have been recipients of 'expert' care for generations and are historically mistrustful of 'experts' or authority figures (Kruske & Murakami-Gold, 2008).

Aboriginal health workers are an important component of the maternity care team. There are a number of models that promote working in partnership with Aboriginal workers. One such model is the Aboriginal Maternal Infant Health Strategy (AMIHS) in NSW that was commenced in 2001. This strategy allows midwives to work alongside Aboriginal health workers or education officers to provide outreach services to Aboriginal women and their families throughout pregnancy and postnatally. The AMIHS has been positively evaluated with demonstrated improvement in antenatal and postnatal care provisions and perinatal morbidity and mortality rates (Murphy & Best, 2012). There are over 40 AMIHS sites in NSW, delivering services to mothers of Aboriginal babies in over 80 locations.

To date, the AMIHS program provides continuity of care across the antenatal and postnatal periods but unfortunately does not yet include birthing, despite the benefits of models that include birth. The Malabar Midwifery

---

A MIDWIFE'S STORY
Sue Kruske, Remote Area Nurse Midwife, Arnhem Land

I was on call one weekend when the phone rang. A 16-year-old primipa was having 'baby pains'. She lived on an outstation, about an hour's drive away. I hurried down to the health centre to check her notes. 'Last seen 4 weeks ago, gestation now 36 weeks.' I grabbed the delivery bundle, some synto [sic], our emergency packs and the oxygen and headed out of town with a sleepy health worker, having woken her up just before dawn.

We arrived an hour later and found the girl in strong labour, surrounded by women. A quick palp and VE revealed she was 8 cm with the head well down. When I tried to explain my findings to the girl and her support team, the aunties and grannies smiled and told me they knew this. One of the senior women had birthed a lot of babies in the old days and she had been with the girl all night.

I was instantly reassured and we had discussions over where the girl should have the baby. This was a long and slow process with many conversations in language where the old women spoke together (not involving the young girl who was labouring quietly alongside them). The Aboriginal health worker was very quiet, deferring to the authority of the older women. Lots of young kids milled about, but seemed respectfully quiet, smiling, moving on, coming back, never too close to get in the way. While I was trying to control my nervousness and suggest that maybe it was better to have this baby back at the health centre, the young girl started to bear down. So much for discussions on getting her to the health centre.

The aunties and grannies turned their attention to the young girl and set off in action. Several women were behind her, one woman supporting the girl like an armchair, arms around her massaging the abdomen, several others at her side. They were quiet and nurturing, murmuring reassuring words in language as the girl recovered from each contraction. She was sitting on her haunches, knees well bent with heels and soles of her feet under her buttocks. They told me later they had instructed her to do this so she would not tear. I felt out of place, and contributed by checking the fetal heart and then quietly withdrew.

I stood in awe of these amazing women, who knew exactly what to do, even though we had been routinely transferring women to the regional hospital for over 20 years. They were in their power. A baby boy was born without any fuss after 15 or 20 minutes. The placenta followed. The Aboriginal health worker and I had not done a thing apart from checking the fetal heart.

Community Link Service in Sydney is an integrated Aboriginal continuity of midwifery care model that has provided continuity of midwifery care with a known midwife in labour, also with demonstrated benefits to the women (Homer et al., 2012).

Another model that has been shown to be effective is the Strong Women, Strong Babies, Strong Culture Program (SWSBSC), where community-based workers work side by side with midwives. This program is more common in remote Australia and particularly in the NT, where it commenced in 1993 (Mackerras, 1998, 2001). These partnerships work best when both knowledge systems are given the same significance. The role of the Aboriginal and Torres Strait Islander workers is not to facilitate the non-indigenous work (though this may be a byproduct), but rather to provide the cultural care that is important in its own right. These types of models are being established in some places around the country (Herceg, 2005).

CRITICAL THINKING EXERCISE

Aboriginal (or Torres Strait Islander) health workers are an essential asset to all non-indigenous midwives. Consider the skills and attitudes you would require when working in partnership with an Aboriginal health worker. How would the roles be determined? How could you complement each other for the benefit of the woman? What could you do to convey your acknowledgement and respect for the Aboriginal health worker's role?

REFLECTIVE THINKING EXERCISE

An Aboriginal woman presents to an urban facility in established labour. She has two children under 3 years of age, and says she had nobody to look after them. What would you do?

Barriers to working in partnership

The attitudes of healthcare providers are often more important to women than is their level of competence. The vast majority of midwives would not believe themselves to be racist. However, the reality for many Aboriginal and Torres Strait Islander women is that they commonly suffer judgment, discrimination and prejudice when accessing mainstream healthcare services (Dietsch et al., 2010). Healthcare staff members are often completely unaware of the offence they have caused. If challenged, their response is most commonly to blame the complainant as the woman with the 'chip on her shoulder'.

Arguably, the most significant way in which non-indigenous Australians can affect Aboriginal and Torres Strait Islander people's health and wellbeing is to examine their own values, beliefs and behaviours and how these may negatively affect the women and families who come into their care.

Healthcare services are largely made up of personnel from the mainstream dominant group (Western, white and middle class) and were designed to meet the needs of this group of people, whose values and beliefs therefore become the norm against which all behaviours and practices are measured (McDonald, 2004). Misunderstanding of behaviours and beliefs that do not conform to this dominant worldview will easily result in individual, professional and institutional prejudice.

The majority of maternity services providers would not consider themselves as racist, prejudiced or judgmental. Indeed many of them choose to work with Aboriginal and Torres Strait Islanders or other vulnerable groups through their desire to 'make a difference'. However, without support and appropriate education many providers unknowingly bring a paternalistic approach to their work that obstructs community members from taking greater control of their health and their community (McDonald, 2004).

REFLECTIVE THINKING EXERCISE

You are the only student midwife in the tea-room and you overhear a conversation where colleagues are talking in a disparaging way about an Aboriginal woman who has presented in pre-term labour. What would you do?

All of us are 'cultural' beings. 'Culture' actually means the *values, beliefs and attitudes* of a group. Yet we are all individuals, with values and beliefs that are developed over a lifetime of experiences. This 'culture' (i.e. the values, beliefs and attitudes) is determined by our gender, social class, sexual orientation, age and religion or spiritual beliefs. These broad categories are not the only things that influence our culture. Our political persuasion, our profession, our sporting activities, our personal experiences with people and events—many things will have an impact on our values, beliefs and attitudes. So, in fact, we each belong to many 'cultural' groups. Some groups we cannot choose (such as ethnicity or gender); others we can move into or out of (such as social class); yet others we can consciously embrace or reject (such as our spiritual beliefs).

Our values and beliefs are commonly played out by our *behaviours* and are sometimes only tested, or recognised, when we come across others who behave or seem different from us. Our 'multicultural' Australia ensures that we do encounter people who behave differently from ourselves, and these differences are even more obvious when we become the *minority*. This could be on a trip to India as a backpacker, a holiday in Japan, working in an Aboriginal community, or working in a healthcare service with high numbers of a particular group (be it intravenous drug users, refugee women or wealthy women accessing in-vitro fertilisation).

Being ethnocentric

We tell ourselves we '**respect**' everybody's right to be different and, at an intellectual level, most of us genuinely think we do. Our unconscious response, however, is often very different. The reality is that when confronted with an 'other' way of thinking or behaving we naturally believe that the way *we* think or behave is the '*best*' way. If we thought that the *other* person behaved or believed in something that we genuinely thought was better, then we would adopt that behaviour or belief, and our values would change.

This is called ***ethnocentrism:***

Ethnocentrism refers to the belief that the values and practices of one's own culture are superior and of greater worth than those of an alternative culture.

(Weller, 1991, p. 31)

In its mildest form, ethnocentrism presents as subconscious disregard for cultural differences; in its most severe form, it presents as authoritarian dominance over groups different from one's own.

(Sutherland, 2002, p. 280)

This is a *natural response* that occurs in all of us, and results in the dynamic and ever-changing nature of the values and beliefs of all societies. All societies change, all of the time. In Australia we don't parent the way our parents did, and our young people of today behave in a vastly different way from young people in the 1960s or 1970s. This indicates our capacity to adapt and adopt values and beliefs that make sense to us. The strange thing is that we seem to resist it, or not want to recognise that it happens.

Accepting that we all are instinctively ethnocentric is only the beginning. The real challenge is preventing ethnocentrism from becoming prejudice.

Prejudice is an unreasonable negative attitude held by people because of their membership of a particular group (Fishbein, 2002). In other words, we *pre-judge*. Prejudice is not a cognitive or intellectual response. Indeed, at a cerebral level, most of us do not hold prejudices towards other groups, as we know that there is no logical or sensible reason we should dislike someone just because they are a bit different from us. The thing about prejudice is that it involves *emotional* responses, sometimes very *powerful* emotional responses.

So when we think that a particular Aboriginal woman is too uneducated to understand some component of her care, or if you think that she will or won't breastfeed based on your other experiences (direct or otherwise) of Aboriginal women, you are *pre-judging* her. These thoughts are ill-informed assumptions and there can be several consequences. We are reinforcing the stereotype and that young girl who may be actually thinking she could breastfeed gets the message (even unconscious to you) that we don't think she can so she doesn't. The other potential consequence is that this young Aboriginal

girl picks up that you do not respect her, and disengages from the midwife and the service. So one small and often unidentified assumption can actually compromise the health of both the woman and her infant by the care provider's erroneous thinking and doing.

This does not mean that we treat all women as if they are well informed—it just means that we have to remind ourselves to *check* with the woman what *her* needs are. That means we *individualise* care in *partnership* with her.

Another strange thing we do is to expect there to be lots of variation among our own cultural group—because there is. Think about all your friends. Some will be anxious, some will be shy, some will be assertive, some will be highly educated and some not. But with minority groups we tend to lump their characteristics all together. Aboriginal women are not all shy, uneducated, victims of domestic violence and poor. Yes, some Aboriginal women are these things—*but not all*, and the risk of categorising all Aboriginal women into one 'type' is that we will *pre-judge*.

White privilege

There is increasing recognition by both black and white scholars of the *privilege* that is automatically afforded to Caucasian Australians. As Mellor et al. (2001) contend, subtle racism occurs in the context of everyday living, such as shopping, using public transport and eating in restaurants—and, importantly, accessing mainstream services, be they healthcare, welfare, education or justice.

For individuals who have never experienced discrimination because of their skin colour or ethnic background, it is often difficult to appreciate the frequent prejudice that individuals from ethnic minority groups encounter. Termed '**white privilege**' (McIntosh, 1988), this racial marker of whiteness is invisible to many who wear it because it is part of the acceptable norm of mainstream Australia (Moreton-Robinson, 2006). Without recognition of this racial marker, individuals of the mainstream group are unaware of the privilege they hold and how this is played out within mainstream Australia. Mainstream individuals and systems need to become aware of this privilege before racism is addressed in our society. When and if this occurs through the critical support of Aboriginal and Torres Strait Islander peoples, we may see the health gap close and a reduction in systematic violence, racism and internalised injury.

THE WAY FORWARDS

The first thing each of us can do is to recognise that prejudice and racism exist—in ourselves, in our profession and in our institutions. By becoming aware of our ethnocentrism and the judgments we make about people every day, we can then try to reduce it.

We used to be told to 'treat everybody the same'. But that is actually impossible—we are human and our response, as we have discussed in this chapter, differs from client to client and is informed by our assumptions and stereotypes. Even if we *could* treat everyone the same, this

203

is also not appropriate—there are some members of our society who actually *need* to be treated differently. Similarly, we are obliged to try to ameliorate some of the disadvantage suffered by many groups in our society. This requires what is termed by some as 'proportionate universalism' (Bennett et al., 2005)—giving disadvantaged people a 'leg up' by offering specific support or resources to help improve access to services, including healthcare and education.

Remember: the vulnerable are those without power, and societies are judged by the way they treat their most vulnerable citizens. Ways for midwives to reduce the power imbalance could include the following:

- Being mindful of our symbols of power—our uniform, the stethoscope, the office or clinic structure (placement of chairs, etc.).
- Sitting alongside, not opposite, quiet or shy clients (e.g. Aboriginal women, young women, refugee women, etc.). Remember, these women are not shy at home—they are shy in front of you because they have no power. Each of us can create an environment where the disempowered can take some power back.
- Determining what the client knows about a particular subject before you 'educate' her. Don't assume she has no knowledge or experience.
- Questioning the assumptions you have about the woman—are any of them negative? If they are, then there is a risk of you passing judgment—and the woman will sense this judgment. For example, an assumption of the woman might be that she is an Aboriginal woman from a remote community, therefore birth is women's business and she will not want her partner with her for birth—but increasingly, young Aboriginal women do want their male partners with them. *All* our assumptions must be checked because not all clients from a particular group will behave in the same way.
- Finally, if clients do behave differently from you (and many of them will), and have different values and beliefs, it is really important that we question our right to disagree with these when the values and beliefs are not causing harm to the woman or her baby. We all like to be treated with respect, and the best thing we can do to reduce power imbalance is to genuinely respect each woman—if it is genuine, the woman will feel that and will be much more likely to trust you, tell you more of her experience and accept your advice.

'Working with' versus 'doing to'

Australia has a long history of carrying out research *on* Aboriginal people. This has been not only in healthcare but also in other services. As Dodson (2003, p. 27) states:

Since their first intrusive gaze, colonising cultures have had a preoccupation observing, analysing, studying, classifying and labeling Aborigines and Aboriginality. Under that gaze, Aboriginality changed from being a daily practice to being 'a problem to be solved'.

Aboriginal and Torres Strait Islander peoples have long requested to participate in decisions regarding their own people, including research and the delivery of healthcare services. Attempts by government to support Aboriginal and Torres Strait Islander programs are often restricted by funding agreements that are structured around Western frameworks. This does not allow communities to develop programs that are informed, run and evaluated within their own Aboriginal knowledge systems. As a result, the programs rarely continue because their success is measured by mainstream models.

To improve relationships, non-indigenous healthcare professionals must have access to 'the diversity, complexity, and richness of Indigenous cultures' (Hurst & Nader, 2006, p. 294). The current lack of awareness has significant implications for both the healthcare providers and their clients. It places the non-indigenous healthcare professional in a state of 'unease and unknowing'. This in turn will have a negative impact on their level of confidence and self-esteem regarding working in the area of Aboriginal health, be it rural, remote or urban (Larson et al., 2007; Mobbs, 1991). This unease is transferred onto their Aboriginal clients, who will respond with a reciprocal unease (Hurst & Nader, 2006; McCoy, 2008; Paradies et al., 2008). Finally, these experiences of unease open a floodgate of misleading information for both clients and healthcare professionals to accept as truths regarding each other (Memmi, 1965).

These 'truths' become stereotypes, are reinforced through stories told by friends or relatives, the radio, television, newspapers or books and are reported in research articles (Langton, 1993; Memmi, 1965). They become the 'truths' of those who accept them, as they have no reason to question their validity; they fit with their experiences and those sources they trust (Sherwood, 2010). They become the 'reality' for the non-indigenous person, embedded in their values and hence part of their 'culture'.

It is important to acknowledge that these beliefs are supported by the 'expert' model of medicine, in which healthcare professionals look for problems and deficits to 'fix' (Davis et al., 2002). Coupled with our colonial history, which has consistently problematised Aboriginal and Torres Strait Islander Australians, these beliefs become embedded in society even without the reality of a personal experience.

Appreciating that these practices are historically and institutionally contrived and hence embedded in the ways of knowing of non-indigenous Australians does not make them less damaging. It is imperative to explore the reasons for these beliefs in order to shift and prevent continuation. This requires the utilisation of a '*decolonisation*' method. This method critiques the historical underpinnings of the present and critically analyses the constitution of a white, Western cultural dominant paradigm, which maintains the continued construction of the 'problematic indigenous person':

Decolonisation requires a respectful awareness of multiple ways of knowing and different systems of truths. Part of this process is acknowledging that colonisation continues to impact on our identities and world views. It requires a balance of many different stories and ideas to contextualise the present through the past.

Decolonisation is an ongoing process that requires critical reflective practice examining the way we perceive the world. Critical reflective thinking is a valuable skill that can be used across multiple disciplines. It starts with the self, supporting notions of self awareness. Being self aware is when we recognise that we all hold biases, prejudices and assumptions that inform our points of view or world view. Learning to think critically will assist us to engage with the ideas presented, to explore many perspectives and to have control over the ways in which we take on board new information.

(Sherwood & Keech, 2011, p. 108)

The organisational level

Health systems must acknowledge that institutional and interpersonal racism exists within its own doors, impacting significantly on indigenous health outcomes (Sherwood, 2009). There are many ways to improve the **cultural competence** of an organisation, listed in Box 10.4. (See also Ch. 17 for a discussion of the terms 'cultural competence' and '**cultural safety**'.)

Cultural competence requires that organisations have a defined set of values and principles, and demonstrate behaviours, attitudes, policies and structures that enable them to work effectively cross-culturally … Cultural competence is a developmental process that evolves over an extended period. Both individuals and organisations are at various levels of awareness, knowledge and skills along the cultural competence continuum.

(Dudgeon et al., 2010, p. 34)

REFLECTIVE THINKING EXERCISE

A woman you are seeing does not speak English and her aunty often speaks for her. How do you ensure that the woman is being informed? What challenges could arise if you were to engage the use of a qualified interpreter?

SUMMARY OF IMPORTANT POINTS

Successful services

Common factors identified in successful midwifery services are:
- community-based and/or community-controlled services
- a specific service location intended for women and children

---

Box 10.4 Cultural competence in maternity services

Key characteristics of culturally competent maternity care are:
- physical environment is culturally appropriate and acceptable
- specific Aboriginal maternal health programs and initiatives
- Aboriginal workforce inclusion and development
- continuity of care and carer
- collaborating with Aboriginal organisations and other agencies promoting integrated care and health networks
- effective and privileged communication, information sharing and transfer of care between health services
- staff attitudes are respectful and cross-culturally aware and sensitive
- cultural education and competency programs
- supportive relationships with Aboriginal individuals, co-workers and partnership with the community
- informed choice and right of refusal
- tools to measure cultural competence
- culture specific guidelines
- culturally appropriate and effective health promotion and behaviour change activities
- engaging with the Aboriginal community consumers and inclusion in clinical governance processes.

(Adapted from Kruske, 2011, p. 8)

- provision of continuity of care and a broad spectrum of services
- integration with other services (e.g. hospital liaison, shared care)
- outreach activities
- home- or community-based services
- a welcoming and safe service environment
- flexibility in service delivery and appointment times
- a focus on communication, relationship building and development of trust
- respect for Aboriginal and Torres Strait Islander peoples and their culture
- respect for family involvement in healthcare issues and child care
- having an appropriately trained workforce
- valuing Aboriginal and Torres Strait Islander staff and female staff
- provision of transport
- provision of child care or playgroups (Herceg, 2005).

Relationship is everything

- Many Aboriginal and Torres Strait Islander peoples will introduce themselves by referring to the groups to which they belong and the land from which they come.

- Families are extensive, so don't deny the importance of involving the wider family unit where appropriate.
- Emphasis is placed on personal relationships, so introduce *who* you are and where you come from.
- Relationship is reinforced through obligations—sharing resources, including financial—and through rituals and ceremony, e.g. birth, death. So, respect the need for Aboriginal women and staff to be available for these obligations.

Culturally safe childbirth

- Try to ensure the presence of female caregivers.
- Promote support people being present.
- Use professional interpreters or Aboriginal health workers.
- Create a non-threatening environment.
- Avoid using the bed.
- Use the elder women to encourage traditional practices.
- Don't presume that the woman doesn't want her partner present.

Key principles

- Changing attitudes will change behaviour.
- Understand the organisational and provider's own cultural influences.
- Culturally responsive action is required at all levels: organisational, systemic and individual practice.
- Genuine partnerships must exist between healthcare service organisations and the communities they serve.
- There is strong evidence to support consumer participation in healthcare planning.
- Increasing evidence exists that a lack of control over one's life and ineffective self-management are important determinants of health in disadvantaged populations.
- 'All this consulting is insulting if nothing ever changes.'
- Midwives must learn to work with women's social systems and address emotional wellbeing.
- Integrated systems of care improve physical and social outcomes.
- Morbidity, including social and emotional morbidity, must be 'counted'.
- Ensure that you regularly participate in a specific Aboriginal and Torres Strait Islander cultural safety training program.

Conclusion

There has been much work and still much more to be done in 'Closing the Gap' in the disparate health outcomes of Aboriginal and Torres Strait Islander mothers and babies, and midwives have a core role. Midwives working with Aboriginal and/or Torres Strait Islander women require a cultural awareness and most importantly cultural competency and cultural safety (CATSINaM, 2017). It is essential that all understand how colonisation and past policies continue to impact on the lives of indigenous peoples in contemporary Australia. Effective midwifery practice begins with a focus on communication, relationship building and development of trust. Respect for Aboriginal and Torres Strait Islander peoples and their cultures must include valuing Aboriginal co-workers. Non-indigenous midwives cannot be cultural experts and they require cultural mentoring to be effective in engaging women. Culturally responsive action is required at all levels—organisational, systemic and individual practice—but each of us can make a difference, one woman at a time.

Review questions

1. Briefly describe how midwives can contribute to 'closing the gap' in the differences between morbidity and mortality between Aboriginal and Torres Strait Islander women and children and non-indigenous Australians.
2. Name four of the key characteristics of working with women in partnership.
3. Define ethnocentrism.

NOTES

a. The term 'indigenous' is used when talking generally, for example, about indigenous peoples of more than one land, or when quoting the work of others. In Australia it is more acceptable to use the term 'Aboriginal and Torres Strait Islander peoples' or 'Aboriginal peoples', and in some circumstances we have used either 'Aboriginal' or 'Torres Strait Islander' depending on the context.

b. Aboriginal people from a remote desert region in Western Australia.

c. Aboriginal people from East Arnhem Land.

Online resources

Australian Indigenous Health Infonet: http://www.healthinfonet.ecu.edu.au/.

Australian Institute of Health and Welfare. The health and welfare of Australia's Aboriginal and Torres Strait Islander people: https://www.aihw.gov.au/reports-statistics/health-welfare-overview/indigenous-health-welfare/overview.

Birthing Business in the Bush: http://pandora.nla.gov.au/pan/45070/20050711-0000/www.maningrida.com/mac/bwc/.

Break the silence: short film on respectful maternity care: https://www.youtube.com/watch?v=K105F9o3HtU.

Maternity remote emergency care resources: https://crana.org.au.

National Rural Health Alliance: http://www.ruralhealth.org.au.

References

Australian Bureau of Statistics (ABS). *Aboriginal and Torres Strait Islander Population.* 2016, Cat: 2071.0. 2017a. https://www.abs.gov.au/ausstats/abs@.nsf/Lookup/2071.0main+features102016

Australian Bureau of Statistics (ABS). *3301.0—Births, Australia, 2016—Aboriginal and Torres Strait Islander Births and Fertility.* 2017b. Online: http://www.abs.gov.au/ausstats/abs@.nsf/Latestproducts/3301.0Main%20Features62016?opendocument&tabname=Summary&prodno=3301.0&issue=2016&num=&view=.

Australian Bureau of Statistics (ABS). *3301.0—Births, Australia, 2016—Aboriginal and Torres Strait Islander Births and Fertility.* 2021. Online: https://www.abs.gov.au/statistics/people/population/births-australia/2020.

Australian College of Midwives (ACM), CATSINaM, CRANAplus. *Birthing on Country Position Statement.* 2016. Online: http://catsinam.org.au/static/uploads/files/birthing-on-country-position-statement-endorsed-march-2016-wfaxpyhvmxrw.pdf.

Australian College of Rural and Remote Medicine (ACRRM) and Rural Doctors Australia Queensland (RDAQ). *Joint ACRRM/RDAQ Submission to the Review of Maternity Services in Queensland, November 2004.* Brisbane: ACRRM, Brisbane and RDAQ; 2004.

Australian Indigenous HealthInfoNet. *Overview of Australian Indigenous and Torres Strait Islander health status, 2016.* Perth, WA: Australian Indigenous HealthInfoNet; 2017. Online: http://www.healthinfonet.ecu.edu.au/uploads/docs/2016-overview.pdf.

Australian Institute of Health and Welfare (AIHW). *Comparing Life Expectancy of Indigenous People in Australia, New Zealand, Canada and the United States: Conceptual, Methodological and Data Issues.* Cat. no. IHW 47. Canberra: AIHW; 2011.

Australian Institute of Health and Welfare (AIHW). *The Health and Welfare of Australia's Aboriginal and Torres Strait Islander peoples 2015.* Cat. no. AIHW 147. Canberra: AIHW; 2017a.

Australian Institute of Health and Welfare (AIHW). *Australia's Mothers and Babies 2015—in Brief. Perinatal statistics series no. 33.* Cat no. PER 91. Canberra: AIHW; 2017b. Online: https://www.aihw.gov.au/getmedia/728e7dc2-ced6-47b7-addd-befc9d95af2d/aihw-per-91-inbrief.pdf.aspx?inline=true.

Bartlett B. *Origins of Persisting Poor Aboriginal Health. Public Health and Community Medicine.* Sydney: University of Sydney; 1998.

Bennett M, Davis H, Roberts S. The way forward—positive discrimination or positive action? *IJDL.* 2005;6(3):223–249.

Bhatia K, Anderson P. *An Overview of Aboriginal and Torres Strait Islander Health: Present Status and Future Trends.* Canberra: Aboriginal and Torres Strait Islander Health Unit, Australian Institute of Health and Welfare; 1995.

Bird Rose D. *Dingo Makes us Human.* Cambridge: Cambridge University Press; 2000.

Briscoe G. *Counting, Health and Identity: A History of Aboriginal Health and Demography in Western Australia and Queensland 1900–1940.* Canberra: Aboriginal Studies Press for the Australian Institute of Aboriginal and Torres Strait Islander Studies; 2003.

Broome R. *Aboriginal Australians, Black Responses to White Dominance, 1788–2001.* Sydney: Allen & Unwin; 2002.

Browne R. *Figures expose soaring rate of Aboriginal women in prison.* Sydney Morning Herald. Sydney: Fairfax Media; 2012. Online: https://www.smh.com.au/national/figures-expose-soaring-rate-of-aboriginal-women-in-prison-20121206-2ay9b.html.

Callaghan H. Traditional Aboriginal birthing practices in Australia: past and present. *Birth Issues.* 2001;10(3/4):92–99.

Carter B, Hussen E, Abbott L, et al. Borning: pmere laltyeke anwerne ampe mpwaretyeke, congress alukura by the grandmothers law. *Aust Aborig Stud.* 1987;1:2–33.

CATSINaM https://catsinam.org.au/

Congress of Aboriginal and Torres Strait Islander Nurses and Midwives (CATSINaM). *Position statement: embedding cultural safety across Australian nursing and midwifery.* Canberra: CATSINaM; 2017.

Congress of Aboriginal and Torres Strait Islander Nurses and Midwives (CATSINaM). *CATSINaM definition of Cultural Safety.* 2018. Online: https://www.catsinam.org.au/policy/cultural-safety.

Connor J. *The Australian Frontier Wars 1788–1838.* Sydney: University of New South Wales Press; 2003.

Czyzewski K. Colonialism as a broader social determinant of health. *Int Indig Policy J.* 2011;2(1/5):1–14.

Darbyshire P, Jackson D. Using a strengths approach to understanding resilience and build health capacity in families. *Contemp Nurse.* 2004;18(1–2):211–212.

Davis H, Day C, Bidmead C. *Working in Partnership With Parents: The Parent—Advisor Model.* London: Psychological Corporation; 2002.

Department of Prime Minister and Cabinet. *Aboriginal and Torres Strait Islander Health Performance Framework 2017 Report.* Canberra: Council of Australian Governments; 2017. Online: https://www.pmc.gov.au/sites/default/files/publications/Aboriginal_and_Torres_Strait_Islander_HPF_2014%20-%20edited%2016%20June2015.pdf.

Department of Prime Minister and Cabinet. *Closing the Gap: The Next Phase Public Discussion Paper.* Canberra: Council of Australian Governments; 2020. Online: https://www.pmc.gov.au/news-centre/indigenous-affairs/closing-gap-2020.

Dietsch E, Shackleton P, Davies C, et al. 'You can drop dead': midwives bullying women. *Women Birth.* 2010;23(2):53–59. doi:10.1016/j.wombi.2009.07.002.

Dodson M. The end in the beginning. In: Grossman M, ed. *Blacklines: Contemporary Critical Writing by Indigenous Australians.* Melbourne: Melbourne University Press; 2003:25–42.

Dudgeon P, Wright M, Coffin J. Talking it and walking it: cultural competence. *J Aust Indig Issues.* 2010;13(3):29–44.

Durie M. The health of Indigenous peoples. *BMJ.* 2003;326:510–511.

Ermine W, Sinclair R, Jeffery B. *The Ethics of Research Involving Indigenous Peoples. Report of the Indigenous Peoples' Health Research Centre to the Interagency Advisory Panel on Research Ethics.* Saskatoon, SK: Indigenous Peoples' Health Research Centre; 2004:1–272.

Fishbein H. *Peer, Prejudice and Discrimination: The Origins of Prejudice.* Mahwah, NJ: Lawrence Erlbaum; 2002.

Haebich A. *For Their Own Good: Aborigines and Government in the Southwest of Western Australia.* Nedlands: University of Western Australia Press; 1988.

Herceg A. *Improving Health in Aboriginal and Torres Strait Islander Mothers, Babies and Young Children: A Literature Review*. Canberra: Australian Government Department of Health and Ageing; 2005.

Hirst C. *Re-Birthing: Report of the Review of Maternity Services in Queensland*. Brisbane: Queensland Government; 2005. Online: https://www.health.qld.gov.au/__data/assets/pdf_file/0024/435660/maternityreview.pdf.

Homer CS, Foureur MJ, Allende T, et al. 'It's more than just having a baby': women's experiences of a maternity service for Australian Aboriginal and Torres Strait Islander families. *Midwifery*. 2012;28(4):E449–E455. doi:10.1016/j.midw.2011.06.004.

Human Rights and Equal Opportunity Commission. *Bringing them Home: Report of the National Inquiry into the Separation of Aboriginal and Torres Strait Islander Children from Their Families*. Sydney: HREOC; 1997. Online: http://www.humanrights.gov.au/sites/default/files/content/pdf/social_justice/bringing_them_home_report.pdf.

Hume L. *Ancestral Power: The Dreaming, Consciousness and Aboriginal Australians*. Melbourne: Melbourne University Press; 2002.

Hurst S, Nader P. Building community involvement in cross-cultural Indigenous health programs. *Int J Qual Health Care*. 2006;18(4):294–298.

Jackson Pulver L, Haswell MR, Ring I, et al. *Indigenous Health—Australia, Canada, Aotearoa New Zealand and the United States—Laying Claim to a Future That Embraces Health for us all. World Health Report. Background Paper, 33*. Geneva: WHO; 2010. Online: http://www.who.int/healthsystems/topics/financing/healthreport/IHNo33.pdf.

Johnston E. *Royal Commission into Aboriginal Deaths in Custody. National Report Volume One*. Canberra: Commonwealth of Australia; 1991. Online: http://www7.austlii.edu.au/au/other/IndigLRes/rciadic/national/vol1/.

Kidd R. *Black Lives, Government Lies*. Sydney: University of New South Wales Press; 2000.

Kildea S. *And the Women Said … Report on Birthing Services for Aboriginal Women From Remote Top End Communities*. Darwin: Territory Health Service; 1999.

Kildea S. Risky business—contested knowledge over safe birthing services for Aboriginal women. *Health Sociol Rev*. 2006;(Special Issue)15(4):387–396.

Kildea S, Lockey R, Roberts J, et al. *Guiding Principles for Developing a Birthing on Country Service Model and Evaluation Framework, Phase 1*. Brisbane: Midwifery Research Unit, MRI-UQ, The University of Queensland; 2016.

Kleinert S, Neale M, eds. *The Oxford Companion to Aboriginal Art and Culture*. Melbourne: Oxford University Press; 2000.

Kruske S. *Characteristics of Culturally Competent Maternity Care for Aboriginal and Torres Strait Islander Women. Report prepared on behalf of the Maternity Services Inter-Jurisdictional Committee for the Australian Health Ministers Advisory Council*. Canberra: Australian Government Department of Health; 2011.

Kruske S, Murakami-Gold L. Working in partnership with Aboriginal families (invited workshop). Australian Association of Infant Mental Health Conference, 5–8 November, Adelaide. Double Bay, NSW: AAIMHI; 2008.

Kruske S, Schultz T, Eales S, et al. A retrospective, descriptive study of maternal and neonatal transfers, and clinical outcomes of a Primary Maternity Unit in rural Queensland, 2009–2011. *Women Birth*. 2015;28(1):30–39. doi:10.1016/j.wombi.2014.10.006.

Kunitz SJ. *Disease and Social Diversity: The European Impact on the Health of Non-Europeans*. New York: Oxford University Press; 1996.

Kwaymullina A. Seeing the light: Aboriginal law, learning and sustainable living in country. *Indig Law Bull*. 2005;6(11):12–15.

Langton M. *Well I Heard it on the Radio and Saw it on the Television: An Essay for the Australian Film Commission on the Politics and Aesthetics of Film-Making by and About Aboriginal People and Things*. Sydney: Australian Film Commission; 1993.

Larson A, Gillies M, Howard PJ, et al. It's enough to make you sick: the impact of racism on the health of Aboriginal Australians. *Aust N Z J Public Health*. 2007;31(4):322–328.

Mackerras D. *Evaluation of the Strong Women, Strong Babies, Strong Culture Program*. Darwin: Menzies School of Health Research; 1998.

Mackerras D. Birthweight changes in the pilot phase of the Strong Women Strong Babies Strong Culture Program in the Northern Territory. *Aust N Z J Public Health*. 2001;25(1):34–40.

McCoy BF. *Holding Men: Kanyirninpa and the Health of Aboriginal Men*. Canberra: Aboriginal Studies Press; 2008.

McDonald H. *Culture in health research and practice. Beyond bandaids: exploring the underlying social determinants of Aboriginal health*. Adelaide: Papers from the Social Determinants of Aboriginal Health Workshop, Cooperative Research Centre for Aboriginal Health; 2004 (July).

McIntosh P. *White Privilege and Male Privilege: A Personal Account of Coming to See Correspondences Through Work in Women's Studies*. Wellesley: Wellesley College Center for Research for Women; 1988.

Mellor DBG, Bynon G, Maller J, et al. The perception of racism in ambiguous scenarios. *J Ethn Migr Stud*. 2001;27:473–488.

Memmi A. *The Colonizer and the Colonized*. Boston: Beacon Press; 1965.

Mills K, Roberts J. *Remote Area Birthing Discussion Paper*. Darwin: Territory Health Services; 1997.

Mobbs R. In sickness and health: the sociocultural context of Aboriginal well-being, illness and healing. In: Reid J, Trompf P, eds. *The Health of Aboriginal Australia*. Sydney: Harcourt Brace; 1991:292–325.

Monk A, Tracy M, Foureur M, et al. Evaluating Midwifery Units (EMU): a prospective cohort study of freestanding midwifery units in New South Wales, Australia. *BMJ Open*. 2014;4(10): e006252. doi:10.1136/bmjopen-2014-006252.

Moreton-Robinson A. Towards a new research agenda? Foucault, whiteness and Indigenous sovereignty. *J Sociol*. 2006;42(4): 383–395.

Murphy E, Best E. The Aboriginal Maternal and Infant Health Service: a decade of achievement in the health of women and babies in NSW. *N S W Public Health Bull*. 2012;23(3–4):68–72. doi:10.1071/nb11051.

National Aboriginal and Torres Strait Islander Health Council (NATSIHC). *National Aboriginal and Torres Strait Islander Health Strategy, Consultation Draft*. Canberra: NATSIHC; 2000.

Neidjie B, ed. *Story About Feeling*. Broome: Magabala Books; 1989.

Paradies Y, Harris R, Anderson I. *The Impact of Racism on Indigenous Health in Australia and Aotearoa: Towards a Research Agenda*. Discussion Paper Series No. 4. Darwin: Cooperative Research Centre for Aboriginal Health/Flinders University; 2008.

Pincus T, Esther R, DeWalt MD, et al. Social conditions and self-management are more powerful determinants of health and access to care. *Ann Intern Med*. 1998;129(5):406–411.

Prentis M. *A Study in Black and White: The Aborigines in Australian History*. 3rd rev. ed. Sydney: Rosenberg; 2009.

PriceWaterhouseCooper Australia. *Indigenous Incarceration; Unlock the Facts*. 2017. Online: https://www.pwc.com.au/indigenous-consulting/assets/indigenous-incarceration-may17.pdf.

Rawlings L. Traditional Aboriginal birthing issues. *Birth Gaz*. 1998;14(1):6–13.

Reconciliation Australia, 2021. https://www.reconciliation.org.au/

Reid J, Lupton, D, eds. Introduction. *The Health of Aboriginal Australia*. Sydney: Harcourt Brace Jovanovich; 1991.

Roberts J. The Northern Territory Remote Area Birthing Project. 4th National Women's Health Conference, Australian Women's Health Network, 19–21 February. Adelaide: 2001.

Saggers S, Gray D. *Aboriginal Health and Society: The Traditional and Contemporary Aboriginal Struggle for Better Health.* Sydney: Allen & Unwin; 1991.

Sherwood J. Who is not coping with colonisation? Laying out the map for decolonisation. *Australas Psychiatry.* 2009; 17(1):s24–s27.

Sherwood J. Do no Harm: Decolonising Aboriginal Health Research (PhD thesis). Sydney: UNSW; 2010.

Sherwood J, Keech S. Building respect and dialogue through critical reflective teaching and learning in indigenous studies. *J Aust Indig Issues.* 2011;14(2–3):104–120.

Steering Committee for the Review of Government Service Provision (SCRGSP). *Overcoming Indigenous Disadvantage: Key Indicators 2009.* Canberra: SCRGSP Productivity Commission; 2009. Online: https://www.pc.gov.au/research/ongoing/overcoming-indigenous-disadvantage/2009.

Sutherland L. Ethnocentrism in a pluralistic society: a concept analysis. *J Transcult Nurs.* 2002;13:274–281.

Swan P, Raphael B. *Ways Forward, National Aboriginal and Torres Strait Islander Mental Health Policy, National Consultancy Report.* Canberra: Commonwealth of Australia; 1995.

Toussaint S. Our shame, blacks live poor, die young: indigenous health practice and ethical possibilities for reform. In: Liamputtong P, Gardner H, eds. *Health, Social Change and Communities.* Melbourne: Oxford University Press; 2003:241–256.

Trudgen R. *Why Warriors Lie Down and Die.* Darwin: Aboriginal Resource and Development Services; 2000.

United Nations (UN) General Assembly. Report of the Special Rapporteur on the Rights of Indigenous Peoples on her Visit to Australia. Human Rights Council, 36th session, 11–29 September 2017. Agenda item 3. New York: UN; 2017. Online: https://www.ohchr.org/en/issues/ipeoples/srindigenouspeoples/pages/sripeoplesindex.aspx.

Van Wagner V, Osepchook C, Harney E, et al. Remote midwifery in Nunavik, Quebec, Canada: outcomes of perinatal care for the Inuulitsivik health centre, 2000–2007. *Birth.* 2012;39(3):230–237.

Weller B. Nursing in a multicultural world. *Clin Anthropol.* 1991;5(30):31–32.

Wild R, Anderson P. *Ampe Akelyernemane Meke Mekarle 'Little Children are Sacred'. Report of the Northern Territory Board of Inquiry Into the Protection of Aboriginal Children From Sexual Abuse.* Darwin: Northern Territory Government; 2007.

Wilkinson R, Marmot M, eds. *The Solid Facts, Social Determinants of Health.* Geneva: World Health Organization; 1998.

World Health Organization (WHO). Primary Health Care. International Conference on Primary Health Care, Alma-Ata, USSR, 6–12 September. Geneva: WHO; 1978. Online: https://www.who.int/teams/social-determinants-of-health/declaration-of-alma-ata.

World Health Organization (WHO). *Social determinants of health.* Geneva: WHO; 2018. Online: http://www.who.int/social_determinants/sdh_definition/en/.

Yunupingu G, ed. *From the Bark Petition to Native Title. Our Land is our Life.* Brisbane: University of Queensland Press; 1997.

Further reading

Access Economics. *Indigenous Health Workforce Needs.* Canberra: Australian Medical Association; 2004.

Australian Medical Association (AMA). *Report Card Series: Aboriginal and Torres Strait Islander Health Cycle of Vulnerability: The Health of Indigenous Children.* Canberra: AMA; 2008:1–8.

Coffin J, Drysdale M, Hermeston W, et al. Ways forward in Indigenous health. In: Liaw ST, Kilpatrick S, eds. *A Textbook of Australian Rural Health.* Canberra: Australian Rural Health Education Network; 2008:14–63. Online: http://www.arhen.org.au/.

Eckermann A, Dowd T, Chong E, et al. *Binan Goonj: Bridging Cultures in Aboriginal Health.* 2nd ed. Sydney: Elsevier; 2006.

Gray M, Hunter B, Taylor J, et al. *Health Expenditure, Income and Health Status Among Indigenous and Other Australians.* Canberra: Centre for Aboriginal Economic Policy Research, Australian National University; 2002.

Herceg A. *Improving Health in Aboriginal and Torres Strait Islander Mothers, Babies and Young Children: A Literature Review.* Canberra: Australian Government Department of Health and Ageing; 2005.

Kildea S. *And the Women Said … Report on Birthing Services for Aboriginal Women from Remote Top End Communities.* Darwin: Territory Health Service; 1999.

Kildea S. Maternal deaths high for Indigenous women. *Women Birth.* 2008;21:175–176.

Kildea S, Van Wagner V. 'Birthing on Country,' Maternity Service Delivery Models: A Review of the Literature. Canberra: Evidence Check/Sax Institute/Maternity Services Inter-Jurisdictional Committee for the Australian Health Minister's Advisory Council; 2012. Online: https://www.saxinstitute.org.au/wp-content/uploads/Birthing-on-Country1.pdf.

Kildea S, Wardaguga M. Childbirth in Australia: Aboriginal and Torres Strait Islander women. In: Selin H, Stone P, eds. *Childbirth Across Cultures, Ideas and Practices of Pregnancy, Childbirth and the Postpartum.* Amherst, MA: Springer; 2009:275–287.

Kildea S, Magick-Dennis F, Stapleton H. *Birthing on Country Workshop Report. Alice Springs, 4th July.* Brisbane: Australian Catholic University and Mater Medical Research Institute; 2013.

Mellor D. Contemporary racism in Australia: the experiences of Aborigines. *Pers Soc Psychol Bull.* 2003;29(4):474–486.

Smith J. *Australia's Rural and Remote Health: A Social Justice Perspective.* Melbourne: Tertiary Press; 2004.

CHAPTER 11

Locating Māori as Tangata Whenua of Aotearoa (New Zealand) in the midwifery partnership

Hope Tupara, Megan Tahere and Kaniwa Kupenga-Tamarama

LEARNING OUTCOMES

Learning outcomes for this chapter are:

1. To describe determinants of health and understand how they affect the health of Tangata Whenua
2. To describe the historical and sociopolitical contexts that underpin the overall health status of Tangata Whenua compared to Tangata Tiriti
3. To recognise that Tangata Whenua have distinct knowledge systems that inform their views of optimal wellbeing and how it is measured
4. To consider how legislation, health systems, structures, policies and midwives contribute to achieving **equality** and **equity** for Tangata Whenua that uphold Te Tiriti o Waitangi.

CHAPTER OVERVIEW

This chapter recognises Māori[a] as the **Tangata Whenua** ('first' people of the land) and a partner signatory of **Te Tiriti o Waitangi**—an agreement with the Crown. All other citizens of Aotearoa, represented by the Crown partner, are referred to as Tangata Tiriti (people of the Treaty).

The term 'Tangata Whenua' appears in Tiriti o Waitangi legislation to settle breaches of Te Tiriti o Waitangi by the Crown (*Waikato Raupatu Claims Settlement Act 1995; Ngāi Tahu Claims Settlement Act 1998*). Māori as the Tangata Whenua are the indigenous people of Aotearoa New Zealand (Aotearoa) that have a societal structure of **whānau** (kin), hapū (collective kin) and iwi (tribes). The language of Tangata Whenua is widely referred to as te reo Māori. Statistical data and narratives use the word Māori when referring to Tangata Whenua, which explains the interchangeable use of the terms in this chapter.

This chapter aims to equip midwives to have a beginning understanding of Tangata Whenua as the Tiriri Partner, and the determinants of holistic health that are relevant to the wellbeing of **wāhine**[b] and whānau. Authors Hope Tupara, Megan Tahere and Kaniwa Kupenga-Tamarama are Tangata Whenua midwives.

KEY TERMS

colonisation
equality
equity
mana enhancing midwifery partnerships and practice

partnership
Tangata Whenua (indigenous, first peoples, Māori)
Tangata Tiriti (non-indigenous citizens of Aotearoa)

Te Tiriti o Waitangi
wāhine
whānau

INTRODUCTION

Midwives in Aotearoa contribute to Tangata Whenua health outcomes. They need a sound knowledge of the drivers of inequality and inequities experienced by Tangata Whenua, an understanding of their own sociocultural beliefs and biases, and the maturity to apply this knowledge and understanding, toward the development of **mana enhancing midwifery partnerships and practice** when caring for wāhine and whānau.

The health and tertiary education systems in Aotearoa are in the midst of significant reforms (New Zealand Government, 2021; Tertiary Education Commission, 2021). This chapter highlights opportunities and challenges for midwives working in partnership with wāhine and whānau. It signals how midwives can make intuitive, intelligent and professional contributions to the health sector that can make a positive difference to the health and wellbeing of wāhine and whānau that enhances the overall health of society in Aotearoa.

Tangata Whenua, Te Tiriti o Waitangi and Colonisation

After the arrival of British explorers to Aotearoa in the 1800s, the British Government took steps to regulate the growing numbers of disorderly comrades that arrived, and at the same time, secure commercial benefits for themselves and thwart French interests in the country. The first major step was He Whakaputanga o te Rangatiratanga o Nu Tīreni (the Declaration of Independence of the United Tribes of New Zealand [He Whakaputanga]), written in English and Māori language (see Appendix 11.1). The Māori language version was signed by 52 Māori chiefs between 1835 and 1839 (Manatū Taonga, 2017a). In time, He Whakaputanga was considered not a powerful enough mechanism for the British to assert complete control over the entire country. Total domination became the main driver for the drafting of a new agreement, Te Tiriti o Waitangi (te Tiriti), that takes its name from the place where it was first signed (see Appendix 11.2). Te Tiriti traversed the country and was signed by British representatives on behalf of the Crown, and 540 Māori chiefs on behalf of their own people (Manatū Taonga, 2017b).

Both He Whakaputanga and te Tiriti were intended to provide for a mutually beneficial relationship between Tangata Whenua and the British Government. Tangata Whenua understood they were active participants in the governance of their own lands, and they were equal members of society (Walker, 1989). But te Tiriti was interpreted by the British as the mechanism needed to dominate Tangata Whenua (Martínez Cobo, 1987; Smith, 2005; Wilmer, 1993). Following the signing of te Tiriti, the *Constitution Act 1852* made provision for a parliamentary system in Aotearoa that was based on the British Westminster model of governance. The first elections were held in 1853 and Parliament sat for the first time in 1854. The right to vote was based on the possession of individual property. Tangata Whenua were collective landowners and therefore they were excluded from voting for Parliament (Manatū Taonga, 2017c).

Indigenous rights are recognised by the United Nations and the governments in Aotearoa and Australia (Macklin, 2009; New Zealand Government, 2010; United Nations, 2008). Tangata Whenua are indigenous to Aotearoa by virtue of an internationally accepted definition (Martínez Cobo, 1987; United Nations, 2008). They have, in common with other indigenous societies, an experience of **colonisation** and they have come to represent a minority in their own lands (Smith, 2005; Wilmer, 1993). Colonisation refers to the cumulative effect of domination by one society over another. It is characterised by imposed structures, processes and practices upon indigenous culture, its social institutions, legal, intellectual, ethical and moral systems (Martínez Cobo, 1987; Smith, 2005; Wilmer, 1993). Colonisation is attributed with creating the platform from which inequalities between Tangata Whenua and **Tangata Tiriti** have emerged.

Determinants of health and wellbeing

Inequalities in health between Tangata Whenua and Tangata Tiriti have become too common in Aotearoa (Robson & Harris, 2007), and it is a characteristic that Tangata Whenua share with the First Peoples of other nations including Australia. Three major contributors to the status of Tangata Whenua health are macropolitical, ecological, and indigenous determinants (Durie et al., 2005). Each determinant has a bearing on the lives of wāhine and their whānau because the systems, structures and conventions that arise from each determinant influence midwives' engagement with them and vice versa.

Macropolitical determinants constitute legislative and policy frameworks across public (e.g. government) and private (e.g. community and commercial) sectors that influence issues like the distribution of resources. Public health policy that prioritises antenatal resources to women most at risk of becoming unwell in pregnancy is more likely to have a positive effect on wāhine, who are often represented in the groups of women most at risk. Health policy that targets equity of health outcomes, rather than equity of access to services for all women, is more likely to advance the health of wāhine, because the effect of such policy is to respond to women in greatest need.

Whānau Ora is government policy that has a core goal to empower whānau to reach their full potential according to their aspirations in their own context. Whānau Ora was launched in 2010 in recognition by Government that standard ways of delivering services to whānau were not working for whānau.

A report to Government in 2009 provided the framework for Whānau Ora development throughout Aotearoa and it was later supported by a high-level partnership of government ministers and iwi leaders in 2015 who

211

co-designed a framework for improving whānau outcomes mapped over 25 years (Te Puni Kōkiri, 2017). Programs that support whānau to reach their goals are funded through a commissioning process and success is determined by the goals whānau reach. Whānau Ora assumes that integration and the joined-up infrastructure of government agencies already exists. But government sectors have a history of working in silos that has created a burden for those members of society who engage with government agencies. In addition, Whānau Ora has traditionally been supported from Te Puni Kōkiri, and it remains to be seen whether the larger government agencies, with their bigger pot of resources, will invest in Whānau Ora in a sustained way. As a range of disparities for Tangata Whenua become more and more apparent over time, the infrastructure of government is being forced to challenge and undo decades of behaviour, policies and practices to address disparities and inequities amongst the most underserved members of Aotearoa society (Te Puni Kōkiri, 2017).

Midwives who familiarise themselves with Whānau Ora policy, initiatives, provider groups and workforce practitioners like Whānau Ora navigators will be equipping themselves with greater knowledge of the networks in their region available to wāhine and their whānau. Whānau Ora responds to the needs of whānau, not the needs of agencies and therefore whānau should be encouraged to contact Whānau Ora providers if they need support.

Ecological determinants are the social, economic, cultural and environmental factors that affect daily health and wellbeing. For example, midwifery care has been shown to reduce smoking in pregnancy and the postpartum period, particularly for wāhine under the age of 25 (Dixon et al., 2009). It is important to describe the various characteristics of midwifery practice models that achieve smoking cessation success with wāhine, which can be replicated to influence other long-term lifestyle changes and health outcomes.

Indigenous determinants recognise that wellbeing is closely linked to cultural identity. As midwives, our role is to work with the unique identity of each woman. Researchers have identified distinct markers of Tangata Whenua identity such as language and social structures (Durie et al., 2005). For example, evidence has shown that whānau can make a positive difference to wellbeing because whānau are a link to the culture of wāhine (Ellison-Loschmann, 1997; Walker, 2006; Williams, 2011). Midwifery practice should therefore be informed by research undertaken by Tangata Whenua researchers because they are exploring issues that are important to Tangata Whenua.

COLONISATION AND ASSIMILATION

New Zealand midwives often look back on their history to reflect on the development of their profession and individual practice. The same approach is necessary to understand the health status of wāhine in Aotearoa.

Historical relationships between Tangata Whenua and representatives of the British Crown, which later established Aotearoa as a British Colony, reveal numerous conflicts (Belich, 1988; Walker, 1989). Land was a major source of the Tangata Whenua economy, with loss of land occurring mainly by compulsory acquisition legislated by the government. Consequently, Tangata Whenua lost much of their economic independence and economic decision power, which is fundamental to the access and privilege to control their own destiny.

In 1857–58 a Census of the Tangata Whenua population, based on an actual headcount was 56,049 people, about one-third of the reported number in 1800. The Census was by no means accurate, but it was consistent with other observed trends of a steadily declining Tangata Whenua population that was suffering from the implications of land loss, like starvation and diseases amongst other causes (Durie, 1997, 2005).

The colonisation of Aotearoa brought with it Western medicine that contributed to scrutiny of Tangata Whenua healers or tohunga who have innate skills and expert knowledge. The *Tohunga Suppression Act 1907* is often cited for prohibiting Tangata Whenua from exercising traditional practices. Although the Act was later revoked and it contained no specific reference to traditional healing, it cast aspersions upon legitimate tohunga (Dow, 1999). At two pages in length and made up of just four clauses the main purpose of the Tohunga Suppression Act was to stop imposters who were attributed with causing many deaths amongst Tangata Whenua because of delays in getting medical treatment for infectious diseases that were introduced by new settlers from abroad. Tangata Whenua politicians and leaders who supported the Act would not have contemplated the enduring impact the law would have and there was likely little care by Courts to distinguish between frauds and genuine tohunga. The Tohunga Suppression Act states:

Every person who gathers Maoris around him by practising on their superstition or credulity, or who misleads or attempts to mislead any Maori by professing or pretending to possess supernatural powers in the treatment or cure of any disease; or in the foretelling of future events, or otherwise, is liable on summary conviction before a Magistrate to a fine not exceeding twenty-five pounds or to imprisonment for a period not exceeding six months in the case of a first offence, or to imprisonment for a period not exceeding twelve months in the case of a second or any subsequent offence against this Act.

(clause 2, p. 1)

Another example of quite discriminatory legislation was the *Native Land Act 1909*, which made it unlawful for Tangata Whenua to adopt a child by native custom, otherwise known as whāngai. It was unlawful for the Native Land Court, which had jurisdiction to register Tangata Whenua adoptions and approve adoptions, or any Magistrate of a Court, to make an order under the *Infants Act 1909* for the adoption of a child by Tangata Whenua. A husband and wife, presumably not Tangata

Whenua, could apply to adopt a child and a Court could rule in favour of one or both. But for Tangata Whenua:

No person other than a Native or a descendant of a Native shall be capable of being adopted by a Native.

(clause 164, p. 196)

Mission schools run by churches and private enterprises were the first English model of education introduced into Aotearoa, bringing with it the instruction of reading and writing, with missionaries as the teachers. Christianity was introduced in the school system and it provided a different belief system which underpinned common law and teachings (Mikaere, 2003; Pihama, 2001). Tangata Whenua easily related to the principles of Christianity because they were consistent with their own values (Newman, 2006). However, teachings of Christianity in the education system that promote one god and biblical origins of mankind conflicted with the knowledge, traditions, values and identity of Tangata Whenua, which included multiple atua, spiritual and creation beliefs that connected them to the land and wider cosmos. Tangata Whenua knowledge was completely absent from the school curriculum (Jenkins & Matthews, 1998).

The Education Ordinance of 1847 provided for the first government funding of mission schools (Waitangi Tribunal, 2009) and schools were required to teach in English in order to benefit from State subsidies. Under the *Education Act 1877*, the government took the first step towards centralised control of education (Waitangi Tribunal, 2009). The curriculum was primarily designed to provide for the education of Tangata Tiriti children. Tangata Whenua tamariki were prevented from speaking their native language (Grace et al., 2001) and the education system was a key instrument of colonisation through a process of assimilation of all tamariki to English lore (Mead, 2003). The implication of a monolingual education system is that by the mid-20th century, use of the native language of Tangata Whenua declined so significantly that it was in danger of becoming extinct (Te Taura Whiri i Te Reo Māori, n.d.).

In 1961, gaps between Tangata Whenua and Tangata Tiriti with respect to housing, university study, vocational apprenticeships, death rates and crime were identified by a commissioned report to the Department of Māori Affairs (Hunn, 1961). The report recommended social reform including the relocation of Tangata Whenua from rural to urban areas that became official government policy (Meredith, 2015).

Concerns about the health of wāhine were highlighted by the findings of research conducted by Te Rōpū Wahine Māori Toko i te Ora (1984). This was the first quantitative research conducted by Tangata Whenua, for Tangata Whenua and about Tangata Whenua. Violence in the home was a significant finding arising from an abusive relationship, insecurity and inability to cope with the stressful environment resulting from abuse. Obesity, smoking and, to a lesser degree, alcohol were also identified as common concerns for wāhine, predisposing them to preventable illnesses (Te Rōpū Wahine Māori Toko i te Ora,1984).

Reasons for diminishing health status and wellbeing amongst Tangata Whenua were explained by the 1988 report of the Royal Commission on Social Policy. The report emphasised the ongoing impact of earlier legislation and government policies to explain the differences in health, justice, employment and education between Tangata Whenua and Tangata Tiriti. Differences were found to have a basis in breaches of Te Tiriti o Waitangi, and the Commission emphasised the importance of three principles arising from te Tiriti: 'partnership, participation and protection'. Today, te Tiriti is the only convention that sanctions a place for Tangata Tiriti in Aotearoa (Jackson, 2006; Sykes, 2007) and it continues to be fundamental for relationships between Tangata Whenua and midwives.

Te Tiriti o Waitangi provides for the interests of Tangata Whenua. It is not the solitary mechanism by which indigeneity can be recognised in law when attempting to define the extent of indigenous rights (Durie, 2003). In Aotearoa the government has endorsed the United Nations Declaration on the Rights of Indigenous Peoples (UNDRIP) that recognises indigenous peoples globally and their right to exist in their own societies, thus reinforcing Te Tiriti o Waitangi in the constitutional framework of Aotearoa.

The challenge faced by the State is the reconciliation of the Crown's dual obligation of fairness to all citizens whilst endorsing indigeneity. The way in which citizenship is understood by the majority is part of the solution (Durie, 2003). An enabling constitutional framework for Tangata Whenua to participate in their own society, culture, social structures, customary resources and political voice, shows indigeneity is valued. This is not to say that special rights be provided to Tangata Whenua, as this would run counter to the democratic principle that all people are equal. Rather, it highlights the need for both Tangata Whenua and Tangata Tiriti to be afforded the same rights to participation in society (Durie, 2003).

Citizenship is more than the simple fostering of individual liberties. Partnership between Tangata Whenua and the Crown needs to be reflected in law and government policies; for example, the provision of publicly funded midwifery care policy assumes access to midwifery care is equal across all women (Manatū Hauora Ministry of Health, 2007). However, the policy does not resolve inequities in health for wāhine and the additional barriers faced by wāhine in situations of high deprivation and vulnerability.

OVERVIEW OF TANGATA WHENUA HEALTH

In 2018 Tangata Whenua (people who identified as being of Māori descent) in Aotearoa were 18.5% or 869,850 of the 4,699,755 total population (Tatauranga Aotearoa, 2019). Projections indicate the Tangata Whenua population will continue to grow by another 16% by 2030 (Manatū Hauora Ministry of Health, 2019).

Of approximately 60,000 births a year in Aotearoa, wāhine account for about 25% of all women who have a baby, and they tend to be younger than women of other ethnicities when they give birth, with a median age of 27.1 years in 2018 (Tatauranga Aotearoa, 2019).

Tangata Whenua have a much younger age structure compared with most other Tangata Tiriti ethnicities (Tatauranga Aotearoa, 2015). Growth of the Tangata Whenua population over the last century has primarily been propelled by high rates of birth. The total fertility rate (an indication of how many births women will have during their lifetime) in 2020 was 2.05 for wāhine, in comparison to 1.63 for all other women in Aotearoa (Tatauranga Aotearoa, 2021).

Ethnic intermarriage or parents with different ethnicities also contributes to the Tangata Whenua population growth and approximately one-quarter of births where the child is identified as Tangata Whenua had a non-Māori mother and a Māori father (Tatauranga Aotearoa, 2015).

Across all socioeconomic indicators, Tangata Whenua are more disadvantaged than Tangata Tiriti. It is important for student midwives to have background information and know the social, economic and cultural landscape in which wāhine, in their care, may be positioned, because each will have a profound impact on the **partnership** success a midwife has with wāhine.

Tangata Whenua have lower rates of school completion, much higher rates of unemployment, are more likely to have less employment opportunities, more likely to have little access to telecommunications (including internet access) and motor vehicles, and more likely to be in rental accommodation, although a growing number of pregnant homeless women is emerging (E Tipu E Rea Whānau Services, 2019; Tokalau, 2018).

Tangata Whenua have lagged behind their peers in educational outcomes for a long time (Te Tāhuhu o te Mātauranga, 2009) with some improvements in school leavers' attainment of National Certificate of Educational Achievement (NCEA) level 2 qualifications (Tumuaki o te Mana Arotake, 2016). In Māori language medium education schools, success rates compared to mainstream schools are better and learners in Māori medium education are more likely to excel in education irrespective of traditional risk factors like poverty and prior education of their parents (Te Tāhuhu o te Mātauranga, n.d.). Educational achievement factors are important to provide the scaffold to build the Māori midwifery workforce.

People with low incomes, poor housing and few qualifications are likely to have disproportionately poorer health (Howden-Chapman & Tobias, 2000; Tatauranga Aotearoa, 2020b).

Wāhine are at greatest risk of being a victim of a crime than any other group (Mayhew & Reilly, 2007). Being Tangata Whenua, female, younger and having a lower socioeconomic position are all associated with an increased prevalence of mental disorder. Wāhine experience greater severity of serious disorders and common mental disorders than do non-Māori women. They are also more predisposed to postnatal depression than other women

(Webster et al., 1994). Women with a history of mental disorder are significantly more likely to have a recurrence during the first few weeks of the postnatal period (Oakley et al., 2006). Mortality rates rise with increasing socioeconomic deprivation and wāhine are disproportionately represented in the most deprived areas and are therefore at higher risk of illness and death overall compared with non-Māori women (Robson & Harris, 2007).

Wāhine generally have poorer access to maternity care and maternity information including antenatal education. They often have low and late referral for antenatal screening, and they are likely to have inadequate coordination of their maternity care. Reasons include inadequacies of the maternity workforce to respond to the cultural needs of wāhine (Ratima & Crengle, 2013), poor information systems and poor communication systems between maternity providers in high-deprivation areas (Counties Manukau District Health Board, 2012), and difficulties monitoring a woman's wellbeing because of transience or frequent changes of address, a characteristic of lower-socioeconomic households (Tāhū o te Ture, 2010). Conventional communication methods will not always work with whānau. Understanding whānau social networks is a contributing factor to successfully linking up with women and the development of one-to-one relationships. It is imperative therefore that midwives are a part of the community and do not work in silos, that they know the whānau connections within their community and can leverage that knowledge to connect with wāhine. Working alongside community service providers will productively enable midwifery practice to have far-reaching impact.

Over a 40-year period, a return to birthing away from hospital among wāhine has increased from 5% in 1967 (Simmonds, 2011) to 9% between 2006 and 2007 (Hunter et al., 2011) then decreased to 4% in 2018 (Manatū Hauora Ministry of Health, 2020). Research in Counties Manukau Health found that a greater proportion of wāhine planned to birth at home (17.4%) or in a primary birthing unit (27.2%), and were more likely to present to the primary birthing unit (Farry, 2015). Results also indicated that primary birthing units offer low-risk women and babies of low-risk women a level of protection for adverse outcomes (Farry, 2015). Outcomes for low-risk women birthing in high-technology facilities are not as good as for those low-risk women who birthed at home or in a primary maternity facility (Davis et al., 2011). Farry's (2015) findings echo this by concluding that if low-risk women of Counties Manukau Health present to a freestanding primary midwifery-led birthing unit in labour, they are significantly more likely to have a normal vaginal birth and healthy baby. In 2018, 15.2% of all wāhine across Aotearoa birthed in a primary unit (Manatū Hauora Ministry of Health, 2020).

Perinatal conditions (including premature birth and sudden unexpected death in infancy (SUDI)[c]) are consistent major causes of death among pēpi (Pomare et al., 1995; Robson & Harris, 2007). One study analysed singleton live births and stillbirths for 1980–2001 to understand the relationship between the effects of young motherhood on Tangata Whenua birth outcomes, the prevalence of small babies (both pre-term and small for gestational age (SGA)) and the influence of economic deprivation on obstetric parameters (Mantell et al., 2004). The study found that the younger age of wāhine does not appear to have an impact on their reproductive outcomes, but there are few initiatives aimed at reducing the impact of motherhood on their education and social development. The study also confirmed the significance of antenatal support with greater focus on wider health and social needs of wāhine, because 'the sensitivity of Māori SGA rates to socioeconomic deprivation suggests that broader social and policy interventions are needed' (Mantell et al., 2004, p. 540). Early initiation and engagement in antenatal care and the provision of antenatal care specific to cultural groups, such as wāhine and teenage women, is thought to be particularly beneficial to reducing adverse birth outcomes (Counties Manukau District Health Board, 2012; Quinlivan & Evans, 2004).

The declining fertility rates in Aotearoa are linked with increased access to fertility interventions such as efficient contraception, lower infant mortality rates and women attaining higher education and pursuing careers, thus accounting for the raising of the median age wāhine are giving birth (Tatauranga Aotearoa, 2019).

In 2017, the median age of all women giving birth in Aotearoa was 30 years old, with wāhine having a younger median age of 26 years old. Of all women younger than 20 years old who gave birth in 2017, wāhine featured highly (Manatū Hauora Ministry of Health, 2019).

Between 2007 and 2019, wāhine represented almost one-quarter of all women in Aotearoa enduring a medically induced termination of pregnancy (Tatauranga Aotearoa, 2020a). Lee (2016) predicts that one in four women in Aotearoa will undergo a termination of pregnancy during their lifetime. Long-acting reversible contraception (LARC) devices have been recognised in significantly reducing the overall rate of pregnancy terminations (Whitley, 2018).

In a publication from 1938, Papakura (1938) advises that wāhine exclusively breastfed their infants, and well past today's standard recommendations with solids often introduced at 9 months of age. Furthermore, wāhine had approximately the same age gap between tamariki and breastfeeding appears to have been a factor in the spacing of tamariki. Exclusively breastfeeding delays the return of fertility and menstrual periods, which provides physiological protection against pregnancy (Van der Wijden & Carol Manion, 2015).

Prior to colonisation, pēpi were exclusively breastfed (Hayes Edwards, 2014). Pēpi have the right to be breastfed and receive the inherited, live rongoā from their māmā that protectively cloaks the whakapapa with the korowai of her breastmilk, promoting life-long health and wellbeing of her pēpi and future mokopuna (grandchildren).

Between 2009 and 2017, pēpi had a national exclusive breastfeeding rate at two weeks of age, at just under 70%. In 2018, the exclusive breastfeeding rate at two weeks of age for pēpi was 70.1%. Between 2012 and 2018, pēpi had the second highest exclusive breastfeeding rates nationally at two weeks of age, following behind European babies (Manatū Hauora Ministry of Health, 2020a).

The breastfeeding practices for Tangata Whenua have undergone an ideological shift from being an assumed continuation of traditional infant caring practices, to a lifestyle choice. The process of colonisation introduced foreign infant care practices, such as the establishment of infant welfare organisations that spread the use of artificial infant milk and foods that greatly impacted upon wāhine and pēpi, attributing to the decline in breastfeeding as a normal infant caring practice (Glover & Cunningham, 2010).

A number of barriers to breastfeeding success for Tangata Whenua are discussed by McBride-Henry (2004), Ellison-Loschmann (1997), Reinfelds (2015) and Glover et al. (2007a, 2007b). Ellison-Loschmann (1997) concluded that while maternity services may be open to wāhine, much of the support being offered is provided in a Tangata Tiriti context that may not draw wāhine to services. Glover et al. (2007a) found the intent to breastfeed amongst wāhine was strong and breastfeeding was the norm in many whānau.

It was detrimental if wāhine experienced interruptions or difficulties in establishing feeding within the first six weeks from birth and lacked professional maternity support for breastfeeding—the switch to formula feeding and solids occurred early. This occurred because of other influences, including a lack of knowledge about how breastfeeding changes over time, which led wāhine to perceive they had an inadequate milk supply at 3–4 months. The pressure to return to work offers an infant feeding practice that is based with the pēpi and separated from the māmā. The researchers suggest that the diversion influences represent potential points of intervention to promote breastfeeding to Tangata Whenua.

The *Native Health Act 1909* is often cited by researchers and academics as forbidding wāhine from breastfeeding in public. There is no evidence that such a law existed (Ellison-Loschmann, 1997). The perpetuation of the myth continues to cause confusion around the actual reasons for the decline in breastfeeding practices amongst wāhine. Wāhine continue to experience contemporary intimidations when breastfeeding in public (Te Ao Māori News, 2019). A 1908 report by the Native Health Officer, Te Rangihiroa, who was also a medical doctor, provides us with documented insights into Tangata Whenua breastfeeding as follows:

Infant Mortality

The mortality amongst infants is very high. The old-time Māori has excellent laws for nursing-mothers as regards diet and cleanliness. Also, in a country devoid of the larger mammals, infants were fed entirely at the breast. Since the advent of the cow, tinned milk, and feeding bottles, much trouble has come upon them. Though the Māori mother does not neglect her children to attend social functions, many have forsaken breastfeeding for a different reason. They have in very many cases copied the example of the European, because what the learned pakeha does is right. The introduction of the feeding bottle into the Māori home has caused as many deaths as the guns of Hongi. Flour and warm water placed in the miracle-working feeding bottle has been given to delicate infants. The cow is a rare animal in many of the Māori villages, so tinned milk is largely used. As to qualities and mixing, the vast majority are woefully ignorant. Any warm liquid of a whitish appearance is milk of the requisite strength. Miss Rochfort in her Rotorua tour, and my addresses in the various villages, have given the people instruction in this important subject. But the practical work lies in a scheme of district nursing. I would place the care of infants as the most important of the duties. The preparation of humanised milk is beyond the reach of the Māori, for we are too scattered to have corporations to prepare it. In our case we should get the maximum results if the mothers were practically instructed in cleanliness and right proportions of cow's milk and water with the other practical rules of infant-feeding and infant care. A Health Officer speaks and passes on, but a nurse would visit and see that instructions were being carried out, for the Māori is liable to weary of new things and to lapse.

(Appendix to the Journals of the House of Representatives, 1908; H31:128–135)

There is direct evidence from New Zealand that links self-reported experience of interpersonal racial discrimination to poorer health outcomes (Harris et al., 2006a). Tangata Whenua are more likely to experience being treated unfairly by a healthcare professional because of their ethnicity. They are also more likely than non-Māori to be victims of ethnically motivated physical or verbal attack (Harris et al., 2006b). Evidence suggests that non-clinical factors may be contributing to ethnic differences in caesarean sections in New Zealand, and although deprivation contributes to this difference it does not fully explain it (Talamaivao et al., 2020). Harris and colleagues' research (2007) questions the equity of access to caesarean section for wāhine based on evidence of racism within the New Zealand healthcare system. Further work is needed to better understand the factors that contribute to ethnic differences in caesarean section rates.

Midwifery services overall can help to achieve health gains, but midwives should understand what is possible in their role and their limitations. Notwithstanding morbidity and mortality evidence that shows Tangata Whenua health is poorer when compared with data of other groups, it is important to view Tangata Whenua health in perspective with the total Tangata Whenua population, because many wāhine and their families are healthy, independent and thriving (Māori Reference Group for the Taskforce for Action on Violence within Families, 2013). In some instances, improvements in wellbeing for Tangata Whenua have been greater than for the total population including life expectancy, participation in tertiary education and employment (Taskforce on Whānau Centred Initiatives, 2010).

CRITICAL THINKING EXERCISE

You have received the results of an anatomy scan for Maraea at 20 weeks gestation that highlights significant concerns about her baby's growth and development. Although you gave Maraea a lab form to have antenatal bloods, you find the lab has no record of any tests being done. Maraea has changed address twice. Your colleague advises you she bumped into Maraea and her two tamariki in the local supermarket and they are now living with an aunt 45 minutes out of town. Maraea is in the middle of a separation from the father of her baby. She has no car and is reliant on her whānau for transport. She has missed several antenatal appointments. You have twice phoned the mobile number she gave you, but it appears to be no longer in use.

What are your obligations and responsibilities to Maraea as her midwife?

CULTURAL COMPETENCE

The Tangata Whenua midwifery workforce in Aotearoa remains disproportionate to the Tangata Whenua childbirthing population, affecting the ability of wāhine to have a choice of midwife of their own ethnicity.

Cultural competence is a construct introduced by legislation in Aotearoa for all regulated health practitioners such as midwives. The aim is to ensure wāhine and their whānau are culturally safe by being cared for by a culturally competent midwife. It requires the midwife to have a strong sense of their own identity first. Second, the midwife needs to recognise similarities and differences between themselves and wāhine. Concentration on the culture of wāhine often neglects a midwife's worldview. Approaching the partnership with humility requires a midwife to embark on the development of self-awareness, an attitude of respect for different worldviews and a relationship where investigation of the woman's goals occurs, as opposed to a tick box of particular needs, beliefs and behaviours (Hunt, 2001; Tervalon & Murray-Garcia, 1998). Self-reflection is not sufficient if the midwife is the main benefactor and is unable to determine whether wāhine and their whānau feel safe 'culturally'. An example is a midwife's attitude to te reo Māori. Although knowledge of and proficiency in te reo Māori is helpful, the respect that a midwife shows wāhine and her whānau through the correct pronunciation of te reo Māori words and names can make a positive difference to the way her professional integrity is viewed by the whānau. A midwife who takes care in the use of another language demonstrates a respect for the culture to which the language belongs.

CRITICAL THINKING EXERCISE

This exercise explores your knowledge of the Tangata Whenua community where you practise. The following questions will help you understand the depth and breadth of your knowledge.

1. What is the demographic make-up of the Tangata Whenua community in your area?
2. What is the specific demographic of wāhine who are pregnant and giving birth?
3. What are the names of the iwi organisations who have mana whenua status in your practice area and what organisations do they have that might support the work of a midwife?
4. Where are the local marae and what are the names of those marae and their associated hapū?
5. Who are the iwi and/or other Tangata Whenua healthcare providers in your practice area, what services do they provide and who do they provide services for?
6. Where are the kōhanga reo, kura kaupapa, whare kura and whare wānanga in your practice area located, if any, and what is their purpose?
7. What professional Tangata Whenua organisations, community groups and significant events are you aware of that support wāhine in your practice area?

The purpose of this exercise is to help inform you about your own community. As an example, Tangata Whenua health providers are not all the same and it is a misconception that they are exclusively for Tangata Whenua. Tangata Tiriti around the country choose to access health services provided by Tangata Whenua organisations as their preferred provider.

MĀORI MIDWIFERY WORKFORCE DEVELOPMENT

Tangata Whenua have the right to access a culturally competent midwifery workforce. This means that they should have the choice of a midwife from their own ethnicity or the choice of a midwife with whom they are culturally safe. In Aotearoa, we have a significant workforce challenge because:

1. We do not have enough midwives to adequately meet the needs of maternity services.
2. We do not have a Tangata Whenua midwifery workforce to ensure there are sufficient numbers for Māori women to have a choice of midwife from their own ethnicity (Tupara & Tahere, 2020) when evidence indicates that a match between women and midwives from the same ethnic group can improve clinical outcomes (Gurung & Mehta, 2001; Huriwai et al., 1998).
3. We do not have a cultural competence framework that is monitored to ensure that midwives are culturally competent as they are required to be by legislation.

Growing the number of Tangata Whenua midwives requires a vision, a strategy and dedicated resources, and must be driven by Tangata Whenua midwifery leadership. Since the regulation of midwifery began in 1904, the Tangata Whenua midwifery workforce has been determined and dependent on Tangata Tiriti leaders in the profession, who are the dominant decision makers in employing institutions within the midwifery sector including clinical settings and midwifery schools.

In 2020, there were 3382 (end of March) and 3273 (end of April) midwives with an annual practising certificate (APC) (Te Tātau o te Whare Kahu Midwifery Council, 2020). The Midwifery Council does not normally publicise the breakdown of the ethnicities of midwives with an APC despite collecting this data as part of its annual survey. However, the total number of Māori midwives has been relatively unchanged since 2015 with around 9.2% in 2015 to 9.83% in 2019 (Calvert, 2020; Te Tatau o te Whare Kahu Midwifery Council, 2015, 2016, 2017, 2018, 2019a, 2020). The workforce data for 2020 shows Māori represent 11.27% of the midwifery workforce (Te Tātau o Te Whare Kahu Midwifery Council, 2021).

Recruitment and retention of Tangata Whenua into midwifery requires planning and commitment. Tangata Whenua are more likely than non-Māori to encounter barriers to success in midwifery education. They are likely to have less experience of secondary or tertiary education, they are more likely to be a single parent and face childcare challenges, and they are more likely to be on a low income, making financing tertiary study problematic.

To ensure successful completion of the midwifery program, students need to have strong social support. The smaller the social network around them, the more isolated are the students, and the less social resources they have to overcome difficulties (Policy Research Initiative, 2005).

Students need a number of strategies in place to deal with unforeseen circumstances that affect personal responsibilities like childcare, or their study may be burdened by the weight of their own anxiety about their whānau at home. In addition to this, time taken away from their wider whānau, which may include iwi, marae or other collective roles, is a recurring compromise over and above their personal responsibilities.

There is a range of ways to achieve success for Tangata Whenua midwifery workforce development (Curtis et al., 2012a). Not all potential candidates will have an impressive academic record to gauge their ability to cope with undergraduate study. All students should have access to a pre-enrolment pathway. Tangata Whenua generally thrive in a cohort where there is collective support. Some will benefit from academic and pastoral advisors who can provide accurate information to help make strategic choices about tertiary study including the application process, preparation and readiness for entry to a university environment. Tailored wrap-around support throughout the study journey enables advice to continue with the aim to reduce attrition rates of Tangata Whenua from tertiary study. Connecting Tangata Whenua students to other Tangata Whenua individuals in the institution, and a Tangata Whenua academic mentor with whom they can reflect on their academic content and personal development, is a successful pastoral care model already in use at tertiary level (Te Rau Puawai, 2017).

Tertiary study should enhance a student's cultural identity. Midwifery institutions are potential sites for colonising students by assimilation, because of the dominance of Western scientific paradigms and pedagogies. It is important that education curricula are developed to integrate Tangata Whenua pedagogies that are delivered by experts who have practical understanding of midwifery. If the connection between Tangata Whenua worldviews and midwifery is not made, students can struggle to see value and they may well view Tangata Whenua knowledge as an imposition, rather than a valid body of knowledge.

Education programs must be proactive and champion behaviours, attitudes, support systems and curricula that promote success by all students. Institutions have a responsibility to ensure that increased Tangata Whenua enrolments driven by key performance indicators result in the desired optimal outcome of increased Tangata Whenua completion rates.

The midwifery education program is demanding. The dedication required to succeed to a high standard requires time management and negotiation constantly to ensure the student's holistic wellbeing and whānau remain intact. This occurs throughout their tertiary journey and as they transition to practice.

Educators can positively influence a student's success indirectly by engaging the student's whānau in the learning process (Williams, 2011). Tertiary study is a natural progression for some students. For others, tertiary study may be a new experience and their whānau may have no understanding of the associated demands and pressures. Tangata Whenua students are often in a minority in their class, and during learning sessions on historical issues involving Tangata, they can experience significant discomfort that often goes unnoticed by their peers and teachers (Curtis et al., 2012b). Beyond the education system, the profession needs to develop succession across all midwifery sectors in hospitals, midwifery schools, and government appointments to ensure that a depth of leadership for Tangata Tiriti and Tangata Whenua is planned early and deliberately. This will provide younger midwives with optimism for a career path in midwifery in which leadership succession is embraced and expected. Otherwise, midwifery will continue to lose exceptional talent to other sectors or disciplines.

Preparation for all midwives

The *Health Practitioners Competence Assurance Act 2003* (New Zealand Government, 2003) makes it a requirement for all healthcare practitioners in Aotearoa to demonstrate cultural competence. In 2020, the *Health Practitioners Competence Assurance Act 2003* was amended, and Section 118 (i) of the Act now includes competencies that will enable effective and respectful interaction with Tangata Whenua. Te Tatau o te Whare Kahu Midwifery Council (2011, p. 3) says cultural competence is:

the ability to interact respectfully and effectively with persons from backgrounds different to one's own. Cultural competence is more than awareness of or sensitivity to other cultures. For midwives, cultural competence means both recognizing the impact of their own culture and beliefs on their midwifery practice and being able to acknowledge and incorporate each woman's culture into the provision of individualized midwifery care. It means having the knowledge, skills and attitudes to understand the effect of power within a healthcare relationship and to develop respectful relationships with people of different cultures.

Cultural competence recognises the limitations of midwives in Aotearoa to provide for the cultural needs of all women. Education about te Tiriti, Tūranga Kaupapa, cultural safety, the midwifery partnership model for practice, Tangata Whenua health and cultural concepts are all-important knowledge foundations for midwives (Te Tatau o te Whare Kahu Midwifery Council, 2011).

The Wai 2575 Health Services and Outcomes Inquiry was established to hear claims concerning grievances relating to health services and outcomes for Tangata Whenua. The Wai 2700 Mana Wāhine Inquiry will hear claims that allege prejudice to wāhine as a result of Tiriti breaches by the Crown, spanning areas of Crown policy, practice, acts and omissions, both historical and contemporary, and associated legislation, service provision and state assistance.

Ngā Māia Māori Midwives Aotearoa[d] is a Tangata Whenua midwifery organisation established in Aotearoa in 1993 with a key objective to protect Māori childbirth knowledge and practices derived from Māori intellectual discourse (Tupara & Tahere, 2020). More recently, Te Wakahuia o Hine was established to ensure the integrity and quality of maternity and midwifery services to achieve the intent of te Tiriti to serve all citizens equally, privileging the equal relationship of Tangata Whenua and Tangata Tiriti, and the guarantees of te Tiriti for all (Te Wakahuia o Hine, 2021).

Tangata Whenua knowledge has much to offer childbirth theory. In 2006, members of Ngā Māia created a set of kaupapa Māori principles, Tūranga Kaupapa, to provide guidelines for working with Tangata Whenua in midwifery partnerships and practice (Ngā Māia Māori Midwives Aotearoa, 2017a, 2017b; Te Tatau o te Whare Kahu Midwifery Council, 2011). As a result of the recognised benefits for wāhine and their whānau, Tūranga Kaupapa were introduced into the professional and regulatory frameworks for midwifery partnerships and practice in 2007 (New Zealand College of Midwives, 2015; Te Tatau o te Whare Kahu, 2011). The ten principles of Tūranga Kaupapa are listed in Table 11.1.

By embedding Tūranga Kaupapa into frameworks for midwifery partnerships and practice, Aotearoa is the first country in the world to recognise the constitutional place of its indigenous peoples within professional and regulatory systems (NZCOM, 2008). The integration and application of Tūranga Kaupapa into midwifery partnerships and practice is a prerequisite to the provision of culturally competent midwifery care in New Zealand (Te Tatau o te Whare Kahu Midwifery Council, 2011). The next phase of

Table 11.1 Tūranga Kaupapa

Tūranga Kaupapa	
Whakapapa	The wahine and her whānau is acknowledged.
Karakia	The wahine and her whānau may use karakia (words chanted to obtain spiritual benefit or provide protection).
Whanaungatanga	The wahine and her whānau may involve others in her birthing program.
Te Reo Māori	The wahine and her whānau may speak Te Reo Māori.
Mana	The dignity of the wahine, her whānau, the midwife and others involved is maintained.
Hau Ora	The physical, spiritual, emotional and mental wellbeing of the wahine and her whānau is promoted and maintained.
Tikanga Whenua	Maintains the continuous relationship to land, life and nourishment; and the knowledge and support of kaumatua and whānau is available.
Te Whare Tangata	The wahine is acknowledged, protected, nurtured and respected as Te Whare Tangata (the 'House of the People').
Mokopuna	The mokopuna is unique, cared for and inherits the future, a healthy environment, wai u and whānau.
Manaakitanga	The midwife is a key person with a clear role and shares with the wahine and her whānau the goal of a safe, healthy, birthing outcome.

(Sources: Ngā Māia, 2017a)

development needed is agreement on curriculum that will effectively cultivate a culturally competent midwifery workforce, and the framework that will measure, assess and evaluate how cultural competence is being applied in practice by midwives.

REFLECTIVE THINKING EXERCISE

Applying Tūranga Kaupapa principles

The following exercise requires you to apply Tūranga Kaupapa principles in a potential real-life situation.

Tira has been excited about her first pregnancy. She has waited a very long time to get pregnant and she is in the first trimester. She was admitted to the secondary care hospital overnight because of low abdominal pain that has increased in severity in the past 24 hours. She has just been diagnosed with an ectopic pregnancy. You call in to see how she is and you find her sobbing with her husband and her mother. Describe how Tūranga Kaupapa principles will guide your contact with Tira and her whānau at this time.

REFLECTIVE THINKING EXERCISE

Tūranga Kaupapa in midwifery partnerships

The following exercise requires you to think about the integration and application of cultural safety, cultural competency and Tūranga Kaupapa (see Ch. 17 for further discussion of these terms) into midwifery partnerships and practice and come to new understandings. As a midwife:

1. How does Tūranga Kaupapa support midwives to identify the similarities and differences between themselves and the women they are caring for?
2. How does Tūranga Kaupapa support women to maintain or reclaim their identity?
3. How can Tūranga Kaupapa be utilised to effect change in the maternity sector?
4. How can Tūranga Kaupapa support your professional development and contribute to you being a change agent for positive Tangata Whenua health outcomes?

Tāngata Whenua childbirth knowledge

Tāngata Whenua have ancient bodies of knowledge pertaining to pregnancy and childbirth. Like any knowledge system, Tangata Whenua knowledge exists in many different forms. It is expressed in symbolism such as in Te Whare Tapa Whā (a traditional house), Te Wheke (octopus) and Te Pae Mahutonga (constellation of stars known as the Southern Cross).

Tangata Whenua knowledge exists in oral traditions such as mōteatea (chant), whakataukī (proverbs) and whakatau-ā-kī (sayings). It exists in tīkanga (rituals); in whakairo (carvings), and in technology for fishing, navigation, weaving, food preparation and building waka (sea vessels) (Durie, 1984, 1999; Pere, 1984; Te Rōpū Wahine Māori Toko i te Ora Māori Womens Welfare League, 1984).

Hine te Iwaiwa, Hinauri, Hina, Rona, Hine-kōtea, Hine-kōrito, Hine-mākehu and Hine-kōrako are the ancestral atua in Tangata Whenua cosmology associated with the procreation of life and the rhythms of life (Tupara, 2017). Tangata Whenua knowledge is dynamic and living. It is not static and suspended in a time warp, nor is it monolingual or singular in nature, because it could not possibly survive. Instead, the traditions that flow from Tangata Whenua knowledge are constantly reimagined and adapted by each generation, each whānau, that uses them.

Underpinning all Tangata Whenua knowledge is philosophy or a set of assumptions. Two assumptions of Tangata Whenua knowledge that are common to knowledge of other indigenous societies are:

1. The world is a whole. In a pregnancy and childbirth context, the women and baby are part of a whole whānau and universe that is culturally constructed. Their wellbeing is interdependent on inter-related factors of the past, present and future, which are all important and all need attention concurrently.

2. All phenomena are explained by the natural world. In a pregnancy and childbirth context, there are multiple explanations for events that manifest in our daily lives of pregnant women and their whānau, which have symbolic meaning and explanations that are also culturally constructed. (Barnhardt & Kawagley, 2005; Durie, 1985; Jackson, 1987; Kawagley, 2006; Marsden, 1989)

Pre-1800s, Tangata Whenua childbirth knowledge was transmitted from one generation to another, by way of a combination of oral, art and practice traditions. Hapū wāhine, for example, were supported by tribal and hapū birth experts, who were trained to recognise and respond to the needs of hapū wāhine and their pēpi, through having gained their skills and knowledge from other learned tribal experts. They lived in a very different environment. They lived in communal settings with kin close by, to support them throughout their hapūtanga and after the birth especially if they had other tamariki. They had access to food sources on land, the sea and the sky. They built their own shelters on well-draining soil, and close to clean, running water, and they used natural resources to make their own clothing and to keep warm.

Tribal and hapū childbirth experts practised into the 1930s and remnants of the knowledge they carried are held in the memories of wāhine they cared for. It is possible they were unable, or unwilling, to pass on their knowledge to the next generation, for fear that they might be convicted of a crime by continuing to provide maternity services to wāhine which had become regulated with the passing of the Midwives Act in 1904. It is equally possible that they had no idea there were legal restrictions on who could practise, because most iwi and hapū were still living on tribal lands and very little if any health services reached them. By the late 1930s, wāhine from iwi and hapū were increasingly going to hospitals to give birth, partly to replicate the practices they were seeing from Pākehā women, and partly because of increasing influence of advice from government or hospital paid district nurses assigned to work with iwi and hapū.

The history of colonisation in Aotearoa represents a concurrent shift away and active suppression of Tangata Whenua knowledge in favour of the dominant knowledges of childbirth brought to Aotearoa by early colonisers and maintained by their descendants.

Tangata Whenua practices, rather than knowledge, are recognised at a generic and very superficial level. Tikanga (rituals) are sometimes written into policy documents or included into student midwives' learning experiences, without any pre-existing purpose, strategic intent, depth of expertise or transformation in organisational practices to guide their implementation. Without sustained Tangata Whenua leadership in an organisation, tikanga policies are most likely to be removed if the majority of people in an organisation do not understand them. Alternatively, some organisations use counter arguments to resist adoption of Tangata Whenua policies by claiming that all groups of women would be disadvantaged if there were not policies for them as well.

Tangata Whenua childbirth knowledge is add-on learning rather than foundation learning for student midwives. Any inclusion of Tangata Whenua knowledge in midwifery education needs to rigorously be debated, because midwives are not experts in Tangata Whenua knowledge. They risk coming into the care of wāhine who are experts and who may feel unsafe in the care of midwives who profess to presume what her needs are.

The growing body of Tangata Whenua childbirth knowledge increasingly challenges the dominant views and ideas being expressed in New Zealand midwifery and childbirth literature about the needs of Tangata Whenua (Tikao, 2020). Kenney (2011) critiques the use of certain aspects of midwifery discourse to highlight the tensions between deductive Western and holistic Tangata Whenua philosophical positions (Denzin & Lincoln, 2000; Durie, 2004; Tupara, 2009).

Today, wāhine and whānau are reclaiming and recreating childbirth knowledge and traditions according to the worldviews of iwi, hapū and, increasingly, their own whānau. A writing tradition has now been added to the toolkit alongside oral, art and practice traditions, to help preserve new knowledge that is created. Midwives should be reflecting on the way the profession, the health system and organisations enable Tangata Whenua childbirth knowledge to be realised to ensure their wellbeing needs are met.

REFLECTIVE THINKING EXERCISE

Midwifery and wairua

Wairua is a multifaceted Māori construct. Sometimes it is translated as the same Western notion of spirituality, which is insufficient to fully explain it. An imbalance in some aspect of wellbeing can include one's wairua. Wāhine may feel an important desire to fulfil their wairua, a concept that is absent from Western health paradigms.

1. View the links to Māori Television's wairua episodes to broaden your understanding of the concept: http://www.maoritelevision.com/tv/shows/wairua.

2. How could you integrate the principles of Tūranga Kaupapa to support wāhine who view wairua to be important?

Māori Health Strategy and Action Plan

The government's Māori Health Action Plan, Whakamaua, guides the health and disability system to implement the aims of He Korowai Oranga: Māori Health Strategy (Manatū Hauora Ministry of Health, 2020b).

The overall aim of He Korowai Oranga and Whakamaua is to ensure Māori achieve high standards of health and wellbeing. The implementation of the strategy remains the responsibility of the health and disability sector as a whole, including midwives (Manatū Hauora Ministry of Health, 2002, 2014).

The government has announced the establishment of a new health authority, Health New Zealand, that is to replace the District Health boards, alongside an independent Māori Health Authority that will have joint decision-making rights and command the spending on programs for Tangata Whenua, who have historically been, and continue to be, chronically underserved by the current healthcare system (Manch, 2021).

The refreshed *New Zealand Health Strategy: Future Direction* (Manatū Hauora Ministry of Health, 2016) sets the framework and direction for the development of the health system. The strategy aims to address the pressures and significant demands on health services and budget. It pursues equitable outcomes for all New Zealanders and reinforces provisions within the New Zealand *Public Health and Disability Act, 2000* to ensure the recognition and respect of the principles of Te Tiriti o Waitangi. The strategy emphasises that services must be provided more effectively for Tangata Whenua owing to the poorer health experienced by Tangata Whenua (Manatū Hauora Ministry of Health, 2016).

The *Equity of Health Care for Māori: A Framework* document guides health practitioners, health organisations and the health system to achieve equitable healthcare for Tangata Whenua by improving access to healthcare services for Tangata Whenua (Manatū Hauora Ministry of Health, 2014). There are three action points to support this framework: leadership, which focuses on championing the provision of high-quality healthcare so that equitable health outcomes can be delivered for Tangata Whenua; knowledge, which focuses on the development of a knowledge base that informs on ways to effectively deliver and monitor high-quality healthcare for Tangata Whenua; and commitment, which focuses on providing high-quality healthcare that meets the needs and aspirations of Tangata Whenua (Manatū Hauora Ministry of Health, 2014). The aforementioned strategies all require midwives to work in partnership with Tangata Whenua to facilitate improvements in health and achieve the health aspirations for Tangata Whenua.

A range of approaches by healthcare providers will improve the health of wāhine, pēpi and whānau. The *Primary Health Care Strategy*, although somewhat dated, remains useful as it outlines the specific contributions primary healthcare makes to improving health outcomes (Manatū Hauora Ministry of Health, 2001). It expects that healthcare providers will work 'in collaboration, cooperation and coordination across the health sector' (Kizito, 2005, p. 5) with the aim of directing health services at areas that will ensure the best health benefits for the New Zealand population, focusing on addressing inequalities in health (Manatū Hauora Ministry of Health, 2001).

Evidence suggests that non-government organisations (NGOs) such as iwi groups are largely being excluded from involvement in the primary healthcare sector in a range of ways, including equitable funding opportunities to tender for projects and the minimising of inequities for Māori (Kizito, 2005; Manawhenua Hauora, 2002; Manatū Hauora Ministry of Health, 2008; Federation of Primary Health Aotearoa New Zealand, 2020). Such gatekeeping is due in part to a lack of understanding by the primary healthcare sector about the structure, skills and services provided by Māori healthcare organisations (Manawhenua Hauora, 2002; Whānau Ora Iwi Leaders Group, 2016). Whānau Ora is an example of the importance of collaboration between organisations because singular services working in isolation are at times insufficient to effect sustainable intergenerational changes in health. Whānau Ora is an inclusive and culturally anchored service approach based on a Te Ao Māori view of health that assumes changes in an individual's wellbeing can be brought about by focusing on the family collective and vice versa (Boulton et al., 2013). The desired results of an intervention will vary according to particular whānau circumstances (Taskforce on Whānau-Centred Initiatives, 2010).

In a maternity context, inequity of access to healthcare services for Tangata Whenua becomes compounded by actions that prevent the involvement of Māori healthcare organisations to support wāhine throughout the childbirth experience (Manatū Hauora Ministry of Health, 2007). Although all women in New Zealand are entitled to the same level of maternity services, Mantell et al. (2004) alluded to the necessity for broader social and policy interventions for Tangata Whenua. Their conclusions continue to be relevant today because wāhine and pēpi require more than just the support of midwives to realise positive health outcomes. They also need social, financial and educational support that is outside the role of a midwife. The best approach to healthcare disease prevention and health promotion will be strategies that include a variety of approaches for a diverse range of solutions (Manatū Hauora Ministry of Health, 2002).

As midwives are the predominant providers of primary maternity care, they have an obligation to consult, collaborate and be informed about the communities of Tangata Whenua, so as to strengthen rather than compromise other healthcare initiatives. Midwifery and Tangata Whenua health goals are similar. The unique perspectives, skills and strategies contributed by each group provides for a complementary approach to improve Tangata Whenua health outcomes. Co-leadership and co-design by the midwifery profession and its Treaty partner are crucial to realise dual aspirations into the next decades.

Conclusion

The health of wāhine, their pēpi and whānau will be in excellent shape when Tangata Whenua are self-sufficient, maintain wellness, have a sense of their distinctive identity and their cultural systems, and prosper in whatever setting they find themselves (Durie, 1998). Reducing inequalities remains an important challenge for both the healthcare system and wider society in New Zealand (Public Health Intelligence, 2008). Midwives are an important part of the healthcare sector. They have a significant role in advancing the integrity of Tangata Whenua social institutions, the preservation of Te Ao Māori culture, knowledge, language, systems of governance, and models of health and wellbeing that remain under constant threat of demise (Smith, 2005). To shift Te Tiriti o Waitangi principles from rhetoric to reality in midwifery there is still much work to be done. Midwives in Aotearoa have led the way internationally by recognising the constitutional place of Tangata Whenua in professional and regulatory frameworks. We need to continue the momentum in the profession and have courageous conversations across the sector to build the infrastructure in the profession and across maternity services that will embed the profound changes that will achieve equitable health outcomes for Tangata Whenua.

Review questions

These questions should be discussed in groups. Student midwives can learn from each other's knowledge and knowledge gaps and discussion will help them understand each other better.

1. You have a midwifery standards review in 2 weeks. How will you go about applying the principles of Tūranga Kaupapa to your practice reflection in a meaningful and enduring way?

2. While working on shift at the hospital, your midwifery colleague says that the Māori woman and whānau she is providing care for are 'typical Māori'. She continues on to say: 'No wonder they all get pregnant and get their babies uplifted by Oranga Tamariki.' How would you respond to your colleague's stereotyped comment in a professional manner? How would you advocate your partnership obligations as a midwife to this wāhine and her whānau?

3. A colleague has confided in you that they are being bullied by a midwife and they have also witnessed the same midwife bully women. How would you support your colleague and what resolution pathways do you know are available for midwives and women in these situations?

4. You are a locum midwife visiting a woman at 26 weeks gestation in a remote location. What strategies would you put in place to keep yourself safe as a midwife, working in a region that you are unfamiliar with?

5. One of your clients, Jocelyn, has given birth 2 hours ago; she is settled in the postnatal ward and she is breastfeeding her baby. A student midwife tells you Jocelyn is going to whāngai her baby. Her aunty is coming for the baby tomorrow and wants to talk about whāngai ū. What is whāngai? What is whāngai ū?

6. Moana contacts you while she is 12 weeks pregnant. She is new to town and she would like to have a Māori midwife, but there are none in the area. You are happy to care for her. In what ways could you reassure Moana about your cultural competency?

7. You are attending an in-service education program at the hospital. The program is about the Treaty of Waitangi and attendance is compulsory. While walking to the session, you and another colleague confide in each other that you are both sick of hearing about the Treaty, because you both feel that what happened in the past has nothing to do with you now. Why is Treaty of Waitangi education important for midwives' practice? What is the difference between Te Tiriti o Waitangi and the Treaty of Waitangi?

8. Jackie is 34 weeks pregnant. You are discussing the third stage of labour with her when she enquires about using muka (flax) to tie the umbilical cord. What information should you share with Jackie and what are your professional responsibilities?

9. You are providing midwifery care to Bella, an Italian woman whose partner has identified as being of Māori ethnicity. After their baby is born you are completing the paperwork where you are asked to provide the ethnicity of their baby. How would you best ascertain the baby's ethnicity?

10. As a midwife, how would you support professional inter-cultural relationships with another midwife who identifies with a minority ethnicity group such as Tangata Whenua, Pasifika, Indian or Chinese? Or another minority group such as the rainbow community?

NOTES

a. The word 'Māori' is used to describe something normal, usual, common, or ordinary and was first expressed in writing in the 1892 edition of the Williams Dictionary as an adjective. Over time the word Māori has been adopted as a noun to refer to tangata maori, Tangata Whenua, and the indigenous peoples of Aotearoa as a collective.

b. The words 'wahine' (singular), 'wāhine' (plural), and 'whānau' are used to privilege the Indigenous and first official language of Aotearoa and refer only to Tangata Whenua or Māori. Tangata Tiriti are non-Māori citizens of Aotearoa.

c. Sudden unexpected death in infancy (SUDI) was formerly called sudden infant death syndrome (SIDS).

d. Ngā Māia Māori Midwives Aotearoa (Ngā Māia), formerly Ngā Māia o Aotearoa me Te Waipounamu Charitable Trust, was registered with the New Zealand Companies Office in a different name, Ngā Māia Trust, on 19 May 2016.

Online resources

New Zealand

Iwi Chairs Forum: http://www.iwichairs.maori.nz/.

Karanga: the first voice—Māori Television series: http://www.maoritelevision.com/tv/shows/karanga-first-voice.

Kia Ora Hauora: http://www.kiaorahauora.co.nz/.

Manatū Hauora Ministry of Health Foundation Course in Cultural Competency: http://learnonline.health.nz/.

Māori and breastfeeding: http://www.mamaaroha.co.nz/.

Māori health providers funded by Manatū Hauora Ministry of Health: http://www.health.govt.nz/our-work/populations/maori-health/maori-health-providers.

Māori medicinal and curative treatment, Te Kāhui Tāwharautanga Ō Ngā Rongoa: http://www.rongoamaori.org.nz/index.php/Home.

Māori Television: http://www.maoritelevision.com/.

Māori Women's Development Inc.: http://www.mwdi.co.nz/.

Mason Durie—StrategyNZ: Mapping our Future—March 2011: https://www.youtube.com/watch?v=Tt_73vX8aRw.

Moana Jackson—He Manawa Whenua Indigenous Research Conference 2013: https://www.youtube.com/watch?v=lajTGQN8aAU.

National SUDI Prevention Coordination Service, Hāpai Te Hauora: http://sudinationalcoordination.co.nz/welcome.

Ngā Māia Māori Midwives Aotearoa: http://www.ngamaia.co.nz.

Ngā Manukura ō Āpōpō: http://www.ngamanukura.co.nz/.

Ngā Pae o te Māramatanga: http://www.maramatanga.co.nz/about.

Talk Treaty—Kōrerotia te Tiriti: http://talktreaty.org.nz/.

Tame Iti—Mana: The power in knowing who you are, Tame Iti, TEDxAuckland: https://www.youtube.com/watch?v=qeK3SkxrZRI.

Te Kāhui Māngai directory of iwi and Māori organisations, Te Puni Kōkiri: http://www.tkm.govt.nz/.

Te Mangai Paho (Māori broadcasting): https://www.tmp.govt.nz/.

Te Matatini: http://www.tematatini.co.nz/.

Te Pou Matakana North Island Whānau Ora Commissioning Agency: https://www.tepoumatakana.com/.

Te Pūtahitanga o te Waipounamu South Island Whānau Ora Commissioning Agency: http://www.teputahitanga.org/.

Te Rau Matatini. Māori Mental Health Workforce Development: http://teraumatatini.com/.

Te Rōpū Rangahau Hauora a Eru Pōmare: http://www.otago.ac.nz/wellington/departments/publichealth/research/erupomare/.

Te Rōpū Wahine Māori Toko i te Ora Māori Women's Welfare League: http://www.mwwl.org.nz/.

Te whānau tamariki—pregnancy and birth, Te Ara Encyclopedia: http://www.teara.govt.nz/en/te-whanau-tamariki-pregnancy-and-birth.

Wairua—Māori Television series: http://www.maoritelevision.com/tv/shows/wairua.

Waitangi Tribunal Wai 2575 Health Services and Outcomes Inquiry: https://waitangitribunal.govt.nz/inquiries/kaupapa-inquiries/health-services-and-outcomes-inquiry/.

Waitangi Tribunal Wai 2700 Mana Wahine Inquiry: https://waitangitribunal.govt.nz/inquiries/kaupapa-inquiries/mana-wahine-kaupapa-inquiry/.

Indigenous peoples

Aboriginal People Respond to 'Australia Day': https://www.youtube.com/watch?v=G8czHlPYXew.

Congress of Aboriginal and Torres Strait Islander Nurses and Midwives (CATSINaM): http://catsinam.org.au/.

Dawn Martin-Hill—Dismantling the white man's Indian: Dr Dawn Martin-Hill at TEDxMcMasterU: https://www.youtube.com/watch?v=f0DsMrTshcA.

Idle no More: http://www.idlenomore.ca/.

The International Council of 13 Grandmothers: http://www.grandmotherscouncil.org/.

Winona LaDuke—Seeds the Creator Gave Us: https://www.youtube.com/watch?v=WEVg_KMPCmg.

References

Barnhardt R, Kawagley A. Indigenous knowledge systems and Alaska native ways of knowing. *Anthropol Educ Q.* 2005;3(1):8–23.

Belich J. *The New Zealand Wars and the Victorian Interpretation of Racial Conflict.* Auckland: Penguin; 1988.

Boulton A, Tamehana J, Brannelly T. Whānau-centred health and social service delivery in New Zealand: The challenges to, and opportunities for, innovation. *MAI J.* 2013;2(1):18–32.

Calvert S. Personal Communication – Midwifery Council of New Zealand Chief Executive and Registrar: Midwifery Council of New Zealand Māori Data 2015–2019; 15 January 2020.

Counties Manukau District Health Board. *External Review of Maternity Care in the Counties Manukau District*; 2012. Online: http://www.countiesmanukau.health.nz/assets/About-CMH/Reports-and-planning/Maternity/2012-CMH-external-report-maternity-care-review.pdf.

Curtis E, Waikaira E, Lualua-Ati T, et al. *Tātou Tātou/Success for All: Improving Māori Student Success.* Wellington: Ako Aotearoa National Centre for Tertiary Teaching Excellence; 2012a. Online: https://akoaotearoa.ac.nz/download/ng/file/group-1652/tatou-tatou—success-for-all-improving-maori-student-success.pdf.

Curtis E, Wikaira E, Stokes K, et al. Addressing indigenous health workforce inequities: a literature review exploring best practice for recruitment into tertiary health programmes. *Int J Equity Health.* 2012b;2012(11):13. Online: https://www.ncbi.nlm.nih.gov/pmc/articles/PMC3402985/.

Davis D, Baddock S, Pairman S, et al. Planned place of birth in New Zealand: does it affect mode of birth and intervention rates among low-risk women? *Birth.* 2011;38(2):111–119. doi:10.1111/j.1523-536X.2010.00458.x.

Denzin N, Lincoln Y. *Handbook of Qualitative Research.* 2nd ed. California. Thousand Oaks: Sage Publications; 2000.

Dixon L, Aimer P, Fletcher L, et al. Smoke free outcomes with midwife lead maternity carers: an analysis of smoking during pregnancy from the New Zealand College of Midwives Midwifery database 2004–2007. *NZCOM J.* 2009; 30:13–19.

Dow D. *Māori Health & Government Policy 1840–1940.* Wellington: Victoria University Press; 1999.

Durie M. *Te Taha Hinengaro: An Integrated Approach to Mental Health*. Hui Whakaoranga. Auckland: Hoani Waititi Marae; 1984.

Durie M. A Māori perspective of health. *Soc Sci Med*. 1985;20(5): 483–486.

Durie M. Whānau, Whanaungatanga and healthy Māori development. In: Te Whaiti P, McCarthy M, Durie A, eds. *Mai i Rangiātea: Māori Wellbeing and Development*. Auckland: Auckland University Press and Bridget Williams; 1997:1–24.

Durie M. *Te Oru Rangahau—concluding remarks. Te Oru Rangahau Māori Research and Development Conference*. Palmerston North: Te Pūtahi-ā-Toi School of Māori Studies; 1998:408–415.

Durie M. Te Pae Mahutonga: a model for Māori health promotion. *Health Promotion Forum N Z Newsletter*. 1999; 49:2–5.

Durie M. Universal provision, indigeneity and the Treaty of Waitangi. In: Durie M, eds. *Ngā Kāhui Pou: Launching Maori Futures*. Wellington: Huia; 2003:591–601.

Durie M. Understanding health and illness: research at the interface between science and indigenous knowledge. *Int J Epidemiol*. 2004; 33:1138–1143.

Durie M. *Whaiora Māori Health Development*. Melbourne: Oxford University Press; 2005.

Durie M, Black T, Cunningham C, et al. *The Parameters of Wellbeing: A Report Prepared for Te Puni Kōkiri*. Palmerston North: Te Mata o Te Tau Academy for Māori Research and Scholarship, Massey University; 2005.

Ellison-Loschmann L. *Māori Women's Experiences of Breastfeeding (MA thesis)*. Wellington: Victoria University; 1997.

E Tipu E Rea Whānau Services. *Housing teen parents in our communities*. 2019. Online: https://etipuereaws.org.nz/housing-teen-parents-in-our-communities/

Farry A. *A retrospective cohort study to evaluate the effect of 'Place Presenting in Labour' and 'Model of Midwifery Care' on maternal and neonatal outcomes for the low-risk women birthing in Counties Manukau District Health Board facilities 2011–2012. (M Health Sci thesis)*. Auckland University of Technology; 2015.

Federation of Primary Health Aotearoa New Zealand. Federation of Primary Health Statement Regarding Health and Disability Review. 2020. Online: https://fph.org.nz/wp-content/uploads/2020/07/Federation-statement-30-June-2020-review-findings.pdf

Glover M, Cunningham C. Hoki ki te Ūkaipō: Reinstating Māori infant care practices to increase breastfeeding rates. In: Liamputtong P, eds. *Infant Feeding Practices*. Springer, New York, NY. https://doi.org/10.1007/978-1-4419-6873-9_15.

Glover M, Manaena-Biddle H, Waldon J. Influences that affect Māori women breastfeeding. *Breastfeed Rev*. 2007a;15(2):5–14.

Glover M, Manaena-Biddle H, Waldon J. The role of Whānau in Māori women's decisions about breastfeeding. *Alternative*. 2007b;143–159.

Grace P, Ramsden I, Dennis J. *The Silent Migration: Ngāti Pōneke Young Māori Club 1937–1948: Stories of Urban Migration*. Wellington: Huia Publishers; 2001.

Gurung R, Mehta V. Relating ethnic identity, acculturation, and attitudes toward treating minority clients. *Cultur Divers Ethnic Minor Psychol*. 2001;7(2):139–151.

Harris R, Robson B, Curtis E, et al. Māori and non-Māori differences in caesarean section rates: a national review. *N Z Med J*. 2007;120(1249).

Harris R, Tobias M, Jeffreys M, et al. Racism and health: the relationship between experience of racial discrimination and health in New Zealand. *Soc Sci Med*. 2006a;63(6): 1428–1441.

Harris R, Tobias M, Jeffreys M, et al. Effects of self-reported racial discrimination and deprivation on Māori health and inequalities in New Zealand: cross-sectional study. *Lancet*. 2006b; 67:2005–2009.

Hayes Edwards, I. *Ūkaipōtanga: A grounded theory on optimizing breastfeeding for Māori women and the whānau. (Master's thesis)*. Auckland University of Technology; 2014. Online http://hdl.handle.net/10292/7472

Howden-Chapman P, Tobias M, eds. *Social Inequalities in Health: New Zealand 1999*. Wellington: Ministry of Health; 2000.

Hunn J. *Report on Department of Māori Affairs with Statistical Supplement, 24 August 1960*. Wellington: R. E. Owen Government Printer; 1961.

Hunt LM. Beyond cultural competence: Applying humility to clinical settings. *Park Ridge Center Bull*. 2001; 24:134–136.

Hunter M, Pairman S, Benn C, et al. Do low risk women actually birth in their planned place of birth and does ethnicity influence women's choices of birthplace? *NZCOM J*. 2011;44:5–11.

Huriwai T, Sellman J, Sullivan P, et al. A clinical sample of Māori being treated for alcohol and drug problems in New Zealand. *N Z Med J*. 1998;111(1065–1067):145–147.

Jackson M. *The Māori and the Criminal Justice System: A New Perspective: He Whaipaanga Hou*. Wellington: Department of Justice; 1987.

Jackson M. *Te Heteri: constitutional change*. Auckland: Māori Television; 2006.

Kawagley A. *A Yupiaq Worldview: A Pathway to Ecology and Spirit*. 2nd ed. Long Grove, IL: Waveland Press; 2006.

Jenkins K, Matthews KM. Knowing their place: the political socialization of Maori women in New Zealand through schooling policy and practice, 1867–1969. *Women's History Review*. 1998; 7;1:85–105. doi:10.1080/09612029800200163.

Kenney C. Māori Women, maternity services and the Treaty of Waitangi. In: Tawhai V, Gray-Sharp K, eds. *'Always Speaking' The Treaty of Waitangi and Public Policy*. Wellington: Huia Publishing; 2011:127–142.

Kizito H. *Non-Government Organisations (NGOs) and the Primary Health Care Strategy: Developing Relationships with Primary Health Organisations From an NGO Perspective. A Report from the Health & Disability Sector NGO Working Group*. Wellington: Ministry of Health; 2005.

Lee KL. *"Not Another Patient Through the Revolving Door": A Case Study Analysis of Six Women's Experiences with Pregnancy Terminations in New Zealand (Masters thesis)*. University of Waikato, Hamilton; 2016. Online: https://hdl.handle.net/10289/10596.

McBride-Henry K. *Responding to the Call to Care: Women's Experience of Breastfeeding in New Zealand (PhD thesis)*. Auckland: Massey University; 2004. Online: http://mro.massey.ac.nz/bitstream/handle/10179/1810/02_whole.pdf?sequence=1&isAllowed=y.

Macklin JM. *Statement on the United Nations Declaration on the Rights of Indigenous Peoples, 3 April. Minister for Families, Housing, Community Services and Indigenous Affairs*. Canberra: Parliament House; 2009. Online: http://www.un.org/esa/socdev/unpfii/documents/Australia_official_statement_endorsement_UNDRIP.pdf.

Manatū Hauora Ministry of Health. *Primary Health Care Strategy*. Wellington: Ministry of Health; 2001. Online: http://www.health.govt.nz/publication/primary-health-care-strategy.

Manatū Hauora Ministry of Health. *He Korowai Oranga Māori Health Strategy*. Wellington: Ministry of Health; 2002.

Manatū Hauora Ministry of Health. *Maternity Services Notice Pursuant to Section 88 of the New Zealand Health and Disability Act 2000*. Wellington: Ministry of Health; 2007.

Manatū Hauora Ministry of Health. *Primary Health Care Strategy: Accelerating Change (Paper 2)*. Wellington: Ministry of Health; 2008.

Manatū Hauora Ministry of Health. *Equity of Health Care for Māori: A Framework*. Wellington, New Zealand: Ministry of Health; 2014. Online: http://www.health.govt.nz/system/files/documents/publications/equity-of-health-care-for-maori-a-framework-jun14.pdf.

Manatū Hauora Ministry of Health. *New Zealand Health Strategy: Future Direction.* Online: http://www.health.govt.nz/new-zealand-health-system/new-zealand-health-strategy-future-direction, Wellington: Ministry of Health; 2016.

Manatū Hauora Ministry of Health. *Report on Maternity 2017.* Wellington: Ministry of Health. 2019. Online: https://www.health.govt.nz/publication/report-maternity-2017.

Manatū Hauora Ministry of Health. *Percentage of women giving birth at home, by ethnicity 2009–2018.* Online: https://minhealthnz.shinyapps.io/Maternity_report_webtool/.

Manatū Hauora Ministry of Health. *Babies: 2018 breastfeeding status at 2 weeks and year and demographics.* 2020a. Online: https://minhealthnz.shinyapps.io/Maternity_report_webtool/.

Manatū Hauora Ministry of Health. *Whakamaua: Māori Health Action Plan 2020–2025.* 2020b. Wellington: Ministry of Health. Online: https://www.health.govt.nz/system/files/documents/publications/whakamaua-maori-health-action-plan-2020-2025-2.pdf.

Manatū Taonga Ministry for Culture and Heritage. *The Whakaputanga – Declaration of Independence. Page 1: Introduction.* 2017a. Online: https://nzhistory.govt.nz/culture/declaration-of-independence-taming-the-frontier.

Manatū Taonga Ministry for Culture and Heritage. *The Treaty in brief. Page 1: Introduction.* 2017b. Online: https://nzhistory.govt.nz/politics/treaty/the-treaty-in-brief.

Manatū Taonga Ministry for Culture and Heritage. *Treaty Timeline. Treaty Events 1850–99.* 2017c. Online: https://nzhistory.govt.nz/politics/treaty/treaty-timeline/treaty-events-1850–99.

Manawhenua Hauora. *Minimal Specifications for a Pilot Primary Care Organisation (PHO). Advice to Mid-Central District Health Board/Te Pae Hauora o Ruahine o Tararua Regarding Primary Health Organisation.* Manawhenua Hauora: Rangitāne, Ngāti Raukawa, Muaupoko, Ngāti Kahungunu; 2002.

Manch T. *Sir Mason Durie the first Māori Health Authority appointment* 2021, 7 May Stuff. Online: http://www.stuff.co.nz/pou-tiaki/125062280/sir-mason-durie-the-first-mori-health-authority-appointment.

Mantell C, Craig ED, Stewart AW, et al. Ethnicity and birth outcome: New Zealand trends 1980–2001: Part 2. Pregnancy outcomes for Māori women. *Aust N Z J Obstet Gynaecol.* 2004;44(6):537–540.

Māori Reference Group for the Taskforce for Action on Violence within Families. *E Tū Whānau Programme of Action for Addressing Family Violence 2013–2018.* Wellington: New Zealand Government; 2013.

Marsden M. Resource Management Law Reform: Part A. *The Natural World and Natural Resources, Māori Value Systems and Perspectives. Part B. Water Resources and the Kai Tahu Claim.* Wellington: Ministry for the Environment; 1989.

Martínez Cobo JR. *Study of the Problem of Discrimination against Indigenous Populations.* Geneva: United Nations; 1987. Online: https://www.un.org/development/desa/indigenouspeoples/publications/2014/09/martinez-cobo-study/.

Mayhew P, Reilly J. *The New Zealand Crime and Safety Survey 2006: Key Findings.* Wellington: Ministry of Justice; 2007.

Mead HM. *Tikanga Māori: Living by Māori Values.* Auckland, New Zealand: Huia Publications; 2003.

Meredith P. *Urban Māori—urbanisation.* Te Ara—the Encyclopedia of New Zealand; 2015. Online: http://www.teara.govt.nz/en/urban-maori/page-1.

Mikaere A. *The Balance Destroyed: Consequences for Māori Women of the Colonization of Tikanga Māori.* Auckland: International Research Institute for Māori and Indigenous Education; 2003.

New Zealand College of Midwives (NZCOM). *Midwives Handbook for Practice.* 4th ed. Christchurch: NZCOM; 2008.

New Zealand College of Midwives (NZCOM). *Midwives Handbook for Practice.* 5th ed. Christchurch: NZCOM; 2015.

New Zealand Government. *Health Practitioners Competence Assurance Act 2003.* Wellington: Ministry of Health; 2003.

New Zealand Government. *Ministerial statement United Nations Declaration on the Rights of Indigenous Peoples—Government support.* Hansard Reports; 2010. Online: https://www.parliament.nz/en/pb/hansard-debates/rhr/document/49HansD_20100420_00000071/ministerial-statements-un-declaration-on-the-rights-of.

New Zealand Government. *Pae Ora (Healthy Futures) Bill,* 2021. Online: https://www.parliament.nz/en/pb/bills-and-laws/bills-proposed-laws/document/BILL_116317/pae-ora-healthy-futures-bill.

Newman K. *Ratana Revisited: An Unfinished Legacy.* Auckland: Reed Publishing; 2006.

Ngā Māia Māori Midwives Aotearoa (Ngā Māia). *Turanga Kaupapa (poster);* 2017a. Online: http://www.ngamaia.co.nz/turanga.

Ngā Māia Māori Midwives Aotearoa (Ngā Māia). *Toitū te Pae Tawhiti/Resources;* 2017b. Online: http://www.ngamaia.co.nz/resources.

Oakley Browne MA, Wells JE, Scott KM, eds. *Te Rau Hinengaro: The New Zealand Mental Health Survey.* Wellington: Ministry of Health; 2006.

Papakura M. *The old-time Māori.* London: Victor Gollancz Limited; 1938.

Pere R. Te Oranga o te Whānau (The health of the family). *Hui Whakaoranga Māori Health Planning Workshop.* Wellington: Department of Health; 1984.

Pihama L. *Tihei Mauri Ora: Honouring our Voices. Mana Wahine as a Kaupapa Māori Theoretical Framework (Doctoral thesis).* Auckland: University of Auckland; 2001. Online: http://www.academia.edu/2893165/Tihei_Mauri_Ora_Honouring_Our_Voices.

Policy Research Initiative. *Measurement of Social Capital: Reference Document for Public Policy Research, Development, and Evaluation.* Ottawa: Statistics Canada; 2005.

Pomare E, Keefe-Ormsby V, Ormsby C, et al. *Hauora: Māori Standards of Health III. A Study of the Years 1970–1991.* Wellington: Te Rōpū Hauora a Eru Pomare Eru Pomare Māori Health Research Centre; 1995.

Public Health Intelligence. *A Portrait of Health: Key Results of the 2006/07 New Zealand Health Survey.* Wellington: Ministry of Health; 2008.

Ngāi Tahu Claims Settlement Act 1998. Online: https://www.legislation.govt.nz/act/public/1998/0097/latest/DLM429090.html

Quinlivan JA, Evans SF. Teenage antenatal clinics may reduce the rate of preterm birth: a prospective study. *BJOG.* 2004; 111: 571–578.

Ratima M, Crengle S. Antenatal, labour, and delivery care for Māori: experiences, location within a lifecourse approach, and knowledge gaps. *Pimatisiwin.* 2013;10(3):353–366. Online: http://www.pimatisiwin.com/online/wp-content/uploads/2013/02/08RatimaCrengle.pdf.

Reinfelds M. Kia Mau, Kia Ū: *Supporting the breastfeeding journey of Māori women and their whānau in Taranaki.* (Master's thesis). Massey University. Online: https://www.researchgate.net/profile/Marnie-Reinfelds/publication/310461205_Kia_Mau_Kia_U_Supporting_the_Breastfeeding_Journey_of_Maori_Women_and_their_Whanau_in_Taranaki/links/582e628208ae138f1c01dacd/Kia-Mau-Kia-U-Supporting-the-Breastfeeding-Journey-of-Maori-Women-and-their-Whanau-in-Taranaki.pdf.

Robson B, Harris R. Hauora Māori Standards of Health IV. *A Study of the Years 2000–2005.* Wellington: Te Rōpu Rangahau Hauora a Eru Pomare Eru Pomare. Māori Health Research Centre; 2007.

Royal Commission on Social Policy. *The April Report: Report of the Royal Commission on Social Policy.* Wellington: Royal Commission on Social Policy; 1988.

Simmonds N. Mana wahine: decolonising politics. *Womens Stud J.* 2011;25(2):11–25. Online: http://www.wsanz.org.nz/journal/docs/WSJNZ252Simmonds11–25.pdf.

Smith L. *Decolonizing Methodologies Research and Indigenous Peoples.* London: Zeb Books; 2005.

Sykes A. *Native affairs: full and final (episode 30, 25 November).* Auckland: Māori Television; 2007.

Tāhū o te Ture. *Who is Vulnerable or Hard-to-reach in the Provision of Maternity, Well Child and Early Parenting Support Services? Addressing the Drivers of Crime: Maternity and Early Parenting Support.* Ministry of Justice. 2010. Online: https://www.justice.govt.nz/assets/Documents/Publications/vulnerable-and-hard-to-reach-final-report.pdf.

Talamaivao N, Harris R, Cormack D, et al. *Racism and health in Aotearoa New Zealand: a systematic review of quantitative studies.* N Z Med J. 2020. Online: https://www.nzma.org.nz/journal-articles/racism-and-health-in-aotearoa-new-zealand-a-systematic-review-of-quantitative-studies.

Taskforce on Whānau-Centred Initiatives. *Whānau Ora: Report of the Taskforce on Whānau-Centred Initiatives*; 2010. Online: https://www.msd.govt.nz/documents/about-msd-and-our-work/publications-resources/planning-strategy/whanau-ora/whanau-ora-taskforce-report.pdf.

Tatauranga Aotearoa. *How is our Māori Population Changing?* Statistics New Zealand. 2015. Online: http://www.stats.govt.nz/browse_for_stats/people_and_communities/maori/maori-population-article-2015.aspx?gclid=CPnC0u-F_sw-CFQokvQodJKQD7g.

Tatauranga Aotearoa. *Parenting and fertility trends in New Zealand: 2018.* 2019, October 24. Online: https://www.stats.govt.nz/reports/parenting-and-fertility-trends-in-new-zealand-2018.

Tatauranga Aotearoa. *Abortion statistics: Year ended December 2019.* 2020a, June 16. Online: http://www.stats.govt.nz/information-releases/abortion-statistics-year-ended-december-2019.

Tatauranga Aotearoa. *Housing in Aotearoa: 2020.* 2020b, December 8. Online: https://www.stats.govt.nz/reports/housing-in-aotearoa-2020#about.

Tatauranga Aotearoa. *Total fertility rate (Maori and total population) (Annual–Sep).* Statistics New Zealand. 2021, February 21. Online: http://infoshare.stats.govt.nz/ViewTable.aspx?pxID=de020526-0ff7-4576-83af-d5a45fb4f1d3.

Tertiary Education Commission. *Reform of Vocational Education.* 2021. Online: https://www.tec.govt.nz/rove/reform-ofvocational-education/.

Tokalau T. *Pregnant women among the homeless on cold Auckland streets.* 2018. Online: https://www.stuff.co.nz/national/104478559/pregnant-woman-among-the-homeless-on-cold-auckland-streets.

Te Ao Māori News. *Women shouldn't have to second-guess breastfeeding in public – mother.* 2019, January 8. Online: https://www.teaomaori.news/women-shouldnt-have-to-second-guess-breast-feeding-public-mother.

Te Puni Kōkiri. *About Whānau Ora*; Ministry of Māori Development. 2017. Online: https://www.tpk.govt.nz/en/whakamahia/whanau-ora/about-whanau-ora.

Te Rau Puawai. *Te Rau Puawai/Māori Mental Health Workforce Development.* Palmerston North: Massey University; 2017. Online: http://www.massey.ac.nz/massey/maori/maori_research/te-rau-puawai/te-rau-puawai_home.cfm.

Te Rōpū Wahine Māori Toko i te Ora. *Rapuora Health and Māori Women.* Wellington: Māori Womens Welfare League; 1984.

Te Tāhuhu o te Mātauranga. *Māori Education Overview.* n.d. Online: https://www.education.govt.nz/assets/Documents/Ministry/Publications/Briefings-to-Incoming-Ministers/4-1093092-Maori-Education-BIM-Annex-ABC.PDF.

Te Tāhuhu o te Mātauranga. *Ngā Haeata Mātauranga Annual Report on Māori Education 2007/08.* Wellington: Ministry of Education; 2009.

Te Tatau o te Whare Kahu Midwifery Council. *Statement on Cultural Competence for Midwives*; 2011. Online: https://www.

midwiferycouncil.health.nz/sites/default/files/professional-standards/PDF%20cultural%20competence.pdf.

Te Tatau o te Whare Kahu Midwifery Council. *2015 Midwifery Workforce Survey*; 2015. Online: https://www.midwiferycouncil.health.nz/about-us/publications/midwifery-workforce-sur-vey-2015.

Te Tatau o te Whare Kahu Midwifery Council. *2016 Midwifery Workforce Survey*; 2016. Online: https://www.midwiferycouncil.health.nz/about-us/publications/midwifery-workforce-survey-2016.

Te Tatau o te Whare Kahu Midwifery Council. *2017 Midwifery Workforce Survey.* Wellington, NZ: Midwifery Council of New Zealand; 2017.

Te Tatau o te Whare Kahu Midwifery Council. *2018 Midwifery Workforce Survey.* Wellington, NZ: Midwifery Council of New Zealand; 2018.

Te Tatau o te Whare Kahu Midwifery Council. 2019 Midwifery Workforce Survey; 2019.

Te Tatau o te Whare Kahu Midwifery Council. 2020 Midwifery Workforce Survey; 2020.

Te Tatau o te Whare Kahu Midwifery Council. 2021 Midwifery Workforce Survey; 2021.

Te Taura Whiri I Te Reo Māori. *Te Reo Māori*; n.d. The Māori Language Commission; Online: http://www.tetaurawhiri.govt.nz/about-us/history-and-timeline.

Tervalon M, Murray-Garcia J. Cultural humility versus cultural competence: a critical distinction in defining physician training outcomes in multicultural education. *J Health Care Poor Underserved.* 1998;9(2):117–125.

Te Wakahuia o Hine. *Online.* 2021. Online: https://tiekiconsultancy.co.nz/te-wakahuia-o-hine/.

Tikao KW. *Raro Timu Taro Take Ngai Tahu Birthing Traditions (PhD thesis),* Canterbury University; 2020. Online: https://ir.canterbury.ac.nz/bitstream/handle/10092/101118/Raro%20Timu%20Raro%20Take%20Ng%c4%81i%20Tahu%20Birth-ing%20Traditions.pdf?sequence=6&isAllowed=y.

Tumuaki o te Mana Arotake. *Summary of our Education for Māori reports.* Controller and Auditor-General. 2016. Online: https://oag.parliament.nz/2016/education-for-maori-summary/docs/summary-education-for-maori.pdf.

Tupara H. *He Urupounamu e Whakahaerengia ana e te Whanau: Whanau Decision Processes (PhD thesis).* Palmerston North: Massey University; 2009.

Tupara H. *Te whanau tamariki – pregnancy and birth – Birth in Māori tradition, Te Ara – the Encyclopedia of New Zealand.* 1 June 2017. Online: https://teara.govt.nz/en/te-whanau-tamariki-pregnancy-and-birth/page-1.

Tupara H, Tahere M. *Rapua te Aronga-a-Hine: The Māori Midwifery Workforce in Aotearoa, A Literature Review - February 2020.* Wellington: Te Rau Ora; 2020.

United Nations. *United Nations Declaration on the Rights of Indigenous Peoples. Adopted by the United Nations General Assembly 13 September 2007.* Geneva: United Nations; 2008. Online: https://www.un.org/esa/socdev/unpfii/documents/DRIPS_en.pdf.

Van der Wijden C, Manion C. Lactational amenorrhoea method for family planning. *Cochrane Database of Syst Rev.* 10. Online. doi:10.1002/14651858.CD001329.pub2.

Waikato Raupatu Claims Settlement Act 1995. Online: https://www.legislation.govt.nz/act/public/1995/0058/latest/DLM369893.html.

Waitangi Tribunal. *Te Tiriti o Waitangi—The Treaty of Waitangi.* Wellington: New Zealand Government; 2009. Online: http://archives.govt.nz/exhibitions/treaty.

Walker R. The Treaty of Waitangi as the focus of Māori protest. In: Kawharu I, eds. *Māori and Pākehā Perspectives of the Treaty of Waitangi.* Auckland: Oxford University Press; 1989: 263–279.

226

Walker T. *Whanau is Whānau.* Wellington: Families Commission/ Kōmihana a Whānau; 2006.

Webster M, Thompson J, Mitchell E, et al. Postnatal depression in a community cohort. *Aust N Z J Psychiatry.* 1994;28(1): 42–49.

Whānau Ora Iwi Leaders Group. *Report of the Strategic Consultation Hui-a-Iwi*, April–June 2016.

Whitley C. *Improved access to long-acting reversible contraception (LARC) and the declining abortion rate (Master's thesis).* University of Otago. Online: http://hdl.handle.net/10523/7935.

Williams T. It's about empowering the whanau: Māori adult students succeeding at university. *Waikato J Educ.* 2011; 16(3):57–68.

Wilmer F. *The Indigenous Voice in the World of Politics: Since Time Immemorial.* California: Sage, Newbury Park; 1993.

Further reading

Baxter J, Kingi TK, Tapsell R, et al. Prevalence of mental disorders among Māori in Te Rau Hinengaro: The New Zealand Mental Health Survey. *Aust N Z J Psychiatry.* 2006;40(10):914–923.

Kahukiwa R, Pōtiki R. *Oriori: A Māori Child is Born—From Conception to Birth.* Auckland: Tandem Press; 1999.

Kotuku Partners. *A Brief Review of Literature on Māori Pregnancy and Childbirth. Auckland. Report for the Māori Working Group of the Regional Health Authority Maternity Forum,* 1994.

McLeod D, Pullon S, Cookson T. Factors that influence changes in smoking behaviour during pregnancy. *N Z Med J.* 2003; 116:1173.

Maxwell G, Robertson J, Kingi V, et al. *Achieving Effective Outcomes in Youth Justice: An Overview of Findings.* Wellington: Te Manatū Whakahiato Ora Ministry of Social Development; 2004.

Murphy, N. *Te Awa Atua: Menstruation in the Pre-Colonial Maori World.* Te Puna Manawa Ltd; 2013.

Murphy, N. *Waiwhero: He Whakahirahiratanga o Te Ira Wahine.* Te Puna Manawa Ltd; 2014

Mulligan E. *Tihei Mauri Ora The Breath of Life: The Conceptualisation of Tihei Mauri Ora within a Bachelor of Midwifery Programme (Master's thesis).* Wellington: Victoria University; 2003.

Palmer S. *Hei Oranga Mo Ngā Wahine Hapū o Hauraki i Roto i te Whare ora (Doctoral thesis).* Hamilton: University of Waikato; 2002.

Ramsden I. *Cultural Safety and Nursing Education in Aotearoa and Te Waipounamu (Doctoral thesis).* Wellington: Victoria University; 2002.

Tupara H. Māori women: the challenge for midwifery education. *NZCOM J.* 2001; 25:6–9.

Appendix 11.1 The declaration of independence 1835*

This declaration was adopted at Waitangi on October 28, 1835. Thirty-five ariki and rangatira representing iwi and hapu from the far north to the Hauraki Gulf signed the declaration at that hui. Later, other notable leaders added their signatures; those from outside the Tai Tokerau included Te Hapuku of Ngati Kahungunu and Potatau Te Wherowhero of Tainui. The English translation presented here was sent to the Under Secretary of State at the Colonial Office in London by James Busby, British Resident in New Zealand, on 2nd November 1835.

{Signatures or signs of 35 chiefs, from North Cape to the Hauraki Gulf}
Witnessed by: (Signed) Henry Williams, Missionary, C.M.S.
George Clarke, C.M.S.
James C. Clendon, Merchant
Gilbert, Merchant

1. KO MATOU, ko nga Tino Rangatira o nga iwi o Nu Tireni I raro mai o Hauraki kua oti nei te huihui i Waitangi i Tokerau i te ra 28 o Oketopa 1835, ka wakaputa i te Rangatiratanga o to matou wenua a ka meatia ka wakaputaia e matou he Wenua Rangatira, kia huaina, Ko te Wakaminenga o nga Hapu o Nu Tireni.	1. WE, the hereditary chiefs and heads of the tribes of the Northern parts of New Zealand, being assembled at Waitangi in the Bay of Islands on this 28th day of October, 1835, declare the Independence of our country, which is hereby constituted and declared to be an Independent State, under the designation of the United Tribes of New Zealand.
2. Ko te Kingitanga ko te mana i te wenua o te wakaminenga o Nu Tireni ka meatia nei kei nga Tino Rangatira anake i to matou huihuinga, a ka mea hoki e kore e tukua e matou te wakarite ture ki te tahi hunga ke atu, me te tahi Kawanatanga hoki kia meatia i te wenua o te wakawakarite ana ki te ritenga o o matou ture e meatia nei matou i to matou huihuinga.	2. All sovereign power and authority within the territories of the United Tribes of New Zealand is hereby declared to reside entirely and exclusively in the hereditary chiefs and heads of tribes in their collective capacity, who also declare that they will not permit any legislative authority separate from themselves in their collective capacity to exist, nor any function of government to be exercised within the said territories, unless by persons appointed by them, and acting under the authority of laws regularly enacted by them in Congress assembled.
3. Ko matou ko nga tino Rangatira ka mea nei kia huihui ki te runanga ki Waitangi a te Ngahuru i tenei tau i tenei tau ki te wakarite ture kia tika te hokohoko, a ka mea ki nga tauiwi o runga, kia wakarerea te wawai, kia mahara ai ki te wakaoranga o to matou wenua, a kia uru ratou ki te wakaminenga o Nu Tireni.	3. The hereditary chiefs and heads of tribes agree to meet in Congress at Waitangi in the autumn of each year, for the purpose of framing laws for the dispensation of justice, the preservation of peace and good order, and the regulation of trade; and they cordially invite the Southern tribes to lay aside their private animosities and to consult the safety and welfare of our common country, by joining the Confederation of the United Tribes.
4. Ka mea matou kia tuhituhia he pukapuka ki te ritenga o tenei o to matou wakaputanga nei ki te Kingi o Ingarani hei kawe atu i to matou aroha nana hoki i wakaae ki te Kara mo matou. A no te mea ka atawai matou, ka tiaki i nga pakeha e noho nei i uta, e rere mai ana i te hokohoko, koia ka mea ai matou ki te Kingi kia waiho hei matua ki a matou i to matou Tamarikitanga kei wakakahoretia to matou Rangatiratanga.	4. They also agree to send a copy of this Declaration to His Majesty the King of England, to thank him for his acknowledgement of their flag; and in return for the friendship and protection they have shown, and are prepared to show, to such of his subjects as have settled in their country, or resorted to its shores for the purposes of trade, they entreat that he will continue to be the parent of their infant State, and that he will become its Protector from all attempts upon its independence.
KUA WHAKAAETIA katoatia e matou i tenei ra i te 28 Oketopa, 1835, ki te aroaro o te Reireneti o te Kingi o Ingarani.	AGREED TO unanimously on this 28th day of October, 1835, in the presence of His Brittanic Majesty's Resident.
I certify that the above is a correct copy of the Declaration of the Chiefs, according to the translation of Missionaries who have resided ten years and upwards in the country; and it is transmitted to His Most Gracious Majesty the King of England, at the unanimous request of the chiefs.	
(Signed) JAMES BUSBY British Resident of New Zealand	

Appendix 11.2 Te Tiriti o Waitangi / The Treaty of Waitangi*

Te Tiriti o Waitangi (Maori version)	The Treaty of Waitangi (English version)
KO WIKITORIA te Kuini o Ingarani i tana mahara atawai ki nga Rangatira me nga Hapu o Nu Tirani i tana hiahia hoki kia tohungia ki a ratou o ratou rangatiratanga me to ratou wenua, a kia mau tonu hoki te Rongo ki a ratou me te Atanoho hoki kua wakaaro ia he mea tika kia tukua mai tetahi Rangatira—hei kai wakarite ki nga Tangata Maori o Nu Tirani—kia wakaaetia e nga Rangatira Maori te Kawanatanga o te Kuini ki nga wahikatoa o te wenua nei me nga motu—na te mea hoki he tokomaha ke nga tangata o tona Iwi Kua noho ki tenei wenua, a e haere mai nei. Na ko te Kuini e hiahia ana kia wakaritea te Kawanatanga kia kaua ai nga kino e puta mai ki te tangata Maori ki te Pakeha e noho ture kore ana. Na kua pai te Kuini kia tukua a hau a Wiremu Hopihona he Kapitana i te Roiara Nawi hei Kawana mo nga wahi katoa o Nu Tirani e tukua aianei amua atu ki te Kuini, e mea atu ana ia ki nga Rangatira o te wakaminenga o nga hapu o Nu Tirani me era Rangatira atu enei ture ka korerotia nei.	HER MAJESTY VICTORIA Queen of the United Kingdom of Great Britain and Ireland regarding with Her Royal Favour the Native Chiefs and Tribes of New Zealand and anxious to protect their just Rights and Property and to secure to them the enjoyment of Peace and Good Order has deemed it necessary in consequence of the great number of Her Majesty's Subjects who have already settled in New Zealand and the rapid extension of Emigration both from Europe and Australia which is still in progress to constitute and appoint a functionary properly authorised to treat with the Aborigines of New Zealand for the recognition of Her Majesty's Sovereign authority over the whole or any part of those islands—Her Majesty therefore being desirous to establish a settled form of Civil Government with a view to avert the evil consequences which must result from the absence of the necessary Laws and Institutions alike to the native population and to Her subjects has been graciously pleased to empower and to authorise me William Hobson a Captain in Her Majesty's Royal Navy Consul and Lieutenant-Governor of such parts of New Zealand as may be or hereafter shall be ceded to her Majesty to invite the confederated and independent Chiefs of New Zealand to concur in the following Articles and Conditions.
Ko te tuatahi	Article the First [Article 1]
Ko nga Rangatira o te wakaminenga me nga Rangatira katoa hoki ki hai i uru ki taua wakaminenga ka tuku rawa atu ki te Kuini o Ingarani ake tonu atu—te Kawanatanga katoa o o ratou wenua.	The Chiefs of the Confederation of the United Tribes of New Zealand and the separate and independent Chiefs who have not become members of the Confederation cede to Her Majesty the Queen of England absolutely and without reservation all the rights and powers of Sovereignty which the said Confederation or Individual Chiefs respectively exercise or possess or may be supposed to exercise or to possess over their respective Territories as the sole sovereigns thereof.
Ko te tuarua	Article the Second [Article 2]
Ko te Kuini o Ingarani ka wakarite ka wakaae ki nga Rangitira ki nga hapu—ki nga tangata katoa o Nu Tirani te tino rangatiratanga o o ratou wenua o ratou kainga me o ratou taonga katoa. Otiia ko nga Rangatira o te wakaminenga me nga Rangatira katoa atu ka tuku ki te Kuini te hokonga o era wahi wenua e pai ai te tangata nona te Wenua—ki te ritenga o te utu e wakaritea ai e ratou ko te kai hoko e meatia nei e te Kuini hei kai hoko mona.	Her Majesty the Queen of England confirms and guarantees to the Chiefs and Tribes of New Zealand and to the respective families and individuals thereof the full exclusive and undisturbed possession of their Lands and Estates Forests Fisheries and other properties which they may collectively or individually possess so long as it is their wish and desire to retain the same in their possession; but the Chiefs of the United Tribes and the individual Chiefs yield to Her Majesty the exclusive right of Preemption over such lands as the proprietors thereof may be disposed to alienate at such prices as may be agreed upon between the respective Proprietors and persons appointed by Her Majesty to treat with them in that behalf.
Ko te tuatoro	Article the Third [Article 3]
Hei wakaritenga mai hoki tenei mo te wakaaetanga ki te Kawanatanga o te Kuini—Ka tiakina e te Kuini o Ingarani nga tangata Maori katoa o Nu Tirani ka tukua ki a ratou nga tikanga katoa rite tahi ki ana mea ki nga tangata o Ingarani.	In consideration thereof Her Majesty the Queen of England extends to the Natives of New Zealand Her royal protection and imparts to them all the Rights and Privileges of British Subjects. (signed) William Hobson, Lieutenant-Governor.

Continued

Appendix 11.2 Te Tiriti o Waitangi / The Treaty of Waitangi*—cont'd

Te Tiriti o Waitangi (Maori version)	The Treaty of Waitangi (English version)
Na ko matou ko nga Rangatira o te Wakaminenga o nga hapu o Nu Tirani ka huihui nei ki Waitangi ko matou hoki ko nga Rangatira o Nu Tirani ka kite nei i te ritenga o enei kupu, ka tangohia ka wakaaetia katoatia e matou, koia ka tohungia ai o matou ingoa o matou tohu. Ka meatia tenei ki Waitangi i te ono o nga ra o Pepueri i te tau kotahi mano, e waru rau e wa te kau o to tatou Ariki.	Now therefore We the Chiefs of the Confederation of the United Tribes of New Zealand being assembled in Congress at Victoria in Waitangi and We the Separate and Independent Chiefs of New Zealand claiming authority over the Tribes and Territories which are specified after our respective names, having been made fully to understand the Provisions of the foregoing Treaty, accept and enter into the same in the full spirit and meaning thereof in witness of which we have attached our signatures or marks at the places and the dates respectively specified. Done at Waitangi this Sixth day of February in the year of Our Lord one thousand eight hundred and forty. (512 signatures, dates and locations)

*Macrons are not used in Te Tiriti o Waitangi to preserve historical accuracy.

Appendix 11.3 Glossary of Māori terms

Aotearoa	Translated as 'Land of the Long White Cloud' and attributed to the sighting of a cloud by the canoe party captained by Māori explorer Kupe, which led to the discovery of land now known as New Zealand
Hapū	Extended kin group made up of smaller collectives. Also, the word for pregnant. The derivative, hapūtanga, meaning 'pregnancy'
Hauora	Literally translated as 'breath of life'—hau meaning 'wind' or 'breath' and ora meaning 'life'. Also, the word for health
Hui	Gathering or meeting
Iwi	Tribal group identified by a common ancestor
Kaupapa	A topic of interest
Māori	Tangata Whenua of Aotearoa. The indigenous peoples of New Zealand
Marae	Traditional settlement
Pākehā	Non-Māori or foreigner
Pēpi	Baby born with Māori whakapapa
Pōwhiri	Formal welcome ceremony
Mana whenua	Authority over the land
Tamariki	Children with Māori whakapapa
Tangata Whenua	Person or people of the land
Te ao Māori	Māori world, Māori worldview
Te reo Māori	Māori language
Tikanga	Etiquette, norm, tradition
Tohu	Sign, symbolic
Tohunga	Skilled in the significance of tohu, a visionary
Tūranga Kaupapa	Foundation principles or concepts, developed by Ngā Māia o Aotearoa Māori Midwives
Waka	Vessel
Whakapapa	Ancestry, genealogy marked by generations and people/places
Whāngai	To take care of, a Māori childcare tradition likened to adoption
Whare	House structure
Whānau	Social unit likened to a family. It can be kin based or kaupapa based
Whānau Ora	Collective wellbeing
Whanaunga	Relative, not necessarily blood relative but common connection, e.g. Pacific nations or indigenous
Whanaungatanga	Relationship/s
Whenua	Land, placenta

There is no 's' in the Māori alphabet and words can thus have singular or plural meaning.
(Source: all translations by Hope Tupara.)

CHAPTER 12

Options for women around fertility and reproduction

Sally K Tracy

LEARNING OUTCOMES

Learning outcomes for this chapter are:

1. To introduce national and international background data on fertility and reproduction
2. To explore the meaning of fertility and infertility
3. To identify key aspects of assisted reproduction
4. To discuss the importance of age and motherhood.

CHAPTER OVERVIEW

This chapter offers a brief introduction to fertility and reproductive issues faced by women who may not achieve pregnancy without assistance. It will introduce you to some of the physical methods of assisted reproduction, and some of the ethical dilemmas associated with fertility and reproduction technology.

KEY TERMS

fecundity
fertility
gamete intrafallopian transfer
 (GIFT)

infertility
intracytoplasmic sperm injection
 (ICSI)
in vitro fertilization (IVF)

luteal support
older women
population
total fertility rate (TFR)

INTRODUCTION

Throughout most of human history, the pace of growth of world **population** has been extremely slow. World population did not reach 1 billion until around 1800, and it took another century and a quarter to reach 2 billion. But the world is currently in the midst of a period of substantially faster population growth, having increased from 3 to 7 billion within the space of the past half-century. Population growth patterns are linked to nearly every challenge confronting humanity, including poverty reduction, urban pollution, energy production, food and water scarcity, and health. With world population now having reached 7.9 billion in 2021 and projected to surpass 9 billion by 2050, these issues and the desire to raise living standards at the same time will create a huge challenge.

WORLD POPULATION TRENDS

In 1968 the United Nations' Population Division predicted that the world population would grow to at least 12 billion by 2050. Since then it has regularly revised its estimates downwards (UN, 2015) (Fig. 12.1). It now expects world population to plateau at around 9 billion in 2050. We are experiencing a profound demographic shift as a result of two forces: increasing longevity and declining fertility (Fig. 12.2). The best-known example of shrinkage is in Italy, where women were once symbols of **fecundity** (able to produce many children). By 2000, Italy's fertility rate was Western Europe's lowest, at 1.2 births per woman.

(The level required by a population to replace itself in the long term, without migration, is 2.1 births per woman.)

Globally, women are having fewer babies, but fertility rates remain high in some parts of the world. The global fertility rate declined from 3.2 live births per woman in 1990 to 2.5 in 2019. In sub-Saharan Africa, the region with the highest fertility levels, total fertility fell from 6.3 births per woman in 1990 to 4.6 in 2019. Over the same period, fertility levels also declined in Northern Africa, Western Asia, Central and Southern Asia, Eastern and South-Eastern Asia, Latin America, the Caribbean, and in Oceania excluding Australia and New Zealand (4.5 to 3.4).

In Australia and New Zealand and in Europe and Northern America, fertility in 1990 was already below 2.0 live

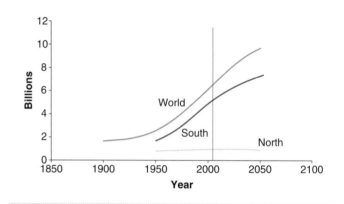

FIGURE 12.1 Growth in world population projected to 2050 (Source: Bongaarts, 2009. Human population growth and the demographic transition. *Philos Trans Roy Soc B.* 364:2985–2990, doi:10.1098/rstb.2009.0137, by permission of the Royal Society)

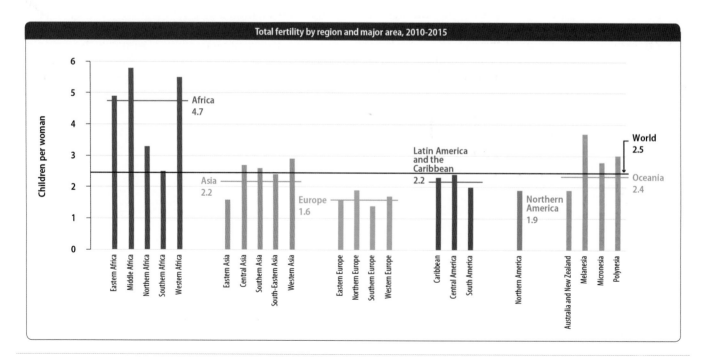

FIGURE 12.2 World fertility by region 2010–15 (Source: United Nations Department of Economic and Social Affairs (UNDESA), Population Division. *World Fertility Patterns 2015*. Data Booklet ST/ESA/SER.A/370. 2015:3. ©United Nations 2015. Reprinted with the permission of the United Nations)

births per woman, and it remained so in 2019, with an average of 1.8 births per woman in Australia and New Zealand, and 1.7 in Europe and Northern America (UNDESA, 2020).

There is a projected rise in world population to 11.2 billion in 2100, representing an increase of 3.8 billion over the 2021 population of 7.9 billion. Nearly all of this future growth is predicted to occur in the 'South'—that is Africa, Asia (excluding Japan, Australia and New Zealand) and Latin America—where population size is projected to increase from 6.1 billion to 9.9 billion between 2015 and 2100. In contrast, in the 'North' (Europe, Northern America, Japan and Australia/New Zealand), This occurs because population growth follows what is known as *demographic transition* (Bongaarts, 2009). Demographic transition refers to the shift from relatively high fertility rates and high mortality rates, to relatively low mortality rates, and subsequently to relatively low fertility rates. The transition usually reflects changes in societies as they move from being dependent on agriculture to becoming industrial societies. At the beginning of the demographic transition, population growth (which equals the difference between the birth and death rate in the absence of migration) is near zero as high death rates more or less offset the high birth rates typical of agrarian societies before an industrial revolution. Then, as the society develops through industrialisation, the population growth moves towards zero as birth and death rates reach low levels and again begin to balance out. Fig. 12.2 reflects the differences between the already industrialised nations and the slower industrialisation occurring in countries such as Africa, Asia and Latin America (UNDESA, 2015).

However, the assumption that demographic transition from high to low birth rates occurs only as a result of exogenous social and economic forces is contested through our clearer understanding of childbearing within a human rights framework. When viewed through this framework, the opportunity to slow population growth draws on a number of scientific disciplines such as ecology, climate change and peace and conflict studies—disciplines that have not traditionally played a large part in the debates on population and family planning (Bongaarts, 2016). Contraception and safe abortion together have lowered family size even in poor, illiterate communities. The strongest predictors of a woman's desired family size are her income, her education level and her infant's chances of surviving—hence the counter-argument that development dollars will be far more effective if they're spent on schooling girls, not on family planning. For many countries the demographic transition has already ended, and as the global fertility rate has now halved, we know that the world as a whole is approaching the end of rapid population growth (UNDESA, 2020).

CRITICAL THINKING EXERCISE

Look into the writings of feminist economists such as Marilyn Waring and determine how population change affects the economy of New Zealand or Australia.

FERTILITY

The **total fertility rate (TFR)** refers to the average number of babies a woman could expect to bear if she experienced current age-specific fertility rates throughout her childbearing life if she survived through to the end of the reproductive age span (see Box 12.1).

The word **'fertility'** used in its broadest colloquial sense denotes the reproductive capacity of a couple. Aside from some medically determined causes of sterility, the reproductive capacity of a couple is usually assessed by predicting the probability of different outcomes given different circumstances in relation to whether pregnancy occurs and how long it takes the couple to conceive (Sallmen et al., 2005).

An awareness of fertility rates is crucial for describing the demographic profile of a country, opportunities for development and change in population size, and for assessing challenges to women's reproductive health. The ability to preserve fertility with various methods has become a key issue for some women. Although the need is most pressing among women with cancer, the same therapeutic options may be available for many other women who are reaching an advanced reproductive age.

The reasons for the fall in fertility in high-income countries are moderately well described. Some attribute the fall to the fact that married women were entering the workforce in larger numbers than before and, as in low- and middle-income countries, there were better contraceptives and their use had become respectable. Thus the world's annual number of births in the late 1990s was only 129 million, well below the 206 million that would have been the situation if the fertility levels of the early 1960s had been maintained. Others speculate that the transition from high to low fertility (the first demographic transition) has resulted primarily from the declining incidence of higher parity births (i.e. births to women who already have two or more children). Large families (or high-parity births) are generally seen as diluting the parental resources that are available to each child and thus threatening children's full potential.

Box 12.1 Total fertility rate (TFR)

- The TFR is equivalent to the average number of children that would be born to a woman over her lifetime were she to experience current age-specific fertility rates through her lifetime. It is a simple (non-weighted) sum of these rates divided by 1000.

- In any given year, fertility rates can be calculated for women of different ages. These 'age-specific' fertility rates are calculated for women from 15 to 49 years (with any births to women outside these ages being included in the fertility rates of 15-year-olds and 49-year-olds respectively).

(Source: Lattimore & Pobke, 2008)

Morgan & Taylor (2006, p. 7) summarise the low-fertility phenomenon in the following ways:

- Fertility timing (the age at which women have children) may have consequences for the number of children that individual women will bear.
- Parents incur high direct and indirect costs in having and rearing children in most contemporary contexts.
- Limiting families through active birth control is currently seen as both a legitimate and cultural norm.
- Given the high costs of having children it has become increasingly rare for women to have many children. In fact high parity births may be viewed as disadvantageous for parents, siblings and society more generally.

CRITICAL THINKING EXERCISE

1. How important is it to consider the changed age structure of the population, rather than population growth itself?
2. Why does having a higher ratio of working-age adults to dependents matter?
3. How will this affect women?

The trend for fertility to drop below replacement level is occurring in most developed, and some developing, countries. Aided by effective and available methods of fertility control, Australian and New Zealand women are increasingly delaying childbearing for a number of social, economic and cultural reasons.

Demographics of New Zealand women

In New Zealand the age of mothers has changed over the past 20 years, with the number of women giving birth over 30 years of age steadily increasing while births among younger women have decreased. The reducing rate for teenage women is a result not of a declining fertility rate but of an increasing abortion rate, and the birth rate in women under the age of 19 remains high by international standards. Young pregnant women—especially those without sufficient family support—require significant support from health and social services. Although the age distribution of mothers may have changed over time (Fig. 12.3), the percentage of births among each ethnic group has changed very little.

The total fertility rate for New Zealand women in 2021 is 1.60 births per woman, down from 1.99 in 2015 (Stats NZ, 2021). Fertility rates of close to or higher than 2.1 births per woman need to be sustained over many years before 'replacement level' fertility can be claimed. Since 1980, fertility in New Zealand has been slightly below replacement level. Demographers say the reasons for the decline include women delaying having children, choosing to have no children due to an increasingly precarious economic environment coupled with high house prices, a growing societal acceptance of child-free lifestyles, and the increasing accessibility of contraceptives (Spoonley, 2021) (Fig. 12.4.)

Demographics of Australian women

In Australia in 2020 the total fertility rate was 1.66 births per woman, and for Aboriginal and Torres Strait Islander women, the total fertility rate was 2.32 births per woman (ABS, 2021). After its long downward trend after the Second World War, Australia's fertility rate may have stabilised (Fig. 12.5). The current trend in fertility rates appears to be similar to that observed in other low-fertility countries including the United Kingdom, Norway and Sweden (ABS, 2021). (See also Fig. 12.4 for comparisons.)

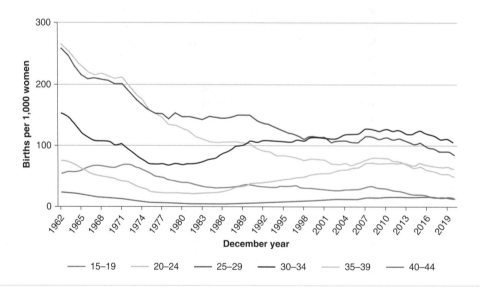

FIGURE 12.3 Age-specific birth rates in New Zealand 1962–2020
(Source: Stats NZ, 2021)

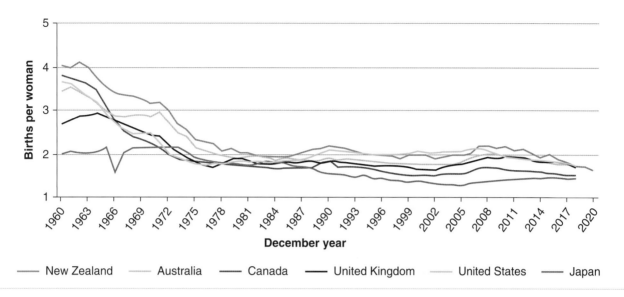

FIGURE 12.4 Total fertility rates for New Zealand and Australia 1960–2020
(Source: Stats NZ, 2021)

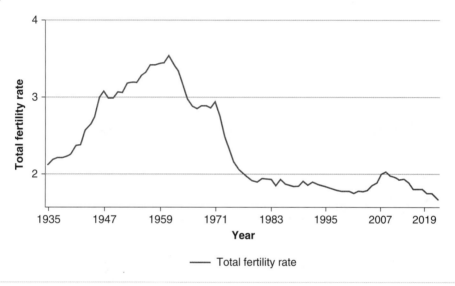

FIGURE 12.5 Australia's fertility rate 1935–2020
(Source: Australian Bureau of Statistics, 2021)

CRITICAL THINKING EXERCISE

Globally, the net reproduction rate is 1.1 surviving daughters per woman. In all regions in the world, the net reproduction rate is at or below this level, except for Africa, where the net reproduction rate is 1.9.

1. Give five reasons for this dramatic shift.
2. How strongly do these phenomena exist in Australia and New Zealand?

Delayed pregnancy

The choice of delaying pregnancy has become the norm for many women in high-income countries. Among some women, however, achieving pregnancy may be difficult or impossible at a later time. Australian and New Zealand women, like women in most high-income countries, are delaying childbirth until their thirties and forties.

The average age of first-time mothers has risen considerably in both Australia and New Zealand (Fig. 12.6).

The reasons that women and their partners elect to delay childbearing are complex and include a wide range of personal, situational and social factors (Bewley et al., 2005). They may include a lack of social and structural support for women to have their children at a time in their lives when their fertility is likely to be more viable without compromising their educational and economic goals and aspirations (Daniluk et al., 2012). Given the nature of women's emancipation and their presence in the workforce, there is a relationship between public

235

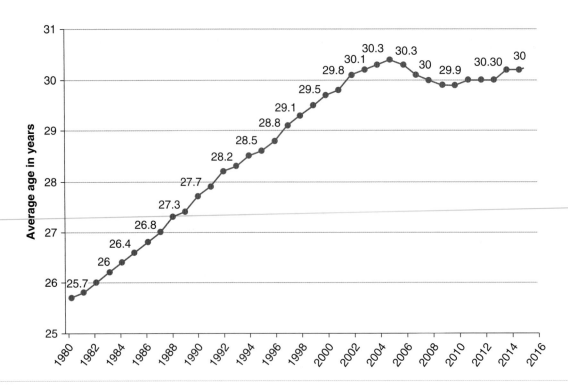

FIGURE 12.6 The median age of mothers at the birth of their first child in New Zealand, 1980–2018
(Source: Stats NZ, 2021)

policies (maternity leave, income tax regulations), workplace conditions (part-time opportunities and the flexibility of work hours) and the availability of affordable non-parental child care that enables mothers to participate in the workforce (Hank & Kreyenfeld, 2003). A growing body of research suggests a changing, now positive, relationship between women's education or employment and fertility with the advent of social contexts that allow women to combine childrearing and employment. Access to affordable child care is essential for this to occur (Hank & Kreyenfeld, 2003).

Women in Australia and New Zealand, along with women elsewhere in the developed world, have had the opportunity to delay childbearing since effective contraception became available in the 1960s. However, because fertility decreases with increasing maternal age, a slow but steady decrease in fertility is observed in women aged between 30 and 35 years, followed by an accelerated decline among women aged over 35 years. This combination of delayed childbearing and reduced fecundity with increasing age has resulted in an increased number and proportion of women greater than or equal to 35 years of age seeking assisted reproductive technology (ART) treatment (Alviggi et al., 2009). At the same time, advances in ART have improved pregnancy rates among infertile couples, adding to the growing group of primiparous women aged 35 years and older.

There were 16,140 babies born (including 15,980 liveborn babies) following ART treatment in 2018. Of these, 14,355 (88.9%) were from Australian clinics and 1785 (11.1%) from New Zealand clinics. Of the liveborn babies, 80.2% (13,018) were singletons at term (gestational age of 37–41 weeks) with normal birthweight (≥ 2,500 grams). The multiple birth rate was 3.2% (Newman et al., 2020).

In 2004, two significant studies suggested that there were higher risks associated with ART that may include poorer neonatal outcomes such as pre-term birth, low birth weight, stillbirth and neonatal deaths (Helmerhorst et al., 2004; Jackson et al., 2004). It was uncertain, however, whether the increased risks were caused by ART directly or by an association of the underlying factors causing **infertility**. The common medical definition of 'infertility' is the failure to achieve a clinical pregnancy after 12 or more months of regular unprotected sexual intercourse (Zegers-Hochschild et al., 2017).

DoPierala et al. (2016) recently found that a history of subfertility per se, rather than ART, was associated with the increased risk of adverse outcomes, at least in singleton pregnancies. Moreover, subfertile women delivering twins were at a higher risk of being delivered by emergency caesarean section. An Australian study confirmed both to be true (Barua et al., 2017); it showed that, although ART is associated with increased risk of pregnancy complications, the risk appeared greatest for women whose underlying infertility involved ovulatory dysfunction, a disorder that predisposes towards diabetes and hypertension, which is then exacerbated by pregnancy.

Time to pregnancy refers to the number of menstrual cycles it takes a couple to conceive. *Fecundability*, in turn, is a couple-specific probability of conceiving a recognised pregnancy per menstrual cycle, given no contraception

(Sallmen et al., 2005). The characteristics of 'infertile' and 'infertility' are made in reference to couples who try for more than a year to conceive. Many infertile couples will eventually conceive, but a sterile subset cannot conceive without medical intervention (Sallmen et al., 2005).

Physiological factors affecting fertility

The peak number of oocytes in the female infant occurs at about 20 weeks gestation, when there are somewhere between 6 million and 7 million oocytes. Then, by the time of birth, the number has reduced to 1 million to 2 million oocytes; by puberty 400,000 oocytes remain and by the time a woman is 37 years old she reportedly has approximately 25,000. This number drops over the years until at menopause (around 50 years of age for most women) a woman will have about 1000 remaining in her body (Lobo, 2016).

As a woman grows older, there is an ongoing rate of atresia of oocytes. The mechanism underlying this process is poorly understood and involves multiple factors encoded by genes on the X chromosome, as well as on autosomes (Simpson, 2000; Stolk et al., 2012; Vichinsartvichai, 2016). In healthy women, at approximately 37.5 years of age an accelerated atresia of the oocytes occurs (Lobo, 2016). Though poorly understood, it is often associated with a small monotrophic rise in the level of follicle-stimulating hormone (FSH), resulting in more activin production leading to enhanced FSH action and decreased fecundity and increased risk of aneuploidy (Alviggi et al., 2009; Lobo, 2016; Scott et al., 1989). The subtle increase in the level of FSH is thought to increase atresia, which is coupled with an accelerated loss of follicles and a further increase in FSH, resulting in a positive-feedback loop (Erickson, 2000).

It is estimated that natural fertility ceases on average 10 years before menopause (Lambalk et al., 2009). Therefore, women who are destined to go through menopause at the age of 45 years (10% of the population) might be expected to have accelerated atresia and reduced fecundity from the age of 32 years. As atresia continues, both the number and the quality of oocytes fall below a critical level. It is well recognised that there is a decrease in the quality of the oocytes with advancing maternal age, as shown by the higher incidence of chromosomal anomalies such as aneuploidies, which in turn reduce the chances of successful fertilisation, implantation and early embryo development (Nwandison & Bewley, 2006). This increase in the rate of aneuploidy is related at least in part to problems of the meiotic spindle resulting in nondisjunction, and this process leads to a greater risk of spontaneous abortion once pregnancy occurs.

Menopause timing has a substantial impact on infertility. Although environmental factors are important, genetic factors predict 44%–87% of the variance in the age at menopause (de Bruin et al., 2001; Schoenaker et al., 2014; van Asselt et al., 2004). Primary ovarian insufficiency (POI), traditionally known as premature ovarian failure, which is defined as menopause before the age of 40 years or hypergonadotrophic amenorrhoea, occurs in up to 0.9% of women in the general population and has multiple causes, including the involvement of several genes. Once POI has been established, fertility is usually lost, although spontaneous pregnancies may occur. Familial POI and environmental factors that may deplete ovarian follicles define this risk category.

Epigenetics (changes in gene expression caused by the environment) may also affect the age at menopause (Ge et al., 2015; Kanherkar et al., 2014). Many genes are known to be involved in the menopause process—such as those implicated in DNA repair and immune function (Kanherkar et al., 2014; Stolk et al., 2012). Environmental factors have been shown to cause epigenetic changes associated with DNA methylation and histone proteins (Joehanes et al., 2016) and have also been reported to shorten the functional life span of a woman's ovaries. Poor diet may play a role in the occurrence of early menopause (Baird et al., 1998; Sapre & Thakur, 2014), as well as cigarette smoking, which is one of the most common and important factors that affects follicle maturation, owing to the compounds in tobacco which exert a deleterious effect (Freour et al., 2008; Plante et al., 2010; Soares & Melo, 2008).

Pelvic diseases—such as endometriosis, neoplasms and infection—may require surgery, which by removing and destroying cortical tissue depletes the follicular or oocyte reservoir and may lead to early menopause. In addition, pelvic surgery may lead to the formation of adhesions, which may affect the ability to conceive naturally. Among the women at greatest risk for the inability to reproduce are those undergoing treatment for cancer, because of the effects of multidrug chemotherapy.

Physiological factors affecting age-related male fertility are summarised in Box 12.2).

The body fat connection

That excessive exercise or undernutrition can postpone puberty, reduce fertility or prevent menstruation was first discovered by Rose Frisch in her pioneering studies beginning in the late 1960s (Box 12.3). Her work describing the reproductive consequences of an altered mass of fat was largely ignored or treated with scepticism. Her hypothesis—that a critical mass of body fat is the crucial trigger of gonadotrophin secretion, both in developing girls and in mature women during reproductive life—was initially based on detailed analysis of worldwide demographic data and was later supported by highly focused clinical investigation (Reichlin, 2003).

In otherwise healthy young women, a critical mass of body fat is the essential trigger of cyclical pituitary–ovarian function. A successful pregnancy requires approximately 50,000 calories stored in the form of fat. A critical body fat mass determines the onset of menses. Excessive leanness, as in people with anorexia nervosa and some competitive athletes and professional dancers, delays the onset of puberty; after menarche has been established,

Box 12.2   Men, ageing and fertility

- Age-related changes occur in the testes. Leydig cells decrease in number and changes also occur in the basal membranes, seminiferous tubules and tunica albuginea. These result in changes in spermatogenesis, both reduced sperm count and increased genetic abnormalities.

- Those genetic abnormalities associated with abnormal sperm tend to result in early abortion rather than live birth. Chromosomal anomalies that are known to be due to paternal origin, such as the XYY karyotype and 45XO (Turner's syndrome), have not been shown to be related to paternal age.

- It is becoming clearer that with advancing paternal age (50 years or more) the risk of early or late fetal loss is almost double compared with that of younger fathers after adjusting for maternal age and other maternal variables.

- The risk of early pregnancy loss is compounded if both maternal age is over 35 years and paternal age is over 40 years.

(Source: Nwandison & Bewley, 2006. What is the right age to reproduce? *Fetal Matern Med Rev*. 17(3):185–204, doi:10.1017/S0965539506001781. Reproduced with permission)

Box 12.3   The body fat connection

Rose Frisch was the scientist who discovered during her studies on weight gain in populations around the world that poor rural girls had their peak rate of growth at an older age than well-nourished urban girls. Since it was known at the time that a period of rapid growth precedes the onset of menarche, she analysed several large population studies in the United States in which the rate of growth and the age of menarche had been assessed, and found that the average weight at menarche was 47 kg whether girls matured early or late. She realised that body weight was a more accurate predictor than chronological age of the age at onset of menstruation.

(Source: Reichlin, 2003)

excessive leanness can cause impaired ovulation, infertility and amenorrhoea. Oestrogen deficiency induced by excessive exercise (and decreased fat mass) is associated with premature osteoporosis, even in runners in whom bone formation has been stimulated by exercise. On the positive side, women who have been extremely active athletically have a much-reduced risk of breast cancer, presumably because they have been exposed to lower levels of oestrogen over time. These insights have been invaluable for the evaluation of women with delayed puberty and amenorrhoea, and they have important social and medical implications for dancers and athletes.

Critical body fat mass is probably also important in determining pituitary gonadal activity in men, though it is less well documented (Reichlin, 2003, p. 870).

OLDER WOMEN AND CHILDBIRTH

Many women over age 35 have healthy pregnancies and healthy babies. Very advanced maternal age, defined as maternal age of 45 years or greater at the time of birth, has important consequences for both mother and baby. Currently, 0.35% of all Australian and 0.2% of all New Zealand women giving birth are in this age category (ABS, 2021; Stats NZ, 2021). Given the trend towards delayed childbearing and the increasing availability of assisted reproductive techniques, women aged 45 and over may increasingly seek advice about the risks of embarking on a pregnancy (Callaway et al., 2005).

The effect of maternal age on the outcome of pregnancy may be best assessed by examining five specific factors (Heffner, 2004) that can negatively affect the desired outcome of a pregnancy—a healthy mother and baby. These are:

- declining fertility
- miscarriage
- chromosomal abnormalities
- hypertensive complications
- stillbirth.

It is not unusual for a woman in her mid thirties or older to take longer to conceive than a younger woman. Age-related *decline in fertility* may be due, in part, to less-frequent ovulation or to problems such as endometriosis, in which tissue similar to that lining the uterus attaches to the ovaries or fallopian tubes and interferes with conception. While women over age 35 may have more difficulty conceiving, they also have a greater chance of bearing twins. The likelihood of naturally conceived (without fertility treatment) twins peaks between ages 35 and 39, then declines.

Miscarriage is defined as 'spontaneous pregnancy loss before the 20th week of gestation' in Australia and New Zealand and before 24 weeks of gestation in the UK and Europe (Jurkovic et al., 2013). Chromosomal abnormalities are the most common cause of first-trimester miscarriage and are detected in 50%–85% of pregnancy tissue specimens after spontaneous miscarriage. Trisomies account for about two-thirds of these, and the risk of trisomy increases with maternal age (Jurkovic et al., 2013). There is a strong relationship between maternal age and miscarriage rates (Fig. 12.7). A prominent Danish study found that about 9% of recognised pregnancies for women aged 20–24 ended in miscarriage. The risk rose to about 25% at age 35–9, and to more than 50% by age 42 (Andersen et al., 2000). It increases to a high of more than 90% among women aged 45 years or older. This high miscarriage rate contributes significantly to decreasing fertility among **older women** (Heffner, 2004). Most miscarriages occur in the first trimester for women of all ages.

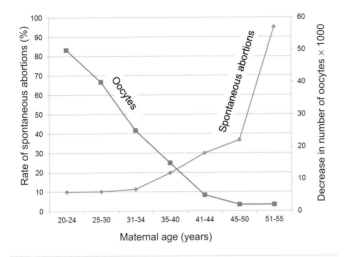

FIGURE 12.7 The maternal age-related decline in fertility is accompanied by a significant decrease in oocytes and an increased percentage rate of spontaneous abortion

(Source: The American College of Obstetricians and Gynecologists Committee on Gynecologic Practice and The Practice Committee of the American Society for Reproductive Medicine, 2016. Female Age-related Fertility Decline: https://www.acog.org/Clinical-Guidance-and-Publications/Committee-Opinions/Committee-on-Gynecologic-Practice/Female-Age-Related-Fertility-Decline)

The success rate in using donor eggs from younger women for in vitro fertilisation supports the hypothesis that deterioration occurs in the quality of the ova with advancing maternal age (Heffner, 2004).

The risk of giving birth to a baby with certain *chromosomal abnormalities* also increases as a woman ages. The most common of these disorders is Down syndrome, a combination of mental retardation and physical abnormalities caused by the presence of an extra chromosome 21 (humans have 23 pairs of chromosomes) (Fig. 12.8). Most pregnant women who are 35 or older are offered the option of prenatal testing (with amniocentesis or chorionic villus sampling) to diagnose or, more likely, rule out

Down syndrome and other chromosomal abnormalities. About 95% of women who undergo prenatal testing find that their baby does not have one of these disorders. If prenatal testing rules out chromosomal defects and the mother is healthy, the baby probably is at no greater risk of birth defects than if the mother were in her twenties.

Both chronic *hypertension* (that antedates pregnancy) and pregnancy-induced hypertension usually occur during the second half of a pregnancy and include both hypertension without proteinuria and the many variants of the disorder preeclampsia. All forms of hypertension can complicate pregnancies by restricting fetal growth and may necessitate premature delivery when the health of either the mother or the fetus is in jeopardy. 'The risk of hypertensive complications of pregnancy increases steadily as women age; such complications are twice as likely among women aged 40 years or older as among younger women' (Heffner, 2004, p. 1928).

Besides the increased risk of diabetes and high blood pressure, women over 35 have an increased risk of placental problems. The most common placental problem is placenta praevia, in which the placenta covers part or all of the opening of the cervix. First-time mothers over age 40 were up to eight times as likely as women in their twenties to have this complication. Some studies suggest that women having their first baby at age 35 or older are at increased risk of having either a low-birth-weight or a pre-term baby (born at less than 37 full weeks of pregnancy). These risks rise modestly but progressively with a woman's age, even if she does not have age-related chronic health problems such as diabetes and high blood pressure. A Danish study also found that women over age 35 had an increased risk of ectopic pregnancy (in which the fertilised egg implants in the fallopian tube) (Andersen et al., 2000).

How should we counsel young women when they ask about their reproductive choices? Generally speaking, the decade between 25 and 35 years of age would seem to be ideal. A woman's education is typically complete, she has usually gained some experience in her professional arena, and pregnancy is at its safest. For women between 35 and

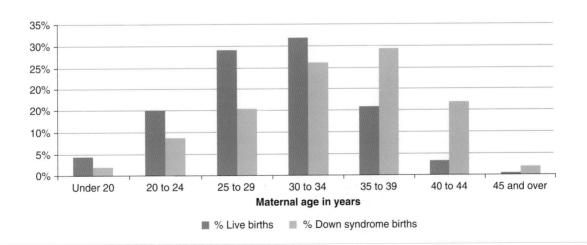

FIGURE 12.8 Prevalence of Down syndrome related to mother's age at time of birth

45 years of age for whom earlier childbearing was not an option, this decade remains safe enough that maternal age alone should not be a contraindication to childbearing. However, women do face decreasing fertility and a moderate increase in the risks of miscarriage and chromosomal abnormalities as they pass 40 years of age (Wood et al., 1992). Perimenopausal and postmenopausal pregnancy remains an option for those women who are lucky enough to find themselves healthy and sufficiently wealthy to pursue it (Heffner, 2004).

TEENAGE PREGNANCIES

In many industrialised countries, teenage pregnancy and teenage parenthood (regardless of marital status) have in recent years been identified as social and public health problems that need to be tackled, though the level of concern varies by context (Shaw et al., 2006). Among teenage mothers in Australia and New Zealand the birth rate continues to decline. This decline is thought to be due to increased access to sex education, contraception and abortion (Shaw et al., 2006).

Teenage parents tend to remain poor and be relatively socially and economically disadvantaged, especially compared with older mothers. This has been substantiated by recent research into the outcomes of teenage pregnancy in Australia, which found that the socioeconomic circumstances of young mothers was more indicative of health outcomes than young maternal age alone and suggested that, whereas health policy tends to focus on maternal age and reducing the number of births to teenagers, interventions 'aimed at reducing maternal poverty and increasing support among those from the most deprived backgrounds may be more effective ways of improving childhood psychological, cognitive, behavioural and health outcomes than would interventions aimed solely at reducing rates of teenage pregnancy and parenthood' (Khatun et al., 2017; Shaw et al., 2006).

Thirty years ago, a study of 37 developed countries including Denmark, Finland, Norway and Sweden showed a relationship between low fertility rates and openness about sexual matters, government policy for providing contraceptives for young unmarried women, well-organised teaching about contraception in schools, and a high percentage of the population living in large cities (Jones et al., 1985).

It is believed that the main reason for a drop in abortion rates worldwide is increased use of contraceptive methods (Chescheir, 2017). In the Netherlands a national emphasis on the importance of contraceptive methods, ongoing positive sex education in schools and easily accessible, low-cost and friendly contraceptive services are the main reasons for low fertility and abortion rates (Ketting & Visser, 1994). In Sweden, accessible contraceptive services for young people were introduced through the development of teenage clinics, run by midwives, which now comprise over 200 nationwide (Bender et al., 2003). The link between fertility and use of contraception, and its preventive effect regarding abortion, was recognised.

Sweden also developed an effective link between sex education in schools and contraceptive services for young people (Bender et al., 2003). The early onset of sexual activity indicates that it is important to ensure that all young people have information about contraception and disease prevention *before* they begin their sexual careers and not simply in their final years of schooling (Rissel et al., 2003). Health promotion, including mandatory sex education, is essential for all young people, male as well as female, and those under as well as over 16 years of age. Studies comparing sexual health outcomes in young people who are subject to sex educational policies in the Netherlands, the United States, France and Australia found that in France and the Netherlands, where there is mandatory secondary school sex education, there are fewer sexually transmitted infections than in Australia and far fewer than in the United States, where sex education is patchy (Weaver et al., 2005).

In Western industrialised countries, *Chlamydia trachomatis* is the predominant infectious agent causing pelvic inflammatory disease that, as a result of damage to the fallopian tubes, accounts for up to half of all ectopic pregnancies. Australian prevalence surveys have shown that chlamydia is a significant health problem in Australia and that prevalence is higher among young women aged 16–24 years (Lewis et al., 2012; Vajdic et al., 2005) and more so in the indigenous population (Bright, 2015; Lewis et al., 2012). The notification rate was over three times higher in the Aboriginal and Torres Strait Islander populations in the Northern Territory, Queensland, South Australia and Western Australia than in the non-indigenous population (Bright, 2015; Kirby Institute, 2016). The substantial financial costs of genital chlamydial infections result from hospital treatment for pelvic inflammatory disease, ectopic pregnancy and infertility, which may indirectly include in vitro fertilisation.

ASSISTED REPRODUCTIVE TECHNOLOGY (ART) OR ASSISTED HUMAN REPRODUCTION (AHR)

Assisted reproductive technology (ART) is a group of procedures that involve the in vitro (outside of body) handling of human oocytes (eggs) and sperm or embryos for the purposes of establishing a pregnancy. Each ART treatment involves a number of stages and is generally referred to as an ART treatment cycle. The embryos transferred to a woman can either originate from the cycle in which they were created (fresh cycle) or be frozen (cryopreserved) and thawed before transfer (thaw cycle) (Newman et al., 2020).

With an increasing number of women electing to delay childbearing, there is a critical need for public education regarding age-related fertility declines and the availability, costs and limitations of assisted human reproduction.

Women who delay pregnancy until they are in their middle to late 30s often regret waiting and wish they had started their families earlier. The long-term psychosocial and societal implications of this increasing trend, which include unintentional childlessness and smaller and more socially complex families, have yet to be fully understood. In 2011 Metwally & Ledger published a paper outlining the key points relating to the known long-term complications of assisted reproduction. They stated in their conclusion:

> ARTs have been linked to several long-term complications affecting both the mother and the child. It is essential that those who provide this form of fertility treatment are fully aware of these complications and that information and support are available to couples during, and well after, their fertility treatment. As new ARTs are introduced, it is imperative that follow-up studies are conducted to determine the long-term safety of these technologies and that national registries are designed to make the appropriate data accessible.
>
> (Metwally & Ledger, 2011, p. 84)

The main complications discussed in this review (Metwally & Ledger, 2011) included the potential for rare but serious risk of thromboembolic disease particularly in the upper half of the body and a higher risk of pregnancy complications including abnormal placentation, miscarriage, gestational diabetes and hypertensive disorders. A link between assisted conception and a number of genital cancers, particularly of the breast, ovary and endometrium, is also reviewed showing that the evidence is currently inconclusive. A number of fetal and neonatal complications including imprinting disorders, low birth weight, congenital malformations and growth disorders were also considered (Metwally & Ledger, 2011).

METHODS OF ASSISTED REPRODUCTION

Conception depends on a woman releasing an egg each month. The egg enters the fallopian tube where it meets the sperm. A sperm cell penetrates the egg in the process known as fertilisation. The resulting embryo is transported down the tube to the uterus, where it implants into the uterine lining (endometrium) a few days later. In general, 75% of couples will achieve a spontaneous pregnancy within 6 months of exposure, 90% by a year and 95% by 2 years. Three major factors determine the chances of a natural conception: female age, sperm quality and duration of exposure.

Common first-line investigatory tests for infertility are:

For women:
- cervical smear test
- urinalysis for *Chlamydia trachomatis* (which may block the fallopian tubes)
- blood test to measure progesterone (7 days before a menstrual period is due)
- test for rubella (if contracted within first 3 months after conception, it can cause harm to the fetus)

- blood test at the time of menstruation to check hormone imbalances such as
  - FSH (follicle-stimulating hormone)
  - LH (luteinising hormone)
  - oestradiol
- anti-Mullerian hormone (AMH; AMH is produced by follicles in the ovaries which contain the eggs and can indicate the ovarian reserve, or how many eggs remain. This is often used as a test for subfertility due to onset of menopause.)
- pelvic ultrasound to examine the patency and health of the fallopian tubes and other pelvic organs

For men:
- semen analysis checking sperm for:
  - motility—how many sperm can swim
  - morphology—the shape of the sperm
  - count—how many individual sperm are present in the sample
  - vitality—how healthy the sperm are and their chance of survival
- urine test for *Chlamydia trachomatis*, which, in addition to being a known cause of infertility in women, can also affect sperm function and male fertility.

It is well known that the risk of an adverse outcome after in vitro fertilisation (IVF) is attributable in large part to the greatly increased rate of multiple births. As such, in 2013 a Cochrane review was carried out to evaluate the effectiveness and safety of the number of embryos transferred in couples who undergo ART (Pandian et al., 2013). The review concluded that repeated single embryo transfer (SET) (two cycles of fresh SET or one fresh SET followed by one frozen SET) was the best option as it may minimise the risk of multiple pregnancies compared with other embryo transfer policies without substantially reducing the likelihood of achieving a live birth. Today SET utilisation has increased globally, now representing more than half of all ART cycles in Japan, Australia and New Zealand (Kushnir et al., 2017).

Over the last five years the proportion of cycles where all oocytes or embryos were cryopreserved for potential future use (freeze-all cycles) has doubled from 13% of initiated fresh cycles in 2014 to 26.7% in 2018. This practice is used for a variety of reasons, including reducing the risk of ovarian hyperstimulation syndrome (OHSS), improving endometrial–embryo synchronicity, as part of a pre-implantation genetic testing (PGT) cycle or for fertility preservation (Newman et al., 2020).

Higher risks of pre-term birth and low birth weight (LBW) are associated with singletons conceived by IVF and have been attributed at least in part to parental characteristics associated with infertility, such as high maternal age and nulliparity (Sunderam et al., 2017; Thurin et al., 2004). In Australia and New Zealand, pre-term birth and LBW are, respectively, 1.3 times and 1.5 times more likely to occur among singletons conceived by transfer of fresh embryos, compared with transfer of frozen embryos. Pre-term birth and LBW are, in addition, more common among couples who had female factor infertility compared with male factor infertility (Newman et al., 2020; Wang et al., 2009).

In vitro fertilisation

In vitro fertilisation (IVF) involves four basic steps: ovarian stimulation, egg recovery, insemination and, finally, embryo replacement. Although IVF was originally devised for women with tubal damage or dysfunction, in combination with intracytoplasmic sperm injection (ICSI) it is a very effective method to treat male factor infertility. In vitro fertilisation treatment may be used in selected instances with donated eggs, sperm or embryos.

It is important to establish the cause of infertility before proceeding to IVF. Investigations would usually include checks of ovulation, tubal patency and an ultrasound for the female partner. A semen analysis is required for the male partner.

Ovarian stimulation

During a natural unstimulated cycle, a follicle containing a single egg develops to maturity. To produce more eggs it is necessary to stimulate the ovaries with a group of drugs known as gonadotrophins. Ovarian hyperstimulation (an excessive response) is a major and potentially life-threatening complication associated with gonadotrophins (see Abandoned cycles).

It is safest to monitor the response of the ovaries by daily oestrogen measurements and ultrasound. Ultrasound scans are used to see the number and size of the follicles and to judge when to do the egg recovery. The oestrogens are necessary to determine the ovarian response to stimulation. By interpreting the results of ultrasound and oestrogen, the specialist will determine the best time to perform the egg collection. About 36 hours before the egg collection is due, an injection of human chorionic gonadotrophin (hCG) is given to initiate the final process of egg maturation. Precise timing is necessary, as the eggs will be suitable for recovery 34–6 hours after the hCG injection.

Egg collection

This is done under sedation or general anaesthetic using a vaginal ultrasound probe. A needle is guided through the top of the vagina into the ovary. Each follicle is aspirated through the needle using a suction device.

Insemination and fertilisation

The eggs are identified in the laboratory and placed in culture medium. They are then placed in dishes in an incubator. The male partner produces a semen sample by masturbation and this is prepared in the laboratory. A number of motile sperm are extracted and used to inseminate the eggs some hours later. It takes about 18 hours for fertilisation to be completed, and about 12 hours later the embryo starts to divide. Two or three days after egg collection, when the embryos have reached the 2- to 6-cell stage, they are ready to be replaced into the woman's uterus.

Embryo transfer

This is a most important step and is best performed under ultrasound guidance. A maximum of two embryos may be replaced. Couples should consider the replacement of a single embryo to prevent a twin pregnancy. There is no evidence that bed rest makes a difference to the outcome and most units recommend resuming normal activities.

Luteal support

Hormone supplementation in the form of hCG injections, or progesterone pessaries or injections, is usually recommended after embryo transfer, to support the uterine lining.

Embryo freezing

Most IVF clinics offer embryo freezing and storage for spare embryos. However, not all surplus embryos are suitable for freezing, not all survive the procedure and the implantation rate after transfer is lower than with fresh embryo transfer.

Abandoned cycles

The abandoned cycle rate varies considerably between units. Cycles may be abandoned before egg recovery as the ovarian response is either inadequate or excessive, and before embryo replacement if no eggs are recovered, or the eggs fail to fertilise or the embryos don't divide. In many instances it will be possible to try again using alternative drugs or methods, such as ICSI for failed fertilisation.

Occasionally IVF cycles are abandoned because of a high risk of ovarian hyperstimulation. (The risk of ovarian hyperstimulation is increased in women with polycystic ovaries.) In these circumstances the cycle may be cancelled during ovarian stimulation and restarted with a lower dose of drugs, or allowed to proceed but with all the embryos frozen and replaced when the ovaries have returned to normal.

The ovarian hyperstimulation syndrome is potentially life threatening. This syndrome occurs in about 2%–3% of cases and consists of severe nausea and vomiting, a rapid gain in weight, abdominal swelling and shortness of breath. The fluid and electrolyte imbalance needs careful management in experienced centres. It starts a week after the hCG injection and is made worse by pregnancy.

Support when undergoing treatment

It is well recognised that undergoing assisted conception treatment, particularly IVF, is both emotionally and physically stressful for couples. It is essential that women and their partners fully understand the proposed treatment program and the commitment in time required for monitoring the cycle. Most clinics have information sheets and some have support groups to help in times of stress. All licensed centres are obliged to offer independent counselling to patients considering IVF treatment. This may prove helpful, as it gives the opportunity for the partners to discuss their infertility and treatment confidentially with an impartial person.

Gamete intrafallopian transfer

Gamete intrafallopian transfer (GIFT) can be considered both a sophisticated form of artificial insemination and a simplified form of IVF. The management of a patient in a GIFT treatment cycle is usually exactly the same as for an

IVF cycle, up until the point at which the oocytes (eggs) have been recovered. A number of drug regimens are used to stimulate the ovaries to produce multiple oocytes, and these are always discussed with the couple at the time the treatment is started.

The growth of the ovarian follicles in which the eggs are developing is always monitored with a combination of serial ultrasound scans and often blood or urine tests. When the follicles are considered to be mature enough, arrangements are made for the patient to receive an injection of hCG and the egg recovery procedure is planned for some 34–6 hours later.

Most clinics now will recover the oocytes by the transvaginal ultrasound-directed technique, as for IVF. Some clinics will, however, recover the eggs laparoscopically. Once the oocytes have been collected and identified, the best two or three are selected. A preparation of the partner's or donor's sperm is taken into a fine catheter, together with the eggs; the tube is gently inserted under direct vision through the laparoscope into the outer ends of one or both fallopian tubes; then the egg/sperm mixture is injected into the tube(s). At the end of this procedure, the woman is returned to the ward to recover, and will go home the same day. Most women are given either injections or pessaries of the hormone progesterone, and some 15 days later a pregnancy test is carried out to determine whether there is early evidence of a pregnancy.

GIFT is generally found to be slightly more successful than IVF in most clinics. This is probably because the fallopian tube is a more physiological environment for fertilisation to occur in than is a laboratory culture dish. However, the procedure does require a laparoscopy, and most clinics now do not generally believe that the extra inconvenience of and potential discomfort of a laparoscopy makes the slightly increased pregnancy rates worthwhile. If a clinic is achieving good results with IVF, then it will generally not do GIFT. Clinics achieving poorer success rates with IVF may find that GIFT is considerably more successful and therefore recommend it. Pregnancy rates are commonly quoted as being in the range of 15%–30% for IVF and 25%–30% for GIFT.

Intracytoplasmic sperm injection

Intracytoplasmic sperm injection (ICSI) was introduced into clinical treatment for certain types of infertility in 1992. It is a type of IVF treatment that involves the injection of a single sperm straight into each egg. The fertilised egg (embryo) can then be transferred into the womb of the woman as in a normal IVF cycle. ICSI quickly became the favoured technique for cases of male factor infertility, as it was discovered that the basic semen parameters, such as having a low sperm count or less motile sperm (Oehninger, 2001), had little impact on its success.

The live-birth rates for ICSI and conventional IVF are similar—about 25% per cycle, in the most recently published Human Fertilisation and Embryology Authority (HFEA) data from the United Kingdom (Human Fertilisation & Embryology Authority, 2016).

What does ICSI involve?

Intracytoplasmic sperm injection is similar to conventional IVF in that gametes (eggs and sperm) are collected from each partner. To achieve fertilisation, a single sperm is taken up in a fine glass needle and is injected directly into an egg. The eggs are then incubated and examined. Usually one or two embryos may then be transferred back into the womb of the woman 2–3 days after fertilisation. Some eggs may not survive the injection process, and not all eggs collected will be of a high-enough quality or mature enough to be suitable for injection.

When is ICSI used?

In conventional IVF the eggs and the sperm are mixed together in a dish and the sperm fertilise the eggs naturally. ICSI bypasses the natural processes involved in a sperm penetrating an egg, and is therefore used when there are problems that make it difficult to achieve fertilisation naturally or by conventional IVF. It is used when:

- the sperm count is very low
- the sperm cannot move properly or are in other ways abnormal
- the sperm have been retrieved directly from the epididymis (PESA) or the testicles (TESA/TESE, see Box 12.4), from the urine, or by electro-ejaculation
- there are high levels of antibodies in the semen
- there have been previous fertilisation failures.

Men who have very few sperm (oligozoospermia) or no sperm (azoospermia) in their semen, or who have high numbers of abnormal sperm that are unable to fertilise an egg, would previously have had little or no chance of fathering their own genetic offspring.

Like IVF, ICSI is an invasive procedure. However, unlike IVF, ICSI involves injecting a sperm directly into an egg, therefore allowing the use of sperm that might not otherwise be able to fertilise an egg. For these reasons, concerns about the potential risks to children born as a result of ICSI have been raised, and several follow-up studies have been published.

As the number of children born from ICSI procedures has exponentially increased, greater attention has focused on the safety of the procedure (Davies et al., 2012; Pereira et al., 2017; Wong & Ledger, 2013). Follow-up studies are extremely important. The complexity of the process of egg and sperm production means that even if

---

> ### Box 12.4 Terms used in assisted reproductive technology
>
> - PESA—percutaneous epididymal sperm aspiration, involving sperm being retrieved directly from the epididymis using a needle.
> - TESA—testicular sperm aspiration, involving sperm being retrieved directly from the testes using a needle.
> - TESE—testicular sperm extraction, involving sperm being retrieved from a biopsy of testicular tissue.

an individual possesses a normal number of chromosomes, their gametes could potentially have an abnormal number. Babies born after ICSI have been reported to have new chromosomal abnormalities in up to 3% of cases compared with the general population of 0.6%. However, it is uncertain whether these abnormalities linked with ICSI were caused by the treatment itself or the underlying infertility (Human Fertilisation & Embryology Authority, 2016).

The ICSI procedure

The woman is stimulated for follicle production, as in conventional IVF. Egg recovery is identical to that for routine IVF, but sperm treatment differs according to individual patient circumstances and, even if obtained from ejaculate, often requires a modification of the procedures used for IVF. This modification uses a high-centrifugation method to concentrate the contents of the seminal plasma into the size of a tiny fraction of a teardrop from which just a few sperm can be obtained and extracted. In certain circumstances microinjection needles are used (approximately 12 times thinner than a strand of human hair) to isolate single sperm from the seminal plasma.

Whichever method is used—centrifugation or single sperm isolation—it is essential that the sperm be washed free of the seminal plasma. The human egg aspirated from the follicle is surrounded by thousands of specialised cells—the cumulus cells (these perform a 'nursing' role while the egg is in the follicle). These cumulus cells are removed by treatment with hyaluronidase, a natural enzyme that is produced by the sperm during its passage through the cumulus cells while in the fallopian tube. In less than a couple of minutes the enzyme digests away the cells, leaving the egg encased in a few layers of another type of specialised cells. These are mechanically removed by the embryologist using gentle suction into a very finely pulled glass tube. The egg denuded of almost all its surrounding cells is then accessible for ICSI.

The ICSI procedure per se begins by first immobilising the sperm. This is often performed by transferring the sperm into a viscous solution, which dramatically slows down its motility. In its sluggish state the single sperm has its tail permanently immobilised—this has been shown to be an extremely important part of the process. The sperm is then aspirated into the tiny microinjection needle and carefully maintained at its tip. The needle is manipulated using a micromanipulator, which has extremely fine control capabilities. The egg itself is held onto another microtool by gentle suction to keep it firmly positioned. The needle containing the sperm is pushed gently up against the outer shell (zone pellucida) and then through the shell, through the outer membrane of the egg and directly into the egg's cytoplasm.

Once the needle is inside the egg, a tiny amount of cytoplasm is aspirated into the microinjection needle to mix with the sperm and ensure that the egg has been properly penetrated. Despite the tiny size of the egg (approximately seven times smaller than the average full stop), the membrane is a very elastic structure and can be extensively stretched without actually being ruptured. Once the embryologist is certain that the egg has been penetrated, the sperm and cytoplasmic mixture is injected back into the egg. This procedure rarely causes residual damage to the egg, and has no lasting effects on further development. The whole procedure is performed under a high-powered microscope. In some cases, immotile but living sperm is used. It is therefore important for the embryologists to be able to distinguish between dead and living immotile sperm. In this situation a solution is used that causes the tail of a living but immotile sperm to curl. The curled tail indicates which sperm are actually living, and the embryologist selects these with the microinjection needle. Once isolated, the sperm can then be transferred to the viscous solution and treated in the same way for the ICSI procedure.

At the end of the injection procedure the microinjection needle is carefully withdrawn and the suction on the egg is released. The egg is washed through a few changes of normal culture medium, and left overnight in an incubator at 37°C in conditions similar to routine IVF culture. The subsequent culture procedures, checking for fertilisation, cleavage of the fertilised egg and transfer of any embryos to the womb, occur in the same routine manner as for conventional IVF.

⚲ CLINICAL POINT

The first IVF baby, Louise Brown, was born in the United Kingdom in 1978, and France had its first *bébé éprouvette* in 1982, called Amandine.

LAWS ABOUT DONATION

Laws around donation in ART vary within and between Australian states and also between New Zealand and Australia. In New Zealand and parts of Australia, the identity of donors is recorded. Knowing about our genetic heritage can help us to understand who we are. This can be important for the following reasons:

- *For the psychological and emotional wellbeing of donor-conceived people*—many of them, like people who have been adopted, are naturally curious about their genetic origins.
- *For medical reasons*—inherited characteristics may predispose the offspring to certain medical conditions. Knowing the medical history may help to get an early diagnosis and effective treatment for an inherited disease.
- *For family relationships*—family secrets can undermine trust and lead to conflict and stress. They can also suggest to children (and others) that their parents are ashamed of how they were conceived.
- *For donor-conceived people's future relationships*—there is a small but real risk that two people who are genetic siblings could have children together without realising they were related. If parents tell their children they were donor conceived, they will be able to check this out.

• *For donors*—donors are often curious about the children they may have created. Under the law in New Zealand and some states in Australia they are able to find out from the clinic how many children were born as a result of their donation. They will not be able to identify them by name, however, although children will be able to find out who the donor was and may wish to contact them.

REFLECTIVE THINKING EXERCISE

1. What are some of the ethical dilemmas around knowing the identity of a donor:
   a. for the offspring?
   b. for the donor parent?
2. Reflect on the approach to egg donation. Should the process be anonymous? If so, why?

DEMOGRAPHICS OF ASSISTED REPRODUCTION

Data on ART in Australia and New Zealand

Since 1979, ART has been used in Australia to help couples achieve pregnancy. The main procedures used in ART treatment cycles include IVF, ICSI and GIFT. The most recent national estimates indicate that 4.9% of all women who gave birth in Australia in 2018 received some form of ART treatment (AIHW, 2021).

Data on treatment cycles and outcomes of pregnancy are collected annually and are collated into an Australian and New Zealand Assisted Conception Data Collection (ACDC). The data collection is funded by the Fertility Society of Australia and is maintained at the National Perinatal Statistics Unit (NPSU). Results of treatments and outcomes of pregnancies in previous years' treatments were reported annually in the past, from the ACDC. With the implementation of the Australian and New Zealand Assisted Reproduction Database (ANZARD), the results of the treatments and their pregnancy outcomes can be reported as a single cohort in the same year in the AIHW Assisted Conception series (see Newman et al., 2020; Online resources). See Fig. 12.9.

Birth outcomes following ART

In vitro fertilisation was introduced into practice with little formal evaluation of its effects on the health of the children conceived with this procedure. Following the introduction of ICSI in 1992, there was a concern that infants conceived with the use of ART might have an increased risk of birth defects (Davies et al., 2017; Hansen et al., 2002; te Velde et al., 1998). A study published in the *New England Journal of Medicine* (Hansen et al., 2002) found that infants conceived with ART were more than twice as likely as naturally conceived infants to have major birth anomalies diagnosed during the first year of life, and were also more likely to have multiple major anomalies. The increase in the risk of a major birth anomaly associated with assisted conception remained significant when only singleton or term singleton

	Number of initiated ART cycles	Percentage of treatment types	Number of clinical pregnancies	Number of live births	Number of liveborn babies	Number of liveborn singletons at term with normal birthweight
Autologous	79,072	94.1	18,440	14,626	15,103	12,334
Fresh	*48,048*	*57.2*	*7,399*	*5,799*	*5,994*	*4,803*
Thaw	*31,024*	*36.9*	*11,041*	*8,827*	*9,109*	*7,531*
Oocyte recipient	2,950	3.5	801	629	649	500
Embryo recipient	548	0.7	168	132	139	104
Oocyte donation	1,078	1.3	0	0	0	0
GIFT[a]	4	0.0	2	2	2	2
Surrogacy arrangement cycles	412	0.5	103	86	87	78
Commissioning cycles[b]	*137*	*0.2*	*0*	*0*	*0*	*0*
Gestational carrier cycles[c]	*275*	*0.3*	*103*	*86*	*87*	*78*
Total	**84,064**	**100.0**	**19,514**	**15,475**	**15,980**	**13,018**

(a) GIFT cycles were classified separately from autologous cycles.
(b) A variety of cycle types undertaken as part of surrogacy arrangements, e.g. cycles undertaken by intended parents or women donating their oocytes or embryos for use by the gestational carrier.
(c) A cycle undertaken by a women who carries, or intends to carry, a pregnancy on behalf of the intended parents with an agreement that the child will be raised by the intended parent(s).

FIGURE 12.9 Number of initiated ART treatment cycles by treatment type, Australia and New Zealand, 2018
(Source: Newman et al., 2020, p. 4)

infants were considered, as well as after adjustment for maternal age and parity, the sex of the infant and correlation between siblings. Furthermore, the estimates of the prevalence of anomalies reported to the registry by 1 year of age in the assisted-conception groups were well in excess of the 6% prevalence of major birth anomalies in the general population (Hansen et al., 2002). Although there have been small reductions in recent data, consistent reporting of increased risk of adverse perinatal outcomes and birth defects following ART persists in recent studies (Chambers et al., 2014; Davies et al., 2017; Hansen et al., 2013; Wang et al., 2017).

More recently, a population-based study from China analysing the relationship between assisted reproductive technology (ART) and birth defects also found that after adjusting for confounding factors, ART use was still associated with an increased risk of any birth defect (5.4% vs 3.5% in ART and non-ART group, adjusted RR (aRR), 1.43, 95% CI 1.08 to 1.90), especially for chromosomal abnormalities. There were non statistically significant increases in circulatory system and musculoskeletal system malformations in singleton births to mothers less than 35 years old. Interestingly the associations between ART and birth defects were not detected in multiple births or mothers ≥35 years (Zhang et al., 2021).

An excess risk of major birth anomalies in infants conceived with ART is plausible owing to the usually older age of the couple concerned as well as the underlying cause of their infertility. The increased risk of anomalies may also be associated with medications used to induce ovulation or to maintain the pregnancy in the early stages and with factors associated with the procedures themselves. However, most outcomes appear better for frozen-thawed than with fresh embryo transfers (Hansen et al., 2013; Marino et al., 2014; Wennerholm et al., 2013).

In 2012, researchers from South Australia published their results of a large population-based cohort comparing the risks of birth anomalies (diagnosed before a child's fifth birthday) among pregnancies in women who received treatment with ART compared with those who did not (Davies et al., 2012). They found that there appeared to be an increased risk even after controlling for known confounders amongst those infants who were born following ICSI (Davies et al., 2012), although Wong & Ledger (2013) argued that the study did not show whether the risks associated with ICSI are related to the procedure or to inherent sperm abnormalities. Davies et al. (2017) suggest that there is a hierarchy of risk associated with treatment strategies, with adverse outcomes more likely when children are conceived with more invasive treatments, and challenge current practitioners to identify the safest, minimal treatment strategy of known conception benefit to a couple before considering more invasive options such as ICSI. Associations between ART and autism spectrum disorder (ASD) have been anticipated because ART shares common risk factors with ASD such as multiple pregnancies, pre-term delivery, and LBW. Consequently, this field has attracted scientific interest and a large number

of studies have attempted to investigate and determine the potential correlation between ART and ASD (Andreadou et al., 2021). A systematic review by Andreadou et al., 2021 found after controlling for confounding factors there appeared to be a degree of correlation between ART and ASD (RR = 1.11, 95% CI 1.03–1.19, $p = 0.009$). However, this correlation was not detected in singletons, suggesting that multiple pregnancies may be an independent direct risk for ASD. Consequently, more large studies are needed to better identify factors leading to ASD and whether the increased risk is due to the underlying cause of infertility or advanced parental age, or if it is due entirely to ART interventions. The authors also noted that epigenetic changes might be a conceivable molecular mechanism linking ART with ASD (Andreadou et al., 2021).

In assisted reproduction, several studies have shown that children born after transfer of frozen-thawed embryos (FET) have a lower risk of pre-term birth, low birth weight, and SGA compared with singletons born after fresh transfer but also a higher risk of being born with a *high gestational age and high birth weight*. Due to high success rates, FET of vitrified/warmed blastocysts has increased dramatically in recent years, including the 'freeze all' technique, where all available embryos of good quality are cryopreserved for later use in a natural or programmed cycle (see Newman et al., 2020 for New Zealand and Australian data on 'freeze all' techniques). The short-term perinatal outcomes for babies of high birth weight and being LGA are mainly associated with problems related to mode of birth and the results of these interventions such as asphyxia, shoulder dystocia, hypoglycemia, respiratory problems, caesarean section and obstetric injuries. For long-term outcomes, linked studies and cohort studies have shown associations between high birth weight and child malignancies, breast cancer, psychiatric disorders and cardiometabolic diseases, however, the current evidence is not conclusive (Magnusson et al., 2021).

Complication rates for women

Complication rates in subfertile women have been ascribed to increased maternal age, lower parity and multiple births resulting from fertility treatment. Studies have found that women who have received such treatment are more likely to develop complications of pregnancy including pre-eclampsia and antepartum haemorrhage than the general obstetric population, after adjustment for confounders such as age and parity (Kallen et al., 2005; Qin et al., 2016; Thomson et al., 2005; Wang et al., 2016). Although the calculated relative risks for placental abruption and placenta praevia are high for subfertile women, the absolute increase in risks is extremely small. Fertility treatment is also a risk for higher rates of caesarean section (Harris, 2016; Newman et al., 2020)—although this could be partially attributed to the anxiety surrounding these pregnancies, which may lower obstetricians' thresholds for intervention. The association between rates of complications and obstetric intervention by obstetricians has been noted before (Bell et al., 2001).

Cost associated with ART

In 2007 the main finding from a national Australian study of the admission costs for women having singleton and multiple-gestation ART babies compared with non-ART babies was that the ART baby admissions were 89% more costly than non-ART infant admissions. ART twins and higher-order multiples (HOMs) were 3 and 11 times more costly respectively than single ART babies and were therefore a substantial contribution to these costs; single ART babies were 31% more costly than non-ART single babies (Chambers et al., 2007). A more recent study of mean hospital costs during the first 5 years of life based on the West Australian population for data collected from 1993 to 2008 found those of a singleton, twin and HOM child to age 5 were US$2730, $8993 and $24,411 respectively, and almost 15% of inpatient costs for multiple births would have been avoidable if ART twins and HOMs had been born as singletons (Chambers et al., 2014). Poorer neonatal outcomes and the high costs associated with ART multiple births add to the overwhelming clinical and economic evidence in support of single-embryo transfer.

A systematic review performed by Petrou et al. (2001) also highlighted the immense ongoing burden on health, education, social services and families arising from preterm birth and low-birth-weight (LBW) infants, for which multiple gestation is a significant risk factor. For example, even those LBW children without a disability use healthcare resources 4.7 times more up to the age of 8–9 years compared with non-LBW children (Chambers et al., 2007).

SURROGACY

It is now estimated that 1 in 7 couples have difficulty conceiving (National Health Service (NHS), 2017). Many such couples attempt several means of ART techniques such as ovulation induction (OI), GIFT, IVF and ICSI. Couples who are unable to conceive for reasons other than those related to fertility, such as same-sex couples or those with medical conditions which make pregnancy dangerous, may not find fertility treatments a universal solution, and adoption and surrogacy are alternatives. For some, the desire to parent a child with a genetic link to one's self can mean surrogacy is the preferred option.

Surrogacy is an age-old method of reproduction that has been practised since biblical times. It can be a very low-tech procedure performed without medical assistance using a simple turkey baster (Ciccarelli & Beckman, 2005). Surrogacy has become controversial in the past 25 years in part because of the emphasis on commercialisation of surrogate mothering.

The World Health Organization (WHO) defines surrogacy in the following way:

A gestational carrier is a woman in whom a pregnancy resulted from fertilization with third-party sperm and oocytes. She carries the pregnancy with the intention or agreement that the offspring will be parented by one or both of the persons that produced the gametes.

(WHO, 2002)

Surrogacy involves a couple—the intended parents—contracting another woman to carry a child for them and agreeing to relinquish the baby to them following the birth. The intended couple then adopt the child. There are two major types of surrogacy arrangements:

- *Partial surrogacy, traditional or genetic surrogacy* is where the surrogate mother provides the egg and the sperm is provided by the intended father. In this case, the impregnated woman is both the genetic and birth (i.e. gestational) mother and the intended father is also the genetic father.
- *Full surrogacy, gestational carrier surrogacy* is where an embryo with gametes of both the intended parents is implanted in the uterus of a surrogate mother through IVF. This is the method used when the female partner has viable eggs but does not have the capacity to carry the pregnancy. In gestational surrogacy, the woman who carries the child has no genetic connection to the child and the intended parents are also the genetic parents (Ciccarelli & Beckman, 2005).

Surrogacy, like abortion, is controversial. It has the potential to divide communities. The following statements are designed to invoke thoughtful debate and discussion on the subject of surrogacy.

- The concept of surrogacy challenges basic concepts about family, motherhood and gender roles (Ciccarelli & Beckman, 2005; Teman, 2008).
- Conservative groups are fearful that surrogacy will undermine traditional cultural values about the two-parent family with the wife primarily responsible for childcare and the husband as provider and patriarch (Ciccarelli & Beckman, 2005).
- Surrogacy defies mainstream assumptions that the woman who gives birth must have an indissoluble mother–child bond (Teman, 2008).
- Feminists are alarmed about the commodification of women and may hold some objection to the social construction of the woman who carries a child as the *surrogate* or *surrogate mother*. The contention arises because the terms do not accurately reflect the reality of contractual parenting since the pregnant woman is the *actual* mother—that is, the gestational or birth mother (Ciccarelli & Beckman, 2005).
- Current terminology may minimise the value of the gestational mother's role and delegitimise her right to a continuing relationship with the child.
- The birth mother may have strong feelings on the matter of how she perceives herself and her role.
- Should babies be sold?
- Is a limitation of women's reproductive freedom (in surrogacy) similar to the curtailment of women's reproductive rights by groups that oppose access to abortion and contraception?
- Is it the 'centrality of motherhood and family'—the basic cornerstones of our Western society—that make it difficult to accept that surrogates may not necessarily be unhappy to voluntarily relinquish a child they bear to relative strangers (Teman, 2008)?
- Motherhood tends to be perceived as biological, whereas fatherhood can be learned (van den Akker, 2007).

247

Box 12.5   Issues in surrogacy

The first case involved Lu and John B, who used IVF with donor eggs and donor sperm. The embryos were subsequently implanted in a genetically unrelated woman (the 'surrogate' mother) for gestation and birth. The Bs intended to rear the resulting child as their own. Before the child, Jay, was born, the couple separated and John wanted to have nothing to do with the child.

In the first trial in this case the judge found that Jay was parentless [regardless of the fact that six adults had been involved in her 'production']. This decision was reversed on appeal, and the appeals court decided that because, under California law, a husband who consents to his wife's artificial insemination becomes the legal father of the child, a husband and wife [should be] deemed the lawful parents of a child after a surrogate bears a biologically unrelated child on their behalf ... [since] in each instance a child is procreated because a medical procedure was initiated and consented to by intended parents. Thus, the court concluded that Lu and John were Jay's legal parents.

To make sure no one missed the analogy, the court expanded on it, stating that gestational surrogacy and artificial insemination are exactly analogous in this crucial respect: both contemplate the procreation of a child by the consent to a medical procedure of someone who intends to raise the child but who otherwise does not have any biological tie. The court did not like the idea of people who are responsible for the creation of a child turning around and disclaiming any responsibility after the child is born. As the court believed that John 'caused' the birth of Jay simply by signing a contract, the court had no problem concluding that the same logic that made him the legal father made Lu (his wife at the time the contract with the surrogate mother was signed) the legal mother, as she agreed to the 'procreative project' at the start. The appeals court nonetheless concluded that 'things might work out for the best'. The court conceded that John may have agreed to the surrogate-mother arrangement simply 'as an accommodation to allow Lu to surmount a formality' but observed that 'human relationships are not static; things done merely to help one individual overcome a perceived legal obstacle sometimes become much more meaningful'. There is no legal basis for such musings, according to George J Annas, writing in the *New England Journal of Medicine* (1998).

(Sources: Annas,1998; *Buzzanca v Buzzanca*, 61 Cal. App. 4th 1410, 1998)

- Is current research into surrogacy framed by the cultural assumption that 'normal' women do not voluntarily become pregnant with the premeditated intention of relinquishing the child for money, together with the assumption that 'normal' women 'naturally' bond with the children they bear (Teman, 2008)?

Issues in surrogacy are summarised in Box 12.5.

The legality of surrogacy

In the United States there are four states that explicitly ban surrogacy (New York, New Jersey, Indiana and Michigan), there are also 14 states where surrogacy is expressly allowed and regulated (including California, Texas, Florida, Maine and Virginia) as well as states where surrogacy is not clearly addressed either by legislation or through case law (Massachusetts, Tennessee and Oregon) (Finkelstein et al., 2016).

Surrogacy in a modern form started in the United States in the late 1970s and first appeared in France in 1984. In its current form, surrogacy may be practised with or without the involvement of IVF, as it was practised before the invention of modern medicine. Surrogacy is outlawed in France, however, because French law forbids persons to sell their body parts (Reineke, 2008). In the UK, non-commercial surrogacy has been legal since 1985 (Teman, 2008).

Australia

The Commonwealth Government of Australia does not universally legislate for reproductive technology practice.

Therefore, each state and territory is responsible for designing and implementing separate legislation. This has resulted in laws and practices that differ from state to state. The Australian Government publishes a fact sheet for prospective couples seeking surrogacy (International Surrogacy Arrangements https://immi.homeaffairs.gov.au/citizenship/become-a-citizen/by-descent/international-surrogacy-arrangements).

- In Queensland, under the *Surrogacy Act 2010*, any form of commercial surrogacy in state or internationally is prohibited and attracts criminal sanctions. Queenslanders are permitted to enter into a non-commercial surrogacy arrangement where no money changes hands.
- In New South Wales (NSW), commercial surrogacy (paying a fee or giving a reward for surrogacy services) is outlawed under the *Assisted Reproductive Technology Act 2007*, but altruistic surrogacy (where there is no financial gain or reward involved) remains legal. The laws outlaw commercial surrogacy and render all surrogacy agreements void. This means a commissioning parent cannot approach a court to force a birth mother to give up a child.
- In the Australian Capital Territory (ACT), surrogacy is permitted and parents are entitled to be recognised as the legal parents.
- In Western Australia (WA), altruistic surrogacy became legal under the *Surrogacy Act 2008*. Intended parents can apply to the Family Court for a parentage order between 28 days and 6 months after birth.

- In Victoria (VIC), under the *Assisted Reproductive Treatment Act 2008*, singles and same-sex and heterosexual couples who are unable to conceive or give birth to their own biological children, or will pass on a severe genetic defect, can be considered for surrogacy. The birth mother must meet stringent requirements including being over the age of 25, having at least one live child and having no genetic link to the intended mother (i.e. she cannot use her own eggs). Commercial surrogacy is illegal. Children born in Victoria through altruistic surrogacy arrangements in another Australian state or the ACT now have their parentage legally recognised here.
- In South Australia (SA), commercial surrogacy is an offence and contracts are illegal and void. Strictly governed conditions are in place controlling who has access to surrogacy. All parties must be over 18, living in SA, be legally married or in a de facto relationship for at least 3 years, and the woman must be infertile, be deemed to be at great risk for pregnancy or birth, or be at risk of passing on a serious genetic defect to her unborn child.
- The Northern Territory does not have surrogacy legislation.
- In Tasmania, a birth mother may choose to relinquish a baby to another person under the *Surrogacy Act 2012*. As with other states, the agreement must be made in writing before the pregnancy and signed by both parties after each has sought legal advice.

In most states (including NSW), the surrogate mother (and her partner, if any) will be the legal parents and there are very few avenues for having the child legally recognised as the child of the intended parent(s). This is the case even if the surrogacy arrangement goes to plan and the parties are all in agreement. In such states, the best option for the intended parents is a parenting order from the Family Court awarding them parental responsibility; however, this does not grant all the rights of full legal parentage. The surrogate mother and her partner, if any, remain the legal parents to the child (e.g. for inheritance reasons, accident compensation, state- and federal-based legal rights, etc.) for the remainder of their child's life. In other states and territories (e.g. ACT, VIC, WA), the intended parents can get a court order in some circumstances transferring the legal parentage from the surrogate mother (and her partner, if any), if the surrogate mother consents. This effectively allows the intended parents to 'adopt' their child, if all parties agree, the agreement satisfies the conditions of the law, and the court determines that a parentage order would be in the best interests of the child. In other words, the child is fully recognised as the child of the intended parents—and not the child of anyone else.

Canada and New Zealand

Commercial surrogacy has been illegal since 2004, although 'altruistic' surrogacy is allowed.

MIDWIFERY CARE FOR WOMEN WHO HAVE PREGNANCIES FOLLOWING ART

In 2013, Allot & Dann published an excellent review informing midwives of the issues for which they need to be mindful, when caring for women with pregnancies following ART. The review highlighted the adverse maternal and perinatal outcomes associated with ART pregnancies due in part to the underlying reduced fertility condition, the drugs and the procedures involved, which have the potential to threaten maternal and neonatal wellbeing. The advice they gave midwives as the main care givers for pregnant women in New Zealand was the need to be well informed, 'mindful of the potential risks to the mother and her baby whilst providing care that is the most appropriate and supportive, to enable these women to achieve a safe and satisfying childbirth experience' (Allot & Dann, 2013, p. 13).

Conclusion

Wide disparities exist in the availability, quality and delivery of infertility services between the resource-rich and resource-poor nations of the world. Infertility is estimated to affect up to 186 million people worldwide (Inhorn & Patrizio, 2015).

Most countries in the industrialised West have declining fertility rates marked by late marriage, postponed childbearing and primary infertility. In contrast, in the developing world there is little voluntary effort to postpone childbearing, and early first marriage is common. However, a high prevalence of sexually transmitted infections and infections acquired as a result of inadequate healthcare result in increased rates of secondary infertility (Nachtigall, 2006). In developing societies, childlessness is often highly stigmatised and leads to profound social suffering for infertile women in particular, yet most infertile people in the developing world have virtually no access to effective fertility treatment.

In countries such as New Zealand and Australia, however, in just over two decades, ART techniques have evolved from a laboratory curiosity to a commercialised, industrialised technology responsible for thousands of births. Human reproduction has always been a matter of philosophical debate and social controversy. In resource-rich nations, the debate has grown more complicated through continued technical evolution. Both hopes and concerns have been raised simultaneously about

249

the legitimacy of pre-embryo research, the slippery slope of preimplantation embryo diagnostic testing and eugenic implications, and the fundamental and philosophical problem of the status of the embryo (Box 12.6).

Among the resource-poor women of the world, an estimated 250 million years of productive life are lost every year as a result of reproductive health problems (UNFPA, 2005). The inability to determine when and how many children to have limits a woman's life choices (UNFPA, 2016). More than two decades after the 1994 Cairo International Conference on Population and Development (ICPD), and a global consensus that reproductive rights are central to human rights, sustainable development, gender equality and the empowerment of women (UNFPA, 2016), millions of women still do not have access to contraceptive services. Maternal mortality rates remain essentially unchanged and many women still die from complications of unsafe abortions. Both fertility and reproductive health problems remain the greatest burden of the world's poorest women.

Box 12.6 Preimplantation genetic screening (PGS)

PGS is a relatively new and little researched technique where one or more cells are removed from the embryo and analysed for chromosomal disorders or genetic diseases.

Aneuploidy is widely recognized as a leading embryonic cause for both implantation failure and pregnancy loss in natural and assisted conceptions. The intention of preimplantation genetic screening (PGS) is to prevent aneuploid embryo transfers in infertile patients undergoing IVF. By identifying euploid embryos for transfer, PGS is expected to increase implantation and live birth rates and reduce miscarriage rates per transfer cycle.

(Sources: Weissman et al., 2017, p. 2; see also Rubio et al., 2017)

Review questions

1. Name four reasons for infertility in women.
2. Name five major reasons for 'subfertility' or infertility in men.
3. What tests would both women and men undergo to establish the reasons for infertility? Why are these significant?
4. Does surrogacy perpetuate the objectification and commodification of women's reproduction by defining women as 'breeders'?
5. What is the difference between GIFT, IVF and ICSI?
6. Do you think there should be a register of sperm donors? If so, what are the ethical issues associated with donor insemination?
7. Describe the issues identified in question 6 from the point of view of a male donor (father's point of view).
8. Describe the issues identified in question 6 from the point of view of an adolescent wanting to trace her biological parents. Address the implications of the importance of genetic information.
9. What are some of the adverse outcomes of assisted reproduction for women? Have these changed over the past 10 years? If so, what has changed?
10. What are the risks of multiple births following assisted reproduction? Are these significantly different from those of multiple births following unassisted reproduction?

Online resources

Australian Government Department of Immigration and Citizenship. Fact Sheet International surrogacy arrangements: https://immi.homeaffairs.gov.au/citizenship/become-a-citizen/by-descent/international-surrogacy-arrangements.

Centers for Disease Control and Prevention. National Public Health Action Plan for the Detection, Prevention, and Management of Infertility. June 2014: https://www.cdc.gov/reproductivehealth/infertility/pdf/drh_nap_final_508.pdf.

National Health and Medical Research Council (NHMRC). Ethical Guidelines for Assisted Reproductive Technology (ART). 2021: https://www.nhmrc.gov.au/art.

New Zealand population statistics: https://www.stats.govt.nz/topics/population.

Reproduction Technology Council: https://www.rtc.org.au/.

United Nations Department of Economic and Social Affairs, Population Division World Fertility and Family Planning 2020: https://www.un.org/development/desa/pd/.

World Health Orgnization. Fertility and Infertility: http://www.who.int/topics/infertility/en/.

World Health Orgnization. Infertility fact sheet: https://www.who.int/news-room/fact-sheets/detail/infertility.

Assisted reproductive technology

For statistics relating to Australian and New Zealand women who underwent ART, the National Perinatal Epidemiology Unit of

Australia publishes yearly reports using ANZARD data: https://npesu.unsw.edu.au/data-collection/australian-new-zealand-assisted-reproduction-database-anzard

Much information is available on websites such as that of the Human Fertilisation and Embryology Authority (HFEA) in the UK: https://www.hfea.gov.uk/. (Note that variations occur between and within countries.)

References

Allot L, Payne D, Dann L. Midwifery and assisted reproductive technologies. *NZCOM J.* 2013;47:10–13.

Alviggi C, Humaidan P, Howles CM, et al. Biological versus chronological ovarian age: implications for assisted reproductive technology. *Reprod Biol Endocrinol.* 2009;7:101. doi:10.1186/1477-7827-7-101.

Andersen NAM, Wohlfahrt J, Christens P, et al. Maternal age and fetal loss: population based register linkage study. *BMJ.* 2000;320:1708–1712.

Andreadou MT, Katsaras GN, Talimtzi P, et al. Association of assisted reproductive technology with autism spectrum disorder in the offspring: an updated systematic review and meta-analysis. *Eur J Pediatr.* 2021 Sep;180(9):2741–2755. doi: 10.1007/s00431-021-04187-9. Epub 2021 Jul 19.

Annas GJ. The shadowlands—secrets and lies and assisted reproduction. *N Engl J Med.* 1998;339(13):935–939.

Australian Bureau of Statistics (ABS). *Births, Australia.* 2021. Online: https://www.abs.gov.au/statistics/people/population/births-australia/latest-release#data-download.

Australian Institute of Health and Welfare. *Australia's mothers and babies.* Canberra: AIHW; 2021. Online: https://www.aihw.gov.au/reports/mothers-babies/australias-mothers-babies/contents/about.

Baird DD, Tylavsky FA, Andersen JJB. Do vegetarians have earlier menopause? *Am J Epidemiol.* 1998;1:907–908.

Barua S, Hng TM, Smith H, et al. Ovulatory disorders are an independent risk factor for pregnancy complications in women receiving assisted reproduction treatments. *Aust N Z J Obstet Gynaecol.* 2017;57(3):286–293.

Bell J, Campbell DM, Graham WJ, et al. Do obstetric complications explain high caesarean section rates among women over 30? A retrospective analysis. *BMJ.* 2001;322:894–895.

Bender SS, Geirsson RT, Kosunen E. Trends in teenage fertility, abortion, and pregnancy rates in Iceland compared with other Nordic countries, 1976–99. *Acta Obstet Gynecol Scand.* 2003;82:38–47.

Bewley S, Davies M, Braude P. Which career first? The most secure age for childbearing remains 20–35. *BMJ.* 2005;331:588–589.

Bongaarts J. Human population growth and the demographic transition. *Philos Trans Roy Soc B.* 2009;364:2985–2990. doi:10.1098/rstb.2009.0137.

Bongaarts J. Development: slow down population growth. *Nature.* 2016;530(7591):409–412.

Bright A. National notifiable diseases surveillance system surveillance report: sexually transmissible infections in Aboriginal and Torres Strait Islander people. *Commun Dis Intell Q Rep.* 2015;39(4):E584–E589.

Buzzanca v Buzzanca, 61 Cal. App. 4th 1410, 1998. Online: https://www.supremecourt.gov/DocketPDF/17/17-878/24277/20171218151547560_USSC%20Petition%20for%20Writ%20of%20Certiorari%20without%20Appendix.pdf.

Callaway LK, Lust K, McIntyre HD. Pregnancy outcomes in women of very advanced maternal age. *Aust N Z J Obstet Gynaecol.* 2005;45:12–16.

Chambers GM, Chapman MG, Grayson N, et al. Babies born after ART treatment cost more than non-ART babies: a cost analysis of inpatient birth-admission costs of singleton and multiple gestation pregnancies. *Hum Reprod.* 2007;22(12):3108–3115.

Chambers GM, Hoang VP, Lee E, et al. Hospital costs of multiple-birth and singleton-birth children during the first 5 years of life and the role of assisted reproductive technology. *JAMA Pediatr.* 2014;168(11):1045–1053.

Chescheir NC. Worldwide abortion rates and access to contraception. *Obstet Gynecol.* 2017;129(5):783–785.

Ciccarelli JC, Beckman LJ. Navigating rough water: an overview of psychological aspects of surrogacy. *J Soc Issues.* 2005;61:21–43.

Daniluk JC, Koert E, Cheung A. Childless women's knowledge of fertility and assisted human reproduction: identifying the gaps. *Fertil Steril.* 2012;97(2):420–426.

Davies MJ, Moore VM, Willson KJ, et al. Reproductive technologies and the risk of birth defects. *N Engl J Med.* 2012;366(19):1803–1813.

Davies MJ, Rumbold AR, Moore VM. Assisted reproductive technologies: a hierarchy of risks for conception, pregnancy outcomes and treatment decisions. *J Dev Orig Health Dis.* 2017;8(4):443–447.

de Bruin JP, Bovenhuis PAH, van Noord PA, et al. The role of genetic factors in age at natural menopause. *Hum Reprod.* 2001;16:2014–2018.

DoPierala AL, Bhatta S, Raja EA, et al. Obstetric consequences of subfertility: a retrospective cohort study. *BJOG.* 2016;123(8):1320–1328.

Erickson GF. Ovarian anatomy and physiology. In: Lobo RA, Kelsey J, Marcus R, eds. *Menopause: Biology and Pathobiology.* San Diego, CA: Academic Press; 2000:13–32.

Finkelstein AMDS, Kintominas A, Olsen A. *Surrogacy Law and Policy in the U.S.: A National Conversation Informed by Global Lawmaking.* New York: Columbia Law School Sexuality and Gender Law Clinic; 2016. Online: http://www.law.columbia.edu/sites/default/files/microsites/gender-sexuality/files/columbia_sexuality_and_gender_law_clinic_-_surrogacy_law_and_policy_report_-_june_2016.pdf.

Freour T, Masson D, Mirallie S, et al. Active smoking compromises IVF outcome and affects ovarian reserve. *Reprod Biomed Online.* 2008;16:96–102.

Ge ZJ, Schatten H, Zhang CL, et al. Oocyte ageing and epigenetics. *Reproduction.* 2015;149(3):R103–R114.

Hank K, Kreyenfeld M. A multilevel analysis of childcare and women's fertility decisions in Western Germany. *J Marriage Fam.* 2003;65:584–596.

Hansen M, Kurinczuk JJ, Bower C, et al. The risk of major birth defects after intracytoplasmic sperm injection and in vitro fertilization. *N Engl J Med.* 2002;346:725–730.

Hansen M, Kurinczuk JJ, Milne E, et al. Assisted reproductive technology and birth defects: a systematic review and meta-analysis. *Hum Reprod Update.* 2013;19(4):330–353.

Harris KFO, Paul RC, Macaldowie A, et al. *Assisted Reproductive Technology in Australia and New Zealand 2014.* Sydney: National Perinatal Epidemiology and Statistics Unit; 2016.

Heffner LJ. Advanced maternal age—how old is too old? *N Engl J Med.* 2004;351:1927–1929.

Helmerhorst FM, Perquin DA, Donker D, et al. Perinatal outcome of singletons and twins after assisted conception: a systematic review of controlled studies. *BMJ.* 2004;328(7434):261.

Human Fertilisation and Embryology Authority (HFEA). *Fertility Treatment 2014 Trends and Figures.* London: HFEA; 2016. Online: https://www.hfea.gov.uk/.

Inhorn MC, Patrizio P. Infertility around the globe: new thinking on gender, reproductive technologies and global movements in the 21st century. *Hum Reprod Update.* 2015;21(4):411–426.

Jackson RA, Gibson KA, Wu YW, et al. Perinatal outcomes in singletons following in vitro fertilization: a meta-analysis. *Obstet Gynecol.* 2004;103(3):551–563.

Joehanes R, Just AC, Marioni RE, et al. Epigenetic signatures of cigarette smoking. *Circ Cardiovasc Genet.* 2016;9(5): 436–447.

Jones EF, Forrest JD, Goldman N, et al. Teenage pregnancy in developed countries: determinants and policy implications. *Int Fam Plan Perspect.* 1985;17:53–63.

Jurkovic D, Overton C, Bender-Atik R. Diagnosis and management of first trimester miscarriage. *BMJ.* 2013;346:f3676. doi:10.1136/bmj.f3676.

Kallen B, Finnstrom O, Nygren KG, et al. In vitro fertilisation in Sweden: obstetric characteristics, maternal morbidity and mortality. *BJOG.* 2005;112(11):1529–1535.

Kanherkar RR, Bhatia-Dey N, Csoka AB. Epigenetics across the human lifespan *Front Cell Dev Biol.* 2014;2:49.

Ketting E, Visser AP. Contraception in the Netherlands: the low abortion rate explained. *Patient Educ Couns.* 1994;23: 161–171.

Khatun M, Al Mamun A, Scott J, et al. Do children born to teenage parents have lower adult intelligence? A prospective birth cohort study. *PLoS ONE.* 2017;12(3):e0167395.

Kirby Institute. *HIV, Viral Hepatitis and Sexually Transmissible Infections in Australia. Annual Surveillance Report.* Sydney: The Kirby Institute, UNSW; 2016.

Kushnir VA, Barad DH, Albertini DF, et al. Systematic review of worldwide trends in assisted reproductive technology 2004–2013. *Reprod Biol Endocrinol.* 2017;15(1):6.

Lambalk CB, van Disseldorp J, de Koning CH, et al. Testing ovarian reserve to predict age at menopause. *Maturitas.* 2009;63(4): 280–291.

Lattimore R, Pobke C. *Recent Trends in Australian Fertility. Productivity Commission Staff Working Paper.* Canberra: Productivity Commission; 2008.

Lewis D, Newton DC, Guy RJ, et al. The prevalence of *Chlamydia trachomatis* infection in Australia: a systematic review and meta-analysis. *BMC Infect Dis.* 2012;12:113.

Lobo RA. Menopause and care of the mature woman. In: Lobo RAG, Lentz GM, Valea FA, eds. *Comprehensive Gynecology.* Philadelphia, PA: Elsevier; 2016:258–293.

Magnusson Å, Laivuori H, Loft A, et al. The association between high birth weight and long-term outcomes—implications for assisted reproductive technologies: a systematic review and meta-analysis. *Front Pediatr.* 2021 9:675775. doi:10.3389/fped.2021.675775.

Marino JL, Moore VM, Willson KJ, et al. Perinatal outcomes by mode of assisted conception and sub-fertility in an Australian data linkage cohort. *PLoS ONE.* 2014;9(1):e80398.

Metwally M, Ledger WL. Long-term complications of assisted reproductive technologies. *Hum Fertil.* 2011;14(2):77–87.

Morgan SP, Taylor MG. Low fertility at the turn of the twenty-first century. *Annu Rev Sociol.* 2006;32:375–399.

Nachtigall RD. International disparities in access to infertility services. *Fertil Steril.* 2006;85:871–875.

National Health Service (NHS) [UK]. *Infertility.* 2017. Online: https://www.nhs.uk/conditions/Infertility/.

Newman JE, Paul RC, Chambers GM. *Assisted reproductive technology in Australia and New Zealand 2018.* Sydney: National Perinatal Epidemiology and Statistics Unit, the University of New South Wales; 2020.

Nwandison M, Bewley S. What is the right age to reproduce? *Fetal Matern Med Rev.* 2006;17(3):185–204. doi:10.1017/S0965539506001781.

Oehninger S. Place of intracytoplasmic sperm injection in management of male infertility. *Lancet.* 2001;357(9274): 2068–2069.

Pandian Z, Marjoribanks J, Ozturk O, et al. Number of embryos for transfer following in vitro fertilisation or intra-cytoplasmic sperm injection. *Cochrane Database Syst Rev.* 2013;(7): CD003416, doi:10.1002/14651858.CD003416.pub4.

Pereira N, O'Neill CL, Lu V, et al. The safety of intracytoplasmic sperm injection and long-term outcomes. *Reproduction.* 2017;154(6):F61–F70. doi:10.1530/REP-17-0344.

Petrou S, Sach T, Davidson L. The long-term costs of preterm birth and low birth weight: results of a systematic review. *Child Care Health Dev.* 2001;27:97–115.

Plante BJ, Cooper GS, Baird DD, et al. The impact of smoking on antimullerian hormone

Qin J, Liu X, Sheng X, et al. Assisted reproductive technology and the risk of pregnancy-related complications and adverse pregnancy outcomes in singleton pregnancies: a meta-analysis of cohort studies. *Fertil Steril.* 2016;105(1):73–85, e1–6. doi:10.1016/j.fertnstert.2015.09.007.

Reichlin S. A review of female fertility and the body fat connection (*Women in Culture and Society* by Rose E. Frisch. Chicago: University of Chicago Press). *N Engl J Med.* 2003;348(9): 869–870.

Reineke S. In vitro veritas: new reproductive and genetic technologies and women's rights in contemporary France. *Int J Fem Approaches Bioeth.* 2008;1(1):91–125. doi:10.1353/ijf.0.0028.

Rissel CE, Richters J, Grulich AE, et al. Sex in Australia: first experience of vaginal intercourse and oral sex among a representative sample of adults. *Aust N Z J Public Health.* 2003;27: 131–137.

Rubio C, Bellver J, Rodrigo L, et al. In vitro fertilization with pre-implantation genetic diagnosis for aneuploidies in advanced maternal age: a randomized, controlled study. *Fertil Steril.* 2017;107(5):1122–1129.

Sallmen M, Weinberg CR, Baird DD, et al. Has human fertility declined over time? Why we may never know. *Epidemiology.* 2005;16(4):494–499.

Sapre S, Thakur R. Lifestyle and dietary factors determine age at natural menopause. *J Midlife Health.* 2014;5(1):3–5.

Schoenaker DA, Jackson CA, Rowlands JV, et al. Socioeconomic position, lifestyle factors and age at natural menopause: a systematic review and meta-analyses of studies across six continents. *Int J Epidemiol.* 2014;43(5):1542–1562.

Scott RT, Toner J, Muasher X, et al. Follicle-stimulating hormone levels on cycle day 3 are predictive of in vitro fertilization outcome. *Fertil Steril.* 1989;51:651–654.

Shaw M, Lawlor DA, Najam JM. Teenage children of teenage mothers: psychological, behavioural and health outcomes from an Australian prospective longitudinal study. *Soc Sci Med.* 2006;62:2526–2539.

Simpson JL. Genetic programming in ovarian development and oogenesis. In: Lobo RA, Kelsey J, Marcus R, eds. *Menopause: Biology and Pathobiology.* San Diego, CA: Academic Press; 2000:77–94.

Soares SR, Melo MA. Cigarette smoking and reproductive function. *Curr Opin Obstet Gynecol.* 2008;20:281–291.

Spoonley P. *The New Open Zealand: Facing demographic disruption.* Massey University Press NZ 2021)

Statistics New Zealand (Stats NZ). *Births and deaths statistics.* Wellington, NZ: Statistics New Zealand; 2021. Online: https://www.stats.govt.nz/information-releases/births-and-deaths-year-ended-march-2021-infoshare-tables.

Stolk L, Perry JR, Chasman DI, et al. Meta-analyses identify 13 loci associated with age at menopause and highlight DNA repair and immune pathways. *Nat Genet.* 2012;44(3):260–268.

Sunderam S, Kissin DM, Crawford SB, et al. Assisted reproductive technology surveillance—United States, 2014. *MMWR Surveill Summ.* 2017;66(6):1–24.

te Velde ER, van Baar AL, van Kooij RJ. Concerns about assisted reproduction. *Lancet.* 1998;351:1524–1525.

Teman E. The social construction of surrogacy research: an anthropological critique of the psychosocial scholarship on surrogate motherhood. *Soc Sci Med.* 2008;67:1104–1112.

Thomson F, Shanbhag S, Templeton A, et al. Obstetric outcome in women with subfertility. *BJOG.* 2005;112:632–637.

Thurin A, Hausken J, Hillensjo T, et al. Elective single-embryo transfer versus double-embryo transfer in in vitro fertilization. *N Engl J Med.* 2004;351:2392–2402.

United Nations (UN). *World Population Prospects: The 2015 Revision, Key Findings and Advance Tables. Working Paper No. ESA/PWP.241.* Geneva: United Nations, Department of Economics and Social Affairs, Population Division; 2015.

United Nations, Department of Economic and Social Affairs (UNDESA), Population Division. *World Fertility Patterns 2015 – Data Booklet (ST/ESA/SER.A/370).* Geneva: UNFPA; 2015. Online: http://www.un.org/en/development/desa/population/publications/pdf/fertility/world-fertility-patterns-2015.pdf.

United Nations, Department of Economic and Social Affairs (UNDESA), Population Division. *World Fertility and Family Planning 2020: Highlights (ST/ESA/SER.A/440).* Online: https://www.un.org/development/desa/pd/.

United Nations Population Fund (UNFPA). *State of World Population 2005. The Promise of Equality—Gender Equity, Reproductive Health and the Millennium Development Goals.* Geneva: UNFPA; 2005.

United Nations Population Fund (UNFPA). *State of World Population 2016. 10 – How our Future Depends on a Girl at this Decisive Age.* Geneva: UNFPA; 2016.

Vajdic CM, Middleton M, Bowden FJ, et al. The prevalence of genital *Chlamydia trachomatis* in Australia 1997–2004: a systematic review. *Sex Health.* 2005;2:169–183.

van den Akker O. Psychological trait and state characteristics, social support and attitudes to the surrogate pregnancy and baby. *Hum Reprod.* 2007;22:2287–2295.

van Asselt KM, Kok HS, Pearson PL, et al. Heritability of menopausal age in mothers and daughters. *Fertil Steril.* 2004;82:1348–1351.

Vichinsartvichai P. Primary ovarian insufficiency associated with autosomal abnormalities: from chromosome to genome-wide and beyond. *Menopause.* 2016;23(7):806–815.

Wang AY, Chughtai AA, Lui K, et al. Morbidity and mortality among very preterm singletons following fertility treatment in Australia and New Zealand, a population cohort study. *BMC Pregnancy Childbirth.* 2017;17(1):50.

Wang ET, Ozimek JA, Greene N, et al. Impact of fertility treatment on severe maternal morbidity. *Fertil Steril.* 2016;106(2):423–426.

Wang YA, Chambers GM, Dieng M, et al. *Assisted Reproductive Technology in Australia and New Zealand 2007. Assisted reproduction technology series no. 13. Cat. no. PER 47.* Canberra: AIHW; 2009. Online: www.aihw.gov.au/publications/per/per-47-10753/per-47-10753.pdf.

Weaver H, Smith G, Kippax S. School-based sex education policies and indicators of sexual health among young people: a comparison of the Netherlands, France, Australia and the United States. *Sex Educ.* 2005;5:171–188.

Weissman A, Shoham G, Shoham Z, et al. Preimplantation genetic screening: results of a worldwide web-based survey. *Reprod Biol Med Online.* 2017;35(6):693–700. doi:10.1016/j.rbmo.2017.09.001.

Wennerholm UB, Henningsen AK, Romundstad LB, et al. Perinatal outcomes of children born after frozen-thawed embryo transfer: a Nordic cohort study from the CoNARTaS group. *Hum Reprod.* 2013;28(9):2545–2553.

Wong M, Ledger WL. Is ICSI risky? *Obstet Gynecol Int.* 2013;2013:473289. doi:10.1155/2013/473289.

Wood C, Calderon I, Crombie A. Age and fertility: results of assisted reproductive technology in women over 40 years. *J Assisted Reprod Genet.* 1992;9:482–484.

World Health Organization (WHO). Medical, ethical and social aspects of assisted reproduction. In: Vayena E, Rowe PJ, Griffin PD, eds. *Current Practices and Controversies in Assisted Reproduction: Report of a WHO Meeting.* Geneva: WHO; 2002.

Zegers-Hochschild et al., The International Glossary on Infertility and Fertility Care, *ASRM.* 2017;108(3):393–406. Online: https://www.fertstert.org/article/S0015-0282(17)30429-6/fulltext.

Zhang L, Zhang W, Xu H, et al. Birth defects surveillance after assisted reproductive technology in Beijing: a whole of population-based cohort study. *BMJ Open.* 2021;11:e044385. doi:10.1136/ bmjopen-2020-044385.

Further reading

Gougeon A, Ecochard R, Thalabard JC. Age-related changes of the population of human ovarian follicles: increase in the disappearance rate of non-growing and early growing follicles in aging women. *Biol Reprod.* 1994;50:653–663.

Henshaw SK, Singh S, Haas T. Recent trends in abortion rates worldwide. *Int Fam Plan Perspect.* 1999;25:44–48.

Kessler B. Recruiting wombs: surrogates as the new security moms. *Womens Stud Quart.* 2009;37(1&2):167–182.

Potts M. Where next? *Philos Trans Roy Soc B.* 2009;364:3115–3124. doi:10.1098/rstb.2009.0181.

Rosenfield A, Schwartz K. Population and development—shifting paradigms, setting goals. *N Engl J Med.* 2005;352(7):647–649.

Sheiner E, Shoham-Vardi I, Hershkovitz R, et al. Infertility treatment is an independent risk factor for cesarean section among nulliparous women aged 40 and above. *Am J Obstet Gynecol.* 2001;185(4):888–892.

United Nations, Department of Economic and Social Affairs (UNDESA). *United Nations Department of Economic and Social Affairs Population Division: World Population 2017.* 2017. Online: https://esa.un.org/unpd/wpp/Publications/Files/WPP2017_Wallchart.pdf.

The midwife

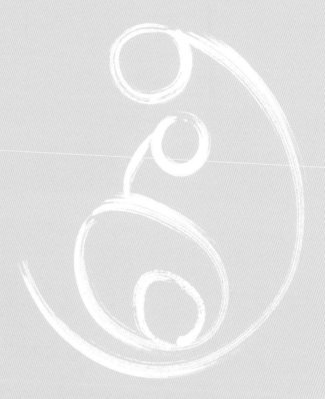

CHAPTER 13

Professional frameworks for practice in Australia and New Zealand

Sally Pairman and Michelle Gray

LEARNING OUTCOMES

Learning outcomes for this chapter are:

1. To explain the development of the midwifery profession in New Zealand and Australia, with respect to role, functions and structure
2. To describe the links between definition and scope of practice of a midwife, philosophy, code of ethics and standards for practice with midwifery standards review and recertification (New Zealand), and continuing professional development and midwifery practice review (Australia)
3. To describe the role and function of the respective regulatory authorities of New Zealand and Australia
4. To explain the relationship between regulatory and professional frameworks and their application to continuing midwifery practice (registration renewal/recertification).

CHAPTER OVERVIEW

This chapter outlines current and evolving professional and regulatory frameworks guiding midwifery practice in Australia and Aotearoa New Zealand. Regulatory frameworks, governed by legislation, protect the public by ensuring that health practitioners provide safe and competent care. They provide the statutory boundaries for midwifery practice and define the extent of professional autonomy each country affords to midwifery. Professional frameworks, developed by the midwifery professional associations in each country, set out the profession's expectations of midwives and provide a guide to professional practice, including articulation of philosophy, values, standards and professional behaviour. Regulatory frameworks and professional frameworks both contribute to ensuring high-quality midwifery care for women and their newborns. This chapter explains the relationships between legislation, regulatory frameworks and professional frameworks in both countries, and how these frameworks affect midwifery practice.

KEY TERMS

competencies
continuing professional development
legislation
midwifery education

professional frameworks
registration
regulation
regulatory framework

scope of practice
standards of practice

INTRODUCTION

As a healthcare profession, midwifery in both Australia and New Zealand is governed by **legislation** that determines, to a greater or lesser extent, the scope of midwifery practice, the level of midwifery autonomy, the expected standards for entering the profession (**competencies**), the processes for entering the profession (**registration**), and the mechanisms for maintaining competence (recertification) and for accountability. The purpose of this **regulatory framework** is to protect the public from harm by ensuring that midwives are appropriately qualified, competent and safe to practise midwifery. The legislation reflects society's understanding of and assumptions about midwifery at the time the legislation was enacted (Abbott, 1988). Regulatory legislation does not necessarily reflect current midwifery practice or, indeed, women's views of the kinds of midwifery services they wish to receive. It may well reflect the interests of other professional groups such as medical practitioners (Baerlocher & Allen, 2009), or those of the state, in determining the direction of maternity services (Dean, 1999). According to Tully (1999, p. 3), 'as both a licensing authority and a source of funding, the state can enhance or diminish the control that an occupation or profession has at any given time over the provision of particular services'.

While legislation provides a regulatory framework for midwifery practice, midwives in both Australia and New Zealand also operate under **professional frameworks** that guide and determine practice. The New Zealand College of Midwives (NZCOM) and the Australian College of Midwives (ACM) are the midwifery professional organisations in their respective countries. Both provide direction for midwifery practice through setting philosophy, standards for practice, and ethics and practice guidelines that midwife members are expected to follow. Both organisations also have a political role in working on behalf of midwives to strengthen and protect midwifery and in working to ensure that maternity services meet the needs of childbearing women.

Regulatory and professional frameworks are complementary. Regulation focuses on public safety to ensure a competent and safe midwifery workforce and regulatory authorities work within the parameters of the legislation. Professional organisations generally have wider concerns, developing and implementing guidelines for midwifery practice and mechanisms to maintain midwifery competence, supporting and advising midwives, advocating for midwives and for women in relation to maternity services, contributing midwifery expertise to policy and advising the government about midwifery services.

Midwives internationally recognise that a strong autonomous midwifery profession requires integration of 10 key elements: midwifery philosophy, essential competencies for midwifery practice, **midwifery education**, midwifery regulation, midwives' association, research, midwife-led continuity of care model of practice, midwifery leadership, enabling environment, and a commitment to gender equality and justice, equity, diversity and inclusion (International Confederation of Midwives (ICM), 2021). The ICM's Professional Framework for Midwifery represents the core beliefs of midwifery and what makes midwifery unique and different to other health professions. It sets out the essential elements that need to be in place to enable quality midwifery services, enhanced sexual and reproductive health for women, their newborns and their families and for more fulfilling careers for midwives. The elements of the framework are interwoven and interdependent; strengthening one can strengthen all others, just as destabilising one destabilises all.

The Australian and New Zealand midwifery professions have both worked to develop strong midwifery professions and they have paid attention to strengthening these same essential elements, but the way in which the regulatory and professional frameworks have developed in each country reflects their unique historical, social, political, cultural and economic contexts.

Australia and New Zealand share a common history of colonial settlement from Britain in the early 19th century and both countries have indigenous peoples who have suffered and continue to suffer owing to the effects of colonisation (see Chs 1, 10 and 11). However, for all their commonalities, Australia and New Zealand have evolved differently into the modern nations they are today. So too have their professions of midwifery. This chapter outlines the development of midwifery regulatory and professional frameworks in both countries.

DEVELOPMENT OF THE MIDWIFERY PROFESSION IN AUSTRALIA

The Australian College of Midwives

The Australian College of Midwives is the peak 'professional' body for midwives in Australia with articulated national standards for midwifery practice, education and regulation consistent with the International Confederation of Midwives (http://www.midwives.org.au). It is the national professional body representing all midwives in Australia, with members in every state and territory. In 2014, the ACM became a single national entity through a process of unification of nine associations, some of whom were incorporated (ACM, n.d.a). Unification occurred in a bid to strengthen governance and to consolidate the ACM as the peak national professional organisation for midwifery in Australia.

In 1978, three midwives[a] founded the National Midwives Association, as a 'special interest group' of what was then called the Royal Australian Nursing Federation (RANF), the chief industrial body for nursing in Australia. Their visionary efforts led to Australia becoming a member of the ICM. In 1979 the National Midwives Association hosted an inaugural conference in Adelaide and successfully bid to host the ICM Congress in Sydney in 1984. Moves to consolidate a specific professional organisation and identity for midwifery nationally saw the group break away from the RANF to become the ACM in 1983 (*Australian Midwifery News*, 2007).

As of 11th August 2021 there were 36,045 midwives registered with the Nursing and Midwifery Board of Australia (NMBA); 6309 of these hold single registration as a midwife (single registration numbers are up 10.2% since 2020) (NMBA, 2022).

Membership of the ACM is voluntary and estimated to comprise of 4460 members (ACM 2020; ACM communication, August 2021c) Although the ACM speaks on behalf of all midwives, in comparison to some of our international counterparts (Royal College of Midwives, Canadian Association of Midwives and NZCOM) the ACM has a fractional proportion of members from the population of Australian midwives. As a result, funding for college work is limited and the money raised from membership fees is supplemented by sponsorship and voluntary time contribution from members on committees and working parties.

The structure of the ACM

The ACM has a Chief Executive Officer (CEO) who is in a paid position and responsible for the operational management of the organisation. The ACM is governed by a constitution and bylaws that outline the aims of the organisation, the terms and categories of membership status, and the functions and powers of the Board of Directors. Constitutional review has seen the ACM move from a National Executive Committee structure to a National Board of Directors. State and territory branches maintain essential grass roots representation, but unification means that all membership fees are paid directly to the centralised organisation.

The CEO is delegated as Company Secretary and is responsible to the Board of Directors for the strategic direction of the college. The CEO manages the organisation of the college including employing and managing the staff (ACM, 2021e). The CEO is supported by many voluntary positions such as the President, Vice President and an eight-member Board of Directors. The Board comprises five midwife members who are elected by the membership for a 3-year term, and an additional three community directors appointed by the Board based on the needs of the organisation (ACM, 2020). Together these volunteers govern the ACM.

Governance involves setting the strategic and financial direction of the organisation and ensuring that professional membership contributions are used wisely. The National Board of Directors meets up to four times per year either face to face or online to fulfil this governance role. National Directors are elected from each state and territory with staggered 3-year terms maintaining both continuity and succession requirements of the organisation. The President is elected by the members and towards the end of each 3-year term nominations are sought and an election held to coincide with the national conference. The Vice President is appointed by the Board from within the Board membership.

The ACM also has an eight-member Council comprising an elected member from each state and territory. The Council has the specific role of managing the ACM Awards program. The Council also informs the Board, President and CEO of issues at local state and territory levels. The Chair of the Council also holds a position on the Board of Directors.

In 2020 a post-unification review was commissioned to identify how to optimise the work of the national Board, Council, and Branches moving forward with the implementation of the new strategic plan (ACM, n.d.b).

Each state and territory branch of the ACM must fulfil the aims and objectives of the college set out in the Strategic Plan, in its operations. Branch committees are made up of a chair, a secretary and a treasurer with additional positions as required. There is usually one branch for each jurisdiction but sub-branches can be organised with agreement. The branches implement the national strategic direction at a local level.

The ACM also has many advisory committees, working groups and liaison midwives who provide feedback to the college on what is happening in the wider community and practice. These advisory groups and individuals are the eyes and ears of the College and support the work of the organisation. Box 13.1 identifies the advisory committees and working groups of the ACM in 2020. However, as identified earlier a review of the structure and purpose of councils and committees is in progress at the time of publication.

The ACM has always sought to establish alliances and effective working relationships with women and maternity consumer groups. However, maternity reform processes at the start of the last decade have strengthened these relationships and their importance is recognised through constitutional changes within state and territory

---

Box 13.1 Advisory committees and working groups for the Australian College of Midwives (2020)

Aboriginal and Torres Strait Islander Advisory Committee

Baby Friendly Health Initiative (BFHI) Advisory Committee

Consumer Advisory Committee

International Confederation of Midwives (ICM) Advisory Committee

Midwifery Education Advisory Committee

Private Practice Midwives Advisory Committee

Safety and Quality Advisory Committee

Scientific Review Advisory Committee

Midwifery Practice Review Working Group

(Source: Australian College of Midwives.)

branches that now enable women consumers to be members of the ACM.

Role and functions

The ACM aims to be the unified political voice for the midwifery profession in Australia. It has strong strategic relationships with the Nursing and Midwifery Board of Australia (NMBA), the Australian Nursing and Midwifery Accreditation Council (ANMAC), the Australian Health Practitioner Regulation Agency (AHPRA), all state and territory Chief Nursing and Midwifery Officers (CNMOs) and the Commonwealth's Nursing and Midwifery Strategic Reference Group (NMSRG). Most recently, the College entered into a Memorandum of Understanding with RANZCOG, agreeing to have respectful conversation in matters of mutual interest so that agreed joint statements can be released whenever possible (NMBA, 2022). The ACM wishes to set professional practice and education standards and support midwives to reach their full potential of working with childbearing women to ensure they have access to continuity of care (COC) by a known midwife.

The national approach to ensuring consistency is the shared vision and mission and the implementation of the strategic plan. The ACM's Vision is 'Enabling strong and confident midwives', and its Mission is stated as 'Midwifery is the primary profession for quality maternity care' (ACM, 2021d). Its strategic priorities are summarised in Box 13.2.

The ACM influences national health policy through acting as a consultant to government bodies and seeks to have midwifery recognised as an essential public health strategy. The ACM also provides information and networks with midwives throughout Australia and other organisations working to improve maternal and newborn health services. Other activities include: supporting governance for the Baby Friendly Hospital Initiative (BFHI) in Australia; enabling a forum for professional midwifery discussion and debate; disseminating current information via the quarterly *Women and Birth* journal, *Australian Midwifery News*, national midwifery conferences, and through state and territory branches and the media; producing Midwifery Guidelines, Midwifery Practice Standards and Position Statements; and providing scholarships for midwives to undertake research and to assist in the promotion of the education and practice of midwifery through administration of the Australian Midwifery Scholarship Foundation and promotion of the Rhodanthe Lipsett Indigenous Midwifery Charitable Trust.

The role and functions of the ACM are summarised in Box 13.3.

ACM supporting continuing professional development

The ACM is involved in the provision of continuing education programs for midwives through MidPLUS, Midwifery Practice Review (MPR), conferences and through provision of online webinars.

The MidPLUS **continuing professional development** (CPD) tool assists midwives to reflect on their midwifery practice, identify their learning needs, and to plan and record their CPD activities. It comprises a flexible CPD program based on the Midwife Standards for Practice (NMBA, 2018[1]b). Midwives complete an individual professional portfolio framework and an online points system encouraging a range of educational and practice activities. Midwives define and accrue a minimum of 30 MidPLUS points (1 hour CPD = 1 MidPLUS point) of activity each year. Activity is specific to the midwife's context of practice or desired area of development, and based on individualised learning requirements. An annual certificate of accomplishment is issued aligned with the national registration renewal period using details recorded in each midwife's online log and reflective practice activities.

Midwifery Practice Review was launched in 2007 and is a national, confidential peer-review process for midwives in clinical practice. It was developed initially with funding from the Australian Commission for Safety and Quality in Health Care (ACSQHC). The express objective was to develop a national process to enable Australian midwives to demonstrate their competence, confidence and capacity to provide safe, high-quality care within the full scope of midwifery practice by demonstrating how they meet the Midwife Standards for Practice (NMBA, 2018b).

MPR is flexible and is available to midwives working in a variety of midwifery practice contexts. It involves a three-stage process: preparation of a synopsis of midwifery philosophy and practice that is context specific, including detailed reflection and examples of how the midwife meets the Midwife Standards for Practice (NMBA, 2018b); face-to-face review and discussion with trained midwife and consumer reviewers, including reflection on relevant practice statistics; and planning and support in relation to professional goals and development (ACM, 2018). Acknowledgement of completion and written feedback are provided to the midwife in addition to an allocation of 30 MidPLUS points (ACM, 2018.).

Box 13.2 The four strategic priorities of the Australian College of Midwives (ACM) Strategic Plan 2021–2023

- Lead the midwifery profession.
- Engage with midwives Australia wide.
- Support midwives to thrive and succeed across their professional lives.
- Influence the transformation of maternity services to enable more satisfying careers for midwives

(Source: https://www.midwives.org.au/common/Uploaded%20files/_ADMIN-ACM/ACM%20Strategic%20Plan%202021-2023%20Public.pdf © Australia College of Midwives.)

Box 13.3 Australian College of Midwives (ACM)—role and functions

Philosophy

Midwife means *'with woman'*: this underpins midwifery's philosophy, work and relationships.

Midwifery:

- is founded on respect for women and on a strong belief in the value of women's work, bearing and rearing each generation
- considers women in pregnancy, childbirth and early parenting to be undertaking healthy processes that are profound and precious events in each woman's life; these events are also inherently important to society as a whole
- protects and enhances the health and social status of women, which in turn protects and enhances the health and wellbeing of society
- is a woman-centred, political, primary healthcare discipline founded on the relationship between a woman and her midwife
- focuses on a woman's health needs, her expectations and aspirations
- encompasses the needs of the woman's baby, and the woman's family, her other important relationships and community, as identified and negotiated by the woman herself
- is holistic and recognises each woman's social, emotional, physical, spiritual and cultural needs, expectations and context as defined by the woman herself
- recognises every woman's right to self-determination in attaining choice, control and continuity of care from one or more known caregivers
- recognises every woman's responsibility to make informed decisions for herself, her baby and her family with assistance, when requested, from health professionals
- is informed by scientific evidence, by collective and individual experience, and by intuition
- aims to follow each woman through pregnancy, labour and birth and the postnatal period, across the transition between institutions and the community, so she remains connected to her social support systems; the focus remaining on the woman, not on the institutions or the professionals involved
- includes collaboration with and consultation between health professionals.

(Inspired by work from: New Zealand College of Midwives, Nursing Council of New Zealand, Nursing and Midwifery Council UK (formerly UKCC/ENB), Royal College of Midwives, College of Midwives of British Columbia, College of Midwives of Ontario, Australian College of Midwives, Nurses Board of Victoria, Nursing Council of Queensland, World Health Organization, Guilliland & Pairman (1995), Leap (2004).)

Midwifery continuity of care

Knowing your midwife—being cared for by, and able to build a trust and rapport with, the same midwife during pregnancy (or even pre-conception), through labour and birth, and into the early weeks of mothering—has benefits for mothers, babies and society.

(Source: https://www.midwives.org.au/midwifery-philosophy)

ACM values

The ACM work is guided by the following values:

Ethical practice:

- applying evidence to everything the College does
- following code of ethics, conduct, practice and standards.

Collaboration:

- working cooperatively with external groups and respecting their role and interaction
- listening, hearing, discussing and passing the agreed message on
- protecting those who are not present and talking to the source.

Trusting and respectful relationships:

- treating each other as we would wish to be treated.

Respect diversity:

- respecting a person's right to have a different opinion.

Innovation:

- be open to new ideas and understand that there is always another way and that anything is possible
- striving for continuous improvement.

Other functions are:

- to provide continuing education programs for midwives through online and face-to-face continuing professional development
- to act as a consultant to government bodies in the development of health policy that makes midwifery a public health strategy
- to provide an information network for midwives throughout Australia and all organisations affiliated with the International Confederation of Midwives
- to provide a forum for professional midwifery discussion and debate
- to disseminate current information via the ACM journal, national newsletter, biennial national midwifery conferences, and through state branches and the media
- to provide scholarships for midwives to undertake research and to assist in the promotion of the education and practice of midwifery through administration of the Australian Midwifery Scholarship Foundation and the national midwifery biennial conferences, and through state branches and the media (ACM, 2008)
- to engage in projects to improve maternity services for women such as the Birthing on Country Project and the Reconciliation Action Plan (ACM, 2017b).

(Sources: New Zealand College of Midwives, Nursing Council of New Zealand, Nursing and Midwifery Council UK (formerly UKCC/ENB), Royal College of Midwives, College of Midwives of British Columbia, College of Midwives of Ontario, Australian College of Midwives, Nurses Board of Victoria, Nursing Council of Queensland, the World Health Organization, Guilliland & Pairman (1995), Leap (2004))

Review is recommended on a 3-yearly basis. MPR forms one of the six regulatory requirements of the NMBA for midwives to establish eligibility for the purpose of notation on the national register as an 'endorsed midwife'. Endorsement annotation will be discussed further later in the chapter. The original design of MPR drew heavily on the NZCOM's Midwifery Standards Review process as well as the Midwifery Council of New Zealand's Recertification program.

Other organisations

Like New Zealand, Australia has a number of organisations that support midwives providing continuity of care. These include:

- Midwives Australia—provides advice and guidance to midwives wishing to set up in private practice (https://www.midwivesaustralia.com.au/about-us/)
- Midwives in Private Practice (MIPP) based in Victoria
- Private Practice Midwives Advisory Committee—the ACM provides advice and recommendations on matters that pertain to midwifery private practice and maternity care (https://www.midwives.org.au/committees/private-practice-midwives-advisory-committee).

These organisations add important infrastructure and communication networks to the community of midwives looking for support in development of caseload midwifery practice in Australia.

In public healthcare facilities throughout Australia, the majority of midwives, as employees of the state, have had no collective salary agreements that are independent of the eight state/territory-based nursing awards under whose conditions, terms and pay structures they are employed. Predominantly, individual-enterprise bargaining arrangements or collective salary agreements for newly emerging midwifery caseload care or expanding midwifery group practices continue to be negotiated between area health services or local health networks and the Australian Nursing and Midwifery Federation (ANMF).

DEVELOPMENT OF THE MIDWIFERY PROFESSION IN NEW ZEALAND

Redefining professionalism in New Zealand

The current status of midwifery as a profession in New Zealand is somewhat different to that in Australia. New Zealand midwives are an autonomous and distinct professional group. They were granted a social mandate for autonomous practice in 1990 through the Nurses Amendment Act and subsequently have established midwives as the main providers of maternity services based on a model of autonomous caseload practice and midwifery partnership (Guilliland & Pairman, 2010a).

Largely through the influence of the midwifery profession, New Zealand's maternity service has been reshaped to be a woman-centred and midwife-led service in which each woman can access one-to-one continuity of midwifery care from early pregnancy through to 6 weeks postpartum, no matter what the course of her childbirth experience and which other providers need to be involved, and no matter where she chooses to give birth (Guilliland & Pairman, 2010b; Pairman & Guilliland, 2003). New Zealand midwives, perhaps more than in any other country, most closely meet the *International Definition of the Midwife* and *Definition of Midwifery* by being able to practise across the full scope of midwifery practice (ICM, 2017a, 2017b; NZ Gazette, 2010).

For the New Zealand midwifery profession, these achievements are the culmination of years of planned political and professional activity to bring about the necessary changes to legislation, to societal understandings of birth and midwifery, and to midwives' understandings of midwifery as a profession that is deeply intertwined with women. The central tenet of New Zealand midwifery's professional identity is that midwifery *is* the partnership between women and midwives (Guilliland & Pairman, 1995, 2010b; NZCOM, 2015; Pairman, 2005). By constituting midwifery practice as 'midwifery partnership', New Zealand midwives have sought to replace traditional notions of professionalism with one in which relationships between midwives and women are negotiated and where power differentials are acknowledged and actively shifted from the midwife to the childbearing woman (Pairman, 2005).

This recognition that midwifery is a partnership between a woman and a midwife resulted from the combined political activity of maternity consumer groups and the New Zealand College of Midwives (NZCOM), which led to the Nurses Amendment Act 1990 and the one-to-one caseload model of midwifery practice that developed subsequently (Guilliland & Pairman, 2010a, 2010b).

Although New Zealand has had a regulated midwifery workforce since the Midwives Act 1904, the scope of midwifery practice diminished as a result of increasing hospitalisation and medicalisation of childbirth from the early 1920s onwards (Donley, 1986; Guilliland & Pairman, 2010a; Mein Smith, 1986; Pairman, 2002, 2005; Pairman & Guilliland, 2003; Papps & Olssen, 1997). Women were encouraged to give birth in hospitals to avoid the risks of puerperal infection in the home and so that they could access 'pain-free' birth. Claims by doctors that hospitals were safer than home were later shown to be unfounded (Mein Smith, 1986) and it is well documented that hospitalisation led to fragmented maternity care, loss of control for women and their families, increased medical intervention and use of technology, loss of confidence in women's bodies and increased fear of birth (Donley, 1986; Donnison, 1988; Kitzinger, 1988; Mein Smith, 1986; Papps & Olssen, 1997; Tew, 1990). Institutional organisational power structures also affected midwives, who lost their one-to-one community-based practice with women to become 'doctor assistants' and 'specialists' in aspects of maternity care. By 1971, midwifery was no longer visible as a separate profession and was incorporated into nursing as 'specialist nursing practice'. Legislative changes in 1983 and 1986 further undermined the definition and **scope of practice** of midwifery, which reached an all-time low where only a handful of home-birth midwives remained practising in a way that bore any resemblance to the *ICM Definition of Midwifery* (Donley, 1986; ICM, 2017b).

It was this near-demise of midwifery that led to its rebirth. In reclaiming their identity as separate from nursing, midwives used their professional group, the Midwives Section of the New Zealand Nurses Association, as a vehicle for political action. Initially this activity was focused on reclaiming the ICM definition of a midwife as a 'person' rather than a 'nurse' (as the Nurses Association had redefined it) and on separating midwifery education from nursing (Pairman, 2002, 2005). However, midwives soon realised that their interests were divergent from those of nursing and could never be served by the (larger) nursing professional organisation. Midwives disbanded the Midwives Sections and in 1989 formed a separate midwifery professional organisation, the New Zealand College of Midwives (Donley, 1989; Guilliland, 1989; Guilliland & Pairman, 2010a).

Maternity consumer groups were also active at this time, seeking to gain control over their birth experiences and to decrease the dominance of the medical model over maternity services (Strid, 1987). These women had faith in midwifery and argued for a return of the autonomous midwife, who they believed would be more likely to share power with women through a more woman-centred and normal-birth philosophy of practice (Dobbie, 1990; Strid, 1987).

Recognising that their aims were mutual, midwives and women joined together in a combined political strategy that would firstly reinstate midwifery autonomy, secondly enable women to have a choice of midwifery care, and thirdly enable the development of direct-entry midwifery education to produce the new type of midwife that would be required for this autonomous scope of practice.

A key outcome was that midwives recognised the benefit to themselves and to women of their political partnership, and they gave meaning to this partnership by incorporating partnership constitutionally into every aspect of the NZCOM. Midwifery 'consciously recognises that the only real power base we have rests with the women we attend' (Guilliland, 1989, p. 14). The active involvement of women in the NZCOM has continued to strengthen midwifery. 'Women's participation in the midwifery profession has given midwives a public, legal and socially sanctioned mandate for practice' (Guilliland & Pairman, 1995, p. 19). This social mandate carries with it a moral obligation for the midwifery profession to provide the kind of service women want. The continued involvement of women (consumers) in the policy formation and processes of the NZCOM ensures that midwives uphold the needs and wishes of women (Guilliland & Pairman, 1995, 2010a).

It was this understanding of the link between professional autonomy and women's need to have control over their birthing experiences that was the basis of New Zealand midwives' determination to redefine professionalism. Although not attracted by the traditional 'power over' model of professionalism, they recognised the potential benefit of professional autonomy. As Oakley & Houd (1990, p. 114) contend, 'the exclusion from childbirth of autonomous midwifery restricts the care options available to childbearing women and inevitably promotes the definition of childbearing as a pathological medicalised event'. New Zealand midwives and women believed that, if midwifery autonomy was reinstated, then midwives would have the ability to once again practise within their traditional role as a guardian of normal birth (Strid, 1987). Each midwife who worked in this way would be a 'positive presence who focuses on the childbearing woman and the baby, with the knowledge and skills required, but also with a sensitivity and respect for the individuality and uniqueness of each woman and her choices for birthing' (Strid, 1987, p. 15). Writers such as Barbara Katz Rothman supported these beliefs; she stated:

> I have come to see that it is not that birth is managed the way it is because of what we know about birth. Rather, what we know about birth has been determined by the way it has been managed. And the way childbirth has been managed has been based on the underlying assumptions, beliefs and ideology of medicine as a profession.
>
> (Katz Rothman, 1984, p. 304)

The determination to provide women and midwives with the opportunity to co-create new knowledge and understandings of childbirth that would lead to women regaining control and choice in childbirth, and to society once again recognising childbirth as a normal life event rather than an illness, was the impetus for political activity to reinstate midwifery autonomy. Through the experience of this political partnership, midwives were able to conceptualise a 'new' model of professionalism:

> By redefining the professional–client relationship as one of 'partnership' in which each partner contributes knowledge and experience, it also embraces feminist criticisms of the hierarchical power relations inherent in the doctor–patient relationship and the consequent devaluing of women's knowledge.
>
> (Tully & Mortlock, 1999, p. 175)

In recognising the knowledge and experience of women/clients as well as midwives, midwifery partnership does not afford midwifery expertise and knowledge the same epistemological priority it held in the 'old' model of professionalism (Tully, 1999). In midwifery partnership, both midwives and women have recognised authority and the midwife's role moves from 'expert' to 'reflective practitioner' whose task is to support, guide and accompany a woman within a more equitable, interdependent and empowering relationship (Tully, 1999). In redefining midwifery practice as partnership, New Zealand midwives have differentiated midwifery services from maternity services offered by other providers and claimed jurisdiction over 'normal' birthing services. Thus partnership with women is an effective professionalising strategy for midwives (Pairman, 2005; Tully, 1999).

The challenge for midwifery is to maintain its partnership relationships with women and, as will be discussed, the professional and regulatory frameworks of New Zealand midwifery both aim to ensure that this occurs. By articulating midwifery as a partnership, New Zealand midwives have redefined traditional notions of professionalism. However, midwives need to understand this definition and the implications of this 'new' style of professionalism for midwifery practice so that midwives do not abuse their power and authority.

> *Instead of seeking to control childbirth, midwifery seeks to control midwifery, in order that women can control childbirth. Midwifery must maintain its women-centered philosophy to ensure that its control of midwifery never leads to control of childbirth.*
>
> (Guilliland & Pairman, 1995, p. 49)

REFLECTIVE THINKING EXERCISE

Consider the above quote from Guilliland & Pairman (1995) and think about what it means for your practice as a midwife. In what ways can you support women to control childbirth? What might it mean for women if midwifery controlled childbirth? What can you do to ensure that women remain at the centre of decisions about their care?

Structure and functions of the New Zealand College of Midwives

The New Zealand College of Midwives is the professional organisation for midwifery in New Zealand. Established in 1989, the College has provided a mechanism for midwives to establish themselves as a profession separate from nursing. Membership is voluntary and approximately 90% of the midwifery workforce (both employed and self-employed midwives) as well as consumers and consumer organisations, choose to be members. Midwives' commitment to midwifery partnership has meant that, from its inception, women consumers have been members as of right and the constitution provides for regional and national membership by individual women and consumer groups. The consumer membership votes for four representatives to the National Board from consumer organisations such as the Parents Centre New Zealand, Home Birth Aotearoa, the La Leche League and the Plunket Society. As the voice for midwifery in New Zealand, the College is involved in a wide variety of activities, both professional and political, to meet the needs of individual midwives, the profession as a whole, and birthing women as its

partners and the focus of its interests, by working to maintain a strong and autonomous midwifery profession. The roles and services of the College are listed in Box 13.4 and its objectives in Box 13.5.

The College structure is simple (Fig. 13.1). New Zealand is divided into 10 regions and 5 sub-regions that function autonomously, each with their own regional committee and constitution that aligns with the national NZCOM constitution. The 10 regional chairpersons (all midwives) are members of the 24-member National Board (the governance body of the College), along with the consumer representatives, midwifery student representatives, Māori midwife representatives and Pacifika midwife representatives. The President and the Chief Executive lead the Committee with support from two kuia or elders (one Māori and one Pākehā [non-Māori] and an Education Advisor). The National Committee meets four times a year to fulfil its governance role. An ad-hoc committee of the National Committee forms a Finance Committee to examine financial and other policy issues in depth, in order to assist and inform the National Committee decision-making processes. The College works in a non-hierarchical and woman-centred model that includes extensive consultation processes and consensus decision making. The National Committee employs the Chief Executive, who in turn employs the staff of the National Office. These staff members, some of whom are midwives, carry out the day-to-day work of the College as represented in Box 13.4.

As it has evolved, the College has recognised the need for other midwifery-specific organisations to meet the business and industrial needs of midwives. Considerable thought went into the establishment of these organisations to ensure that their structure, functions and governance mechanisms

---

Box 13.4　New Zealand College of Midwives roles and services

1. Professional practice advice and information for midwives, District Health Boards (DHBs), consumers and community agencies

2. Professional representation, including to Ministry of Health and DHBs

3. Quality assurance, including Midwifery Standards Review and Complaints Resolutions Committees

4. Ongoing education and professional development, including Midwifery First Year of Practice Programme and continuing education

5. Ongoing liaison and consultation

6. Research

7. Communication and promotion, including publications

For more information see https://www.midwife.org.nz/midwives/college-roles-and-services/.

Box 13.5 New Zealand College of Midwives objectives

- To purposefully and continuously develop and maintain a strong autonomous midwifery profession in New Zealand.
- To lead, promote and support partnership-based midwifery practice that conforms to the Code of Ethics and the Standards for Midwifery Practice.
- To lead the development and maintenance of a quality assurance framework to improve maternity outcomes for women and families.
- To advocate for the development and provision of services, policies and programmes that support the improvement of maternity outcomes and health status of women and their families/whānau.
- To provide expert advice to government and other relevant agencies to strengthen and support the midwifery profession.
- To advocate for, promote, and evaluate undergraduate and postgraduate education and provide continuing education for midwives.
- To conduct, promote and disseminate relevant research which provides an evidence base for midwifery practice in New Zealand.
- To commit to upholding the articles of Te Tiriti O Waitangi by recognising Māori as Tangata Whenua of Aotearoa.
- To build and maintain relationships with relevant national and international agencies to the benefit of midwifery in New Zealand, and to contribute to the global midwifery community.
- To operate in an efficient and effective manner to the benefit of its members through the delivery of a comprehensive professional service to its members.

(Source: New Zealand College of Midwives. Online: https://www.midwife.org.nz/midwives/college-roles-and-services/)

---

did not become blurred with the College and dissipate the overall strength and unity of the midwifery voice. The College has therefore created three separate but parallel organisations: the Midwifery and Maternity Provider Organisation, the Midwifery Employee Representation and Advisory Service, and the Joan Donley Midwifery Research Collaboration. Each organisation has its own governance structure and specific role and functions, and its links to the College are maintained through College representation to its governance structure and through the requirement for midwives to be members of the College first before they can access services from any of these organisations.

The Midwifery and Maternity Provider Organisation (MMPO)

The College established the MMPO in 1997 as a separate limited-liability company with its own governance structure. Its purpose is to provide the College's lead maternity carer (LMC) midwife members with a supportive practice management and quality assurance infrastructure and a business framework. In turn this support enables LMC midwives to provide high-quality continuity of care for women throughout New Zealand. The MMPO provides its members with:

- a standardised, peer-reviewed set of maternity notes and a series of individualised reporting templates (paper and electronic)
- access to and ongoing support for an electronic maternity record and practice management system incorporating the NZCOM data set and a suite of records (Midwifery Information System) and integrating with New Zealand's national electronic maternity record
- a reliable maternity service claiming and payment system
- collection of relevant maternity outcome data and maintenance of a midwifery database that enables individual midwives to track their outcomes and benchmark themselves against the profession's standards, the College to provide aggregated clinical information about midwifery practices and outcomes, and a database for midwifery research
- workforce support, including locum support
- business workshops and support, including equipment insurance
- data security.

The linkage between providing midwives with women-friendly maternity notes and collection of data for a midwifery-focused perinatal database has been a significant achievement (Hendry & Guilliland, 2010). Women have access to their notes (hard copy of electronic via an app), midwives maintain their copy as a clinical and legal record, and the MMPO also accesses the notes (hard copy of electronic) to claim fees from the government on behalf of midwives and for clinical data entry into the NZCOM midwifery database. Midwives receive their fee payment together with a report on their clinical outcomes and statistics, which they take to their biennial Midwifery Standards Review.

The majority of self-employed midwives throughout New Zealand use this service, and the MMPO also manages the midwife claims for some District Health Board and Community Trust employers.

NZCOM contracts the MMPO to enter the clinical data from the maternity notes for its midwifery database. It then uses the database to analyse the aggregated and anonymous data and produce national reports on midwifery care activities and outcomes; in 2016 the report represented over half of all registered births in that year (NZCOM, 2016; Stats NZ, 2017).

Locum Services

The Locum Services are a joint venture between NZCOM and the MMPO. Established in November 2009 with funding from the Ministry of Health (MOH), the Rural Midwifery Recruitment and Retention Service (RMRRS) supports and sustains midwifery services for rural

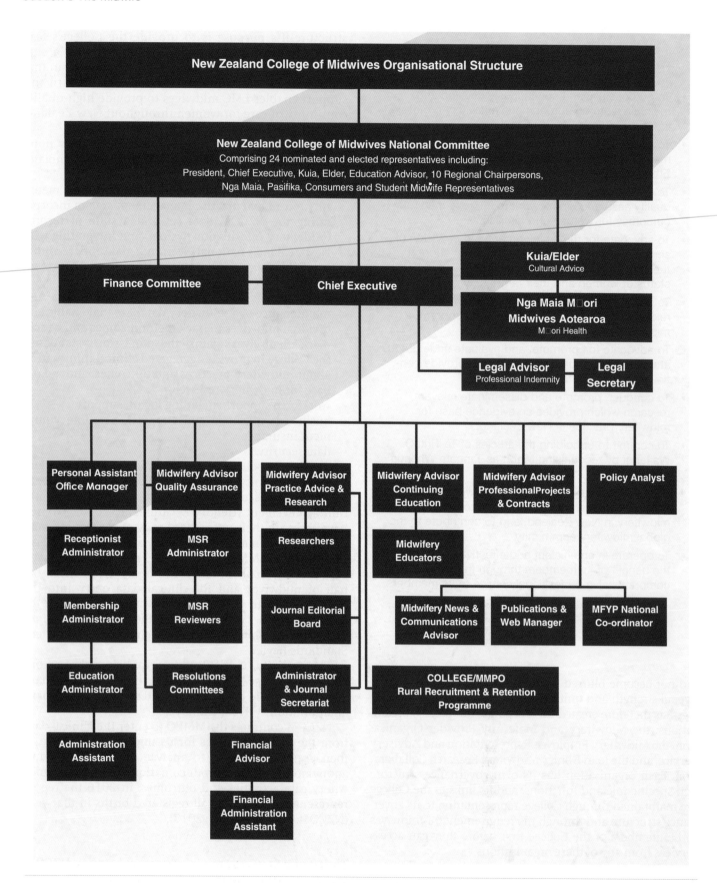

FIGURE 13.1 New Zealand College of Midwives (NZCOM) management and organisational structure. MFYP=Midwifery First Year of Practice; MSR=Midwifery Standards Review; MMPO=Midwifery and Maternity Provider Organisation
(Source: NZCOM, 2018; © New Zealand College of Midwives)

communities, through providing time off for education, annual leave and emergencies. Eligible LMC midwives are provided with nine days of funded locum cover per year and up to five days of locum cover for accident or illness, bereavement, family emergencies or special circumstances. In 2018 the MMPO secured funding to also provide emergency locum support services to urban-based LMC midwives (https://mmpo.org.nz/).

The Midwifery Employee Representation and Advisory Service (MERAS)

MERAS is the union for employed midwives. Its formation arose from the wish of College members for a more midwifery-focused representation in the workplace (Guilliland & McIlhone, 2010). Until 2002, industrial representation for midwives was available only through the New Zealand Nurses Organisation (NZNO), and salaries and conditions to meet the needs of employed midwives and their various practice models could be recognised only through varying the nursing agreement. The establishment of MERAS in 2002 provided a union dedicated to representing midwives and around 90% of employed midwives belong to MERAS.

MERAS negotiates a collective agreement specifically for midwives and links this to the regulatory and professional frameworks of the Midwifery Council of New Zealand and the New Zealand College of Midwives. MERAS's multiple employer collective agreement (MECA) incorporates the Midwifery Quality and Leadership Programme, a national framework that links DHB-required professional development with midwifery professional development and the recertification requirements of the Midwifery Council of New Zealand (MERAS, 2014). For more information see: https://www.midwife.org.nz/wp-content/uploads/2018/08/QLP-Revision-November-2014.pdf.

MERAS represents members in their employment issues, negotiates collective agreements, and supports the professional needs of employed midwives.

The Joan Donley Midwifery Research Collaboration (JDMRC)

The JDMRC is housed in the College and is named after midwife Joan Donley, one of the founders of the NZCOM and midwife author and researcher. The JDMRC provides the framework and secretarial support for all research undertaken by the College and in line with its research strategy. Set up in honour of Joan Donley's commitment to an evidence-based midwifery profession, its core purpose is to promote and facilitate midwifery research and contribute to evidence about New Zealand's unique maternity service context. It provides a mechanism for collaboration between researchers, educators and the profession to evaluate and research the effectiveness and appropriateness of midwifery practice and policy. In collaboration with the College the JDMRC hosts a biennial national research forum to support and promote postgraduate midwifery researchers, to develop expertise, to support a research culture in DHBs and to provide a forum for developing robust research.

The JDMRC website provides access to a database of New Zealand research and to summaries of Cochrane reviews of midwifery care (https://www.midwife.org.nz/midwives/research/joan-donley-midwifery-research-collaboration-jdmrc/).

Professional activities

The leadership of the NZCOM has been a major driver in the development of the midwife-led and women-centred maternity service that New Zealand enjoys today (Guilliland & Pairman, 2010a; Pairman, 2005; Pairman & Guilliland, 2003). Its leadership has also been essential in the development of midwifery as a strong and autonomous profession. There have been many processes through which the College has worked and continues to work with midwives to build their professional identity and enhance professional standards. These include:

- developing its philosophy and setting standards for practice and an ethical framework, first approved in 1990 and subsequently updated periodically (NZCOM, 2015)
- producing consensus statements (https://www.midwife.org.nz/midwives/professional-practice/consensus-statements/) and guidelines to support best practice (https://www.midwife.org.nz/midwives/professional-practice/practice-guidance/)
- providing an extensive range of continuing education opportunities on a range of topics including documentation and record keeping, mentoring, perineal care, postnatal care, the Treaty of Waitangi and bicultural practice and unexpected outcomes (https://www.midwife.org.nz/midwives/education/continuing-midwifery-education/)
- undertaking and publishing research into midwifery practice, including establishing a midwifery database of published New Zealand midwifery research (https://www.midwife.org.nz/midwives/research/)
- managing various grants for student midwives and practising undertaking study (on behalf of Health Workforce New Zealand) (https://www.midwife.org.nz/midwives/college-roles-and-services/grants-available/)
- publishing resources to guide practice and professional development (e.g. *Midwives Handbook for Practice, Midwives Portfolio*)
- advising and monitoring preregistration midwifery education programs
- managing and providing the Midwifery First Year of Practice (MFYP) program (on contract by Health Workforce New Zealand) (https://www.midwife.org.nz/midwives/mentoring/midwifery-first-year-of-practice-mfyp/)
- running biennial national midwifery conferences and research forums (https://www.midwife.org.nz/news/category/midwives)
- publishing a journal and newsletter (https://www.midwife.org.nz/midwives/publications/).

Perhaps one of the College's most innovative and important professional developments is its Midwifery

Standards Review. This, together with its Resolutions process, provides a quality-assurance process for midwifery practice in New Zealand that aims to improve and maintain professional midwifery standards. Each region of the College has standing committees for its MSR process and its Resolutions process. As will be discussed later, the College's MSR process is an essential feature of the compulsory recertification program established in 2005 by the MCNZ for all practising midwives.

Midwifery Standards Review (MSR)

The Domiciliary Midwives Society initially established Midwifery Review in 1988 to review the practice of home-birth midwives. This was in response to moves by obstetric and hospital managers to try to impose hospital practices and protocols on the home-birth service. As more midwives moved into self-employed practice after 1990, the College realised that it needed to provide a similar quality assurance mechanism for all midwives. Consequently, in 1992, the College adopted the domiciliary review process and modified it to include the College's **standards of practice**. Eventually the Domiciliary Midwives Society dissolved and became part of the College, and all midwives are now reviewed under the same criteria (Campbell & Guilliland, 2010).

The Midwifery Standards Review (MSR) is a systematic process that enables the midwife, whatever her practice setting, to reflect on how she works with the MSR committee, using the NZCOM Standards of Practice and Tūranga Kaupapa as a guide.

Each MSR committee comprises one midwife, nominated from the region, and one consumer, nominated from consumer organisations. Each College region endorses all members. All reviewers attend a College-run national training program that seeks to ensure a standardised approach to MSR throughout the country and to help reviewers develop the personal and communication skills necessary for the reviewer role.

Midwives prepare for review by examining their work since their last MSR, analysing their birth outcomes (statistics) or, if employed as a core midwife, those of the facility in which the midwife works, considering feedback from women clients (collected via client evaluations by a third party and provided to the midwife for her review) and from colleagues, undertaking a self-assessment against the NZCOM Standards for Practice, commenting on achievement of the professional development goals set at her last review and how she has met the Midwifery Council requirements for recertification and considering future goals to be discussed and determined at the review (https://www.midwife.org.nz/midwives/midwifery-standards-review/midwifery-standards-review-process/).

Midwives meet individually with the Review Committee and can explore and discuss their midwifery practice through a supportive and educative process. A main outcome is the joint development of a Professional Development Plan that is revisited at the next review.

It was caseloading midwives who initially undertook MSR, usually annually. In 2003, NZCOM began encouraging core midwives (hospital midwives not working in caseload models) to undertake MSR, and since 2005 the Midwifery Council has made it mandatory for all midwives as part of its recertification program. Initially, caseload midwives were reviewed annually and core midwives every 3 years. Then from 2008 the Midwifery Council required all midwives to undergo MSR every 2 years. The Council's 2020–21 recertification program requires all midwives to undertake MSR as follows:

- Midwives in the Midwifery First Year of Practice Programme complete a MSR at the end of their first year and third years of practice; reviews are three yearly thereafter.
- Midwives on a Return to Practice Programme complete a review at the end of their second year of practice. Reviews are three yearly thereafter.
- Internationally Qualified Midwives undertaking the Overseas Competence Programme complete a review at the end of their second year of practice. Reviews are three yearly thereafter.

MSR reviewers have the discretion to require a midwife to complete a review before the required timeframe but they cannot extend any timeframes (https://www.midwiferycouncil.health.nz/common/Uploaded%20files/Annual%20Practising%20Certificates/Recertification%20programme.pdf).

Resolution Committees

While the review process is consciously midwife centred, the College's commitment to partnership with women is reflected in the establishment of Resolution Committees. These focus on consumers, and any woman with concerns about the midwifery care she has received can use this process. One midwife and one consumer make up the committee and also participate in a national training program. The committee helps a woman to resolve her issues through facilitating a meeting with the midwife or by providing a forum in which a woman can have her concerns heard and discussed. If resolution is not possible, the committee helps the woman access other available avenues (https://www.midwife.org.nz/midwives/college-roles-and-services/resolutions-committee/).

Pay equity

The College has also provided significant leadership in ensuring that midwives are appropriately recognised and valued for the important work they do and the responsibilities they hold. LMC midwives identified inadequate payment as a significant issue over several years and despite numerous opportunities the government did not act to remedy the situation. In 2015 the College sought a judicial review by the High Court against the MOH under the Bill of Rights. The College asked the High Court to decide whether lack of equitable funding for LMC midwives was the result of systemic and historic discrimination because midwives were women (NZCOM, 2017b).

After 21 months of discussion the College reached a landmark agreement with the MOH to work together to jointly redesign a funding model that pays community LMC midwives equitably for the work they actually do. This legally binding agreement required funding recommendations to be submitted to the government by August 2018. Continuity of midwifery care was to remain at the heart of the funding model and there were no plans to change New Zealand's remarkable model of maternity care. Rather, the redesign was intended to address the structural barriers that have denied community LMC midwives pay equity and threatened the sustainability of the LMC system (NZCOM, 2017b).

Unfortunately the promise this agreement offered was not honoured by the Ministry of Health, albeit some significant increases were made in some fees under the old structure of Section 88 of the Health and Disability Services Act. This remains the situation at the time of writing in 2022. The Ministry committed to delivering a new national midwifery contract by July 2020, reflecting a blended payment model, alongside determining 'fair and reasonable' pay for LMC midwives. However, this has not been delivered and the College has been again forced to put the government on notice that it intends further Court action to achieve the pay equity promises made in good faith so long ago (NZCOM, 2017b, n.d.).

Midwifery education in New Zealand

Preregistration midwifery education

Since 1992, midwifery students have completed a three-year Bachelor's program to prepare for midwifery registration. The majority of students are direct entry, without a previous nursing registration, but registered nurses can enter the same program and apply for recognition of prior learning as appropriate. Since 2004 the Midwifery Council of New Zealand has set the standards for preregistration midwifery education programs. In 2007 the program was extended to the equivalent of 4 academic years, although still undertaken over 3 calendar years (Pairman, 2010). The Midwifery Council reviewed the education standards in 2019 and provided for two time scales—the extended academic year (4 years delivered in 3 calendar years) or 4 academic years (MCNZ, 2019a). (See later in this chapter.)

Midwifery First Year of Practice (MFYP)

Since 2007, all new graduates have had access to the MFYP program, funded by the government and delivered by the NZCOM. This program provides all new graduates with support from a named mentor as well as paid education and professional development hours to assist midwives develop knowledge and skills to progress from a competent to a confident midwife. The MFYP program is also an important workforce strategy, as support of new graduates is seen as a mechanism to enhance retention and strengthen the capability of midwives. The program

was evaluated in 2008, with excellent outcomes (Oliver, 2008). Research conducted in 2014 and 2016 assessed whether participation in the MFYP program supported the retention of new graduate midwives and explored which elements of the program contributed to retention and development of confidence for the new graduate midwife practitioner; graduates considered each element of the program important, found that it met their needs and identified that it helped them to increase confidence in their first year of practice as a registered midwife (Dixon et al., 2014; Pairman et al., 2016). Support from midwifery colleagues across all settings was particularly important and the MFYP program has successfully fostered a culture within the profession of support and nurturing of new graduate midwives (Kensington et al., 2016). The Midwifery Council in 2016 made the MFYP program compulsory for all New Zealand registered midwifery graduates and the program is fully funded by government.

Postgraduate midwifery education

Postgraduate midwifery programs have been available through various educational institutions since the mid 1990s. However, in 2008 the NZCOM and the MCNZ made joint representation to the Minister of Health for funding for postgraduate education that met identified workforce needs. In 2009, funding was made available for experienced midwives to undertake a postgraduate certificate in complex maternity care. Since 2011, further funding for postgraduate midwifery education has been made available through Health Workforce New Zealand and administered through the NZCOM. Midwives undertaking study at Master's or PhD level are eligible to apply for grants towards the costs of this study. Various criteria apply but the intention of this funding is to help retain midwives in the midwifery workforce by supporting appropriate postgraduate education and building specific skills and expertise (https://www.midwife.org.nz/midwives/college-roles-and-services/grants-available/).

Midwifery as a profession in New Zealand

The NZCOM displays a strong level of commitment to midwifery and to ensuring a midwife-led and women-centred maternity service. Midwives in New Zealand claim a unique body of knowledge and skill as guardians of normal birth that arises from their model of midwifery partnership, and it is this experiential knowledge that may be New Zealand midwives' greatest contribution to the discipline.

The contribution that midwives make to society is recognised by the authority the midwifery profession has been granted over midwifery, and thus pregnancy and childbirth services, through legislative changes. As a result, midwives have wide jurisdiction to make midwifery judgments and provide midwifery care on their own responsibility. Legislative authority means that midwifery as a profession is self-regulating and must therefore ensure that midwives provide appropriate standards of care and are accountable for their midwifery judgments. The control of a sphere of practice is never static, however, and the College needs to be constantly vigilant to maintain the profession's position as the main provider of primary maternity services.

While the midwifery profession in New Zealand can claim to have achieved a great deal, it still faces challenges in consolidating its status as a profession, in maintaining pay equity and in getting its midwifery outcomes publicly recognised (see Ch. 2). Midwifery care makes a positive impact on the health of mothers and their newborns and, within a global context of increasing medicalisation and inappropriate use of technology in high income countries, New Zealand's national maternity care outcomes are better than many countries, including Australia (Guilliland & Pairman, 2010a; Ch. 2). An important ongoing role of the profession is to encourage and assist midwives to act on their personal and professional autonomy and use their midwifery knowledge with confidence in an endeavour to reduce the impact of these global ideologies on childbearing women and their families (Guilliland, 2004; see also Chs 1 and 2).

MIDWIFERY REGULATION IN AUSTRALIA

Historical changes in legislation related to midwifery registration

Midwifery in Australia has been regulated in some form or other since the beginning of the 20th century. The first registration of midwives in Australia occurred in Tasmania in 1911 (Bogossian, 1998). In the same year the 'Nurses Board of Queensland I' commenced registration of nurses on 31st December 1911 (Queensland Government, n.d.a). A day later, on 1st January 1912, the Nurses' Registration Board introduced the requirement that trainee midwives must enter the hospital in order to secure a practice licence certificate (Davies, 2003). South Australia was the first state in Australia to implement legislation that incorporated the registration of nurses, midwives and mental health nurses together (Summers, 1995, 1998).

The 1915 Midwives Act legislated for the first regulation of midwifery in Australia and in 1916 a further Midwives Act protected the title 'midwife', meaning that no one could perform the duties of a midwife without being registered. This bill enabled the establishment of a Midwives Board that was responsible for the registration of both vocational and formally trained midwives (Fahy, 2007). Initially, midwives with a variety of qualifications were permitted entry to the register. For example, the inaugural register included any midwife who could prove

she had practised as a midwife for the previous 'two years in Victoria or any other state in the Commonwealth of Australia or within the Dominion of New Zealand' (Public Record Office Victoria, 2005). This meant that, initially, the register contained midwives with formal training, vocational midwives and lay midwives (Fahy, 2007; *Midwives Act 1915*).

Formally trained midwives also practised at different standards based on their level of preparatory training. Midwives with formal training, or recognised military service, were permitted direct entry to the 1915 register, whereas midwives with only 1 year of recognised midwifery practice could opt to complete an approved examination. These requirements presented the first form of registration standards. By 1 January 1916, 1921 women had provided evidence that permitted them entry to the register as midwives (*Midwives Act 1928*). Registrants were charged an initial registration fee (5 shillings), and a subsequent annual registration renewal charge of 2 shillings and 6 pence; failure to pay resulted in removal from the register (*Midwives Act 1928*).

The 1923 Nurses' Act established the first Nurses Board in Australia. From 1923 to 1928 nursing and midwifery coexisted as separate professions. However, the simultaneous passing of the *Nurses Act 1928* and the *Midwives Act 1928* consolidated the laws regulating nursing and midwifery. The *Midwives Act 1928* repealed all previous legislation regulating midwives and removed midwives' independent registration status by including midwives under the regulation of the Nurses' Board in each respective state and territory (Public Record Office Victoria, 2005). A Register of Midwives was kept under the 1928 Act for single registrants without a nursing qualification who registered in 1915 (*Midwives Act 1928*). However, in most states, the midwives' boards were abolished by the *Nurses Act 1928*. Consequently, for most of Australia's post-federation history, midwifery has been seen as a subsidiary of a nursing qualification (Barclay, 1985).

A Board of Nursing was established in each state and territory by the 1928 legislation and these boards were deemed responsible for registration and training of nurses and midwives (*Nurses Act 1928*). Each board was authorised to determine whether registrants from the midwifery register should complete supplementary training (*Midwives Act 1928*), a measure most likely aimed at standardising the level of midwifery practitioner, based on the initial registration of vocational midwives in 1915. The nursing boards became responsible for midwifery training and determined who could be recruited, and where midwifery training could occur (*Nurses Act 1928*). This governance structure introduced post-nursing registration midwifery training in Australia, and midwifery became an additional certificate or endorsement after initial nurse training (*Nurses Act 1928*). Direct-entry midwifery training ceased to exist.

From 1928 onwards, the various nursing boards transitioned through many name changes. For example, in

Queensland the Nurses Board of Queensland I was responsible for the registration of nurses between 1911 and 1928 and it then became the Nurses and Masseurs Board of Nursing Studies in Queensland (1928–1965) (Queensland Government, n.d.b), then the Nurses Board of Queensland II (1965–1976), and then the Board of Nursing Studies (1976–1993), before becoming the Queensland Nursing Council (1993–2010) (Queensland Government, n.d.c). Nursing boards continued in one form or other from 1928 until 2010 when all state and territory boards were disbanded in a staged approach.

Between 1928 and 1948, several events impacted on the progression of regulatory developments. World War II (WWII) (1939–45) saw nurses either leave to assist in the war effort or support the delivery of short-staffed civilian hospital services. Barclay (2008) acknowledges that regular wages and the hospital working environment became familiar for midwives during WWII, leading to midwives remaining within the hospital system after the war. After WWII, a postwar baby bonus was paid to encourage population growth to build future economic stability. Births moved to hospitals, with women convalescing for up to 12 days (O'Sullivan, 2006). The combination of birth in hospitals, an increase in the birth rate, staff shortages after the war and the incorporation of midwifery into the nursing profession resulted in formalised and regulated practices of maternity care practitioners. Evetts (2011, 2013) suggests that the role of the 'nation-state' plays a pivotal role in granting legitimacy to professional status by licensing professional activity, giving public funds for education and paying for the services provided by practitioners. Thus regulation of health professions ensures that public funds result in health services which provide effective care to users.

Many authors have identified inconsistencies in the way that midwifery was regulated in Australia between 1928 and 2010 (Barclay, 1985; Bogossian, 1998; Brodie & Barclay, 2001; NSW, 2009). Midwifery was a post-nursing qualification with registration as an 'endorsement' to nursing registration. Mechanisms for recognising direct entry midwives from other jurisdictions did not exist, although some states amended legislation to provide for direct-entry midwives from overseas. For example, in Queensland, the Nursing Act (Queensland Government, 1992, section 74 (3)) was amended to mention 'a midwife who was not a nurse' and allowed midwives with a single qualification to register as a nurse with midwifery endorsement, even though they did not have a nursing qualification. The endorsement contained practice restrictions to practise only midwifery (*The Nursing Act 1992*). Recertification requirements also differed between states and in New South Wales (NSW) and Western Australia (WA) there was no mechanism in place to manage poor practice of an individual unless a professional inquiry was initiated into their practice (Brodie & Barclay, 2001; NNNET, 2006; NSW Registration Board, 2010).

The legislation of nursing and midwifery through state and territory jurisdictions remained relatively unchanged until 2009. An analysis conducted in 2006 of the legislation and professional regulation of nursing and midwifery in Australia found that only three jurisdictions provided separate registers for midwives with no nursing qualification—the Australian Capital Territory (ACT), NSW and South Australia (SA) (NNNET, 2006; NSW Registration Board, 2010)—while other states and territories persisted in recognising midwifery qualifications as an endorsement on the nursing register. This regulatory regime meant that practitioners were able to practise only in their state of registration or were required to apply for registration in another state in order to move and practise (NNNET, 2006; Productivity Commission, 2005) thereby compromising workforce mobility.

Transition to nationally agreed standards of midwifery practice

Midwifery was initially a vocational trade where midwives were trained using an apprenticeship approach. The first midwifery school is identified as commencing in Melbourne in 1862 (Barclay, 2008) and training was an endorsement on the nursing register until the introduction of the Bachelor of Midwifery programs in 2002.

Differing preregistration education requirements and standards, and processes for registration, existed between states and territories until 1992 (NNNET, 2006). Lack of recognition between jurisdictions compounded differences and created barriers for movement of midwives across states and territories. Systematic national standards were introduced in 1992 by the Australian Nursing Council (ANC) as the first Australian national nursing body. The ANC introduced professional practice guidelines, codes of ethics and professional conduct and competency standards. Regulatory bodies finally agreed to the national standards and nurses and midwives were able to apply for recognition of qualifications across state and territory borders. Eventually responsibility for preregistration nursing education shifted from state health services to the federally funded higher education sector and standards of competency for both nursing and midwifery were developed. However, despite the nationally agreed competency standards for initial registration, inconsistencies in registration renewal standards persisted.

In 1997, the Queensland Nursing Council (QNC) introduced registration renewal requirements (QNC, 2005, 2008) (these standards were transferred to the NMBA in 2006), which involved nurses making self-declarations to confirm their competence to renew their registration. This declaration process initially applied only to the nursing register and was not extended to the midwifery endorsements until 2007. It wasn't until 2010 when national registration was introduced in Australia that the need to demonstrate competence separately for nursing and midwifery registers commenced.

The move to a nationally consistent registration process: the National Scheme

Variation in education, registration and regulation was not limited to the nursing and midwifery professions and, following reviews of several state, territory and national health services, the Council of Australian Governments (COAG) launched a national investigation into healthcare practitioners in 2004, to be undertaken by the Productivity Commission. The Commission identified inconsistencies in the regulation of health professionals that raised questions about public safety and recommended the introduction of a national registration process supported by profession-specific national boards. In 2006, COAG committed to strategic reform of the health and higher education sectors to improve health practitioner capacity (COAG, 2006). In 2008, COAG members committed to the establishment of a National Registration and Accreditation Scheme (NRAS) (National Scheme) for health Professionals by 1st July 2010 (APHRA, 2011). The NRAS brought about national uniformity of regulatory standards across all health practitioners (AHPRA, 2011). The Health Practitioner Regulation Law Act No. 45 of 2009 (The Act) was enacted to advance the objectives of the NRAS. Details of the aims and objectives of the NRAS can be found in Box 13.6.

The Health Practitioner National Law statute was adopted in each jurisdiction of Australia. Table 13.1 lists the month, year and statutory legislation passed separately in each state and territory.

The *Health Practitioner Regulation National Law Act 2009* aimed to develop a flexible, responsive and sustainable workforce, and to increase the mobility of the healthcare workforce across borders by reducing the administration impact on healthcare practitioners and accommodating the surveillance of overseas-trained health practitioners through rigorous and responsive assessments. Ten health professions (nurses and midwives, medicine, psychology, chiropractic, podiatry, dental, optometry, osteopathy, pharmacy and physiotherapy) amalgamated in May 2010 onto one national register governed by the AHPRA. In 2012 an additional four health professions (Chinese medicine, Aboriginal and Torres Strait Islander health practice, medical radiation, occupational therapy) were added (COAG, 2008). Then in December 2018, paramedicine practitioners were added to the national register for the first time. Of most significance to nursing and midwifery was the addition of the 's' to the legislation (Health Practitioner Regulation National Law (WA) Amendment Bill 2017) which legislatively separates the nursing and midwifery registers.

The single national register means that these health professionals are authorised to practise in any state or

---

Box 13.6   The National Registration and Accreditation Scheme (NRAS)

The aims of NRAS include:

- protecting the public by ensuring that only suitably trained and qualified practitioners are registered
- facilitating workforce mobility across Australia
- enabling the continuous development of a flexible, responsive and sustainable Australian health workforce.

The National Scheme has a number of objectives, including to:

- help keep the public safe by ensuring that only health practitioners who are suitably trained and qualified to practise in a competent and ethical manner are registered
- facilitate workforce mobility for health practitioners
- facilitate provision of high-quality education and training for practitioners
- facilitate the assessment of overseas qualified practitioners
- facilitate access to care provided by health practitioners
- enable the continuous development of a flexible Australian health workforce.

(Source: Australian Health Practitioner Regulation Agency, 2015. *National Registration and Accreditation Scheme Strategy 2011–14*. Online: http://www.ahpra.gov.au/About-AHPRA/What-We-Do/NRAS-Strategy-2015-2020/NRAS-Strategy-2011-2014.aspx)

---

territory, thereby promoting workforce mobility. Each healthcare professional group has a national board that regulates practitioners to the same minimum professional standards, which include annual registration renewal, indemnity insurance for their scope of practice, continuing professional development and a minimum recency of practice hours. The NMBA regulates the nursing and midwifery professions.

Regulation through the Nursing and Midwifery Board of Australia

Midwifery registration

The AHPRA supports the national boards in its regulatory role. Three types of registration are possible: initial or ongoing general (with or without endorsements), non-practising or registration with conditions. Since commencement of the 2010 National Scheme (NRAS) practitioners who hold dual registration as a midwife and a nurse are required to demonstrate current competence and recency of practice in both professions to meet mandatory registration and renewal standards as both a midwife and a nurse. Non-practising registration is available

Table 13.1 The Adoption of the National Law Act in Australia[a]		
Date	Jurisdiction	Statute
2008	National[b]	Health Practitioner Regulation (Administrative Arrangements) National Law Act (accreditation functions assigned to external accreditation councils for all professions)
November, 2009	Queensland	Queensland Health Practitioner Regulation National Law Act 2009 (from 1 July 2014: Ombudsman Act 2013)
November 2009	New South Wales	New South Wales Health Practitioner Regulation National Law (NSW) No 86a 2009
December 2010	Victoria[c]	Victoria Health Practitioner Regulation National Law (Victoria) Act 2009
March 2011	Australia Capital Territory	Australian Capital Territory Health Practitioner Regulation National Law (ACT) Act 2010
March 2011	Northern Territory[d]	Northern Territory Health Practitioner Regulation (National Uniform Legislation) Act 2010
June 2010	Tasmania[e]	Tasmania Health Practitioner Regulation National Law (Tasmania) Act 2010
June 2011	South Australia[f]	South Australia Health Practitioner Regulation National Law (South Australia) Act 2010
October 2011	Western Australia[g]	Western Australia Health Practitioner Regulation National Law (WA) Act 2010

[a]The Health Practitioner Regulation National Law Act was adopted in each state and territory between 2009 and 2010; it resulted in National boards appointed in each jurisdiction. Each jurisdiction statute can be accessed from the AHPRA website: https://www.ahpra.gov.au/About-AHPRA/What-We-Do/Legislation.aspx.
[b]Australian Capital Territory Health Practitioner Regulation National Law (ACT) Act 2010. Online: http://www.legislation.act.gov.au/a/db_39269/current/pdf/db_39269.pdf.
[c]Victoria Health Practitioner Regulation National Law (Victoria) Act 2009. Online: http://www.legislation.vic.gov.au/Domino/Web_Notes/LDMS/PubStatbook.nsf/51dea4977 0555ea6ca256da4001b90cd/02566FDB9453A0CECA25768600149A94/$FILE/09-079a.pdf.
[d]Northern Territory Health Practitioner Regulation (National Uniform Legislation) Act 2010. Online: https://legislation.nt.gov.au/Legislation/HEALTH-PRACTITIONER-REGULATION-NATIONAL-UNIFORM-LEGISLATION-ACT.
[e]Tasmania Health Practitioner Regulation National Law (Tasmania) Act 2010. Online: http://www7.austlii.edu.au/cgi-bin/viewdb/au/legis/tas/consol_act/hprnla2010498/.
[f]South Australia Health Practitioner Regulation National Law (South Australia) Act 2010. Online: https://www.legislation.sa.gov.au/LZ/C/A/HEALTH%20PRACTITIONER%20 REGULATION%20NATIONAL%20LAW%20(SOUTH%20AUSTRALIA)%20ACT%202010.aspx.
[g]Western Australia Health Practitioner Regulation National Law (WA) Act 2010. Online: https://www.slp.wa.gov.au/legislation/statutes.nsf/main_mrtitle_12107_homepage. html.

for midwives who have retired from practice, or may require extended leave, or be practising overseas.

Initial and ongoing annual registration requires the payment of a fee; the guiding principles of the National Law require the National Scheme to operate in a 'transparent, accountable, efficient, and fair way'; and for registration fees to be reasonable 'having regard to the efficient and effective operation of the scheme' (AHPRA, 2013a). Nurses and midwives pay one fee under the current law for one or two registers. Legislation requires that registrants must annually declare that they meet the standards set out in Box 13.7.

REFLECTIVE THINKING EXERCISE

Annual registration renewal requires each practitioner to demonstrate that they meet the standards set out in Box 13.7. The National Board has defined 'practice' as:

> . . . any role, whether remunerated or not, in which the individual uses their skills and knowledge as a nurse or midwife . . . practice is not restricted to the provision of direct clinical care. It also includes working in a direct

non-clinical relationship with clients, working in management, administration, education, research, advisory, regulatory or policy development roles, and any other roles that impact on safe, effective delivery of services in the profession and/or use of their professional skills.

> (http://www.nursingmidwiferyboard.gov.au)

How do you interpret this definition and apply it to your own practice? What does the term 'practice' mean to you?

Notations

Practitioners with ongoing general registration can apply for a notation on their registration. Notations include endorsement to prescribe scheduled medications and eligibility to provide Medicare Benefits Schedule (MBS) and Pharmaceutical Benefits Schedule (PBS) rebates. The term 'eligible midwife' has been used since 2010 to describe a midwife with a notation on the midwife register as an eligible midwife, but from 1st January 2017 the term 'eligible midwife' has been phased out and since June 2018 has no longer been used by the NMBA. Instead, midwives who have completed an accredited pharmacology course can be endorsed on the NMBA register for the prescribing of scheduled medicines under

Box 13.7   Standards required for registration renewal with the Nursing and Midwifery Board of Australia

- A clear criminal record
- Insurance to cover scope of practice
- Completion of 20 hours of continuing professional development for each registration and additional hours for endorsement(s)
- Demonstrate competence through recency of practice—the equivalent of 3 months full-time practice across the past 5 years

(Source: Nursing and Midwifery Board of Australia (2017a), Meeting the registration requirements, http://www.nursingmidwiferyboard.gov.au/Registration-and-Endorsement/International/Meeting-the-registration-requirements.aspx)

the National Law, section 94, to prescribe schedule 2, 3, 4 and 8 medicines, so that they may prescribe subsidised medications, subject to the provisions of interjurisdictional Controlled Substances, Poisons and Drug Acts in accordance with relevant state and territory legislation.

These notations require continuing professional development and will be discussed further, later in the chapter.

Continuing professional development as a midwife

The National Board expects that registered midwives with an endorsement to prescribe scheduled medicines will practise midwifery consistent with:

- the professional practice framework developed by the National Board
- the National Board-endorsed safety and quality framework
- best-evidence clinical guidelines, such as the National Board-endorsed ACM *Guidelines on Consultation and Referral* (2016)
- the best available evidence.

There is the additional requirement that midwives will be mindful of their professional boundaries as outlined in the Midwife Standards for Practice (NMBA, 2018b).

The NMBA regulates the profession through initial and ongoing annual registration renewal and requires all midwives to meet nationally consistent professional practice standards. These include midwifery practice standards, guidelines, codes and competencies as summarised in Box 13.8.

The current Australian Midwife Standards for Practice (NMBA, 2018b) provides details of the skills, knowledge and attitudes expected of a midwife to work within the midwifery scope of practice. They detail what a midwife is expected to know and what she is expected to be capable of doing to define the midwifery scope of practice. As

Box 13.8   Australian national midwifery practice standards, guidelines, codes, competencies

Competency standards
- Midwife *Standards for Practice* (NMBA, 2018b)

Codes: ethics and professional conduct
- The *International Code of Ethics for Midwives* (ICM, 2014) adopted in Australia in 2018
- The new Code of Conduct for Midwives (NMBA, 2018a)

Decision-making framework
- Decision making framework for nursing and midwifery (NMBA 2020)
- Decision making framework summary—midwifery (NMBA, 2020)
- Decision Making Framework—Midwifery Flowchart rebranded* (NMBA, 2020)
- Safety and Quality Framework for Privately Practising Midwives, NMBA (2017b)

Professional practice guidelines
- National Midwifery Guidelines for Consultation and Referral, 3rd edn, issue 2. ACM (2016)

- Guidelines for Professional Indemnity Insurance Arrangements for Midwives, NMBA (2016a)
- Guidelines for Advertising Regulated Health Services, NMBA (2014a)
- Guidelines for Mandatory Notifications, NMBA (2014b)

Registration standards
- Registration Standard: Continuing Professional Development, NMBA (2016b)
- Nursing and Midwifery Criminal History Registration Standard, NMBA (2018c)
- Registration Standard: English Language Skills, NMBA (2015)
- Nursing and Midwifery Professional Indemnity Insurance Arrangements Registration Standard, NMBA (2016c)
- Registration Standard: Recency of Practice, NMBA (2016d)
- Registration standards, NMBA (2017c)
- Registration Standard: Endorsement for Scheduled Medicines for Midwives, NMBA (2017d)

(Sources: ACM, 2016; ANMAC, 2014; NMBA, 2013, 2014a, 2014b, 2015a, 2015, 2016a, 2016b, 2016c, 2016d, 2017b, 2017c, 2017d, 2018a, 2018b, 2018c; ICM, 2014)

a form of professional regulation practice standards are reviewed regularly, usually every 3 years.

In 2016 the NMBA commenced a review of the midwifery scope of practice and new *Midwife Standards for Practice* commenced on 1st October 2018 (NMBA, 2018b). They replaced the *National Competency Standards for the Midwife* and provide a framework for assessing a midwife's competence to practise in Australia. There are seven standards as follows:

- Promotes evidence-based maternal health and wellbeing
- Engages in respectful partnerships and professional relationships
- Demonstrates the capability and accountability for midwifery practice
- Undertakes comprehensive assessments
- Develops plans for midwifery practice
- Provides safe and quality midwifery practice
- Evaluates outcomes to improve midwifery practice.

Midwifery regulation: disciplinary matters

Under National Law the National Board has power to establish health, performance and professional standards panels in its role to protect the public. Where notification of a complaint is received in relation to a midwife's professional conduct, performance, competence or capacity, the board of the NMBA works closely with the relevant state or territory health complaints entity and may refer the matter to a panel. Under the National Law, panels must have a certain number of members from the relevant health profession and community members, drawn from the Board's approved persons list. The panel has the authority to make decisions on matters. This includes dismissing the investigation, imposing conditions on the midwife, suspending the midwife's registration, and applying cautions or reprimands on matters of performance and professional standards.

Midwifery regulation: accreditation of midwifery education programs

The National Registration and Accreditation Scheme also established the Australian Nursing and Midwifery Accreditation Council as the national education accreditation authority (Department of Health (DOH), 2013a) for all education programs leading to registration as a midwife or a nurse. ANMAC was reappointed in this role in 2018. ANMAC midwifery standards exist to support the preparation of the future midwifery profession and to address safety and quality issues in midwifery services nationally (http://www.nursingmidwiferyboard.gov.au).

In the Australian regulatory context, 'midwife' currently describes a registered/regulated healthcare professional who has undertaken either a comprehensive 3-year undergraduate Bachelor of Midwifery degree or an undergraduate Bachelor of Nursing degree with subsequent postgraduate midwifery education and qualifications. In limited jurisdictions, 4-year undergraduate dual-degree programs enabling initial registration as a midwife and a nurse are also offered.

Currently, 34 programs leading to admission to the midwifery register are offered on the AHPRA website (https://www.ahpra.gov.au/Accreditation/Approved-Programs-of-Study.aspx?ref=Midwife&Type=General). These include 8 Graduate Diploma in Midwifery, 15 Bachelor of Midwifery, 8 dual degree programs with one degree being Bachelor of Midwifery, and 3 Master of Midwifery programs. These programs enable nurses and non-nurses to complete education programs leading to entry to the midwives register.

ANMAC and the NMBA set nationally consistent professional practice standards for entry to the Australian register. The Australian curriculum in the education of midwives, in a bid to align with international standards, has seen the transition to 3-year Bachelor of Midwifery Degree programs at Australian Universities over the past decade and a half. The ICM sets the *International Definition of the Midwife* (ICM, 2017a), *Essential Competencies for Midwifery Practice* (ICM, 2019) and *Global Standards for Midwifery Education* (ICM, 2021). These international standards are adopted globally and used to map minimum practice standards in midwifery education programs. The first programs aimed for congruence with the ACM's *Standards for the Accreditation of Bachelor of Midwifery Programs Leading to Initial Registration as a Midwife in Australia* (ACM, 2006). Programs were designed to provide students with 50% theory and 50% practice. A vital part of the inaugural practice component was the introduction of the 'follow-through' experiences to provide midwifery students with experience of caring for women during continuity of care (COC) relationships. Students accompany women to all maternity care interactions with numerous different health professionals that women meet during their childbearing journey. The students' consistent presence has been well received by women (Stulz et al., 2020; Jefford et al., 2020; Tickle et al., 2016; Tickle et al., 2020).

The ANMC Midwifery Framework was amended in 2009 in response to feedback from some academics and students who considered that the requirement to follow 30 women in COC experiences was excessive and caused hardship for students (McLachlan et al., 2013). The continuity of care numbers were then reduced to 20 (ANMC, 2009) and then to 10 (ANMAC, 2014). Nevertheless, research which investigated midwifery students' views of the COC experiences showed midwifery students felt the experiences were educationally beneficial (Foster et al., 2021; Dawson et al., 2015; Gray et al., 2016).

At the time of introduction of the new curriculum, the configuration of the midwifery workforce showed most midwives practised in fragmented services (Homer et al., 2001; Leap et al., 2002) where women saw a different health professional for each visit. The first framework of the curriculum objectives caused tensions within mainstream maternity service models as the majority of midwives had no comparative experience of COC themselves. However, this education strategy aimed to address international parity, industry shortages including an ageing midwifery workforce (Australian

Health Workforce Advisory Committee (AHWAC), 2012; Health Workforce Australia (HWA), 2012), and grow a future workforce ready and able to practise in COC models to meet consumer demand for comprehensive midwifery services. It resulted in a professional paradigm shift in midwifery education in Australia as students are required to meet Standard 3 outlined in Box 13.9. The development of the national midwifery framework aims to prepare graduates with standards comparable with international standards.

Despite national standards for demonstration of initial competence as a midwife (NMBA, 2018), university curricula are still producing graduate midwives with different levels of expertise upon initial registration. Although the ANMAC standards set minimum requirements to complete COC experiences, many midwifery students do not get an opportunity to practise within COC models such as midwifery group practice (MGP). Furthermore, the ANMAC accreditation standards for new courses/programs set minimum requirements which do not include the full scope of practice as defined

by the ICM. Skills such as suturing and cannulation are not universal in all programs. Subsequently, these skills are taught and acquired through postgraduate continuing education. This means that, at the point of registration, graduates of Australian Bachelor of Midwifery programs are not eligible to practise independently until they are able to demonstrate 3 years full-time practice across the full scope of practice (NMBA, 2017e). This contrasts with several other Western countries (e.g. New Zealand, Canada, Netherlands) where preregistration midwifery education programs are designed to equip graduate midwives to work autonomously at the point of registration (Gray et al., 2016). In Australia, although the Trans-Tasman Mutual Recognition Arrangement (TTMRA) provides mutual recognition of, amongst other things, health professional qualifications and registration, the MCNZ requires Australian graduates to complete additional preparation before being eligible to register as a midwife in New Zealand (Daly et al., 2010).

Clinical practice requirements are set as outlined in Box 13.9.

Box 13.9   Australian Nursing and Midwifery Accreditation Council Midwife Accreditation Standards (2021)

Standard 3 Program of study

3.13 The inclusion of periods of midwifery practice experience in the program, so students can complete the following minimum supervised requirements.

Continuity of care experiences (COCE)

a) Experience in woman-centred care as part of continuity of care experiences. The student is supported to:

 i) establish, maintain and conclude a professional relationship while experiencing continuity with individual women through pregnancy, labour and birth, and the postnatal period, regardless of model of care

 ii) provide midwifery care within a professional practice setting and under the supervision of a midwife—in collaborative practice arrangements supervision by other relevant registered practitioners (for example, medical officer qualified in obstetrics, child health nurse or physiotherapist) may be appropriate

 iii) engage with a minimum of 10 women—engagement involves attending four antenatal visits, two postnatal episodes of care and, for the majority of women, the labour and birth

 iv) maintain a record of each engagement incorporating regular reflection and review by the education or health service provider.

Antenatal care

b) Attendance at 100 antenatal episodes of care. This may include women the student is following as part of their continuity of care experiences.

Labour and birth care

c) Under the supervision of a midwife, act as the primary birth attendant for 30 women who experience a spontaneous vaginal birth, which may include women the student has engaged with as part of their continuity of care experiences. This also involves:

 i) providing direct and active care in the first stage of labour, where possible

 ii) managing the third stage of labour, including the student providing care as appropriate if a manual removal of the placenta is required

 iii) facilitating initial mother and baby interaction, including promotion of skin-to-skin contact and breastfeeding in accordance with the mother's wishes or situation

 iv) assessment and monitoring of the mother's and baby's adaptation for the first hour post-birth including, where appropriate, consultation, referral and clinical handover.

Provide direct and active care to an additional 10 women throughout the first stage of labour and, where possible, during birth—regardless of mode.

(Source: Australian Nursing and Midwifery Accreditation Council. *Midwife Accreditation Standards*, 2014, https://www.anmac.org.au/sites/default/files/documents/06920_anmac_midwife_std_2021_online_05_fa.pdf)

Transition to practice programs in Australia

Potential midwifery graduates can commence a process towards initial entry to the register approximately 6 weeks before they complete their studies. Potential new registrants pay their fee and enter their details in anticipation of their university sending the completed transcript affirming that the student has passed the qualification and met ANMAC Midwife Standards (2014).

New graduate transition to practice programs, lasting up to 1 year, run in each state and territory. Jurisdictions recruit new graduates into temporary paid contracts for the duration of their graduate program. New graduate programs typically afford the new midwife the opportunity to rotate around the different areas of the maternity services to consolidate their clinical experiences. Graduate programs are designed to provide support during the transition from student to registered practitioner, thus regular education and debriefing is an important element of the program. Opportunities for new graduates to work in COC models are limited (Cummins et al., 2016).

New registrants are recruited through an application process organised by the state/territory health service, which involves applying for a position at a number of locations which they identify by ranking their preference. Successful applicants are selected for an interview where a panel uses a selection criterion which is graded in response to the candidate's responses. New graduates who are unable to move location must rank their preference from a limited number of hospitals within their region, and the number of graduates outnumbers the places available on each program. However, for new graduates able to move location there is always the option of applying for positions in other jurisdictions.

Continuing professional development as a registered midwife

From endorsement as a midwife on the nursing register to midwife—prescribe scheduled medicines

The introduction of the *Health Amendment (Midwives and Nurse Practitioners) Act 2010* has helped expand midwifery services, facilitating the expansion of initiatives which see midwives working more autonomously. The Act and associated legislation, including implementation of a government-supported indemnification scheme for midwives (Australian Government, 2010a, 2010b), underpinned reforms to fund antenatal care, intrapartum care in hospital and postpartum care by 'eligible' midwives, regulated under the National Law via section 38(2) (Commonwealth of Australia (COA), 2009; DOH, 2013b). In response to the government health and hospital reform agenda (National Health Reform Agreement; COA, 2011, 2012) Australia offers practice opportunities for some midwives to work across their full scope (Hartz et al., 2012; Homer et al., 2008) enabling them the option of being providers under the MBS and PBS, with insurance

cover. Since November 2010, eligible midwives have been able to provide some women in some areas with greater access to privately practised midwifery services where they work in collaboration with medical providers (DOH, 2011, 2013c; Wilkes et al., 2009).

An approved program of study leads to an endorsement for scheduled medicines. Midwives undertake an educational program to develop a midwife's knowledge and skills in prescribing medicines that has been accredited by the ANMAC and approved by the NMBA for the purpose of enabling the midwife to seek endorsement. This was a two-staged process of applying for notation, then endorsement, where midwives were required to complete an assessment (MPR). From 1 January 2017 the *Eligible Midwife Registration Standard* (2010) ceased to apply, and a one-step process of applying for endorsement has now replaced the former two-step process. A transition period ended on 30 June 2018 and the term 'eligible midwife' and notation are no longer used (NMBA, 2017e). As notated midwives who met the previous requirements of this standard transition to an endorsement, the wording on their registration will change to that agreed under the revised *Registration Standard: Endorsement for Scheduled Medicines for Midwives* (NMBA, 2017d), which states:

- An endorsed midwife qualified to prescribe schedule 2, 3, 4 and 8 medicines and to provide associated services required for midwifery practice in accordance with relevant state and territory legislation.

Under the revised *Registration Standard,* midwives must demonstrate all of the following:

- current general registration as a midwife in Australia with no conditions/undertakings relating to unsatisfactory professional performance/unprofessional conduct
- registration as a midwife that is the equivalent of 3 years' full-time clinical practice (i.e. 5000 hours) in the last 6 years (from the date when the application seeking endorsement is received by the NMBA)—either across the continuum of care, or in a specified context of practice
- Successful completion of either an NMBA-approved program of study leading to endorsement for scheduled medicines, or one that is substantially equivalent to such a program of study as determined by the NMBA.

Ongoing endorsement is conditional on the midwife complying with current NMBA-approved registration standards in continuing professional development, recency of practice, criminal history and professional indemnity insurance arrangements, as well as other applicable NMBA-approved codes and guidelines and, for privately practising midwives, the *Safety and Quality Guidelines for Privately Practising Midwives.*

Endorsement for medication prescribing with the NMBA enables access to rebate for midwifery services associated with the Commonwealth MBS and PBS (DOH, 2013c). Passage of Commonwealth legislation enabling endorsed midwives to prescribe subsidised medications, to bill their services to Medicare and to access a government-supported indemnification scheme, whilst now in place, has many continuing tensions and unresolved issues (Maternity Coalition, 2008; Maternity Coalition/Australian Midwives Act Lobby Group (AMALG), 2003; DOH, 2013d). These arrangements currently extend to antenatal and postnatal midwifery services, some telehealth services, and institutionalised/hospital intrapartum options under the 'collaborative arrangement' terms of Commonwealth Determination 2010 and recent amendments. However, the reforms do not encompass the option of Medicare-funded home birth (Dahlen et al., 2011). These are all significant developments in Australia, including service constraint of state-funded, indemnified home-birth access to oversubscribed public health programs.

Collaborative agreements

The journey toward the arrangement of collaborative agreements has been a rocky road. The now historical federal reforms in March 2010 were highly contentious, drawing strong critique in both professional and public domains, and generated two Federal Senate Inquiries. Principal areas of contention included the lack of provision and direct exclusion of midwifery rebates and indemnification for midwifery home-birth access outside current limited public-sector service options, as well as failure to address access and the ability for eligible midwives to admit childbearing women directly to the public hospital system in order to attend women's births.

Initially the National Health Determination (Australian Government, 2010c) required 'eligible' midwives to engage in written collaborative arrangements with individual doctors. This was identified as an attempt to veto the professional scope of midwifery practice in Australia (Barclay & Tracy, 2010; Lane, 2012). Issues and impediments within different states and territories persist, however, nationally the ACM provided guidance through documents such as *Implementing Visiting Access for Medicare Eligible Midwives; A Guide for Hospitals and Health Services* (ACM, 2015). The number of collaborative agreements which facilitate access of private practice midwives to public hospitals has increased. However, in 2019 the ACM issued a response to the latest review of the Collaborative agreements which continues to 'encumber' midwives' practice. The Participating Midwife Reference Group report was supportive of the midwifery principles of continuity of care and women's access to the Medicare Benefits Scheme, however the ACM felt that the failure of the Review Taskforce to abolish the requirement for a collaborative agreement was frustrating. The ACM lodged a request for the government to reconsider this decision; to this date the decision has not been reversed and Australian midwives continue to need a collaborative agreement in place with hospitals for admitting rights.

Collaborative agreements must be set up with the health service and the midwife must undergo a credentialling process by the hospital to ensure she/he is a safe practitioner. This is in addition to the Midwifery Practice Review process and successful completion of a recognised prescribing course. The ACM acknowledges that when midwives have visiting access to a health service (HS):

... women are able to claim some of the costs of private midwifery care from Medicare. This increases options for women and includes increased access to private models of maternity care. Eligibility allows privately practising midwives greater opportunities to extend their practice and work collaboratively with HS. In turn, the advantage of eligibility for the HS is that financial savings are made, midwifery care is at no cost to the HS and reductions in acute care demand are achieved by the continuity of midwifery care model.

(ACM, 2015, p. 6)

Midwives in private practice in a collaborative arrangement with a private medical provider have also been able to bill their services to Medicare Australia.

Indemnity insurance for midwives

Provision of indemnity insurance cover for midwives is sanctioned by the Commonwealth Department of Health. Under Section 39 of the Health Practitioner Regulation National Law Act (the National Law) as in force in each state and territory, midwives must not practise their profession unless they are covered in the conduct of their practice by appropriate professional indemnity insurance (PII) arrangements. The majority of midwives in Australia work as employees. In most cases, this is in public or private health services, or in private medical practices; most midwives who are employees are covered by their employer's insurance. Employed midwives are advised to check their PII arrangements with their employing organisation as there are situations where a civil claim may be made against a midwife as an individual. This includes situations where employer-based liability cover may not apply; for example, the midwife may have acted in a way that a court would find was not within the 'course and scope of their employment'.

Australian Government-supported insurance scheme

Since 1st July 2010, privately practising midwives have had access to Australian Government-supported PII and can purchase insurance from Medical Insurance Group Australia (MIGA).

The Government-supported insurance will not cover the planned delivery of babies in the home. However, midwives in private practice must still have insurance for providing antenatal and postnatal services, regardless of the birth setting, and midwives must ensure that the insurance covers them for a set of specified requirements. PII arrangements that midwives should consider include:
- civil liability cover
- unlimited retroactive cover
- run-off cover.

The Government-sponsored insurance provider has a number of specific requirements that midwives must meet to qualify for the insurance cover. For the PII exemption to apply under the National Scheme and satisfy

NMBA requirements, midwives in private practice will be required to demonstrate they meet all obligations in the NMBA-approved Safety and Quality Framework (SQF) available at: www.nursingmidwiferyboard.gov.au/Codes-Guidelines-Statements/Codes-Guidelines.aspx. Audits of private practising midwives were performed in 2017. The ACM organised support for their members during the SQF audit by facilitating peer support connections.

Although the Standing Council on Health (SCoH) has approved an extended government waiver on mandatory indemnification for midwives attending home births outside public-sector employment, this is not a satisfactory, guaranteed or long-term policy solution for child-bearing women or midwives. The ACM, in collaboration with women, is a significant stakeholder in this discourse.

Maternity reform and regulation—considerations for midwives and women

Changes in legislation since 2010 have increased opportunities for midwives to develop their autonomy through the MBS, PBS, limited insurance for scope of practice, and visiting access to health services. A significant change to legislation, the Health Practitioner Regulation National Law, where midwifery was recognised as a distinct profession, passed through the Queensland parliament on 6th September 2017. (In Australia, national legislation has to pass through all state and territory houses of parliament; it starts in Queensland, which has one house, and the other states and territories adopt it for themselves. See also Ch. 14.) Commonwealth reforms that have introduced Medicare funding for services undertaken by midwives support safe autonomous midwifery practice; however, other ongoing legislative and policy impediments continue to deny Australian women equity in accessing a full suite of midwifery-based services (Teakle, 2013). Issues persist with lack of insurance for home birth for privately practising midwives. Thus, there persists restricted midwifery practice around birthing, which reduces options for women.

Unlike New Zealand, where midwives are reimbursed for services via the Maternity Benefit Schedule, the majority of midwives in Australia work within public or private maternity services, within contracts that determine the ways in which they work. Many different models of midwifery care exist within the maternity services; however, the number of midwives working in midwifery-led COC models remains small. It is estimated that less than 10% of women currently have access to COC from a known carer (Dawson et al., 2016), thus there is gross disparity and inequality with regards to women's choice of care and carer during pregnancy, birth and the puerperium. Government recommendations call for an expansion to the number of midwifery models of care (AHMAC, 2016); however, because many experienced midwives have traditionally worked within maternity services

where care is delivered from separate units, there exists a workforce unprepared for COC—while at the same time, new graduate midwives aspiring to consolidate their COC practice are restricted to practise within hospital services. However, in a couple of small studies performed in Australia where new graduate midwives were transitioned directly into midwifery-led COC models, it was found that the new graduates developed confidence and competence through the supportive relationships established with the midwives they worked alongside (Clements et al., 2013; Cummins et al., 2015).

In 2018 numerous changes occurred to regulation documents that govern midwifery practice; starting 1st March with the adoption of the ICM *Code of Ethics for Midwives*, a new *Code of Conduct for Midwives*, the change in the notation of private-practice midwives, and finally on 1st October the commencement of the new national Midwife Standards for Practice. Professional boundary expectations are included in the new *Code of Conduct for Midwives*, and are no longer a separate document. Midwives will need to stay alert to professional developments to ensure they meet their statutory professional requirements and are able to influence congruence between their professional aspirations and regulatory requirements.

CRITICAL THINKING EXERCISE

As a midwife in Australia with an ambition to become a private-practice midwife, what processes would you need to navigate? What time scales apply to new and experienced midwives in relation to demonstrating sufficient scope of practice? How would you plan your future career pathway to meet your objective of private practice? Which professional and statutory standards are you required to demonstrate to become recognised as proficient to provide safe autonomous care?

MIDWIFERY REGULATION IN NEW ZEALAND

In December 2003 a new regulatory authority, the Midwifery Council of New Zealand (MCNZ), was established with the passing of the *Health Practitioners Competence Assurance Act 2003* (HPCAA) (Fahy, 2007). This historic event provided final recognition that midwifery is a profession in its own right, as the MCNZ took over all regulatory functions and responsibilities from the Nursing Council.

The MCNZ comprises six midwives and two lay members, and its focus is on protecting the public and ensuring that they receive safe and competent midwifery care. It does this by carrying out a number of statutory functions that came into force on 18th September 2004 (see Ch. 14).

Midwifery Scope of Practice

The HPCAA required each profession to define its scope(s) of practice. The *Midwifery Scope of Practice* (Box 13.10) further amended previous modifications made by NZCOM to the ICM definition of a midwife in order to ensure that the *Midwifery Scope of Practice* statement appropriately reflected current midwifery practice in New Zealand (https://gazette.govt.nz/notice/id/2010-gs 142; ICM, 2017a; NZCOM, 2015).

The *Midwifery Scope of Practice* provides a broad statement of the boundaries of what a New Zealand midwife can do on her own professional responsibility. It provides a legal definition of New Zealand midwifery practice. It does not mean that every midwife must practise the full scope all the time. Rather, it is expected that all midwives can demonstrate that they are able to practise the full scope, even if their daily practice is more restricted. The *Midwifery Scope of Practice* reflects what the public expects from anyone holding the title of 'midwife' (MCNZ, 2004b, n.d.a.).

Since 2020 the MCNZ has been reviewing the Midwifery Scope of Practice as part of its Aotearoa Midwifery Project that seeks to 'develop Te Tiriti-honouring ways of working that will meaningfully impact the safety of midwifery care for Māori and all whānau across Aotearoa' (MCNZ, n.d.b.) The project is controversial and the challenge for the MCNZ

will be to stay within the limitations of its legislated regulatory role and ensure it remains focused on ensuring the competence of individual midwives and maintaining the safety of all childbearing women in New Zealand be they Māori or non-Māori.

Competencies for Entry to the Register of Midwives

In setting the competencies required of midwives in order to gain registration in New Zealand, the MCNZ amended competencies initially developed in 1996 by the Nursing Council in collaboration with the NZCOM (MCNZ, 2007b). They were further updated in 2007 in order to integrate Tūranga Kaupapa—guidelines for working with Māori women developed by Ngā Maia, a whānau -based organisation supporting Māori midwives and maternity services for Māori women (MCNZ, 2007a). The *Competencies for Entry to the Register of Midwives* (Box 13.11) provide the detail of the skills, knowledge and attitudes expected of a midwife working within the *Midwifery Scope of Practice*. Whereas the *Midwifery Scope of Practice* provides the broad boundaries of midwifery practice, the competencies provide the detail of how a registered midwife is expected to practise and what she is expected to know and be able to do. These are minimum competence standards required of all midwives who register in New Zealand. Again, not all midwives will necessarily demonstrate all competencies all the time in their everyday practice. However, the MCNZ requires all midwives to make an annual declaration that they are able to meet these competencies (MCNZ, 2007a).

Cultural competence

The HPCAA requires all regulatory authorities to, amongst other things, set standards of cultural competence. The Midwifery Council has integrated cultural competence into its competencies for entry to the register of midwives. Cultural competence for midwives requires the application of the principles of cultural safety to the midwifery partnership and integration of Tūranga Kaupapa (guidelines on the cultural values of Māori as applied to midwifery practice) within midwifery partnership and midwifery practice. In 2012 the Midwifery Council of New Zealand published its *Statement on Cultural Competence for Midwives* and this is available on its website (https://www.midwiferycouncil.health.nz/common/Uploaded%20files/About%20Us/Statement%20on%20cultural%20competence.pdf).

Code of Conduct

The HPCAA requires all regulatory authorities to set standards for conduct and the Midwifery Council published its *Code of Conduct* in December 2010 (MCNZ, 2010). The Code provides a standard by which midwives' behaviour can be measured and it is an important document for the Council's Professional Conduct Committee.

Box 13.10 New Zealand Midwifery Scope of Practice

The midwife works in partnership with women, on her own professional responsibility, to give women the necessary support, care and advice during pregnancy, labour and the postpartum period up to 6 weeks, to facilitate births and to provide care for the newborn.

The midwife understands, promotes and facilitates the physiological processes of pregnancy and childbirth, identifies complications that may arise in mother and baby, accesses appropriate medical assistance, and implements emergency measures as necessary. When women require referral, midwives provide midwifery care in collaboration with other health professionals.

Midwives have an important role in health and wellness promotion and education for the woman, her family and the community. Midwifery practice involves informing and preparing the woman and her family for pregnancy, birth, breastfeeding and parenthood and includes certain aspects of women's health, family planning and infant wellbeing.

The midwife may practise in any setting, including the home, the community, hospitals, or in any other maternity service. In all settings, the midwife remains responsible and accountable for the care she provides.

(Source: MCNZ, 2004a; NZ Government Gazette Notice, 2010. Online: https://gazette.govt.nz/notice/id/2010-gs142)

Box 13.11 Competencies for Entry to the Register of Midwives

Competency 1

The midwife works in partnership with the woman throughout the maternity experience.

Explanation

The word 'midwife' has an inherent meaning of being 'with woman'. The midwife acts as a professional companion to promote each woman's right to empowerment to make informed choices about her pregnancy, birth experience and early parenthood. The midwifery relationship enhances the health and wellbeing of the woman, the baby and their family/whānau. The onus is on the midwife to create a functional partnership. The balance of 'power' within the partnership fluctuates but it is always understood that the woman has control over her own experience.

Competency 2

The midwife applies comprehensive theoretical and scientific knowledge with the affective and technical skills needed to provide effective and safe midwifery care.

Explanation

The competent midwife integrates knowledge and understanding, personal, professional and clinical skills within a legal and ethical framework. The actions of the midwife are directed towards a safe and satisfying outcome. The midwife utilises midwifery skills that facilitate the physiological processes of childbirth and balances these with the judicious use of intervention when appropriate.

Competency 3

The midwife promotes practices that enhance the health of the woman and her family/whānau and which encourage their participation in her healthcare.

Explanation

Midwifery is a primary health service in that it recognises childbirth as a significant and normal life event. The midwife is therefore responsible for supporting this process through health promotion, education and information sharing, across all settings.

Competency 4

The midwife upholds professional midwifery standards and uses professional judgement as a reflective and critical practitioner when providing midwifery care.

Explanation

As a member of the midwifery profession the midwife has responsibilities to the profession. The midwife must have the skills to recognise when midwifery practice is safe and satisfactory to the woman and her family/whānau.

Each of the above competencies has a number of criteria that provide detailed measures of how a midwife would demonstrate her competence against each competency statement. The full list of competencies and criteria can be found on the Midwifery Council of New Zealand website (https://www.midwiferycouncil.health.nz).

In New Zealand the Midwifery Council of New Zealand *Competencies for Entry to the Register* is the document against which all midwives' practice is measured.

(Source: Midwifery Council of New Zealand (MCNZ). *Competencies for Entry to the Register of Midwives.* Wellington: MCNZ; 2007a. Online: http://www.midwiferycouncil.org.nz.)

It includes statements about professional relationships with women, interprofessional relationships and professional behaviour (including appropriate use of social media). The Code is available from the Council's website (https://www.midwiferycouncil.health.nz/common/Uploaded%20files/Registration/Code%20of%20Conduct.pdf).

Registration as a midwife in New Zealand

The MCNZ is responsible for setting policy and managing the process for registration in New Zealand of its own midwifery education graduates, overseas-registered midwives and midwives applying from Australia.

All applicants must provide evidence of fitness for registration, specified qualifications and competence to practise in the *Midwifery Scope of Practice* as measured by the *Competencies for Entry to the Register of Midwives*. Midwives applying from Australia under the *Trans-Tasman Mutual Recognition Act 1997* (see Ch. 14) are deemed to be registered, but along with other overseas applicants are likely to have conditions placed on their practice.

Common conditions that apply to Australian and other overseas midwives are that they work in peer-supported contexts such as maternity hospitals or group practices, and that they cannot prescribe medications until they have completed a course in pharmacology and prescribing. They must also undertake courses that:

- orientate them to New Zealand's maternity and midwifery services
- develop cultural competence in the New Zealand midwifery context
- update skills in newborn assessment and examination. Midwives educated in New Zealand must complete an approved Bachelor of Midwifery program (equivalent of 4 academic years, delivered over 3 calendar years or 4 academic years).

Since 2013, new graduate midwives from overseas, including Australia, have been required to practise under supervision for a period of time. These new graduates are not eligible for the MFYP program.

Preregistration midwifery education standards

Bachelor of Midwifery programs began in 1992 and have been the only route to midwifery registration since 1996. Most midwifery students are 'direct entry' or women without a previous nursing qualification. A small number of nurses choose to change careers and become midwives, and they can access slightly shorter programs through the recognition of prior learning policies of the various educational institutions.

In August 2007, following a 2-year review of preregistration midwifery education, the MCNZ released new standards for preregistration midwifery education programs (MCNZ, 2007b). These standards increased total program hours from 3600 to 4800, thereby requiring delivery of a 4-year (equivalent) degree over 3 years (45 programmed weeks per year). The rationale was to increase both competence and confidence upon graduation by providing more midwifery practice experience for students and by maximising opportunities for practice across the calendar year. Additionally, programs were to be delivered flexibly to increase access to midwifery education for women outside of the main centres. These standards form an important component of a wider midwifery workforce strategy to ensure both access to midwifery education to women from rural, provincial and urban locations in New Zealand and sufficient graduates to meet midwifery workforce needs. All midwifery programs were redeveloped to meet the new standards with the first graduates from South Island programs in 2011 and from North Island programs in 2012. The Midwifery Council reviewed the standards in 2014 publishing the updated standards in 2015. Further amendments in 2019 allowed the 4 academic-year program to be delivered over 3 calendar years or via a traditional 4-year academic pathway (MCNZ, 2019a).

Continuing competence as a midwife

A central tenet of the HPCAA (2003) is that all healthcare practitioners must demonstrate ongoing competence to practise in order to be issued with an annual practising certificate. The MCNZ makes this assessment through its recertification program.

All midwives make a declaration of their competence each year. Over each subsequent 3-year period they must maintain a portfolio to record their activities and reflections and:

- work across all aspects of the *Midwifery Scope of Practice*
- annually complete a Midwifery Emergency Skills Refresher comprising maternal and neonatal resuscitation updates and childbirth emergency skills
- annually complete 8 hours of continuing education that has direct relevance to a midwife's professional role and which enhances and leads to development of their practice
- annually complete 8 hours of professional activity that contribute to professional practice and quality improvement (MCNZ, 2019b).

A key element of the recertification program is that every midwife is required to undergo the NZCOM's Midwifery Standards Review process every three years. As part of the review, the MSR committee focuses on the midwife's ability to meet the NZCOM standards for practice and the MCNZ competencies and assists the midwife to identify a personal development plan for the forthcoming year(s). Midwives are randomly audited to ensure they comply with the requirements of the recertification program.

The Midwifery Council reviews its recertification program regularly with the latest update in 2019 for the 2020–21 period. Up-to-date-information about the content of the recertification program can be found on the Council's website at: https://www.midwiferycouncil.health.nz/common/Uploaded%20files/Annual%20Practising%20Certificates/Recertification%20programme.pdf.

Competence review

Where it has reason to be concerned about a midwife's competence to practise, the MCNZ can carry out a competence review. It establishes a Competence Review Panel to make an assessment of a midwife's competence. If concerns are identified, the Council has various powers, such as requiring the midwife to complete a specific competence program, undertake further education or work under certain conditions. If the MCNZ believes that a midwife poses a risk of serious harm to the public, it has the power to suspend the midwife from practice.

Disciplinary functions

All complaints made by consumers about midwives are investigated by the Health and Disability Commissioner and assessed in relation to the Code of Health and Disability Services Consumers' Rights, and findings are reported to the MCNZ. If the Commissioner decides the matter is a serious professional matter, he or she may refer it on to the Director of Proceedings, who may then decide to lay charges against the midwife. The HPCAA established a separate tribunal—the Health Practitioners Disciplinary Tribunal (HPDT)—to hear allegations of professional misconduct. The HPDT can impose various

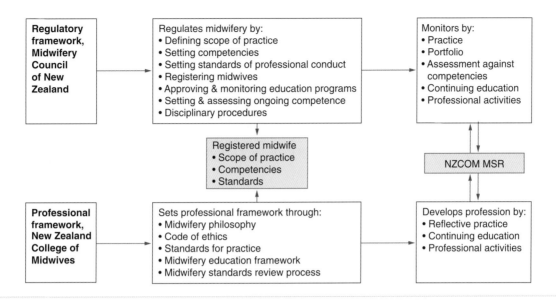

FIGURE 13.2 Relationship between professional and regulatory frameworks for practice in New Zealand. NZCOM MSR = New Zealand College of Midwives Midwifery Standards Review
(Based on Midwifery Council of New Zealand (MCNZ). *Midpoint*. Newsletter of the Midwifery Council of New Zealand, December, 2004c)

penalties, including suspension, fines and cancellation of registration.

The MCNZ has established a Professional Conduct Committee (PCC) to which it can refer matters for investigation. Such matters may include notifications of practice below required standards of competence and conduct, and notification of convictions for certain offences or against certain legislation. The PCC can investigate, call for evidence and receive evidence or submissions. It can make recommendations to the MCNZ and can lay charges before the HPDT.

Other functions

The MCNZ has powers to seek information about any midwife who is notified as being unable to practise appropriately because of some physical or mental condition and to apply conditions to that midwife's practice in order to protect both the public and the midwife. The MCNZ also has an important role in approving and accrediting midwifery education providers, programs and courses.

Relationship between the New Zealand College of Midwives and the Midwifery Council of New Zealand

Although they are separate organisations, the roles of the NZCOM and the MCNZ are complementary. The MCNZ provides the regulatory framework within which midwives must practise, and it sets the minimum standards required for public safety. The NZCOM provides the professional framework in which midwives practise, and it aims to develop and support high standards of midwifery

practice. Both organisations have an interest in ensuring that the regulatory processes for midwives are integrated in a professional framework and that appropriate standards of midwifery practice are maintained so that the public can be assured of safe and competent midwifery care. Fig. 13.2 shows the interface between these professional and regulatory frameworks.

CRITICAL THINKING EXERCISE

According to the International Confederation of Midwives, midwifery in every country needs to be embedded within a strong professional framework to ensure high-quality midwifery services, more fulfilling careers for midwives and enhanced reproductive health for women, their newborns and their families (ICM, 2021). The ICM's Professional Framework for Midwifery identifies 10 elements of this professional framework: midwifery philosophy, essential competencies for midwifery, midwifery education, midwifery regulation, midwives' association, research, midwife-led continuity of care model of practice, midwifery leadership, enabling environment, and commitment to gender equality, justice, equity, diversity and inclusion (ICM, 2021).

Consider the implications if any of these elements of the profession were weak. What can you do as a midwife to ensure the profession is strong?

Both the midwives' association and the midwifery regulatory authority share responsibility for strengthening and developing the midwifery profession, but they have different roles and different priorities. What steps can they take to ensure their objectives are aligned and that they work in partnership for the benefit of the profession and for women, their newborns and families?

Conclusion

This chapter has provided a brief overview of the professional and regulatory frameworks for midwifery practice in Australia and New Zealand. Although midwifery in both countries is claimed to be a profession, New Zealand midwifery has a legal and professional framework that supports greater autonomy. Australian midwifery continues to evolve, and implementation of legislative, professional and policy frameworks that recognise midwifery as a profession separate from nursing has begun with the Health Practitioner Regulation National Law, but continues to face challenges. Professional cohesion, strong partnerships with childbearing women and ongoing detailed attention to systemic health policy and maternity service reforms will support midwifery's professional framework and aspirations in both countries. Although professional frameworks are extremely important, legislated changes are essential if midwifery is truly to be self-determining as a profession.

Review questions

1. What are the main characteristics of a profession and why is it important for midwifery to be a profession?
2. Which historical events in Australia led to midwifery becoming regulated by nursing, and which legislation has acknowledged midwifery as a separate profession once more?
3. What is the purpose of regulation of midwifery and how does it work?
4. What has been the impact of national registration and recent maternity reforms on midwives in Australia?
5. How do the midwifery professions in New Zealand and Australia influence the delivery of maternity services in each country?
6. How do current social/partnership models of birth affect the notion and development of midwifery as a profession in Australia and in New Zealand?
7. How is the midwifery scope of practice (as defined by the International Confederation of Midwives) enabled or constrained in the Australian and New Zealand contexts respectively?
8. What is the relationship between scope of practice and competencies?
9. What is the relationship between the professional and regulatory frameworks in Australia and New Zealand?
10. How does New Zealand's Midwifery Standards Review process work to improve standards of midwifery practice?

NOTES

[a]Pam Hayes from New South Wales, Margaret Peters from Victoria and Jenny Cooling from South Australia.

Online resources

Australian Health Practitioner Regulation Agency: http://www.ahpra.gov.au.

Australian Nursing and Midwifery Accreditation Council: http://www.anmac.org.au.

Australian Private Midwives Association: http://www.australian-privatemidwivesassociation.blogspot.com.au/.

Health Amendment (Midwives and Nurse Practitioners) Act 2010. Act No 29 of 2010 as amended, Australian Government Commonwealth Law: http://www.comlaw.gov.au/Details/C2012C00830.

Medicare Benefits Schedule: http://www.health.gov.au/internet/mbsonline/publishing.nsf/Content/Medicare-Benefits-Schedule-MBS-1.

Midwifery Council of New Zealand: www.midwiferycouncil.health.nz.

Midwifery Employee Representation and Advisory Service: http://www.midwife.org.nz/meras.

Midwifery and Maternity Providers Organisation: http://www.mmpo.org.nz.

Midwife Professional Indemnity (Commonwealth Contribution) Scheme Act 2010—C2010A00030: http://www.comlaw.gov.au/Details/C2010A00030.

Midwife Professional Indemnity (Run-off Cover Support Payment) Act 2010—C2011C00495: http://www.comlaw.gov.au/Details/C2011C00495.

New Zealand College of Midwives: http://www.midwife.org.nz.

Nursing and Midwifery Board of Australia: http://www.nursing-midwiferyboard.gov.au.

References

Abbott A. The System of Professions—An Essay on the Division of Expert Labour. Chicago: University of Chicago Press; 1988.

Australian College of Midwives (ACM). *Midwifery Practice Review.* Canberra: ACM; n.d.a Online: https://www.midwives.org.au/mpr.

Australian College of Midwives (ACM). Strategic Plan 2021–2023. Canberra: ACM; n.d.b. Online: https://www.midwives.org.au/sites/default/files/uploaded-content/field_f_content_file/acm_strategic_plan_2021-2023_public.pdf.

Australian College of Midwives (ACM). *Standards for the Accreditation of Bachelor of Midwifery Education Programs Leading to Initial Registration as a Midwife in Australia 2006.* Canberra: ACM; 2006. Online: http://www.midwives.org.au.

Australian College of Midwives (ACM). 2015. Implementing Visiting Access for Medicare Eligible Midwives; A Guide for Hospitals and Health Services. Canberra: ACM; 2015. Online: http://www.midwives.org.au.

Australian College of Midwives (ACM). (2018). *Information Sheet–Midwifery Practice Review Process*. https://www.midwives.org.au/sites/default/files/uploaded-content/website-content/MPR/general_information_-_mpr_process_0.pdf

Australian College of Midwives (ACM). (2019). Media release 8 April 2019. https://www.midwives.org.au/sites/default/files/uploaded-content/field_f_content_file/20190408_media_release_-_mbs_taskforce_review.pdf

Australian College of Midwives (ACM). (2020) 2019–2020 Annual Report https://www.midwives.org.au/sites/default/files/uploaded-content/field_f_content_file/acm_ar2020_final.pdf.

Australian College of Midwives (ACM). *National Midwifery Guidelines for Consultation and Referral*. 4th ed. Canberra: Australian College of Midwives; 2021a.

Australian College of Midwives (ACM). *Midwifery Philosophy*. Canberra: ACM; 2021b. https://www.midwives.org.au/about-us.

Australian College of Midwives (ACM). 2021c. Communication regarding membership numbers.

Australian College of Midwives (ACM). *ACM Vision and Mission*. Canberra: ACM; 2021d. Online: https://www.midwives.org.au/sites/default/files/uploaded-content/field_f_content_file/acm_strategic_plan_2021-2023_public.pdf.

Australian College of Midwives (ACM). *Staff*. Canberra: ACM; 2021e. Online: https://www.midwives.org.au/governance.

Australian Government. *Midwife Professional Indemnity (Commonwealth Contribution) Scheme Act 2010*—C2010A00030. 2010a. Online: http://www.comlaw.gov.au/Details/C2010A00030.

Australian Government. *Midwife Professional Indemnity (Run-off Cover Support Payment) Act 2010*—C2011C00495. 2010b. Online: http://www.comlaw.gov.au/Details/C2011C00495.

Australian Government. National Health (Collaborative Arrangements for Midwives) Determination 2010—F2010L02105. 2010c. Online: http://www.comlaw.gov.au/details/f2010l02105.

Australian Health Practitioner Regulation Agency (AHPRA). Australian Health Practitioner Annual Report (2010–2011). 2011. Online: http://www.ahpra.gov.au/Publications/Annual-reports/Annual-report-archive.aspx.

Australian Health Practitioner Regulation Agency (AHPRA). Legislation. 2013a. Online: http://www.ahpra.gov.au/About-AHPRA/What-we-do/Legislation.aspx.

Australian Health Practitioner Regulation Agency (AHPRA). Approved Programs of Study. https://www.ahpra.gov.au/Accreditation/Approved-Programs-of-Study.aspx

Australian Health Workforce Advisory Committee (AHWAC). The Midwifery Workforce in Australia 2002–2012. Sydney: AHWAC; 2012.

Australian Midwifery News. Obituary: a legacy of midwifery wisdom—Pam Hayes OAM 15th December 1935–18th February 2007. Aust Midwifery News. 2007;7(1):29.

Australian Nursing and Midwifery Accreditation Council (ANMAC). Midwife Accreditation Standards. 2014. Online: www.anmac.org.au/accreditation-standards.

ANMAC (2020). Annual Report 2019-2020 https://www.anmac.org.au/sites/default/files/documents/anmac_annualreport_2019-20.pdf.

Australian Nursing and Midwifery Council (ANMC). Midwives: Standards and Criteria for the Accreditation of Nursing and Midwifery Courses Leading to Registration, Enrolment, Endorsement and Authorisation in Australia With Evidence Guide. Canberra: ANMC; 2009.

Baerlocher M, Allen S. Professional monopolies in medicine. *J Am Med Assoc*. 2009;301(8):858-860.

Barclay L. Australian midwifery training and practice. *Midwifery*. 1985;1:86-96.

Barclay L. A feminist history of Australian midwifery from colonisation until the 1980s. *Women Birth*. 2008;21(1):3-8.

Barclay L, Tracy SK. Legally binding midwives to doctors is not collaboration. *Women Birth*. 2010;23(1):1-2.

Bogossian F. A review of midwifery legislation in Australia: history, current state and future directions. *Aust Coll Midwives J*. 1998;11(1):24-31.

Brodie P, Barclay L. Issues in the regulation of Australian midwives. *Aust Health Rev*. 2001;24(4):113-118.

Campbell N, Guilliland K. Accountability: midwifery standards review and resolution committees. In: Guilliland K, Pairman S, eds. *Women's Business: The Story of the New Zealand College of Midwives 1986–2010*. Christchurch, NZ: New Zealand College of Midwives; 2010:373-417.

Clements V, Davis D, Fenwick J. Continuity of care: supporting new graduates to grow into confident practitioners. *Int J Childbirth*. 2013;3(1):3-12.

Commonwealth of Australia (COA). *Explanatory Memorandum The Health Legislation Amendment (Midwives and Nurse Practitioners Bill*. Canberra: Government of Australia; 2009. Online: http://www.comlaw.gov.au/Details/C2009B00133?Explanatory%20Memorandum/Text.

Commonwealth of Australia (COA). *Council of Australian Governments National Health Reform Agreement: 1–70*. Canberra: Government of Australia; 2011. Online: http://www.federalfinancialrelations.gov.au/content/npa/health/_archive/national-agreement.pdf.

Commonwealth of Australia (COA). National Maternity Services Plan: 2010–2011. Annual Report: 1–9, Canberra: Government of Australia; 2012. Online: https://www.health.gov.au/internet/main/publishing.nsf/Content/8AF951CE492C799FCA257BF0001C1A4E/$File/maternityplan.pdf.

Council of Australian Government (COAG). *Intergovernmental Agreement for a National Registration and Accreditation Scheme for the Health Professions*. Canberra: COAG; 2006.

Council of Australian Governments (COAG). *Intergovernmental Agreement for a National Registration and Accreditation Scheme for the Health Professions, 26/3/2008*. Adelaide. Canberra: COAG; 2008.

Cummins AM, Denney-Wilson E, Homer CSE. The experiences of new graduate midwives working in midwifery continuity of care models in Australia. *Midwifery*. 2015;31(4):438-444.

Cummins AM, Denney-Wilson E, Homer CSE. The challenge of employing and managing new graduate midwives in midwifery group practices in hospitals. *J Nurs Manage*. 2016;24(5):614-623.

Dahlen H, Jackson M, Stevens J. Homebirth, freebirth and doulas: casualty and consequences of a broken maternity system. *Women Birth*. 2011;24(1):47-50.

Daly J, Speedy S, Jackson D. *Context of Nursing: An Introduction*. Chatswood, NSW: Churchill Livingstone. Elsevier; 2010.

Davies RA. 'She Did What she Could' ... a History of the Regulation of Midwifery Practice in Queensland 1859–1912. (PhD thesis), Brisbane, QLD: University of Technology; 2003. Online: https://eprints.qut.edu.au/15819/.

Dawson K, Newton M, Forster D, et al. Exploring midwifery students' views and experiences of caseload midwifery: a cross-sectional survey conducted in Victoria, Australia. *Midwifery*. 2015;31(2):e7–e15.

Dawson K, McLachlan H, Newton M, et al. Implementing caseload midwifery: exploring the views of maternity managers in Australia—a national cross-sectional survey. *Women Birth*. 2016;29(3):214-222.

Dean M. *Governmentality: Power and Rule in Modern Society*. London: Sage; 1999.

Department of Health (DOH). Extended Medicare Safety Net Review of Capping Arrangements Report 2011: A Report by the Centre for Health Economics Research and Evaluation—Contextual Overview. Canberra: Commonwealth of Australia; 2011. Online: http://www.health.gov.au/internet/main/publishing.nsf/Content/2011_Review_Extended_Medicare_Safety_Net/$File/Final%20Contextual%20Overview%20-%20PDF.pdf.

Department of Health (DOH). *National Registration and Accreditation Scheme.* 2013a. updated 2016. Online: http://www.health.gov.au/internet/main/publishing.nsf/Content/work-nras.

Department of Health (DOH). *Eligible Midwives Questions and Answers.* 2013b. Online: http://www.health.gov.au/internet/main/publishing.nsf/Content/B1E08CEB22092366CA257BF0001A4C4A/$File/midwives_nurse_pract_qanda_01_11_13.pdf.

Department of Health (DOH). *Evaluation of the Maternity Services Reform Budget Package. 2013c:1–13.* Online: http://www.health.gov.au/.

Department of Health (DOH). *Eligible Midwives and Medicare.* 2013d. Online: http://www.health.gov.au/internet/main/publishing.nsf/Content/midwives-nurse-pract-qanda#10.

Dixon L, Pairman S, Tumilty E, et al. *Stepping Forward Into Life as a Midwife in New Zealand/Aotearoa: An Analysis of the Midwifery First Year of Practice Programme 2007 to 2010.* Christchurch, NZ: New Zealand College of Midwives; 2014.

Dobbie M. *The Trouble with Women. The Story of Parents Centre New Zealand.* South Island, Cape Catley: Whatamango Bay; 1990.

Donley J. *Save the Midwife.* Auckland: New Woman's Press; 1986.

Donley J. *Professionalism. The importance of consumer control over childbirth.* NZCOM J. 1989;(Sept):6-7.

Donnison J. *Midwives and Medical Men. A History of the Struggle for the Control of Childbirth.* 2nd ed. London: Historical Publications; 1988.

Evetts J. A new professionalism? Challenges and opportunities. *Curr Sociol.* 2011;59(4):406-422. doi:10.1177/0011392111402585.

Evetts J. Professionalism: value and ideology. *Curr Sociol.* 2013;61(5–6):778-796. doi:10.1177/0011392113479316.

Fahy K. An Australian history of the subordination of midwifery. *Women Birth.* 2007;20(1):25-29.

Foster W, Sweet L, Graham K. Midwifery students experience of continuity of care: A mixed methods study. *Midwifery.* 2021 Jul;98:102966. doi:10.1016/j.midw.2021.102966. Epub 2021 Mar 18. PMID: 33794393.

Gray M, Malott A, Murray B, et al. A scoping review of how new midwifery practitioners transition to practice in Australia, New Zealand, Canada, United Kingdom and The Netherlands. *Midwifery.* 2016;42:74-79. doi:10.1016/j.midw.2016.09.018.

Guilliland K. Maintaining the links. *NZCOM J.* 1989;1:14.

Guilliland K. A hundred years of midwifery and what have we learnt about ourselves? Centenary Oration. *Midwifery News.* 2004;4–6(34):28-29.

Guilliland K, McIlhone B. Industrial representation for midwives: MERAS and NZNO. In: Guilliland K, Pairman S, eds. *Women's Business: The Story of the New Zealand College of Midwives 1986–2010.* Christchurch, NZ: New Zealand College of Midwives; 2010:543-578.

Guilliland K, Pairman S. *The Midwifery Partnership: A Model For Practice.* Department of Nursing and Midwifery Monograph Series 95/1. Wellington, NZ: Victoria University of Wellington; 1995.

Guilliland K, Pairman S. *Women's Business: The Story of the New Zealand College of Midwives 1986–2010.* Christchurch, NZ: New Zealand College of Midwives; 2010a:418-452.

Guilliland K, Pairman S. *The Midwifery Partnership: A Model for Practice.* 2nd ed. Christchurch, NZ: New Zealand College of Midwives; 2010b.

Hartz D, Foureur M, Tracy SK. Australian caseload midwifery: the exception or the rule. *Women Birth.* 2012;25(1):35-46.

Health Amendment (Midwives and Nurse Practitioners) Act. Act No 29 of 2010 as amended, Australian Government Commonwealth Law. 2010. Online: http://www.comlaw.gov.au/Details/C2012C00830.

Health Practitioner Regulation National Law (WA) Amendment Bill 2017, EXPLANATORY MEMORANDUM. Online: https://www.parliament.wa.gov.au/parliament/bills.nsf/34ECFB60383D0C144825817D00404F8D/$File/EM20-2.002.pdf.

Health Workforce Australia (HWA). Health Workforce 2025: Doctors, Nurses and Midwives—Volume I. Adelaide: HWA; 2012:1-178. Online: https://submissions.education.gov.au/forms/archive/2015_16_sol/documents/Attachments/Australian%20Nursing%20and%20Midwifery%20Accreditation%20Council%20(ANMAC).pdf.

Hendry C, Guilliland K. The Midwifery and Maternity Providers Organisation: a strategy for future-proofing midwifery in New Zealand. In: Guilliland K, Pairman S, eds. *Women's Business: The Story of the New Zealand College of Midwives 1986–2010.* Christchurch: New Zealand College of Midwives; 2010:418-452.

Homer C, Brodie P, Leap N. Midwifery Continuity of Care: A Practical Guide. Sydney: Churchill Livingstone; 2008.

Homer C, Davis G, Brodie P, et al. Collaboration in maternity care: a randomised controlled trial comparing community-based continuity of care with standard hospital care. *BJOG.* 2001;108:16-22.

International Confederation of Midwives (ICM). ICM International Definition of the Midwife. London: ICM; 2005.

International Confederation of Midwives (ICM). *Essential Competencies for Midwifery Practice.* London: ICM; 2019. Online: https://www.internationalmidwives.org/assets/files/general-files/2019/02/icm-competencies_english_final_jan-2019-update_final-web_v1.0.pdf.

International Confederation of Midwives (ICM). ICM International Definition of the Midwife. London: ICM; 2011a. (revised). Online: http://internationalmidwives.org/assets/uploads/documents/Definition%20of%20the%20Midwife%20-%202011.pdf.

International Confederation of Midwives (ICM). *Global Standards for Midwifery Education.* 2021. Online: https://www.internationalmidwives.org/assets/files/education-files/2021/10/global-standards-for-midwifery-education_2021_en-1.pdf.

International Confederation of Midwives (ICM). Strategic Directions 2014–2017. London: ICM; 2014. Online: https://internationalmidwives.org/assets/uploads/documents/Governance/ICM_2014_Strategic_brochure_ENG.pdf.

International Confederation of Midwives (ICM). *International Definition of the Midwife.* London: ICM; 2017a. Online: https://www.internationalmidwives.org/assets/files/definitions-files/2018/06/eng-definition_of_the_midwife-2017.pdf.

International Confederation of Midwives (ICM). *Definition of Midwifery.* London: ICM; 2017b. Online: https://www.internationalmidwives.org/assets/files/definitions-files/2018/06/eng-definition_midwifery.pdf.

International Confederation of Midwives (ICM). *Professional Framework for Midwifery, 2021.* Online: https://www.internationalmidwives.org/our-work/policy-and-practice/icms-professional-framework-for-midwifery.html.

Jefford E, Nolan S, Sansone H, et al. 'A match made in midwifery': Women's perceptions of student midwife partnerships. *Women Birth.* 2020;33(2):193-198. https://doi.org/10.1016/j.wombi.2018.11.018

Katz Rothman B. Childbirth management and medical monopoly: midwifery as (almost) a profession. *J Nurse Midwifery.* 1984;29(5):300-306.

Kensington M, Campbell N, Gray E, et al. New Zealand's Midwifery Profession: embracing graduate midwives' transition to practice. *NZCOM J.* 2016;52:20-25. http://dx.doi.org/10.12784/nzcomjnl52.2016.3.20-25.

Kitzinger S. *The Midwife Challenge*. London: Pandora Press; 1988.

Lane K. When is collaboration not collaboration? When it's militarized. *Women Birth*. 2012;25(1):29-38.

Leap N, Sheehan A, Barclay L, et al. Mapping midwifery education in Australia survey: findings of the AMAP Education Survey. Australian Midwifery Action Project Report Vol. 2. 2002.

McLachlan HL, Newton M, Nightingale H, et al. Exploring the 'follow-through experience': a statewide survey of midwifery students and academics conducted in Victoria, Australia. *Midwifery*. 2013;29:1064-1072.

Maternity Coalition. Funding Primary Maternity Care: A Proposal to Address Cost Shifting as an Obstacle to Public, Primary Maternity Services. Australia's National Maternity Consumer Organisation. 2008. Online: www.maternitycoalition.org.au.

Maternity Coalition/Australian Midwives Act Lobby Group (AMALG). Submissions to the Commonwealth Review of the Medicare Funding Agreement. Submission Number 169. 2003. Online: http://www.maternitycoalition.org.au, http://www.aph.gov.au/senate_medicare.

Mein Smith P, Department of Internal Affairs. *Maternity in Dispute in New Zealand 1920–1939*. Wellington: Historical Publications Branch; 1986.

Midwifery Council of New Zealand (MCNZ). n.d.a. Standards of Clinical & Cultural Competence & Conduct. Online: https://www.midwiferycouncil.health.nz/Public/Midwifery-in-Aotearoa--New-Zealand/I-am-a-registered-midwife/Standards-of-Clinical---Cultural-Competence---Conduct/Public/06.-I-am-a-registered-midwife/1.-Standards-of-Clinical---Cultural%20Competence---Conduct.aspx?hkey=b3251793-36c1-46b8-821f-afb858c8b04a.

Midwifery Council of New Zealand (MCNZ). n.d.b. Te Tatau o te Whare Kahu ki Hine Pae Ora Aotearoa Midwifery Project. Online: https://www.midwiferycouncil.health.nz/Public/Midwifery-in-Aotearoa--New-Zealand/Aotearoa-Midwifery-Project/Public/10.-Aotearoa-Midwifery-Project/Aotearoa-Midwifery-Project-Landing.aspx?hkey=4d788699-866e-4b51-ba01-ff5326fa02bc.

Midwifery Council of New Zealand (MCNZ). *Midwifery Scope of Practice*. Wellington: MCNZ; 2004a. Online: http://www.midwiferycouncil.health.nz

Midwifery Council of New Zealand (MCNZ). *Midpoint*. Newsletter of the Midwifery Council of New Zealand; September. 2004b.

Midwifery Council of New Zealand (MCNZ). *Midpoint*. Newsletter of the Midwifery Council of New Zealand: December. 2004c.

Midwifery Council of New Zealand (MCNZ). *Competencies for Entry to the Register of Midwives*. Wellington: MCNZ; 2007a. Online: http://www.midwiferycouncil.health.nz.

Midwifery Council of New Zealand (MCNZ). *Standards for Approval of Pre-registration Midwifery Education Programmes and Accreditation of Tertiary Education Organisations*. Wellington: MCNZ; 2007b.

Midwifery Council of New Zealand (MCNZ). Code of Conduct. Wellington, NZ: MCNZ; 2010. Online: https://www.midwiferycouncil.health.nz/sites/default/files/documents/midwifery%20code%20of%20conduct%20feb%202011.pdf.

Midwifery Council of New Zealand (MCNZ). *Statement on Cultural Competence for Midwives*. Wellington, NZ: MCNZ; 2012. 2015. Online: https://www.midwiferycouncil.health.nz/sites/default/files/documents/PDF%20cultural%20competence.pdf.

Midwifery Council of New Zealand (MCNZ). Standards for Approval of Pre-registration Midwifery Education Programmes and Accreditation of Tertiary Education Organisations. 2nd ed. Wellington, NZ: MCNZ; 2019a. Online: https://www.midwiferycouncil.health.nz/sites/default/files/professional-standards/Midwifery_Standards_2015_web_final.pdf.

Midwifery Council of New Zealand (MCNZ). Recertification Requirements 2020–2021. Wellington, NZ: MCNZ; 2019b. Online: https://www.midwiferycouncil.health.nz/common/Uploaded%20files/Annual%20Practising%20Certificates/Recertification%20programme.pdf 2019.

Midwifery Employee Representation and Advisory Service (MERAS). District Health Boards Quality and Leadership Programme for Midwives covered by the MERAS and NZNO Employment Agreements. 2014. Online: https://www.midwife.org.nz/wp-content/uploads/2018/08/QLP-Revision-November-2014.pdf.

Midwives Act. 1915 (No2773) Agency VA3143 Midwives Board. *Public Record Office Victoria (2005) Online Catalogue*. Online: http://wwwaccess.prov.vic.gov.au/component/daPublicBaseContainer.

Midwives Act. 1928 (No3587) March 1929. *Public Record Office Victoria (2005) Online Catalogue*. Online: http://wwwaccess.prov.vic.gov.au/component/daPublicBaseContainer.

National Nursing and Nursing Education Taskforce (NNNET). Towards Consistent Regulation of Nursing and Midwifery Practice in Australia: A Select Analysis of the Legislation and Professional Regulation of Nursing and Midwifery in Australia. A report prepared by Amanda Adrian and Associates for the National Nursing and Nursing Education Taskforce. 2006. Online: http://www.dhs.vic.gov.au/nnnet/downloads/rec4_mapping_report.pdf.

New South Wales (NSW). Health Practitioner Regulation National Law (NSW) No. 86a. 2009.

New Zealand College of Midwives (NZCOM). *Midwives Handbook for Practice*. 4th ed. Christchurch: NZCOM; 2015.

New Zealand College of Midwives (NZCOM). Report of New Zealand's MMPO Midwives Care Activities and Outcomes 2016. Christchurch, NZ: NZCOM; 2016. Online: https://www.midwife.org.nz/wp-content/uploads/2019/01/MMPO-report-2016.pdf.

New Zealand College of Midwives (NZCOM). *New Zealand College of Midwives management and organisational structure*. Christchurch, NZ: NZCOM; 2017a. Online: https://www.midwife.org.nz/wp-content/uploads/2018/12/Organisational-structure-2018.pdf.

New Zealand College of Midwives (NZCOM). Mediation Report to Members. Christchurch, NZ: NZCOM; 2017b.

New Zealand College of Midwives (NZCOM). n.d. Letter to members – pay equity claim. Online: https://www.midwife.org.nz/news/letter-to-members-pay-equity-claim/.

New Zealand Gazette. Midwifery (Scope of Practice and Qualifications) Notice, 2010. Online: https://gazette.govt.nz/notice/id/2010-gs3828.

Nurses Act. 1928 (Australia). Public Record Office Online Catalogue. Victorian Nursing Council (VA1352). 1928. Online: http://www.access.prov.vic.gov.au/public/component/daPublicBaseContainer?component=daViewAgency&entityId=3144.

Nursing and Midwifery Board of Australia (NMBA). Revised NMBA English Language Skills Registration Standard. Melbourne: NMBA; 2011. Online: http://www.nursingmidwiferyboard.gov.au/News/2011-08-29-New-English-Language-Skills-Registration-Standard.aspx.

Nursing and Midwifery Board of Australia (NMBA). Guidelines for Advertising Regulated Health Services. Melbourne: NMBA; 2014a. Online: http://www.nursingmidwiferyboard.gov.au/Codes-Guidelines-Statements/Codes-Guidelines/Guidelines-for-advertising-regulated-health-services.aspx.

Nursing and Midwifery Board of Australia (NMBA). *Guidelines for Mandatory Notifications*. Melbourne: NMBA; 2014b. Online: http://www.nursingmidwiferyboard.gov.au/Codes-Guidelines-Statements/Codes-Guidelines/Guidelines-for-mandatory-notifications.aspx.

Nursing and Midwifery Board of Australia (NMBA). *Registration Standard: English Language Skills*. Melbourne: NMBA; 2015. Online: http://www.nursingmidwiferyboard.gov.au/News/2011-08-29-New-English-Language-Skills-Registration-Standard.aspx.

Nursing and Midwifery Board of Australia (NMBA). *Guidelines for Professional Indemnity Insurance Arrangements for Midwives*. Melbourne: NMBA; 2016a. Online: http://www.nursingmidwiferyboard.gov.au/News/Newsletters/June-2015.aspx.

Nursing and Midwifery Board of Australia (NMBA). *Registration Standard: Continuing Professional Development*. Melbourne: NMBA; 2016b. Online: http://www.medicalboard.gov.au/Registration-Standards.aspx.

Nursing and Midwifery Board of Australia (NMBA). *Professional Indemnity Insurance Arrangements*. Melbourne: NMBA; 2016c. Online: http://www.nursingmidwiferyboard.gov.au/Registration-Standards/Professional-indemnity-insurance-arrangements.aspx.

Nursing and Midwifery Board of Australia (NMBA). *Registration Standard: Recency of Practice*. Melbourne: NMBA; 2016d. Online: http://www.medicalboard.gov.au/Registration-Standards.aspx.

Nursing and Midwifery Board of Australia (NMBA). Meeting the registration requirements. 2017a. Online: http://www.nursing-midwiferyboard.gov.au/Registration-and-Endorsement/International/Meeting-the-registration-requirements.aspx.

Nursing and Midwifery Board of Australia (NMBA). *Safety and Quality Framework for Privately Practising Midwives*. Melbourne: NMBA; 2017b. Online: http://www.nursingmidwiferyboard.gov.au/Codes-Guidelines-Statements/Codes-Guidelines.aspx.

Nursing and Midwifery Board of Australia (NMBA). *Registration Standards*. Melbourne: NMBA; 2017c. Online: http://www.nursingmidwiferyboard.gov.au/Registration-Standards.aspx.

Nursing and Midwifery Board of Australia (NMBA). *Registration Standard: Endorsement for Scheduled Medicines for Midwives*. Melbourne: NMBA; 2017d. Online: http://www.nursingmidwiferyboard.gov.au/Registration-Standards.aspx.

Nursing and Midwifery Board of Australia (NMBA). *Guideline for Midwives Applying for Endorsement for Scheduled Medicines*. Melbourne: NMBA; 2017e. Online: http://www.nursingmidwiferyboard.gov.au/Registration-and-Endorsement/Endorsements-Notations/Guidelines-for-Midwives-applying-for-endorsement-for-scheduled-medicines.aspx.

Nursing and Midwifery Board of Australia (NMBA). *Code of Conduct for Midwives*. Melbourne: NMBA; 2018a. Online: http://www.nursingmidwiferyboard.gov.au/Codes-Guidelines-Statements/Professional-standards.aspx.

Nursing and Midwifery Board of Australia (NMBA). *Midwife Standards for Practice*. Melbourne: NMBA; 2018b. Online: http://www.nursingmidwiferyboard.gov.au/.

Nursing and Midwifery Board of Australia (NMBA). *Criminal History Registration Standard*. Melbourne: NMBA; 2018c. Online: http://www.ahpra.gov.au/Registration/Registration-Standards/Criminal-history.aspx.

Nursing and Midwifery Board of Australia (NMBA). *Decision-Making Framework for Nursing and Midwifery Practice*. Melbourne: NMBA; 2020. Online: http://www.nursingmidwiferyboard.gov.au/Codes-Guidelines-Statements/Frameworks.aspx.

Nursing and Midwifery Board of Australia (NMBA). *Guidelines for Registration Standards*. Melbourne: NMBA; 2021. Online: http://www.nursingmidwiferyboard.gov.au/Codes-Guidelines-Statements/Codes-Guidelines.aspx.

Nursing and Midwifery Board of Australia (NMBA). 2022. Nursing and Midwifery in 2019/2020 Annual Report. https://www.nursingmidwiferyboard.gov.au/News/Annual-report.aspx.

Oakley A, Houd S. *Helpers in Childbirth. Midwifery Today*. London: Hemisphere Publishing/World Health Organization; 1990.

Oliver P. Midwifery First Year of Practice Pilot Programme Evaluation. Final report for the Clinical Training Agency, July 2008.

O'Sullivan JF. Two hundred years of midwifery 1806–2006. *Ulster Med J*. 2006;75(3):213-222.

Pairman S. Towards self-determination: the separation of the nursing and midwifery professions in New Zealand. In: Papps E, eds. *Nursing in New Zealand. Critical Issues, Different Perspectives*. Auckland: Pearson Education; 2002.

Pairman S. *Workforce to Profession: An Exploration of New Zealand Midwifery's Professionalising Strategies from 1986 to 2005*. (Doctoral thesis). Sydney: University of Technology; 2005.

Pairman S. Educating midwives for autonomous practice. In: Guilliland K, Pairman S, eds. *Women's Business: The Story of the New Zealand College of Midwives 1986–2010*. Christchurch: New Zealand College of Midwives; 2010:480-563.

Pairman S, Guilliland K. Developing a midwife-led maternity service: the New Zealand experience. In: Kirkham M, eds. *Birth Centres: A Social Model for Maternity Care*. London: Books for Midwives; 2003:97–111, [(Ch. 9)].

Pairman S, Dixon L, Tumilty E, et al. The Midwifery First Year of Practice programme: supporting New Zealand midwifery graduates in their transition to practice. *NZCOM J*. 2016;52:12-19. doi:10.12784/nzcomjnl52.2016.2.12-19.

Papps E, Olssen M. *Doctoring Childbirth and Regulating Midwifery in New Zealand*. Palmerston North: Dunmore Press; 1997.

Productivity Commission. Australian Health Workforce Research Report. Canberra: Productivity Commission; 2005.

Public Record Office Victoria. Agency VA3134 Midwives Board 1915–1929. 2005. Online: http://cc.bingj.com/cache.aspx?q=1916+Midwives+Board&d=4607775623090020&mkt=en-AU&setlang=en-AU&w=WMlfzdKsIDQvX-m9PlKqlJimvanh1ObA.

Queensland Government. Department of Science, Information Technology and Innovation. *Register of Nurses, With Examination Results*. Queensland State Archives Series ID17342. n.d.a. Online: http://www.archivessearch.qld.gov.au/Search/SeriesDetails.aspx?SeriesId=17342.

Queensland Government. Department of Science, Information Technology and Innovation. *Nurses and Masseurs Registration Board (22/12/1928–27/7/1965)*. Queensland State Archives Agency ID 1457. n.d.b. Online: http://www.archivessearch.qld.gov.au/Search/AgencyDetails.aspx?AgencyId=1457.

Queensland Government. Department of Science, Information Technology and Innovation. *Queensland Nursing Council*. Queensland State Archives Agency ID1670. n.d.c. Online: http://www.archivessearch.qld.gov.au/Search/AgencyDetails.aspx?AgencyId=1670.

Queensland Government. Nursing Act 1992 No.55, section 74(3). Brisbane: The State of Queensland; 1992. Online: https://www.legislation.qld.gov.au/view/pdf/asmade/act-1992-055.

Queensland Nursing Council. *Registration Renewal Standards*. Brisbane: Queensland Nursing Council; 2005.

Queensland Nursing Council. *Registration Renewal Standards*. Brisbane: Queensland Nursing Council; 2008.

Statistics New Zealand (Stats NZ). Births and Deaths: Year Ended December 2016; 2017. Online: https://www.stats.govt.nz/information-releases/births-and-deaths-year-ended-december-2016-and-march-2017.

Strid J. Midwifery in revolt. *Broadsheet*. 1987;153:14-17.

Stulz V, Elmir, R, Reilly, H. Evaluation of a student-led midwifery group practice: A woman's perspective. *Midwifery*. 2020; 86. doi:10.1016/j.midw.2020.102691.

Summers A. *For I Have Ever so Much More Faith in Her Ability as a Nurse: The Eclipse of the Community Midwife in South Australia 1836–1942*. Adelaide, SA: Flinders University; 1995.

Summers A. The lost voice of midwifery. *Collegian*. 1998;5(3): 16-22.

Teakle B. Have the 2010 national maternity reforms delivered choice, control and continuity to Australian women? *Women Birth*. 2013;26:97-99.

Tew M. *Safer Childbirth? A Critical History of Maternity Care.* London: Chapman & Hall; 1990.

Tickle, N, Gamble, J, Creedy, DK. Women's reports of satisfaction and respect with continuity of care experiences by students: Findings from a routine, online survey. *Women Birth.* 2020;20: 30377–2. doi:10.1016/j.wombi.2020.11.004.

Tickle N, Sidebotham M, Fenwick J, et al. Women's experiences of having a Bachelor of Midwifery student provide continuity of care. *Women Birth.* 2016;29(3):245-251.

Tully E. *Doing Professionalism Differently: Negotiating Midwifery Autonomy in Aotearoa/New Zealand.* (Doctoral thesis). Christchurch, NZ: University of Canterbury; 1999.

Tully E, Mortlock B. Professionals and practices. In: Davis P, Devo K, eds. *Health and Society in Aotearoa New Zealand.* Auckland: Oxford University Press; 1999:175.

Wilkes E, Teakle B, Gamble J. Medicare rebates for midwives: an analysis of the 2009/2010 Federal Budget. *Women Birth.* 2009;22(3):79-81.

Further reading

Aboriginal Women of Central Australia. *Congress Alukura by Grandmother's Law. Model of Healthy Public Policy.* Alice Springs: Congress Alukura; 1985.

Chief Nursing Officer's Office. *Enhanced Role Midwife Project.* Perth: Department of Health, Government of Western Australia; 2001.

Children, Youth and Women's Health Service State Wide Midwifery Caseload Forum. (unpublished discussion paper). Adelaide: Women's and Children's Hospital; 2005.

Department of Health New South Wales. Maternity Services in New South Wales. Final Report of the Ministerial Taskforce on Obstetric Services in NSW (Shearman Report). Department of Health Publication no. (HSU) 89–007. Sydney: Department of Health; 1989.

Fahy K. An Australian history of the subordination of midwifery. *Woman Birth.* 2007;20:25-29.

Hancock H. Pathology protocol—Australian first for midwives in the NT's Home Birth Service. *Aust Midwifery News.* 2006;6(1):22-23.

Health Department of Victoria. Having a Baby in Victoria. Final Report of the Ministerial Review of Birthing Services in Victoria, Melbourne. Melbourne: Victorian Government; 1990.

Hirst C. Re-Birthing: Report of the Review of Maternity Services in Queensland. Brisbane: Queensland Government; 2005. Online: https://trove.nla.gov.au/work/11831656.

Homer C, Passant L, Kildea S, et al. The development of national competency standards for the midwife in Australia. *Midwifery.* 2007;23:350-360.

Jag Films Pty Ltd. *Birth Rites (Film Documentary Produced by Jennifer Gheradi).* Margaret River, WA: JAG Films; 2001. Online: www.jagfilms.com.au/pages.asp?pageid=60&;submenu=60.

Kildea S. And the Women Said ... Reporting on Birthing Services for Aboriginal Women From Remote Top End Communities. Darwin: Women's Health Strategy Unit; 2000. Online: https://healthinfonet.ecu.edu.au/key-resources/publications/?id=6640.

Lane K. Autonomous midwifery in Australia: the safer alternative. *Birth Matters.* 1999;3(2):6-12.

National Health and Medical Research Council (NHMRC). *Options for Effective Care in Childbirth.* Canberra: Australian Government Printing Service; 1996.

Pairman S. Woman-centred midwifery: partnerships or professional friendships. In: Kirkham M, eds. *The Midwife–Mother Relationship.* London: Macmillan; 2000:28-52.

Queensland Health Legislation Amendment Regulation No. 4. 2007. Online: http://www.health.qld.gov.au/ocno/documents/dtphmp.pdf.

Stewart M. *Ngalangangopum Jarrakpu Purrurn: Mother and Child. The Women of Warnum as Told to Margaret Stewart.* Broome, WA: Magabala Books; 2000.

Tracy SK, Hartz D, Tracy M, et al. Caseload midwifery care for women of all risk compared to standard maternity care: a randomized controlled trial. ((Midwives @New Group practice options: M@NGO trial). *Lancet.* 2013;382(9906):1723-1732. doi:10.1016/S0140-6736(13)61406-3.

Turnbull H. *Select Committee on Intervention in Childbirth.* Select Committee on Intervention in Childbirth Report. Perth: Western Australian Legislative Assembly; 1995. Online: http://www.parliament.wa.gov.au/Parliament%5Ccommit.nsf/%28Report+Lookup+by+Com+ID%29/4C8BAD0EFBEFCF4548257831003E942A/$file/report.pdf.

CHAPTER 14

Legal frameworks for practice in Australia and New Zealand

Carla Humphrey and Bashi Kumar-Hazard

LEARNING OUTCOMES

Learning outcomes for this chapter are:

1. To understand key legislative provisions affecting midwives in Australia and New Zealand relating to regulation and control of midwifery practice

2. To understand key legal principles concerning midwives' duties pertaining to consumer rights, privacy, births, deaths and consumer complaints

3. To examine the role and the function of the Coroner's Court relating to midwifery practice

4. To consider the role and appropriate medicolegal response of the midwife in an unexpected outcome.

CHAPTER OVERVIEW

As with all professions today, the law regulates the practice of midwifery and governs the framework that enables the practice of midwifery within appropriate legal and ethical parameters. It also provides the mechanisms for consumer complaints made by persons who were cared for by, or have concerns about, a practitioner. This chapter provides an overview of the law and regulatory oversight in Australia and Aotearoa New Zealand that affects the practice of midwifery.

KEY TERMS

common law[a]
complaints
consent

information giving
legislation
notifications

privacy
regulation
statutes

INTRODUCTION: THE LAW

The primary function of the law is to protect members of the public, to administer and regulate professional and consumer entitlements, and to sanction those who offend against the norms and values of any society, as defined within its legal system. In Australasia the generic term 'law' refers to Acts of Parliament (or **statutes**), the regulations that are made by government and implemented by the administrative arm of government, and the **common law**, which is law made by judges, coroners and tribunals, usually in the context of individual cases brought against practitioners.

Midwives must be familiar with the legislative framework in which they practise, to enable them to fulfil their legal and professional obligations. The law confers both privileges and duties on you (including the right to use the protected title of 'midwife') and provides for the protection of the fundamental rights of healthcare consumers. It is in your interests, as a practitioner, to be familiar with the legal framework, both to deliver safe care and to protect yourself.

A helpful way of classifying the law for health professionals is to examine the remedies it provides for when there are breaches of people's legal rights. This has been explained in a seminal article by Bates (1989) and the remedies are set out in Table 14.1.

Midwifery practice in both Australia and New Zealand is governed by a number of statutes. This chapter summarises key Australian and New Zealand statutes to help you understand your legal responsibilities.

Australia, unlike New Zealand, is a federation with six states and two territories. The Commonwealth can draft legislation and guidelines to regulate professional practice which, in turn, ensures consistency in quality and safety measure across the country. It is, however, up to each state and territory to implement those laws and guidelines that affect midwifery practice. Implementation can result in some variations in the application of the laws at the state level. To prevent too much variation, the Council of Australian Governments, comprising the leadership of each state and jurisdiction as well as the Commonwealth (COAG) will regularly meet to agree (as far as is possible) changes to health regulation in a consistent way. In a chapter such as this, it is impossible to cover all the variation in laws governing the practice of midwifery at the state and territory level. Instead, it provides an overview of certain key pieces of **legislation** and professional guidelines governing midwives, including the most important legal principles underpinning your practice as a midwife. It will encourage you to always investigate governing legislation that could affect your practice or changes in your practice and to keep up to date with the regulatory framework at all times. It is one of the benefits and burdens of joining a profession.

The law discussed in this chapter is divided into three sections: (1) midwifery **regulation**, public safety, **consent** and information giving; (2) **privacy** and personal information; and (3) midwifery practice, first for Australia and then for New Zealand. In the final section, the role of the Coroner is addressed for Australia and New Zealand together, as it is similar in both countries.

THE REGULATION OF MIDWIFERY PRACTICE

Midwifery regulation in Australia overview

Background

On the 1st of July 2010, a new National Registration and Accreditation Scheme came into being as a result of passing legislation in the Queensland Parliament (Beaupert et al., 2014). This legislation established 10 (now 15) health professional registration boards and one overarching management organisation to support the boards and employ the staff who work in the scheme. The Australian Health Practitioner Regulation Agency (AHPRA) is the organisation responsible for supporting the boards and implementing the National Registration and Accreditation Scheme across Australia (AHPRA, 2017a).

Relevant legislation and structure of the scheme

AHPRA's operations are governed by the *Health Practitioner Regulation National Law Act 2009 (Qld)* (hereafter the National Law), as in force in each state and territory (State of Queensland, 2018). This law means that, for the first time in Australia, 16 health professions are regulated by nationally consistent legislation. While nursing and midwifery are governed by one board, the Nursing and Midwifery Board of Australia (NMBA), they are each recognised as a separate profession. This National Law, with the approval of the states and territories, now governs the operation and implementation of the National Registration

Table 14.1 Remedies model as a means of classifying laws that bear on professional liability	
Remedy provided	Area and source of law
To punish offenders and to deter potential offenders	Criminal law
To protect the public against incompetent or grossly deficient moral qualities or technical proficiency	Administrative law (civil) (professional misconduct)
To compensate injured victims	Civil law (negligence/battery)
To provide information and to review decision-making procedures	Administrative law (judicial review)

and Accreditation Scheme across the health professions, including nursing and midwifery (Beaupert et al., 2014).

The object of the National Law is set out in the Schedule Part 1, s3(1) and is as follows (State of Queensland, 2018, p. 55):

... to establish a national registration and accreditation scheme for—
(a) the regulation of health practitioners; and
(b) the registration of students undertaking—
(i) programs of study that provide a qualification for registration in a health profession; or
(ii) clinical training in a health profession).

The scheme also has a number of objectives, set out in s3(2), and these are as follows (p. 55):

(a) to provide for the protection of the public by ensuring that only health practitioners who are suitably trained and qualified to practise in a competent and ethical manner are registered; and
(b) to facilitate workforce mobility across Australia by reducing the administrative burden for health practitioners wishing to move between participating jurisdictions or to practise in more than one participating jurisdiction; and
(c) to facilitate the provision of high quality education and training of health practitioners; and
(d) to facilitate the rigorous and responsive assessment of overseas-trained health practitioners; and
(e) to facilitate access to services provided by health practitioners in accordance with the public interest; and
(f) to enable the continuous development of a flexible, responsive and sustainable Australian health workforce and to enable innovation in the education of, and service delivery by, health practitioners.

The traditional purpose of a professional regulatory scheme is to protect the public. It is usually said that those working in professional regulation exercise a 'protective jurisdiction' (AHPRA, 2015). The new professional regulatory scheme, however, also has a number of added objectives relating to workforce mobility and flexibility. It is a significant new development to explicitly include such objectives in a scheme that has traditionally been about protecting the public—a process that has, on occasions, been criticised for limiting access to certain professions and creating monopolies (Levi-Faur, 2012).

Also for the first time in Australia, midwifery is recognised nationally as a profession distinct from, but professionally aligned with, nursing. This is congruent with many other countries that recognise both direct entry and post-nursing registration pathways into midwifery (World Health Organization (WHO), 2009). The major difference in the new scheme in Australia is that there are now separate registers for nursing and midwifery, which means that people who have a qualification only in midwifery are able to register solely as a midwife. In the Council of Australian Governments (COAG Health Council, 2017) *Summary of the Draft Health Practitioner Regulation National Law Amendment*

Law 2017 (Summary), Australia finally recognised nursing and midwifery as separate professions. The Summary has the following commentary about this recognition (p. 7):

29. *The significant majority of midwives in Australia hold dual registration as nurses and midwives (approximately 30,000). However, there are approximately 3,000 registered midwives who are qualified to practise as midwives only. In recent years, direct entry training programs for midwifery, and the introduction of alternative maternity choices for women, mainly in metropolitan areas, have seen a growth in the proportion of registered midwives who do not hold concurrent registration as a nurse.*

30. *The independent review recommended that the National Law be amended to reflect that nursing and midwifery are two professions regulated by one National Board. The Bill amends the National Law to recognise that nursing and midwifery are separate professions.*

That said, other proposed changes within the governance of midwifery regulation that can ensure greater midwifery input into matters relating to registrations and notifications about midwives have not been made. This is significant. While midwifery is treated as a separate profession, the profession is still being governed by a professional board led by nurses.

To register as a midwife, your application must meet the eligibility requirements set out under s52 of the National Law. Midwives must undertake an approved program of study (s53 of the National Law) and prove the recency of midwifery practice. Registration must be renewed annually. Midwives must do continuing professional development (CPD) relating to midwifery practice to renew their registration, although a midwife also registered as a nurse can use the CPD undertaken for nursing to satisfy CPD obligations for both nursing and midwifery (Nursing and Midwifery Board of Australia (NMBA), 2017a). You cannot practise as or call yourself a midwife without becoming registered with the NMBA.

In addition to the obligation to register as a midwife, major changes have occurred in the Registration Standards for Midwives, stipulated under s94 of the National Law (NMBA, 2017b) over the last 15 years. Every 10 years, the federal government conducts a review of maternity services, together with stakeholders, for the purposes of issuing guidelines for development and improvement of these services. The 2008 review of maternity services, named the *Maternity Services Review* (see Department of Health and Ageing (DOHA), 2008), recommended that consumers cared for by privately practising midwives (PPMs) be able to claim rebates under the Medicare Benefits Schedule (MBS) and Pharmaceutical Benefits Scheme (PBS) rebates. The Maternity Services Review also recommended government-sponsored professional indemnity insurance (PII) for services provided by appropriately qualified and experienced midwives (at that time described as 'eligible midwives' (EMs)). The PII arrangements do not cover planned intrapartum care in the home.

In 2016, a further consultation resulting in the new National Strategic Framework for Maternity Services 2016 (NFMS) was published. The NFMS provides guidance for the planning and delivery of women-centred, safe, high-quality healthcare across the maternity continuum of care. As noted above, the NFMS is a strategic guide for states and territories. Implementation is entirely up to the states and territories.

The process for obtaining scheduled medicines endorsement for midwives, the PII requirements for PPMs, and the PII exemptions for PPMs offering home birth are discussed in turn.

(1) Registration standard for endorsement for scheduled medicines for midwives under s94

Section 94 of the National Law gives registered midwives the opportunity to become 'endorsed' to prescribe certain scheduled medicines and tests for their clients. If you are an endorsed midwife, you will be described in the national register as 'An endorsed midwife qualified to prescribe schedule 2, 3, 4 and 8 medicines and to provide associated services required for midwifery practice in accordance with relevant state and territory legislation' (NMBA, 2017b, p. 1).

To seek endorsement for scheduled medicines as a midwife you must demonstrate all of the following (NMBA, 2017b, p. 2):

1. *Current general registration as a midwife in Australia with no conditions or undertakings relating to unsatisfactory professional performance or unprofessional conduct.*
2. *Registration as a midwife that is the equivalent of three years' full-time clinical practice (5,000 hours) in the past six years that is either:*
   — *across the continuum of care, or*
   — *in a specified context of practice*
      from the date when the complete application seeking endorsement for scheduled medicines is received by the NMBA.
3. *Successful completion of:*
   — *an NMBA-approved program of study leading to endorsement for scheduled medicines, or*
   — *a program that is substantially equivalent to an NMBA-approved program of study leading to endorsement for scheduled medicines as determined by the NMBA.*

There are also ongoing requirements for endorsement. Ongoing endorsement by the NMBA is conditional on the midwife complying with the current (NMBA, 2017b, p. 2):

1. *NMBA-approved Continuing professional development registration standard, Recency of practice registration standard, Criminal history registration standard and Professional indemnity insurance arrangements registration standard*
2. *any other applicable codes and guidelines approved by the NMBA, and*
3. *for midwives who are privately practising, the safety and quality guidelines for privately practising midwives.*

(2) The safety and quality guidelines for privately practising midwives

Under s129 of the National Law, registered health practitioners cannot practise their profession without appropriate PII. PII gives financial protection to both practitioners and patients in circumstances where a patient sustains an injury (or adverse outcome) caused by medical misadventure, malpractice, negligence or an otherwise unlawful act. In Australia, it is compulsory for all registered health professionals to hold medical indemnity insurance under the National Law Act.

Employee midwives are, owing to the doctrine of vicarious liability, covered by their employer's insurance. The situation is more complex for PPMs. Since 2001, PPMs have struggled to obtain total PII cover for services rendered in Australia.

In 2008, limited Commonwealth government-subsidised and other insurance products were made available to PPMs, but only in relation to antenatal and postpartum care. Insurance products are, however, still not available for the provision of intrapartum care at home. Recent government regulations imposing obligations on insurers to offer full PII coverage to medical practitioners and privately practising nurses and PPMs deliberately excluded mandated PII coverage for intrapartum care at home (*Medical and Midwife Indemnity Legislation Amendment Act 2019* (Cth)).

This lacuna is deterring PPMs from practice and restricting access for women who wish to home birth with a skilled practitioner. For this reason, from 1 July 2010, under s284 of the National Law, PPMs were provided a time-limited exemption from the requirement to hold PII for intrapartum care in the home.

To be eligible for the exemption, PPMs must meet four requirements specified in s284(1)(b) and (c). First, PPMs must have insurance coverage for the provision of antenatal and postnatal services, regardless of the birth setting. PII arrangements that midwives are advised to consider include civil liability cover, unlimited retroactive cover and run-off cover (NMBA, 2017c).

Second, a PPM must obtain the 'informed consent' of any woman under her care (s284(1)(b) National Law). This is mandated by the NMBA and is in accordance with the National Health and Medical Research Council (NHMRC)'s *General Guidelines for Medical Practitioners on Providing Information to Patients* (NHMRC, 2004a). If the PPM is also providing home birth services, consent must be obtained in accordance with s284 of the National Law which states: 'written consent given by a woman after she received a written statement by the midwife that includes a statement that appropriate PII arrangements will not be in force in relation to the midwife's practice of private midwifery in attending homebirth' (NMBA, 2017c, p. 3).

Third, the midwife must comply 'with any requirements set out in a code or guideline approved by the National Board under s39 about the practice of private midwifery, including any requirement in a code or

293

guideline about reports to be provided by midwives practising private midwifery' (s284(1)(c)(i) National Law). The Board has published a number of codes and guidelines specifically for midwives, and these documents are detailed in the safety and quality guidelines for PPMs (NMBA, 2017c).

Finally, under S284(1)(c)(ii) requires midwives in private practice to meet the requirements detailed in these guidelines with regard to safety and quality for the PII exemption.

(3) Evidentiary requirements for privately practising midwives

All PPMs must comply with the guidelines and demonstrate that they meet the requirements with supported documented evidence as described in Table 14.2. Note there are additional requirements for PPMs offering home birth. All PPMs in Australia need to meet these evidentiary requirements in order to be exempt from holding PII for home births, under the National Law. In

Table 14.2 Evidentiary requirements for privately practising midwives	
Requirement	**Evidence**
Informed consent	Informed consent must be obtained from women in the care of a PPM in accordance with the NHMRC general guidelines for medical practitioners on providing information to patients. In addition to the above, if the PPM is providing home birth services, the consent must be in accordance with section 284 of the National Law, which states: *written consent given by a woman after she received a written statement by the midwife that includes a statement that appropriate PII arrangements will not be in force in relation to the midwife's practice of private midwifery in attending homebirth.*
Risk assessment	Documented process for identification and evaluation of clinical risk and evidence of correcting, eliminating or reducing these risks. This assessment should be completed with reference to the ACM *National Midwifery Guidelines for Consultation and Referral* (2013). There should be two registered health professionals, educated to provide maternal and newborn care and skilled and current in maternity emergency management and maternal/neonatal resuscitation, one of whom is a midwife, present at a home birth.[a] Consideration of the distance and time to travel to an appropriately staffed hospital service, in case of the need for transfer must be incorporated into the plan of care.
Referral pathways	Clearly articulated referral pathways for consultation and/or referral in line with the ACM *National Midwifery Guidelines for Consultation and Referral* must be documented and followed.
Collaborative arrangements	Demonstrate practice according to the requirements outlined in the NHMRC national guidance on collaborative maternity care including comprehensive documentation.
Submission of reports and data	Evidence of submission of the required data of all births attended as per each state and territory and national perinatal data collection.
Clinical audit	Comprehensive clinical notes including consent forms, management plans, pregnancy record, labour and birth records and postnatal care plan/notes. These should enable data collection in accordance with the AIHW national core maternity indicators where applicable as well as peer and reflective practice review/evaluation.
Adverse event management	Where appropriate, documented processes for notifying and reporting of incidents and adverse events, or the more serious category of sentinel events such as those endorsed by the ACSQHC. Reporting should be in accordance with the relevant state or territory health department requirements.
PPM portfolio	Completion of a minimum of a PPRP.
	Demonstration of annual competencies in adult basic life support and neonatal resuscitation and training in accordance with the NMBA's registration standard: Continuing professional development.

[a]This may include a paramedic who is skilled and current in maternity emergency management and maternal/neonatal resuscitation.
ACSQHC = Australian Commission on Safety and Quality in Healthcare; ACM = Australian College of Midwives; AIHW = Australian Institute of Health and Welfare; NMBA = Nursing and Midwifery Board of Australia; NHMRC = National Health and Medical Research Council; PPM = privately practising midwife; PPRP = professional practice review program.

addition to these evidentiary requirements, the NMBA is auditing all PPMs who provide home birth services against the guidelines in 2017 (NMBA, 2017d).

Notifications and complaints about midwives under the National Law regime

The protection of the public means that the public in general (including other healthcare practitioners (HCPs)) have a right (and in some instances, a duty) to notify the relevant registration authority if they have concerns about a practitioner's or student's conduct, health or performance. They are expected to do so if the midwife / student appears to be putting the public at risk. AHPRA provides advice on the types of conduct, health or performance matters that can result in a notification (AHPRA, 2017b).

When a **notification** is received, AHPRA will, as a first step, assess it to determine whether the NMBA should take immediate action to protect public health or safety. If immediate action is required, the registration status of the student or practitioner may be suspended or subject to conditions. If immediate action is not required, AHPRA will assess the notification and commence an investigation. Each investigation is tailored to the notification received, with complex matters often taking more time to resolve (AHPRA, 2017c).

As discussed above, mandatory notifications are imposed in some situations under the National Law. HCPs and employers must report a registrant they believe has engaged in notifiable conduct. This is a new requirement for midwives. Under s140, notifiable conduct in relation to a registered HCP means that the practitioner has (pp. 166–7):

a. *practised the practitioner's profession while intoxicated by alcohol or drugs; or*

b. *engaged in sexual misconduct in connection with the practice of the practitioner's profession; or*

c. *placed the public at risk of substantial harm in the practitioner's practice of the profession because the practitioner has an impairment; or*

d. *placed the public at risk of harm because the practitioner has practised the profession in a way that constitutes a significant departure from accepted professional standards.*

Notification and complaints handling in New South Wales (NSW)

While registration and accreditation functions for nursing and midwifery continue to be managed centrally by NMBA / AHPRA and the Australian Nursing & Midwifery Accreditation Council (ANMAC) nationally, some states such as NSW and Queensland have opted to retain their **complaints** handling, investigating and prosecuting mechanisms. The NSW Government established a complaints-handling authority called the Health Professional Councils Authority (HPCA), an administrative body that supports the 15 Health Professional Councils to perform their regulatory and legislative functions in NSW.

The HPCA came into existence from 1 July 2010 and is an administrative body of the Health Administration Corporation. The HPCA provides the administrative and secretarial support to each of the 14 NSW Councils in their primary role to protect the public. Whilst the actual processes in terms of who conducts the investigation and prosecution are different, many of the requirements are the same as for the national scheme, including a requirement for mandatory notification. The HPCA website provides valuable and comprehensive advice for nurses and midwives in NSW regarding the NSW processes through a series of FAQs (Health Professional Councils Authority (HPCA), 2018).

Queensland moved to a similar scheme in 2013 and established the Office of the Health Ombudsman (OHO, 2017), although the Queensland scheme uses the services of AHPRA more extensively than the NSW scheme.

Under the *Trans-Tasman Mutual Recognition Act 1997 (Cth)* there is reciprocal recognition of registration for nurses and midwives moving between Australia and New Zealand.

Midwifery regulation in New Zealand overview

Nurses Act 1977 and Nurses Amendment Act 1990

The *Nurses Act 1977* was the governing legislation for nurses and midwives in New Zealand until 2003 and it established the Nursing Council of New Zealand as the statutory body. Part of the Nursing Council's role was to regulate nurses and midwives. The regulation of midwives was transferred from the Nursing Council to the Midwifery Council of New Zealand (MCNZ) as a result of the *Health Practitioners Competence Assurance Act (HPCAA) 2003*. This legislation established the Midwifery Council as the responsible authority to regulate the practice of midwifery.

The enactment of the *Nurses Amendment Act 1990* represented a significant advancement for midwives and women in New Zealand. Prior to this Act, the requirement for a doctor to oversee maternity care and be present at every birth meant that women were limited in the type of care they could access. Women who wanted to birth at home struggled to find a doctor willing to attend the birth. As a profession, midwifery regained its professional autonomy and midwives were given a socially mandated right to practise independently of medical practitioners and medical oversight.

The Amendment Act also enabled midwives (through changes to other legislation) to provide a full range of maternity services, including the right to order laboratory tests and ultrasound scans, to prescribe drugs for antenatal, intrapartum and postnatal care, including the controlled drug pethidine, to refer clients to specialists and to admit women to public hospitals under midwifery care. It also enabled experimental midwifery education programs to be established and paved the way for direct-entry midwifery education, which is now the most common route to midwifery registration in New Zealand.

The Health Practitioners Competence Assurance Act 2003

Professional regulatory authorities

Prior to the HPCAA, there were 11 regulatory statutes in respect of 15 types of health practitioner in New Zealand. The HPCAA established four new autonomous healthcare professions and their respective councils, including the 'profession of midwifery' and the 'Midwifery Council' (MCNZ). It is perhaps the world's first legislation that recognised midwifery as completely separate from nursing and medicine in terms of regulation. This sea change came about partly because of political acceptance that childbirth was not an 'illness' but a natural and normal life event, that many midwives in New Zealand were already practising independently under a 'continuity-of-care model' and that midwives were a cohesive workforce professionally well supported through bodies such as the New Zealand College of Midwives (NZCOM).

All governing bodies of all healthcare professions are now termed 'responsible authorities'. Each responsible authority is 'appointed in respect of the profession' to be 'responsible for the registration and oversight of practitioners' of its particular profession. All responsible authorities must operate under the same provisions and procedures of the HPCAA to ensure there is 'a consistent accountability regime for all health professions'. The principal purpose of the Act is 'to protect the health and safety of members of the public by providing mechanisms to ensure that health practitioners are competent and fit to practise their professions'. It is the legal obligation of the MCNZ to promote the Act's purpose when carrying out its activities. The Midwifery Council website (listed in Online resources at the end of this chapter) contains detailed information on its functions.

Medicolegal aspects of HPCAA

This section discusses the main aspects of the HPCAA where medicolegal concerns tend to arise.

Impairment

Some circumstances require mandatory reporting of a health professional to the MCNZ. Where there is reason to believe 'that a health practitioner is unable to perform the functions' of midwifery because of 'some mental or physical condition', this belief must be notified to the MCNZ promptly. The belief must be both held and reported by any person who (section [s]45):

(a) *is in charge of an organisation that provides health services; or*
(b) *is a health practitioner; or*
(c) *is an employer of health practitioners; or*
(d) *is a medical officer of health.*

Following consideration by the Health Committee of the MCNZ and having regard to any medical reports and submissions, the MCNZ may suspend the midwife's registration or order that conditions be included in the midwife's scope of practice (s50).

The impairment provisions of the Act are not disciplinary in nature.

Competence

Midwives are expected to maintain their competence, including cultural competence as prescribed for by the MCNZ Competencies for Entry to the Register of Midwives (MCNZ, 2007, 2011). The MCNZ may enquire into and review the competence of the midwife of its own motion at any time or, more usually, where (s36):

1. it has received a notification from the Health and Disability Commissioner (HDC) or another health practitioner that either has 'reason to believe' the midwife 'may pose a risk of harm to the public by practising below the required standard of competence'; or
2. it has received a notification from an employer of a midwife who has resigned or was dismissed for reasons relating to competence; or
3. it has received a recommendation to that effect from a Professional Conduct Committee (PCC) following an investigation of a midwife's conduct.

The duty to notify the MCNZ is mandatory only where the HDC or District Health Board (DHB) believes the 'risk of harm' test is met. An individual health practitioner has discretion as to whether to report in such circumstances.

For the year to 31 March 2020, 43 competence referrals were made—largely from other health providers (MCNZ, 2021).

Competence reviews must be carried out according to a defined process including elements of natural justice (s37). If the MCNZ finds the midwife fails to meet the required standard of competence it must make one or more of the following orders (s38):

(a) *that the midwife undertake a competence programme;*
(b) *that 1 or more conditions be included in the midwife's scope of practice;*
(c) *that the midwife sit an examination or undertake an assessment specified in the order;*
(d) *that the midwife be counselled or assisted by 1 or more nominated persons.*

It is not a ground for disciplinary action if a midwife fails to satisfy the requirements of a competence order; however, in such a case the MCNZ may suspend the midwife's registration, impose practice conditions or alter the scope of practice by changing any health services the midwife is permitted to perform (s43).

Conduct/discipline

The MCNZ may refer a midwife to its Professional Conduct Committee to consider a complaint concerning the midwife's conduct for possible disciplinary proceedings in the Health Practitioners Disciplinary Tribunal (HPDT). The HPDT is set up under the HPCAA to hear charges against health professionals brought to it by either the PCC or the HDC.

The role of the PCC is not to determine whether the midwife is guilty of professional misconduct but rather to decide whether there is a prima facie ('on the face of it') case to answer. It investigates a midwife's conduct measured against the MCNZ's *Code of Conduct* (MCNZ, 2010) and the philosophy, standards of practice, consensus statements and practice guidelines of NZCOM. If it considers there is a prima facie case to answer, and it considers the matter serious enough, it may lay charges with the HPDT. As alternatives to laying charges, the PCC must make one or more of the following recommendations to the MCNZ (s80):

1. that the MCNZ review the midwife's competence to practise midwifery
2. that the MCNZ review the midwife's fitness to practise midwifery, i.e. impairment issues
3. that the MCNZ review the midwife's scope of practice
4. that the MCNZ refer the subject matter of the investigation to the police
5. that the MCNZ counsel the midwife
6. that no further steps be taken under the HPCAA against the midwife
7. in the case of a complaint, that the complaint be submitted to conciliation.

The PCC uses an inquisitorial rather than adversarial model to gather the evidence to make its assessment. Any charges laid against a midwife following a PCC hearing will be framed in terms of the grounds for discipline set out in the HPCAA. These are (s100):

1. malpractice/negligence—professional misconduct because of any act or omission that amounts to malpractice or negligence in relation to the practice of midwifery such as, for example, a failure to provide adequate care
2. bringing the profession into disrepute—professional misconduct because of any act or omission that has brought, or is likely to bring, discredit to the profession of midwifery such as, for example, any breach of professional boundaries including breach or abuse of position of trust or unprofessional communications with healthcare colleagues
3. criminal offending—conviction of an offence that reflects adversely on a midwife's ability to practise (Box 14.1 sets out the offending that will attract disciplinary action)
4. failure to practise as authorised by the MCNZ—this includes practising without a practising certificate or outside the authorised scope of practice
5. breaching any order of the HPDT.

Charges before the HPDT are often adversarial in style. The Supreme Court has confirmed that the standard of proof for professional disciplinary bodies is the civil standard of the 'balance of probabilities' which will be 'flexibly applied' to require stronger evidence in cases where the allegations are more serious (*Z v Dental Complaints Assessment Committee* [2008]). If proven guilty, the health practitioner can be ordered to pay costs and expenses of

---

Box 14.1 Criminal offending

Midwives should remember that they are subject to the whole realm of law, just like any other citizen. However, unlike other citizens, a conviction may have the additional result for a midwife of a professional misconduct hearing and a loss of the privilege to practise. Although some of the following scenarios will be more applicable to midwives than others, section 67 of the HPCAA states that the Court Registrar must notify the MCNZ if a midwife is convicted of an offence punishable by imprisonment for a term of 3 months or longer or for any offence against any of the following Acts:

- *Accident Compensation Act 2001*
- *Births Death Marriages and Relationship Registration Act 1995*
- *Burial and Cremation Act 1964*
- *Coroners Act 2006*
- *Health Act 1956*
- *Health and Disability Services (Safety) Act 2001*
- *Human Tissue Act 2008*
- *Medicines Act 1981*
- *Mental Health (Compulsory Assessment and Treatment) Act 1992*
- *Misuse of Drugs Act 1975*
- *Radiation Protection Act 1965.*

---

the investigation and hearing; a fine up to $30,000; other penalties including censure, cancellation of their registration; or suspension for up to 3 years (s101). For the year to 31 March 2020, 6 conduct cases were notified to the MCNZ (MCNZ, 2021).

COMPLAINTS AND PROFESSIONAL ACCOUNTABILITY PROCESSES

Complaint procedures and professional negligence in Australia

Unlike New Zealand, Australia does not have a no-fault liability scheme to compensate injured clients. Following an adverse event, a client may choose to seek redress in a number of ways. They may go directly to the healthcare provider—be that an employer such as a healthcare authority, a group midwifery practice or a self-employed midwife—to state a grievance. Alternatively, they can raise a grievance with a regulatory authority as discussed above, or to a healthcare complaints authority as discussed below.

Table 14.3 Australian health complaints authorities

Legislation	Complaints body
Human Rights Commission Act 2005, ACT	Human Rights Commission
Health Care Complaints Act 1993, NSW	Health Care Complaints Commission
Health and Community Services Complaints Act 2016, NT	Health and Community Services Complaints Commission
Health Ombudsman Act 2013 Qld	Office of the Health Ombudsman
Health and Community Services Complaints Act 2004, SA	Health and Community Services Complaints Commission
Health Complaints Act 1995, Tas	Health Complaints Commissioner and State Ombudsman
Health Complaints Act 2016, Vic	Health Complaints Commissioner
Health and Disability Services (Complaints) Act 1995, WA	Health and Disability Services Complaints Office

Consumers can also bring private legal claims against a midwife or the midwife's employer for negligence, misadventure or malpractice.

Health complaints authorities in Australia

Each state and territory has an independent healthcare complaints body set up under specific legislation to deal with complaints about healthcare providers and / or services (Table 14.3). The healthcare complaints authorities were established to acknowledge and protect patient rights (Reader et al., 2014).

Many aggrieved patients choose not to pursue private litigation through the courts. The legal process is time consuming, expensive and stressful, whether or not a case proceeds to court. They may seek an alternative means of resolution through a healthcare complaints authority, where the patient can make a complaint about the healthcare provider. The legislation varies from jurisdiction to jurisdiction, but in general the aim of the legislation is to provide an independent body for the resolution of complaints between healthcare consumers and providers.

These bodies have the authority to pursue and investigate complaints against unregistered health practitioners and other health services, which gives them a much wider remit than a regulatory authority. The commissioner or director of the healthcare complaints authority has the power to investigate and conciliate a matter arising from a complaint. Both parties must consent to a matter being referred to conciliation. If appropriate, a matter can be referred to the registering authority of the professional for an investigation.

Professional negligence

Negligence is part of the law of civil wrongs, also known as the law of torts, which seeks to compensate persons injured through the act or omission of another. The person bringing the action in negligence is called the plaintiff and it is their responsibility to prove that the HCP (in our case) was negligent and to prove it 'on the balance of probabilities'—in other words, they are required to prove that it was more likely than not that the negligent act or omission occurred and caused the damage complained of (Staunton & Chiarella, 2016, p. 38).

Civil liabilities legislation has been enacted in the states and territories in response to the medical insurance 'crisis' in 2001 (Staunton & Chiarella, 2016). Legislation now regulates the legal principles that make up negligence law, which were initially developed by common or judge made law. To establish negligence, the plaintiff must prove that a duty of care was owed, that there was a breach in the duty of care—that is, the standard of care fell below that of an ordinary reasonable midwife given the circumstances—and that the damage or injury was a reasonably foreseeable consequence of that breach.

There is no question that a midwife owes a client a *duty of care*. To successfully argue otherwise would, in most cases, be extremely difficult. Lord Atkin, in the now famous case of *Donoghue v Stevenson* [1932], established to whom a duty of care is owed:

> *You must take reasonable care to avoid acts or omissions which you can reasonably foresee would be likely to injure your neighbour. Who then in law is my neighbour? The answer seems to be persons who are so closely affected by my act that I ought reasonably to have them in contemplation as being so affected when I am directing my mind to the acts or omissions which are called in question.*
>
> (*Donoghue v Stevenson* [1932] AC 562 at 580)

The statutory duty of care is now regulated by s5B of the Civil Liability Act 2002 (WA); similar provisions exist in other jurisdictions within Australia. Section 5B states:

(1) *A person is not liable for harm caused by that person's fault in failing to take precaution against a risk of harm unless—*
   (a) *the risk was foreseeable (that is, it is a risk of which the person knew or ought to have known);*
   (b) *the risk was not insignificant; and*
   (c) *in the circumstances, a reasonable person in the person's position would have taken those precautions.*
(2) *In determining whether a reasonable person would have taken precautions against a risk of harm, the court is to consider the following (amongst other relevant things)—*

(a) *the probability that the harm would occur if care were not taken;*

(b) *the likely seriousness of the harm;*

(c) *the burden of taking precautions to avoid the risk of harm;*

(d) *the social utility of the activity that creates the risk of harm.*

Once a duty is established, the plaintiff must prove that the midwife breached her duty of care or that it was her fault that the injury occurred. The test used to establish a breach in relation to treatment is one of *reasonableness*. The standard required of a midwife is an objective test according to what a 'reasonable midwife' would or would not have done in the circumstances. In determining whether the standard has been met, the court will consider not only expert evidence but also various documents such as appropriate statutes, hospital policy and the midwife's case notes.

It is important to note that, whilst the standard expected for treatment and care is that of the reasonable midwife, there is a higher standard expected in relation to **information giving** in Australian law as a result of the High Court decision in *Rogers v Whitaker* [1992] where the standard for information giving was based not on the views or needs of the doctor or treating practitioner, but on the need to warn a patient of material risks in a proposed or intended procedure or treatment. The High Court identified two categories of patients for whom a risk might be material and thus information needs might be different. The first was the 'reasonable patient' and the second was the 'particular patient'. In the second case, particular patients might have specific information needs over and above that which would ordinarily be reasonable, based on their particular circumstances.

To prove *causation* the plaintiff must prove that the breach of duty by the defendant caused the injury. In other words, it cannot be too remote. The traditional test in Australia has been the 'but for' test—expressed as 'whether the consequences were a foreseeable result of the breach [of the duty of care]' (*Finch v Rogers*, 2004, pp. 147–8). Civil liabilities legislation now requires a factual causation—that is, whether the harm was caused by the negligence and whether 'it is appropriate to extend the scope of the tortfeasor's (defendant's) liability to the harm so caused (scope of liability)' (s5C Civil Liability Act 2002, WA).

Consumer complaint procedures and professional accountability in New Zealand

The New Zealand legal system was founded on the English legal system. Up until 1974, medical malpractice litigation was the only legal redress for citizens' monetary claims against healthcare professionals, and was based on the common-law tort based on a duty of care. Australia continues to have a similar tort-based system. In 1974, New Zealand replaced the tort-based system with a government-funded 'no-fault' compensation system operated by the Accident Compensation Corporation (ACC). However, the ACC system, limited as it was to cases where injury occurred, was not designed to address consumer complaints about service quality generally. With the introduction of the *Health and Disability Commissioner Act (HDCA) 1994*, it is now the statutory right of every consumer of a healthcare or disability service to complain about a provider in any form appropriate to the consumer according to the Code of Health and Disability Services Consumers' Rights (the Code).

The most common areas of complaint against midwives relate to poor communication, poor documentation, lack of informed consent, failure to recognise and act on deviations from normal (particularly with respect to fetal heart patterns and failure to progress), failure to refer women to a specialist in a timely and appropriate manner, and lack of clarity of roles involving the primary and secondary care interface.

Health and Disability Commissioner Act 1994

The Office of the Health and Disability Commissioner (HDC) was established following calls from consumer groups for an independent person to investigate complaints against healthcare professionals.

The purpose of the HDCA is stated to be 'to promote and protect the rights of health consumers and disability services consumers, and, to that end, to facilitate the fair, simple, speedy, and efficient resolution of complaints relating to infringements of those rights' (s6 HDCA). The HDC is the primary consumer complaints organisation in New Zealand, managing almost all complaints that have not already been resolved between the consumer and the healthcare professional.

For the year to 30 June 2020, the HDC received 2393 new complaints, 60 of which were against individual midwives. The separate 'lower-level' advocacy service of the HDC received another 2754 new complaints, and mostly against GPs and DHBs. (HDC, 2020).

Midwives have obligations imposed under this legislation—the principal obligations being set out in the Code of Health and Disability Services Consumers' Rights (HDC, 1996). There are 10 fundamental legal rights in the Code for any person receiving a healthcare or disability service. These rights cannot be examined in any detail here, but are reproduced in full in Box 14.2. Although the rights are comprehensive, there are also exculpatory provisions. A provider will not be in breach of the Code 'if the provider has taken reasonable actions in the circumstances to give effect to the rights, and comply with the duties in this Code'. The 'circumstances' means 'all relevant circumstances, including the consumer's clinical circumstances and the provider's resource constraints' (Regulation 3, Health and Disability Commissioner (Code of Health and Disability Services Consumers' Rights) Regulations 1996). Circumstances such as workforce shortages or lack of funding will be taken into account.

Box 14.2   The Code of Health and Disability Services Consumers' Rights

1. Consumers have rights and providers have duties:

(1) Every consumer has the rights in this Code.

(2) Every provider is subject to the duties in this Code.

(3) Every provider must take action to—

   (a) Inform consumers of their rights; and

   (b) Enable consumers to exercise their rights.

2. Rights of consumers and duties of providers:

The rights of consumers and the duties of providers under this Code are as follows:

RIGHT 1. Right to be treated with respect

(1) Every consumer has the right to be treated with respect.

(2) Every consumer has the right to have his or her privacy respected.

(3) Every consumer has the right to be provided with services that take into account the needs, values, and beliefs of different cultural, religious, social, and ethnic groups, including the needs, values, and beliefs of Māori.

RIGHT 2. Right to freedom from discrimination, coercion, harassment, and exploitation

Every consumer has the right to be free from discrimination, coercion, harassment, and sexual, financial or other exploitation.

RIGHT 3. Right to dignity and independence

Every consumer has the right to have services provided in a manner that respects the dignity and independence of the individual.

RIGHT 4. Right to services of an appropriate standard

(1) Every consumer has the right to have services provided with reasonable care and skill.

(2) Every consumer has the right to have services provided that comply with legal, professional, ethical, and other relevant standards.

(3) Every consumer has the right to have services provided in a manner consistent with his or her needs.

(4) Every consumer has the right to have services provided in a manner that minimises the potential harm to, and optimises the quality of life of, that consumer.

(5) Every consumer has the right to cooperation among providers to ensure quality and continuity of services.

RIGHT 5. Right to effective communication

(1) Every consumer has the right to effective communication in a form, language, and manner that enables the consumer to understand the information provided. Where necessary and reasonably practicable, this includes the right to a competent interpreter.

(2) Every consumer has the right to an environment that enables both consumer and provider to communicate openly, honestly, and effectively.

RIGHT 6. Right to be fully informed

(1) Every consumer has the right to the information that a reasonable consumer, in that consumer's circumstances, would expect to receive, including:

   (a) An explanation of his or her condition; and

   (b) An explanation of the options available, including an assessment of the expected risks, side effects, benefits, and costs of each option; and

   (c) Advice of the estimated time within which the services will be provided; and

   (d) Notification of any proposed participation in teaching or research, including whether the research requires and has received ethical approval; and

   (e) Any other information required by legal, professional, ethical, and other relevant standards; and

   (f) The results of tests; and

   (g) The results of procedures.

(2) Before making a choice or giving consent, every consumer has the right to the information that a reasonable consumer, in that consumer's circumstances, needs to make an informed choice or give informed consent.

(3) Every consumer has the right to honest and accurate answers to questions relating to services, including questions about:

   (a) The identity and qualifications of the provider; and

   (b) The recommendation of the provider; and

   (c) How to obtain an opinion from another provider; and

   (d) The results of research.

(4) Every consumer has the right to receive, on request, a written summary of information provided.

RIGHT 7. Right to make an informed choice and give informed consent

(1) Services may be provided to a consumer only if that consumer makes an informed choice and gives informed consent, except where any enactment, or the common law, or any other provision of this Code provides otherwise.

(2) Every consumer must be presumed competent to make an informed choice and give informed consent, unless there are reasonable grounds for believing that the consumer is not competent.

(3) Where a consumer has diminished competence, that consumer retains the right to make informed choices and give informed consent, to the extent appropriate to his or her level of competence.

(4) Where a consumer is not competent to make an informed choice and give informed consent, and no person entitled to consent on behalf of the consumer is available, the provider may provide services where:

   (a) It is in the best interests of the consumer; and

   (b) Reasonable steps have been taken to ascertain the views of the consumer; and

Box 14.2 The Code of Health and Disability Services Consumers' Rights—cont'd

(c) Either,

  (i) If the consumer's views have been ascertained, and having regard to those views, the provider believes, on reasonable grounds, that the provision of the services is consistent with the informed choice the consumer would make if he or she were competent; or

  (ii) If the consumer's views have not been ascertained, the provider takes into account the views of other suitable persons who are interested in the welfare of the consumer and available to advise the provider.

(5) Every consumer may use an advance directive in accordance with the common law.

(6) Where informed consent to a healthcare procedure is required, it must be in writing if:

  (a) The consumer is to participate in any research; or

  (b) The procedure is experimental; or

  (c) The consumer will be under general anaesthetic; or

  (d) There is a significant risk of adverse effects on the consumer.

(6) Every consumer has the right to refuse services and to withdraw consent to services.

(7) Every consumer has the right to express a preference as to who will provide services and have that preference met where practicable.

(8) Every consumer has the right to make a decision about the return or disposal of any body parts or bodily substances removed or obtained in the course of a healthcare procedure.

(9) No body part or bodily substance removed or obtained in the course of a healthcare procedure may be stored, preserved, or used otherwise than:

  (a) With the informed consent of the consumer; or

  (b) For the purposes of research that has received the approval of an ethics committee; or

  (c) For the purposes of one or more of the following activities, being activities that are each undertaken to assure or improve the quality of services:

    (i) a professionally recognised quality assurance programme

    (ii) an external audit of services

    (iii) an external evaluation of services.

RIGHT 8. Right to support

Every consumer has the right to have one or more support persons of his or her choice present, except where safety may be compromised or another consumer's rights may be unreasonably infringed.

RIGHT 9. Rights in respect of teaching or research

The rights in this Code extend to those occasions when a consumer is participating in, or it is proposed that a consumer participate in, teaching or research.

RIGHT 10. Right to complain

(1) Every consumer has the right to complain about a provider in any form appropriate to the consumer.

(2) Every consumer may make a complaint to:

  (a) The individual or individuals who provided the services complained of; and

  (b) Any person authorised to receive complaints about that provider; and

  (c) Any other appropriate person, including:

    (i) An independent advocate provided under the Health and Disability Commissioner Act 1994; and

    (ii) The Health and Disability Commissioner.

(3) Every provider must facilitate the fair, simple, speedy, and efficient resolution of complaints.

(4) Every provider must inform a consumer about progress on the consumer's complaint at intervals of not more than 1 month.

(5) Every provider must comply with all the other relevant rights in this Code when dealing with complaints.

(6) Every provider, unless an employee of a provider, must have a complaints procedure that ensures that:

  (a) The complaint is acknowledged in writing within 5 working days of receipt, unless it has been resolved to the satisfaction of the consumer within that period; and

  (b) The consumer is informed of any relevant internal and external complaints procedures, including the availability of:

    (i) Independent advocates provided under the Health and Disability Commissioner Act 1994; and

    (ii) The Health and Disability Commissioner; and

  (a) The consumer's complaint and the actions of the provider regarding that complaint are documented; and

  (b) The consumer receives all information held by the provider that is or may be relevant to the complaint.

(7) Within 10 working days of giving written acknowledgement of a complaint, the provider must:

  (a) Decide whether the provider:

    (i) Accepts that the complaint is justified; or

    (ii) Does not accept that the complaint is justified; or

  (b) If it decides that more time is needed to investigate the complaint:

    (i) Determine how much additional time is needed; and

    (ii) If that additional time is more than 20 working days, inform the consumer of that determination and of the reasons for it.

Continued

Box 14.2   The Code of Health and Disability Services Consumers' Rights—cont'd

(8) As soon as practicable after a provider decides whether or not it accepts that a complaint is justified, the provider must inform the consumer of:

(a) The reasons for the decision; and

(b) Any actions the provider proposes to take; and

(c) Any appeal procedure the provider has in place.

(Source: The Code of Health and Disability Services Consumers' Rights)

The HDC must give the provider midwife an opportunity to respond to any complaint. Many complaints are not formally investigated and, after an initial consideration of the complaint and response, the HDC may decide to take no further action. See *A Guide for Providers: HDC's Investigation Processes* (HDC, 2013).

If, after investigation, a midwife is found to be in breach of the Code, the HDC may make recommendations, may refer the midwife to the MCNZ to consider whether competence is an issue, or may refer the midwife to the Director of Proceedings to consider whether disciplinary or compensation proceedings are warranted.

Responding to a complaint

Midwives have an obligation to have a complaints procedure that complies with the Code. A midwife is required to 'facilitate the fair, simple, speedy, and efficient resolution of complaints'. The midwife must follow a timetable for response and consideration of the complaint and also inform the consumer of any internal and external complaints procedures, including the availability of the Health and Disability Commissioner and independent advocates appointed under the Act.

Being the subject of a complaint is usually stressful and, in line with how other healthcare professionals react, midwives may commonly experience such feelings as shock, shame, guilt, anger and depression while also being fearful of the consequences both professional and financial. A complaint can take months if not years to be resolved, and the same complaint may receive multiple airings or investigations under different jurisdictions—adding to the responsibilities for the midwife concerned. The legal processes themselves create professional responsibilities (such as the need to consult lawyers, draft written statements, attend meetings or appear in court) and it is important that professional indemnity insurance is in place and legal advice is sought at an early stage. Most midwives will seek legal advice when they first become aware of a complaint, or when they anticipate that a complaint may arise. Prompt notification of complaints is a condition of most professional indemnity insurance policies to ensure that the complaint is appropriately managed from an early stage. Support systems for the midwife such as confidential counselling and legal support can be accessed at this time. Low-level resolution of the complaint is the preferred outcome for any provider. Resolution avenues such as prompt and appropriate direct communication or the NZCOM Complaints Resolution Service should be

---

Box 14.3   NZCOM advice on responding to a complaint

If you are involved in a case in which you may be held to account for your practice, the following steps, from the booklet 'Unexpected Outcome?' (NZCOMa), are advised for NZCOM members. Non-members and Australian midwives may wish to adapt the steps to their particular circumstances.

- Contact the Legal Advisor at the earliest possible opportunity and before you provide any written information to any agency.
- The clinical records are vitally important—review them and make additional notated retrospective entries if necessary. Always date and sign your entries. Ask your colleagues to review the records for you.
- Write down your detailed reflections (thoughts) and a separate factual report about the case as soon as possible after the case in separate private records. Sign and date the records and keep them in a safe place.
- Seek the support of your colleagues so you can take time out if you need to and have additional support in your practice for as long as you need it.
- Seek the support of your family and friends to make sure you get the necessary emotional support.
- Ensure that the woman receives ongoing midwifery care or is referred to the most appropriate obstetric service.
- Consider the College's resolutions process if the family wants assistance to resolve any issues.
- The College provides a professional framework, systems and structures to support you.
- Consider taking a special review of the case.
- It may be some time (if at all) before you are held to account for your practice in relation to this case.

(Source: New Zealand College of Midwives. Unexpected Outcome? [Booklet]. Christchurch: NZCOMa)

---

considered. Box 14.3 provides NZCOM advice for midwives responding to a complaint.

Legal standards of care for civil cases

The general standard is variously described as whether the care was 'adequate' or what the majority of midwives would consider as 'reasonable care in the circumstances'.

What is 'adequate' or 'reasonable' in any given situation may give rise to debate. Deciding bodies such as the HDC, Coroner and ACC will often refer such questions to midwifery experts. It is generally the case that expert midwives will comment on midwifery care; however, obstetric opinion is sometimes taken into account or followed. The primary clinical reference points for determining whether care was reasonable are:

- NZCOM Philosophy and Code of Ethics (NZCOM, 2015a)
- NZCOM *Midwives Handbook for Practice* Standards and guidelines (NZCOM, 2015b)
- NZCOM Consensus Statements (NZCOMb)Section 88 *Public Health and Disability Act 2000* including the:
  - Primary Maternity Services Notice 2021 (MOH, 2021a)
  - Guidelines for Consultation with Obstetric and Related Services (Referral Guidelines) (MOH, 2012)
- Multi-disciplinary guidelines (NZCOMc)
- Local hospital policies promulgated with the midwifery profession or any national protocols.

Human Rights Act 1993

The *Human Rights Act 1993* established the Human Rights Review Tribunal (HRRT), previously known as the Complaints Review Tribunal. If a practitioner is found to be in breach of the *Human Rights Act 1993*, the *Privacy Act 2020* or the Code of Rights under the *Health and Disability Commissioners Act 1994*, an 'aggrieved person' or someone acting on their behalf can seek damages of up to NZ$350,000. The claim in the HRRT may cover pecuniary (monetary) loss and expenses reasonably incurred by the complainant and any loss of benefit the person might reasonably have expected to obtain, but for the breach that occurred.

HRRT hearings are generally held in public and witnesses may be summonsed to give evidence.

Accident Compensation Act 2001

This Act enshrines New Zealand's 'no fault' accident and insurance scheme, whereby any person suffering personal injury by accident may receive financial compensation and assistance. A person entitled to cover under the Act is legally barred from bringing a civil claim for monetary damages for their damages except for exemplary damages, also known as punitive damages. Punitive damages are not compensatory in nature but rather are awarded to reform or deter the defendant/others from engaging in the same course of action that caused the injury. The threshold test to warrant an award of exemplary damages is high.

Before 1 July 2005, claimants involved in healthcare still had to prove 'fault' or negligence on the part of a health professional—known under the legislation as 'medical misadventure' claims. Alternatively, it had to be proven that the injury was a rare and severe occurrence—known as 'medical mishap'. From 1 July 2005, amending legislation simplified the criteria and claims process for healthcare cases to be consistent with the rest of the Act's no-fault scheme and the only criteria that now needs to be established is that there was a 'treatment injury'.

A key objective of the amending legislation was to encourage healthcare providers to facilitate the timely provision of assistance by the Accident Compensation Corporation (ACC) to claimants. The view was that, ideally, claims should be made on behalf of the patient by the healthcare professional who provided the treatment that caused the injury; however, in practice, another practitioner will usually assist with the claim. The ACC will usually but not always notify the midwife that there has been a claim and ask for a copy of the notes and/or the provision of some information. Although the scheme is 'no fault', the ACC will report a case to the MCNZ if it believes that the care in any given case discloses a risk of public harm (s284 of the Act). The definition of 'treatment' includes:

- the giving of treatment; diagnosis; choice of treatment including a decision not to treat; failure to provide treatment or to provide it in a timely manner
- failing of any equipment, device or tool used as part of the treatment process
- the application of any relevant support systems, including policies, processes, practices and administrative systems.

A 'treatment injury' is a personal injury that has occurred within the context of treatment provided by, or at the direction of, one or more healthcare professionals. There must be a direct causal link between the injury and the treatment. Cover is for outcomes that are abnormal, unusual or exceptional having regard to the patient's particular circumstances, and such events are not expected to happen often. Claims involving midwifery tend to relate to claims for neonatal encephalopathy including hypoxic birth injuries and hypoxic ischemic encephalopathy (HIE) as well as perineal tears and their management.

Criminal law provisions

The more significant criminal law provisions that may involve health professionals in New Zealand are discussed below.

Manslaughter

In manslaughter cases under the former provisions of the *Crimes Act 1961* (CA), to obtain a conviction it had to be proven that the healthcare professional had failed 'to use reasonable knowledge, skill, and care' to avoid endangering human life (s156 CA). The law was amended in 1997 so that a healthcare professional could not be convicted for 'mere' lack of reasonable care (ordinary negligence in the civil sense). What must be proven now is that the healthcare professional committed 'a major departure from the standard of care expected of a reasonable person' in such circumstances (s150A CA).

Assault

Midwives will also be mindful that it is possible to commit the crime of assault. Assault is defined as (s2):

the act of intentionally applying or attempting to apply force to the person of another, directly or indirectly, or threatening by any act or gesture to apply such force to the person of another, if the person making the threat has, or causes the other person to believe on reasonable grounds that he has, present ability to effect his purpose.

(*CA 1961* and *Summary Proceedings Act 1957*)

Consent

Both Acts recognise that it is not a crime if the proper consent of the person has first been obtained. 'Consent' for these purposes is a simple 'yes' or indication of acquiescence rather than full 'informed consent' as it is described later in this chapter. It is also unlikely that a practitioner will be convicted if consent cannot be obtained and the midwife is carrying out necessary procedures (House of Lords, 1989). In respect of surgical operations, a defence is provided by section 61 of the CA as follows:

> *Everyone is protected from criminal responsibility for performing with reasonable care and skill any surgical operation upon any person for his benefit, if the performance of the operation was reasonable, having regard to the patient's state at the time and to all the circumstances of the case.*

Vulnerable persons—sections 195 and 195A Crimes Act 1961

Under these sections, a 'child' is someone under 18 years and a 'vulnerable adult' means 'a person unable, by reason of detention, age, sickness, mental impairment, or any other cause, to withdraw himself or herself from the care or charge of another person'.

Ill-treatment or neglect of child under 18 or vulnerable adult (ss 2,195 CA)

A vulnerable adult might, for example, include a woman in labour; a woman with acute preeclamptic toxaemia symptoms or one during or following surgery. The Act has yet to be tested in the Courts. Section 195 CA relates to *ill-treatment or neglect of a child or vulnerable adult*. Section 195A relates to *failure to protect a child or vulnerable adult from the acts of others*. Both carry a maximum penalty of 10 years imprisonment. In the midwifery context, Section 195 applies to any self-employed or employed midwife or student who has the 'actual care or charge' of the 'child' or 'vulnerable adult'. This covers many clinical settings both in the community and in hospitals. It also applies to any 'staff of any hospital, institution, or residence' where the 'child' or 'vulnerable adult' 'resides'. The said staff member need not be in a clinical role. The act must be:

- intentional, and can be either conduct or failure to perform a legal duty
- a major departure from the standard of care to be expected from 'a reasonable person'
- likely to cause suffering, injury, adverse effects to health, or any mental disorder or disability to a child or vulnerable adult.

There is no requirement that actual harm be caused to the victim, just that there is a likelihood of it. Nor is it clear that a midwife must even know that the major departure may be likely to cause harm—that is, ignorance is no excuse. Midwives have existing obligations not to place women or whānau at risk or cause harm. Clinical care that is informed by professional standards and evidence-based practice will continue to be the best defence a midwife can have. However, midwives going out on a limb either deliberately or through ignorance and practising in a way that is a 'major departure' from expected standards will potentially be exposed to the above provisions. Changes to the *Crimes Act 1961* on 19 March 2012, by the *Crimes Amendment Act 2011*, created a new criminal offence under section 195A CA, which makes it an offence, in certain circumstances, to fail to protect a child or vulnerable adult from risk of death, grievous bodily harm or sexual assault as a result of an *'unlawful act'* by another person.

Section 195A applies only to a midwife who is a staff member of any hospital, institution, or residence where the child or vulnerable person resides. Whether this includes a child born in a hospital and remaining there in the postnatal period, or a woman in hospital for any length of time, remains to be established by a court. The midwife must also have had frequent contact with the victim and *'know'* that the victim *'is at risk'*. Thus the midwife must have enough knowledge to be able to form a judgment that there is a risk that the 'victim' could die or suffer from serious offending such as grievous bodily harm or sexual assault. The midwife should not consider risk in terms of whether the risk is 'high', 'medium' or 'low', or whether the risk is 'imminent' or not. The only assessment is whether the midwife knows there is a risk of the types of harms listed. She can be liable if she does not take *'reasonable steps'* to prevent the victim from that risk. What is reasonable will be determined on a case-by-case basis and, if time permits, midwives should urgently seek advice / guidance.

The Vulnerable Children Act 2014

The Vulnerable Children (VC) Act aims to improve protection for children at risk of abuse and neglect. The *White Paper for Vulnerable Children*, released by the Ministry of Social Development (2012, p. 6), defined vulnerable children as:

> *... children who are at significant risk of harm to their wellbeing now and into the future as a consequence of the environment in which they are being raised and, in some cases, due to their own complex needs. Environmental factors that influence child vulnerability include not having their basic emotional, physical, social, developmental and/or cultural needs met at home or in their wider community.*

The VC Act does not introduce mandatory reporting of child abuse but does set up frameworks with compulsory elements including:

- the development of a cross-agency plan on vulnerable children between Police, Education, Justice, Social Development, Te Puni Kōkiri (Ministry of Maori Development), Business Innovation and Employment (housing) and Health Ministries

- the development of separate 'child protection policies' for any staff or self-employed persons working with children
- safety checking for the government-funded workforce; this includes a police check and a risk assessment and reassessment
- workforce restrictions on those with certain serious criminal convictions.

Both employed and self-employed midwives are subject to the VC Act. The employers of midwives will be responsible for the organisation's child protection policy. Self-employed midwives must have their own plan and evidence of a safety check in order to claim payments from the Ministry of Health. Plans must be written and contain, at the very least, provisions on the identification and reporting of child abuse and neglect in accordance with section 15 of the *Tamariki Oranga Act 1989*, also known as the *Children's and Young People's Well-being Act 1989* (until 2017 known as the *Children, Young Persons, and Their Families Act 1989*). The New Zealand College of Midwives has developed a Child Protection Policy (2021) for lead maternity carers (LMCs) to use or adapt (NZCOM, 2021).

Health and Safety at Work Act (HSWA) 2015

The HSWA, in force from 4 April 2016, introduced major changes to New Zealand's health and safety legislation and affects midwives whether they work as employees or as LMCs. Persons with responsibilities under the Act are any 'person conducting a business or undertaking', known as 'PCBU' for short. This includes LMCs, DHBs, stand-alone primary birthing units, and visiting tradespersons and contractors making site visits. The PCBU must ensure, so far as is reasonably practicable, that the health and safety of workers and other persons (such as visiting members of the public) are not put at risk from work carried out as part of the PCBU operations. Individual LMCs and staff are also required to ensure their own safety. Larger companies / DHBs may have particular obligations relating to worker participation. PCBUs are required to formulate a health and safety operational plan. The New Zealand College of Midwives has developed a Health and Safety Policy (NZCOM, 2017) for LMCs to adapt or use.

The Health and Safety at Work (General Risk and Workplace Management) Regulations 2016 (and anticipated subsequent regulations) set out guidance for the matters to be set out in a health and safety plan or policy including policies and procedures to:

- acquire / keep updated knowledge of health and safety matters
- understand the PCBU operations and associated hazards and risks
- ensure the PCBU eliminates / minimises risk, obtains information regarding incidents and responds to incidents in a timely way
- ensure there are first aid facilities and adequately trained staff
- address emergency situations, protective equipment and remote work.

Both a self-employed LMC and the DHB accessed by the LMC are PCBUs in their own right and should have their own health and safety policies. All PCBUs who share a worksite, including the example of the LMC / DHB, must consult with each other, cooperate and coordinate for any situations where there are 'overlapping duties'. Some consequences for PCBUs or their officers (e.g. CEOs / Directors) who fail to carry out their duties include conviction and a fine up to $500,000 or imprisonment for up to 2 years together with the payment of reparation. There is no need to establish that actual harm has occurred. Under the HSWA, it is prohibited for any insurance policy to cover and pay for any such fines imposed.

REFLECTIVE THINKING EXERCISE

1. List 10 ways in which you would structure your practice to address your legal obligations. Briefly reference your list to any legal / societal expectations.
2. Reflect and compare on how you see your aspirations as a midwife in relation to society's expectations of you in a legal sense.

LEGAL ASPECTS OF OBTAINING INFORMED CONSENT—INFORMED CHOICE IN AUSTRALIA AND NEW ZEALAND

Overview

It is a fundamental legal requirement in Australia and New Zealand that patients are provided with information and choices upon which to make an informed decision prior to undertaking care or treatment. The original role of consent, which was primarily to avoid a charge of assault and battery, has expanded in recent decades owing to the advancement of consumer rights and the human right to bodily autonomy. The common-law position in Australia and in New Zealand is similar following the High Court of New Zealand's approval in *B v Medical Council of New Zealand* (1996) of the High Court of Australia decision of *Rogers v Whitaker* [1992], which stated at p. 490:

> *The law should recognize that a doctor has a duty to warn a patient of a material risk inherent in the proposed treatment; a risk is material if, in the circumstances of the particular case, a reasonable person in the patient's position, if warned of the risk, would be likely to attach significance to it or if the medical practitioner is or should reasonably be aware that the particular patient, if warned of the risk, would be likely to attach significance to it.*

Obtaining consent and ensuring the patient has adequate information to make an informed decision in the midwifery context is also based on the ethical principles of a woman's human right to autonomous decision making. This is upheld through the partnership model, whereby the midwife is professionally responsible for providing sufficient information to the woman to enable her right to consent or refuse treatment meaningfully. It is your responsibility to provide information in a timely manner, but it is the woman's right to consent. That right must be *voluntarily* exercised, without coercion or pressure. At times, a woman's competence may be at issue. For example, informed consent is unlikely to be obtainable from a woman who is suffering from an acute psychiatric episode. That, however, is not your decision to make. Except in a genuine emergency, you must refer the woman to a specialist in mental health for assessment. If the woman and / or her family members object, the matter may have to be referred to a tribunal or court of law.

Australian legal provisions

As far as the civil law in Australia (and NZ) is concerned, there is a technical distinction to be made between assault and battery, although in common parlance no such distinction is made and the word assault is often (inaccurately) used to embrace both actions. To explain the technical distinction, an assault can be committed merely by putting a person in fear of his or her physical wellbeing; for example, physically threatening to punch the person could well constitute an assault. If such a threat were to be carried out, the actual application of the blow to the person's body would constitute the technical offence of battery. The offence of battery, it was once famously said, 'exists to keep people free from "unconsented-to touchings"' (Kennedy, 1984, p. 460).

Any consideration of the absence or otherwise of consent to treatment must not be confused with negligence. Negligence, on the one hand, and assault and battery on the other are two distinct and separate civil wrongs. It is not necessary for a negligent act to precede a battery in order for a civil action alleging battery to succeed. As far as any treatment given to a patient is concerned, it is quite possible that such treatment was competently given, that the patient suffered no harm and recovered completely, yet the patient can still succeed with an action in battery if the person has not given valid consent. The fact that the specific type of 'touching' occurred without the patient's consent means that a battery has occurred. This is important for you to understand, as the need to ensure that the birthing woman fully understands and has agreed to what you did becomes critical in this light.

What information is available to help women and midwives?

There are many useful documents available to assist healthcare professionals and consumers alike, both to understand the law and to provide the best available information and practices. For HCPs, there is a range of useful information—for example, the National Health and Medical Research Council (NHMRC) publication *General Guidelines for Medical Practitioners on Providing Information to Patients* (NHMRC, 2004a). The NHMRC has also produced a companion document, *Communicating with Patients: Advice for Medical Practitioners* (NHMRC, 2004b). Although these documents inexplicably refer only to medical practitioners, they will be of equal value for midwives who provide information to women. State and territory governments also produce comprehensive policy documents relating to consent for medical treatment. Links to two state policy examples in Western Australia (in 2011) and New South Wales (in 2005) are provided in the Further reading list.

How may consent be given?

The word 'consent' comes from the Latin *consensere*, meaning 'to agree'. Thus, consent is an agreement between two parties and requires a level of common understanding in order for a woman to give a valid consent—to give permission. The use of the term 'valid consent' means the consent given must comprise certain elements; otherwise the consent will be invalid. The elements that comprise valid consent apply regardless of the way in which consent is given. Consent can be given in several ways, as set out in Box 14.4.

'Implied consent' to care can be given in a variety of ways and is most often used to give consent to a simple procedure of common knowledge. For example, a midwife might request a woman to hold out her arm to have her blood pressure taken. Her compliance would imply consent to that procedure. However, the element of common knowledge means that it is not sufficient to make the claim that a person has given consent to a treatment simply by turning up at the hospital or birth centre. It is also not the case that getting into a bed implies consent to a vaginal examination. In the deep sleep therapy (DST) case of *Hart v Herron* (1984), the Supreme Court held that turning up at the hospital was not sufficient to imply consent for treatment, and the defendant was found to be liable in battery for administering the DST. DST does not constitute a simple procedure of common knowledge. It is never possible to consent to a procedure about which you have neither knowledge nor understanding. A person cannot agree to that which they have not contemplated.

Verbal consent is probably the most common form of consent occurring in relation to simple procedures in any

---

Box 14.4 Ways in which consent may be given

- Impliedly
- Expressly—verbally
- Expressly—in writing

setting. Both verbal and written consents are often described as express consent—that is, the woman has expressly indicated that she consents/agrees to the intervention.

Written consent, in the form of either a standard or specialised written consent form, is generally nothing more than documentary evidence of what has already been discussed and consented to verbally. In general terms, therefore, the main function that a written consent fulfils is to express in writing what has been agreed to verbally between the parties. Although there is no general legal principle that states that consent forms must be signed before a patient can be treated, there are now a number of situations where either law, policy or hospital guidelines require consent in writing, such as the requirement for the documentary evidence of consent by a midwife providing home birth in Australia or the requirement to obtain consent before commencing a surgical procedure.

The most significant point about a completed written consent form is that it provides is documentary evidence that consent was given, should a dispute arise over that point. Having said that, a written consent in no way guarantees that the consent given is a valid one—that is another issue completely. In the forced forceps delivery case of *Montgomery v Lanarkshire* (2015), the UK Supreme Court said the use of standardised consent forms as a formality, without adequate discussion or explanation of what treatment is intended, together with a *timely* discussion of the material risks and questions raised by the woman that gives her the opportunity to consider the information before making a decision, does not satisfy the requirement for consent. A consent form is only as good or as valid as the quality of the consent/agreement that has been discussed and that it represents. It is the validity of the consent that goes to the heart of the procedural requirements, and not the signing of a piece of paper.

It also goes without saying that consent is required for each and every treatment offered, however small or significant. Blanket consent forms do not constitute consent. They are, in effect, a waiver of consent which is enforceable if the woman does not know what she is waiving.

What are the elements of a valid consent?

The following three elements, also set out in Box 14.5, must be present before consent is said to be valid.

Consent must be given freely and voluntarily

This means that any consent given by a patient must be given without any fraud, duress or coercion. This includes repeatedly badgering or taunting or harassing the woman to agree to your recommendation.

> ### Box 14.5 Elements of a valid consent
>
> 1. That any consent given is freely and voluntarily given
> 2. That any consent given is properly informed
> 3. That the person giving consent has the legal capacity to give it

---

If it can be established that any coercion or duress was brought to bear on a woman in order to obtain her consent, that consent will be invalid.

The patient is informed 'in broad terms of the nature of the procedure which is intended'

This element probably gives the greatest concern to midwives, largely because of the problems that arise in relation to written consent forms. From a strictly legal perspective, the term 'informed consent', which can be traced to early American decisions, is no longer considered to be appropriate, as it confuses the requirement for consent as a defence to actions in assault and battery with the requirement to give information about material risks to avoid negligence or medical malpractice claims. That said, the phrase 'informed consent' carries legal and human rights significance in international law, particularly in relation to violence against women. Where legislation has been introduced to expressly protect the right to informed consent, such as s17(c) of the *Queensland Human Rights Act 2019*, HCPs have a legal obligation to observe that right. In terms of your practice, it is prudent to apply both: people need not only to be informed in broad terms (thus providing a defence against an action in battery), but also to be informed about the material risks (thus providing a defence against a potential action in negligence).

Perhaps a helpful way to think about the issue is to consider the concept of giving information (and informed consent) in general, everyday terms. On a day-to-day basis, people make decisions on a whole variety of issues which affect their lives—whether it be to buy a house or a new car, take an overseas holiday, take out insurance or change jobs. In making such decisions, people obtain relevant information which can help them decide whether or not to go ahead with a particular proposal—for example, cost, finance available, repayments, access to public transport and schools, career opportunities and so on. The gathering of information needed to arrive at the decision most appropriate for that person constitutes the informed element of the consent process. That information is used to decide whether to go ahead with or reject the proposal. The process is the same when considering whether or not to consent to a particular program of care or treatment. The consequences of making a decision about healthcare, however, are far more serious than deciding whether or not to buy a new car, which only increases your obligation to provide information and care.

How much information does the patient require to make a decision as to whether to consent to treatment?

Invariably, when this issue is considered in healthcare practice, it is done within the confines of negligence law. This is because the High Court of Australia in *Rogers v Whitaker* said that provision of information about a proposed treatment should properly be considered as part of a HCP's duty of care within the context of an action in negligence. Be warned, however, the duty to warn of material risks may not satisfy the consent needed to protect a practitioner from a claim of assault and battery.

Satisfying the obligation to both warn of materials and obtain valid consent can be summarised as follows:

- A woman must be given sufficient information to be able to understand the nature and consequences of the proposed treatment so she can decide whether it is in her best interests to proceed; and
- Failure to advise and inform a woman about the nature and consequences of the proposed treatment as well as its material risks would, in most instances, amount to a breach of the midwife's duty of care, which could, should damage ensue, make the midwife liable in negligence; and
- Consent that is not freely and voluntarily given can expose a midwife to an action in assault and battery.

Legal capacity or competence

The person giving consent must have the legal capacity to give consent. Any woman over 18 years, barring any mental incapacity, can clearly give and withhold consent to treatment. Yet, even with adults, situations arise where the issue of consent to treatment or otherwise needs to be carefully considered.

Legal capacity or competence to give or refuse consent has a number of components, whether it relates to mental capacity or to age. These were identified in the English case of Re C (Adult: Refusal of Treatment (1994)), which addressed the question of whether a man who suffered from a mental illness was capable of refusing treatment to amputate a limb that was gangrenous. Here Thorpe J determined that he had capacity, and defined capacity as a sufficient understanding of 'the nature, purpose and effects of the proffered treatment' (Re C, 295).

It has been argued that the concept of competence has both an ethical and a legal function. From an ethical perspective, 'competenc[e] operates as a gatekeeper' and tells us 'which bioethical principle, respect for autonomy or beneficence, should take precedence in any particular patient's case' (Devereux & Parker, 2006, p. 56). From a legal perspective, competence again acts as a gatekeeper in that it forms one of the elements of a valid consent. Devereux & Parker (2006, p. 58) provide a comprehensive list of abilities generally agreed to be required to be those of a competent individual and these are set out in Box 14.6.

This is a helpful set of criteria with which to evaluate capacity.

Emergency situations

No consent is required where a woman is unconscious or seriously ill and the situation calls for immediate intervention in order to save her life. The overriding duty of care which arises in such emergency situations negates the need for consent on the grounds of the doctrine of emergency or medical necessity. However, the treatment required must be an urgent treatment required to save life or prevent severe and long-lasting deterioration. Kerridge et al. (2013, p. 347) state that 'tort law appears to be more

> **Box 14.6 Abilities agreed to be required for a competent individual**
>
> The competent individual needs to be able to:
>
> - receive, understand and recall relevant information
> - integrate the information received and relate it to one's situation
> - evaluate benefits and risk in terms of personal values
> - rationally manipulate the information in order to select an option, and give cogent reasons for the choice
> - communicate one's choice to others, and
> - persevere with the choice until the decision is acted upon.

settled and clearly requires threat of imminent harm: *London Borough of Southwark v Williams* [1971] Ch 734'.

New Zealand Legal Provisions on informed consent—New Zealand Bill of Rights Act 1990

This Act identifies and enshrines certain fundamental rights into law, including the 'right to refuse to undergo any medical treatment' (section 11). Although the right to refuse treatment must be recognised and upheld, the health professional must also ensure that the right has been exercised based on the principles of informed consent or, in this case, informed choice to refuse. Further considerations of informed choice in the New Zealand context are to be found in the provisions below.

New Zealand College of Midwives Consensus Statement (NZCOM, 2016)

NZCOM's consensus statement: *Informed Consent and Decision Making* is reproduced in Box 14.7 and can be accessed online, as referenced at the end of this chapter.

New Zealand College of Midwives *Handbook for Practice* and Code of Ethics (NZCOM, 2015a, 2015b)

A number of informed consent elements also appear throughout the NZCOM *Handbook for Practice* and Code of Ethics. For example, it is an ethical requirement under the Code that 'Midwives uphold each woman's right to free, informed choice and consent throughout her childbirth experience' and that 'Midwives accept the right of each woman to control her pregnancy and birth experience'. The criterion in Standard Two points to the potential for the midwife and the woman to disagree on aspects of care. To illustrate: if a midwife's 'professional judgement is in conflict with the decision or plans of the woman' the midwife must 'clearly state' her view. However, if the woman's

Box 14.7 NZCOM consensus statement: informed consent and decision making

The New Zealand College of Midwives believes midwifery care takes place in partnership with women.[1,2] It is the midwife's professional responsibility to uphold each woman's right to informed decision making throughout the childbirth experience.

Rationale

Informed decision making involves the exchange and understanding of relevant information. Informed decision making emphasises the autonomy of the individual. It respects the rights of individuals to make decisions about actions which affect them. Making an informed decision is part of a process, which results in either informed consent or refusal.

Practice notes

- Information should be provided in a way that the woman and her family can understand. It must be accurate, objective, relevant and culturally appropriate. It should include:
  - the proposed treatment/intervention
  - the benefits of the treatment/intervention
  - the risks of the treatment/intervention
  - the alternatives to the treatment proposed and their risks and benefits
  - what would happen if no treatment/intervention were used.
- Where there is more than one professional perspective on a given issue this should be acknowledged and information given on, and how to access, this perspective.
- Women should be given time to think about the information and discuss it with others.
- Documentation should include a brief outline of the information given and when this occurred. All decisions

should be clearly documented. Written consent must be obtained where either party requests it.

- Informed consensus is dynamic. If new evidence comes to light, the woman and the family have the right to change their minds.

Ratification

This Statement was originally ratified at the New Zealand College of Midwives AGM May 1996.

The purpose of New Zealand College of Midwives Consensus Statements is to provide women, midwives and the maternity services with the profession's position on any given situation. The guidelines are designed to educate and support best practice.

All position statements are regularly reviewed and up to date.

Bibliography
Title: Midwives Handbook for Practice (5th ed)
Author: New Zealand College of Midwives
Source: Christchurch, 2015
Title: *Code of Health and Disability Services— Consumers Rights*
Author: Health and Disability Commission
Source: www.hdc.org.nz
Title: *Health and Disability Advocacy*
Author: Health and Disability Commission
Source: ww.hdc.org.nz/Advocacy Services in your area
References
1. New Zealand College of Midwives. *Midwives Handbook of Practice*. 5th ed. Christchurch: New Zealand College of Midwives; 2015.
2. Guilliland K, Pairman S. *The Midwifery Partnership, A Model for Practice*. 2nd ed. Christchurch, New Zealand: New Zealand College of Midwives; 2010.

(Source: New Zealand College of Midwives (NZCOM). Consensus Statement: Informed Consent and Decision Making. Christchurch, NZ: NZCOM; 2016. Online: http://www.midwife.org.nz/ quality-practice/practice-guidance/nzcom-consensus-statements/)

decision is an informed one, then the midwife must respect the decision 'even where these decisions are contrary to her own beliefs'. Irrespective of the ultimate decision made by the woman, it is incumbent on the midwife to provide sufficient information for the woman to make an informed choice. This may include providing written educational material or ensuring specialist input occurs as per the Ministry of Health (MOH, 2012) guidelines discussed below.

Ministry of Health Guidelines for Consultation with Obstetric and Related Medical Services (referral guidelines)

These guidelines (MOH, 2012), developed with input from NZCOM, provide LMCs with a list of conditions and

criteria about referring pregnant women for consultations with other clinicians, particularly specialists, as well as transferring care in emergencies. The guidelines are under review (2022), however the key principles of informed consent are unlikely to change substantially. Under 'Guiding Principles', principle three states:

The woman has the right to receive full, accurate, unbiased information about her options and the likely outcomes of her decisions. The woman has a right to make informed decisions on all aspects of her care, including the right to decline care, and to decline referral for specialist consultation or transfer of clinical responsibility.

The referral guidelines set out pathways, including flow diagrams for steps that an LMC is expected to take to facilitate the attainment of informed consent. Section 5

Box 14.8 Ministry of Health Guidelines relating to refusal of consent

5 When a woman declines a referral, consultation, transfer of clinical responsibility, emergency treatment or emergency transport

The right to informed consent, including the right to refuse medical treatment, is enshrined in law and in the Code of Health and Disability Consumers' Rights in New Zealand. This means that a woman can choose to decline treatment, referral to another practitioner, or transfer of clinical responsibility.

If a woman chooses not to be referred or not to consult with a specialist, her LMC may be left operating outside their experience or scope of practice, and/or may feel that they cannot provide the level of care the woman needs for her safety and the safety of her baby. The process maps reflect this possibility.

In the event that a woman declines a referral, consultation or transfer of clinical responsibility, the LMC should:

- advise the woman of the recommended care, including the evidence for that care
- explain to the woman the LMC's need to consider discussing her case with at least one of the following (ensuring that the woman's right to privacy is maintained at all times):
  - another midwife, GPO or GP
  - an appropriate specialist
  - an experienced colleague/mentor
- share the outcomes of the discussion and any resulting advice with the woman
- document in the care plan the process, the discussions, recommendations given and decisions made, and the woman's response.

If, after this process, resolution satisfactory to the LMC and the woman has not been reached, the LMC must decide whether to continue or to discontinue care.

If the LMC decides to continue care, she or he should:

- continue making recommendations to the woman for safe maternity care, including further attempts at referral

- engage other practitioners as appropriate for professional support (e.g. secondary obstetric service, other midwives)
- continue to document all discussions and decisions.

If the LMC decides to discontinue care, she or he should:

- clearly communicate the decision and the reasons for it to the woman
- assist the woman to find alternative care within a reasonable timeframe.

In an obstetric emergency, the LMC cannot refuse to attend the woman. If the woman declines emergency transport or transfer of clinical responsibility while in active labour, the LMC should remain in attendance. The Guidelines recognise that this may result in the LMC being called on to deal with a situation that is not within the LMC's scope of practice. It may be outside the LMC's experience or ability to safely deal with, or require treatment that the LMC cannot perform.

In these situations the LMC should:

- provide care within professional standards
- provide care to the best of their ability
- attempt to access appropriate resources and/or personnel to provide any needed care (dependent on the woman's consent)
- clearly document all discussions and actions
- debrief with clinical colleagues after the event with appropriate support.

When the woman/parents decline care for the baby

In the rare event that a woman or parents decline consent for treatment of her/their baby, LMCs should follow the Guidelines above when discussing the baby's needs and treatment options with the woman or parents, and document all advice given and actions taken.

GP = general practitioner; GPO = general practitioner obstetrician; LMC = lead maternity carer.
(Source: Ministry of Health. *Guidelines for Consultation with Obstetric and Related Medical Services* (Referral Guidelines), 2012:18–19. Online: https://www.health.govt.nz/system/files/documents/publications/referral-glines-jan12.pdf)

---

of the guidelines sets out the expectations 'when a woman declines a referral, consultation, transfer of clinical responsibility, emergency treatment or emergency transport', and is reproduced in Box 14.8.

Ministry of Health Primary Maternity Services Notice 2021

This Notice (MOH, 2021a) sets out the terms and conditions upon which the Ministry of Health will make a payment to a maternity provider for providing primary maternity services, and includes the requirement that 'a maternity provider must ensure that the relationship between the

maternity provider (including the practitioners who work for them) and a woman is based on informed choice and consent and respects the dignity of the woman'. Following an audit of the maternity notes and care, the Ministry has the power to reject a payment to the midwife where informed consent was absent.

Rights 6 and 7, Code of Health and Disability Services Consumers' Rights

Consumer rights concerning informed consent are also recognised in Rights 6 and 7 of the Code, discussed earlier in the chapter and reproduced in full in Box 14.2.

An increasing number of cases before the HDC relate to informed consent. Some complaints, not all of which were upheld, concerned:

- whether the potential risks of choice of birth at home or at a birthing centre were adequately explained
- whether the midwife enabled informed choice by providing the woman with sufficient information on the obstetric referral guidelines (see above) including whether the woman's decision to decline was adequately informed
- whether sufficient antenatal information was provided concerning the risks to the baby of using an amnihook to rupture amniotic membranes
- whether in a high-risk clinical pregnancy, a woman's decision to birth at home was based on informed consent
- whether a midwife correctly managed a woman's refusal to undergo a vaginal examination, abdominal palpation or fetal heart monitoring during labour.

Emergency situations

Right 7(4) of the Code of Health and Disability Services Consumers' Rights (HDC, 1998), reproduced in Box 14.2, permits emergency care in defined circumstances where the consumer is unable to give informed consent. The emergency care must be 'in the best interests of the consumer'; regard must be given to any known views of the consumer with reasonable steps having been taken to ascertain those views; and if there are no known views, the views of 'other suitable persons' if these are available.

CRITICAL THINKING EXERCISE

Hera is a 40-year-old woman pregnant with her fifth child. She has a history of severe postpartum haemorrhage and has experienced a previous obstructed labour. She has refused referral to a secondary care provider or a specialist, and chooses to birth at home.

- What issues does the midwife face?
- What are her legal responsibilities?
- What steps should the midwife take in relation to the legal and ethical ramifications of any decisions?

PRIVACY, CONFIDENTIALITY AND ACCESS TO PERSONAL INFORMATION

Australia

As of 1 March 2018, the NMBA has adopted a new *Code of Conduct for Midwives* in Australia (NMBA, 2018) and there is also the *International Code of Ethics for Midwives* issued by the International Confederation of Midwives (ICM,

2008). The fundamental requirement for midwives to observe a duty of confidentiality is spelt out in both these documents. To deliver appropriate care may require the disclosure of highly sensitive personal and medical information. Clients need to feel secure that any such disclosure, in relation to both the person who is disclosing and the subject matter given in confidence will not be shared without their prior informed consent. Disclosure is permitted with consent, but only to the extent to which consent was given. For example, a woman may consent to sharing information with the team but not with her family. Any disclosure to the family, however incidental, will be considered a breach of the duty.

The requirements for confidentiality and privacy are set out in section 3.5 of the new *Code of Conduct for Midwives* in Australia (NMBA, 2018, p. 10) and are outlined in Box 14.9.

There are exceptions to the duty of confidentiality:

1. where disclosure is mandated or permitted by statute or court order such as, for example, the mandatory reporting of notifiable diseases and suspected child abuse or a court issued subpoena requiring production of medical reports.
2. where disclosure is 'in the public interest'. This obligation tends to fall into two areas—the first being what is sometimes described as the 'iniquity rule' (i.e. the disclosure of a crime or misdeed), and the second the 'balancing rule', where the disclosure must be balanced in the public interest against the need for confidentiality. Disclosure of criminal activity or other civil wrongdoing, even if it involves disclosing information that is confidential, may sometimes be justified on this ground provided the disclosure is in the public interest. If the public interest is not advanced by the disclosure, it will not be permissible to breach confidentiality.

Overall, the expectation is that we will take great care to respect the confidences entrusted to us by our clients. Midwives owe a duty to protect the confidentiality of clients, which the courts have said arises from the midwife / client relationship which is, in nature, built on trust and confidentiality.

The increasing complexity of our society has resulted in the perceived need for a variety of government and private sector agencies to acquire and store information of a personal and often sensitive nature about individuals, which seriously threatens the notion of individual privacy in the conduct of people's daily lives. The need to compile a healthcare record about a client is obvious and the use to which such records are formally put cannot be seriously questioned. The very nature of healthcare records is such that highly personal and sensitive material is often contained in them. Federal, state and territory governments have all imposed some type of legislation to require managers of healthcare records to preserve client confidentiality.

Australian privacy legislation

The *Privacy Act 1988 (Cth)* (Privacy Act) regulates how personal information is handled. The Privacy Act defines personal information as: 'information or an opinion,

Box 14.9 Confidentiality and privacy requirements

The requirements for confidentiality and privacy are set out in s.3.5 of the new Code of Conduct for midwives in Australia (NMBA, 2018) and the basic issues that are addressed in that section are summarised below.

- The primary expectation is that women have the right to expect that midwives will respect both their privacy and their confidentiality.
- The exceptions to that duty of confidentiality are as follows:
  - where the woman consents to have her information shared
  - where there is a legal requirement to provide specific information, either through statute or because of public interest concerns, and
  - where the requirement for consent is overridden in emergency.
- Midwives are expected to provide an environment where a woman can share private information without fear of being overheard.
- Midwives are expected to adhere to policies relating to confidentiality and privacy, including the NMBA social media policy and relevant standards for practice.
- Healthcare records should be accessed by the midwife only on a need-to-know basis and when the midwife has authority to do so.
- Any images, either still or moving, of a woman and/or her family can be reproduced only with the full consent of those involved.
- Midwives must recognise that a woman has a right to access the information in her health records and must both assist the woman to access the records and be available to explain the records.
- Midwives must promptly enable relevant health information to be transferred to any other healthcare provider or managed in accordance with the legislation governing privacy and health records either when requested by the woman in accordance with local policy or when closing or relocating a practice.

whether true or not, and whether recorded in a material form or not, about an identified individual, or an individual who is reasonably identifiable'.

Common examples are an individual's name, signature, address, telephone number, date of birth, medical records, bank account details and commentary or opinion about a person. The Privacy Act includes 13 Australian Privacy Principles (APPs), which apply to some private sector organisations as well as most Australian and Norfolk Island Government agencies. These are collectively referred to as 'APP entities'. The Privacy Act also regulates the privacy component of the consumer credit reporting system, tax file numbers, and health and medical research.

The APPs contained in schedule 1 of the Privacy Act 1988 (Privacy Act) outline how most Australian and Norfolk Island government agencies, all private sector and not-for-profit organisations with an annual turnover of more than $3 million, all private health service providers and some small businesses (collectively called 'APP entities') must handle, use and manage personal information. Although the APPs are not prescriptive, each APP entity needs to consider how the principles apply to its own situation. The principles cover:

- the open and transparent management of personal information including having a privacy policy
- an individual having the option of transacting anonymously or using a pseudonym where practicable
- the collection of solicited personal information and receipt of unsolicited personal information including giving notice about collection
- how personal information can be used and disclosed (including overseas)
- maintaining the quality of personal information
- keeping personal information secure
- the right for individuals to access and correct their personal information (Office of the Australian Information Commissioner, 2017).

The link to the full text of the APPs is included in the Further reading at the end of this chapter.

New Zealand statutes on privacy and information

Health (Retention of Health Information) Regulations 1996

These regulations impose an obligation on midwives to retain original health information about their clients, both mothers and babies, for a minimum of 10 years. The information may be retained in any form the midwife thinks fit. Health information for the purposes of the regulation may include midwifery diaries, travel logs and phone logs if clinical details are noted in such documents. Prior to the 10-year mark, the information can be transferred to the client, or to another provider. Although such transfer is possible, this may have significant legal risk if a claim is later brought against the midwife and the midwife no longer has access to the notes. The 10-year period for retaining clinical information held by DHBs may be reduced or extended under the *Public Records Act 2005* and a General Disposal Authority issued to a DHB by Archives New Zealand. For example, maternal health records, paediatric records and mental health records must be held for a minimum of 20 years; or, for paediatric records, until the child reaches 25 years, whichever is later in time; or, in all cases, for 10 years after the death of the patient.

Privacy Act 2020 / Health Information Privacy Code 2020

The *Privacy Act 2020* (PA) replaced the *Privacy Act 1993* and expanded the set of rules for agencies handling personal information. The PA sets out privacy principles that are widely applicable. The PA applies to every person or organisation in New Zealand in respect of personal information held in any capacity other than for the purposes of their personal, family or household affairs. It controls how agencies collect, use, disclose, store and give access to personal information. Under the authority of the PA the Privacy Commissioner, after consultation with the health sector, issued the Health Information Privacy (HIP) Code 1994, now updated to a 2020 Code, which is a code of practice for the healthcare industry. The Code provides more focused information in the form of 13 'rules' or guidelines for personal information dealt with by healthcare agencies. Complaints alleging a breach of privacy may be made to the Privacy Commissioner. A new requirement in the 2020 Act imposed a duty on agencies, including health providers, to notify the Privacy Commissioner of certain breaches of privacy, additionally creating the offence of failing to notify.

Most midwives who practise in partnership with women will provide a copy of any health information collected, such as clinical notes and scans. Such women-held notes are a progressive and unique feature of midwifery in the New Zealand healthcare landscape. All agencies including LMCs must have a privacy policy that is available to the woman. At registration, the woman should be informed of the purpose for which information is being collected by the midwife; her rights in relation to provision of information including her right to access or correct any information gathered. The PA and Code provide limited circumstances in which the woman's information can be shared without her consent. For example, in cases where there is a safety concern, Rules 10 and 11 of the HIP permit disclosure where there is a 'serious threat' to the life of the woman or another individual, and in general only where the woman's consent to disclosure cannot be obtained or it is not desirable that consent be obtained. For example, it may not be desirable to obtain consent if the act of seeking consent might increase risk to safety. Section 7 of the PA defines 'serious threat' as:

> A threat that an agency reasonably believes to be a serious threat having regard to all the following:
> (a) the likelihood of the threat being realised; and
> (b) the severity of the consequences if the threat is realised; and
> (c) the time at which the threat may be realised.

Disclosure of information—ethical conduct and requests from third parties

In addition to the *Privacy Act 2020*, a woman's right to have the personal information she discloses to the midwife remain private has an ethical basis in midwifery. Her rights are affirmed in the MCNZ Code of Conduct (MCNZ, 2010) and the NZCOM Code of Ethics (2015a). The NZCOM provides guidance in the form of the NZCOM Child Protection Policy (NZCOM, 2021), and an information sheet 'The effect on midwives of the changes to the

information sharing legislation' (NZCOM, 2019). Recent law changes under the *Family Violence Act 2018* and the *Oranga Tamariki Act 1989* have increased the ability and duties to share information in family safety concern cases. However, privacy breaches may still result in professional disciplinary action where justification cannot be demonstrated, therefore midwives should only disclose information with either the consent of the woman which should be sought in all cases where reasonable or practicable; where there is a safety concern and legislation permits it; or under legal requirement.

Some legislative provisions permit, but do not require, a midwife to disclose information. 22C of the *Health Act 1956* (HA), is often cited by the police when seeking information from a midwife; however the HA itself does not provide any protection for the midwife who discloses information without a separate and proper legal basis. Another permissive provision is under section 15 of the *Oranga Tamariki Act 1989* and its associated name the *Children's and Young People's Well-being Act 1989* (formerly the *Child, Young Persons and their Families Act 1989*), where the midwife may make a report of concern to Oranga Tamariki or a constable where she 'believes that a child or young person has been, or is likely to be, harmed, ill-treated, abused, (whether physically, emotionally, or sexually), neglected, or deprived, or who has concerns about the well-being of a child or young person'. Protection from civil, criminal or disciplinary action is given to the midwife who makes proper disclosure in good faith concerning a child's well-being under section 15. Section 20 of the Family Violence Act (FVA) allows family violence agencies—such as DHBs, the police, Oranga Tamariki, Corrections, FV NGOs, health practitioners, teachers and social workers—to request or disclose information about a perpetrator or victim of family violence to each other for all or any of the following purposes:

1. to make, or contribute to a family violence risk or need assessment
2. to make, or contribute to the making or carrying out of, a decision or plan that is related to, or that arises from or responds to, family violence
3. to help ensure that a victim is protected from family violence.

Family violence is defined in wide terms in s9 of the FVA and includes physical, sexual and psychological abuse. It also includes patterns of such behaviour that has coercive or controlling features and causes cumulative harm. Disclosures pursuant to this Act are protected from civil, criminal or disciplinary proceedings. (s25 FVA)

There is no mandatory reporting regime for safety concerns in New Zealand, however the FVA imposes a duty to consider disclosing personal information if (i) they believe on reasonable grounds it will or may ensure protection of a victim from family or (ii) they receive a request made under s20 (as above). In all cases, professional judgment should be exercised taking into account the following:

- the NZCOM Child Protection Policy 2021 (NZCOM, 2021)

- the NZCOM information sheet 'The effect on midwives of the changes to the information sharing legislation' (NZCOM, 2019)
- the Ministry of Health guidance 'Sharing information safely—Guidance on sharing personal information under the Family Violence Act 2018' (MOH, 2019)
- Oranga Tamariki 'Working with children—Information sharing' (OT, 2019).

Disclosure by the midwife is sometimes required by law. These situations include:

1. a subpoena from a court or tribunal or a written notice under section 120 of the *Coroner's Act 2006*
2. a formal written notice from an agency (e.g. a social worker, police) under s66 of the *Oranga Tamaraki Act 1989* for purposes relating to the wellbeing and safety of children and young persons
3. a requirement by the Midwifery Council during a competency review or recertification (section 42 of the HPCAA)
4. certain statutes such as section 11 of the *Social Security Act 1964* regarding investigations into entitlements to benefits—failure to comply with a section 11 request may give rise to a summary offence carrying a fine of up to NZ$2000; however, the request for information must be a valid and legal one and midwives should seek legal advice upon receipt of such a request.

CRITICAL THINKING EXERCISE

John is the partner of Sue, a woman you cared for 2 years ago. He phones and says that he is in a custody and paternity dispute and wants a copy of Sue's midwifery notes to show that he was actively involved in the birth of their son.

- To whom do the notes belong?
- Is John entitled to a copy?
- Is there any circumstance in which you would release the notes?

⚲ CLINICAL POINT

There may be times when a midwife will observe evidence of violence or neglect of a baby and this will lead to concern about the baby's life or safety. If the matter is not urgent, then the midwife should document her concerns and involve social workers, Family Start program support, general practitioners or family/whānau to help the parents and prevent future harm. On rare occasions, however, the midwife may consider that immediate intervention should take place and she will need to urgently report the mother, father or partner to the appropriate agency. Technically this may constitute a breach of confidentiality, but the midwife who acts in good faith and has reasonable grounds to believe that her actions are necessary to prevent serious harm to a child is likely to have a defence.

REFLECTIVE THINKING EXERCISE

You have received a written complaint from the mother of a 17-year-old woman for whom you recently cared. During the antenatal period the woman could not decide whether she would agree to the administration of vitamin K for her baby. You gave her verbal information about the risks of not having vitamin K on one occasion. You did not document this discussion. Shortly after the birth, you raised the matter again with the woman; she declined vitamin K. You wrote in the notes 'declined vit K'. The baby subsequently developed vitamin K deficiency bleeding and suffered brain damage. The grandmother says you should have made more effort to get her daughter to agree to vitamin K administration and, as she was only 17, you should have given the injection to the baby anyway. Discuss the issues relating to:

- adequacy of information / informed consent
- assault
- documentation
- privacy
- professional expectations where the midwife does not agree with the woman's choice.

LEGISLATION ON MIDWIFERY PRACTICE

Australian legislation

Notification of birth

The notification of birth involves the entry of the particulars of a birth into the Births, Deaths and Marriages Register of the state or territory in which a child is born. An HCP present at the birth (i.e. a midwife or doctor) must notify the appropriate authorities of details such as the time and date of birth, sex and gestation.

Each state and territory in Australia has a Births, Deaths and Marriages Act. The definitions of 'birth' and 'child', and the requirements for registration of a stillborn as either a birth and/or a death varies between jurisdictions, but all agree on the gestation and weight parameters of a stillborn:

> A 'stillborn' is a child that exhibits no sign of respiration or heartbeat, or other sign of life, after birth and that:
> (a) is of at least 20 weeks' gestation, or
> (b) if it cannot be reliably established whether the period of gestation is more or less than 20 weeks, has a body mass of at least 400 grams at birth.
>
> (s4, *Births, Deaths and Marriages Registration Act 1995, (NSW)*)

In the Australian Capital Territory (ACT), New South Wales (NSW), South Australia (SA), Victoria (Vic), Tasmania (Tas) and the Northern Territory (NT), a stillborn or stillbirth is registered as a birth but not a death. In Western

Australia (WA) and Queensland (Qld), a stillborn is registered as a birth and a death. In the ACT, Queensland, South Australia, Tasmania and Western Australia, a birth is defined as the expulsion or extraction of a child from its mother; a child is further defined as including a stillborn. In the ACT, New South Wales, the Northern Territory and Victoria, a birth includes a stillbirth.

Health legislation requires the notification of all births, whether stillborn or live birth. Under the respective legislation, a midwife who attends a birth is required to notify the appropriate authority, and a failure to do so is an offence. A prescribed form is specified under respective legislation. The time frame for notification varies from jurisdiction to jurisdiction, but ranges from 2 days in Queensland (s12 *Births Deaths and Marriages Act 2003, Qld*) for live birth to 28 days in Western Australia (s12 *Births, Deaths and Marriages Act 1998, WA*). Tasmania and New South Wales require a stillbirth to be notified within 48 hours.

In Western Australia a neonatal death is defined as 'the death of a live-born child within 28 days after the birth' (s4 *Births, Deaths and Marriages Act 1998, WA*).

In Victoria a perinatal death means:

(a) *the death of a live-born child within 28 days after the birth; or*
(b) *a stillbirth.*

(s4, *Births, Deaths and Marriages Act 1996, Vic*)

In Western Australia, for the purposes of burial under the *Cremation Act 1929, WA* and the *Cemeteries Act 1986, WA*, a dead body 'means the body of a deceased person (who was born alive) and includes the body of an infant of not less than 7 months' gestation that was still-born'.

Adoption laws in Australia

Midwives in Australia do not have a role in the adoption of children. Adoptions must be carried out through an approved agency. For further information, midwives should refer to the respective state and territory legislation dealing with adoptions.

New Zealand legislation

New Zealand Public Health and Disability Act 2000

Under section 88 of the *New Zealand Public Health and Disability Act 2000*, the Crown or a DHB may issue a notice of the terms and conditions under which payment will be made to those providing a public health service. One example is the current Primary Maternity Services Notice 2021, which sets out the terms and conditions for the provision of maternity services (MOH, 2021a). All practitioners who claim payment under this Notice, including employees, are bound by its provisions. Section 88 also promulgates the *Guidelines for Consultation with Obstetric and Related Specialist Medical Services* (MOH, 2012), and the national Access Agreement to enable LMCs access to a Maternity Facility or a Birthing Unit (MOH, 2021b). The Notice also contains general provisions setting out the

expectations concerning matters such as: antenatal, birth and labour and postnatal care; the compulsory engagement in peer review; and the requirement to comply with all relevant laws and professional requirements and to cooperate with others in order to promote a safe and effective primary maternity service. Practitioners are also required under the Notice to cooperate (usually by filling out a form) with the Perinatal Mortality Review Committee, a ministerial committee established in 2005 that aims to reduce the numbers of preventable perinatal and maternal deaths in New Zealand.

Births, Deaths, Marriages, and Relationships Registration Act 1995

Under this Act, the midwife has several legal responsibilities following the birth of a baby. When a baby is born alive or stillborn, a preliminary notice of birth in the prescribed form must be completed and sent to the Registrar under the Act within 5 working days of the birth. Generally this notification is the responsibility of the occupier of the hospital where the birth took place, and a person attending the birth, such as a midwife, endorses it. Where the birth takes place at home, the midwife will complete the notice unless a doctor was present, in which case it is the doctor's responsibility. As soon as practicable, both parents (if both are available and can cooperate on the matter) are required to notify a Registrar of the birth together with their personal details and citizenship information (s5A and s9).

The definition of 'birth' is deemed to include stillbirth, but a miscarriage (which is defined as 'the issue from its mother, before the 21st week of pregnancy, of a dead foetus weighing less than 400 g') is not (s2). The midwife will often be best placed to determine whether the baby is born alive or is stillborn. 'Live birth' is the complete expulsion or extraction from the mother of a baby, irrespective of the duration of pregnancy, which, whether or not the umbilical cord has been severed or the placenta detached, at any time after issuing completely from its mother breathed or showed any other sign of life (such as beating of the heart, pulsation of the umbilical cord, or definite movement of the voluntary muscles). A stillborn child is a dead fetus that has not at any time shown such signs of life, and weighed 400 grams or more when it issued from its mother or issued from its mother after the 20th week of pregnancy (s2).

If a death certificate is signed, it will be by a doctor. Where there was no doctor present at a stillbirth, nor one present to examine the child after the stillbirth, a midwife may be called upon to sign a certificate that the child was born dead—there being a need for such a certificate before a stillborn child can be buried, cremated or disposed of (s46A *Burial and Cremation Act 1964*). However, where a doctor is not present at the birth but examines the stillborn child after 'birth', then the midwife is not permitted to sign the certificate.

Every death must also be notified to the Registrar, generally by a funeral director, 'forthwith' after the disposal of the body (s42). Where a death has been reported to a

Coroner, the Coroner must notify the Registrar forthwith after a Coroner's authorisation in relation to the release of the body with such particulars as are then known to the Coroner, or forthwith after acquiring further information that may be learned from a Coroner's investigation or inquest (s45). There is further commentary below on the *Coroner's Act 2006*. Section 89 of the Act creates various offences for non-compliance with the Act, ranging from fines to imprisonment for up to 5 years.

Adoption Act 1955

From time to time midwives become involved in adoptions, particularly where adoptions take place within an extended family grouping or whānau. Midwives should be aware that the New Zealand *Adoption Act 1955* sets out a statutory procedure that must be followed before an adoption can legally take place. A midwife cannot act as an agent, nor can she broker an adoption arrangement between parties. If a midwife is caring for any woman considering an adoption of her baby, the midwife should ensure that the woman is referred to the appropriate state agencies. This will usually require the early involvement of a social worker. Disciplinary proceedings have ensued from midwives not maintaining appropriate boundaries or procedures in adoption cases.

Contraception, Sterilisation and Abortion Act 1977

The key responsibility of midwives under this Act is to be aware of the referral requirements for any woman seeking abortion. Often it is the midwife to whom a woman will come for diagnosis or confirmation of pregnancy. It is illegal for any midwife to help a woman procure an abortion. If any woman does not want to continue a pregnancy, then the role of the midwife is to refer her to a medical practitioner for further counselling and assessment.

LEGISLATION ON DRUG ADMINISTRATION AND PRESCRIBING

Australia

Each state and territory has legislation dealing with the control of poisons and prescribing medicines. Midwives, particularly PPMs, are advised to consult their local legislation for the storage and administration of medicines.

In Australia, with the passing of the Health Legislation Amendment (Midwives and Nurse Practitioners) Bill 2009 (Commonwealth of Australia, 2010), endorsed midwives now also have prescribing rights to certain medicines under the Pharmaceutical Benefits Scheme (PBS). State and territory legislation has been amended to allow for these changes, but there is still much work to be done to reach national consistency. The requirements for midwives to be endorsed to prescribe are set out under the section on regulation.

New Zealand

Medicines Act 1981 and Regulation

New Zealand midwives have been able to prescribe a range of drugs and medications related to antenatal, intrapartum and postnatal care since 1990. The Medicines Amendment Regulations 2011 changed the ambit of prescription rights from 'antenatal, intrapartum or postpartum care' to any situation within 'the midwifery scope of practice' as determined by an authorisation of the Midwifery Council. Any prescriptions must not exceed 3 months' supply.

Section 41 of the Medicines Regulations 1984 prescribes the form of any prescription, which must include:
- that it shall be legibly and indelibly printed
- the date, address, name, telephone number and personal signature of the prescriber
- the surname, each given name and address of the person for whom the prescription is given
- the name and, if appropriate, strength, dose, dosing frequency and method of administration of the medicine
- the total amount that may be dispensed, or the total period of supply.

Subsequent Regulations under the Medicines Act enable the Director of Health to waive some or all such requirements. Under such waiver, electronic prescribing is authorised if using the New Zealand Electronic Prescribing Service (NZePS) but with restrictions for prescribing controlled drugs. Some temporary exemptions, including for controlled drugs, were introduced to support non NZePS signature exempt prescriptions due to COVID-19 (MOH, 2020).

Whenever a midwife prescribes a medication, there must be a discussion about the reason for the prescription, the effects, side effects and contraindications to that medication, an identification of any allergy or previous problems with the medication, and a clinical assessment of the appropriateness of the medication for that person in the presenting circumstances. Ultimately where the drug is given the practitioner must demonstrate that this was done with the informed consent of the client. An exception to this is an emergency, such as where there is a seriously depressed neonate who might be given naloxone, or where a woman is experiencing an overwhelming postpartum haemorrhage, becomes unconscious and is administered intravenous fluids and possibly blood products. In most cases, however, such scenarios will have been discussed antenatally and the woman's views ascertained prior to this occurring. Where therapeutic products that are not medicines are suggested or recommended by the midwife, the client must be informed whether there is any clinical evidence of the efficacy of such products.

Urgent prescriptions

Section 40A of the Medicines Regulations 1984 enables a registered midwife to request an urgent prescription orally (in person or by phone) from a pharmacist to whom she is known personally. The midwife must then forward a written script of the oral communication within 7 days. The schedule of this Amendment also discusses standing orders with respect to controlled drugs, although in practice it would be unusual for a midwife to use this mechanism because if a controlled drug may be required, the midwife or her back-up should either already be in attendance and considering a transfer to hospital for a prescription; or should immediately attend to assess the woman.

Controlled drugs

The Misuse of Drugs Amendment Regulations 2014 and the *Medicines Amendment Act 2013* enable midwives to prescribe the controlled drugs pethidine, morphine and fentanyl under certain conditions. The regulations set out the frequency with which midwives can prescribe controlled drugs—that is, they may be supplied on two occasions at a specified interval with: (a) the first occasion being not more than 4 days after the date of the prescription, and (b) the second occasion being not more than 4 days after the termination of that interval. The Midwifery Council has determined the scope of practice of a midwife in relation to prescription of opiate analgesia to be for intrapartum use only. Intrapartum is defined as referring to labour, birth and the immediate postnatal period (MCNZ, 2014). Midwives with pre-2014 existing prescribing rights may continue to prescribe pethidine but may prescribe morphine and fentanyl only upon completion of a Council-approved educational program. Fentanyl may be prescribed only by a midwife practising in a secondary or tertiary hospital setting with medical back-up available. Fentanyl may not be prescribed for women in a primary birthing unit or those requiring transfer to another facility. The controlled drug codeine cannot be prescribed although tramadol may be prescribed although the conditions under which this would be warranted are limited. See: NZCOM Prescribing information Reminder and Medsafe Alert re Codeine and Tramadol (NZCOM, 2018).

CORONER'S COURT LEGISLATION AND PROCESS

The office of the Coroner is an ancient one, and each state and territory in Australia and New Zealand has a separate Coroner's Act. The Coroner enquires into those deaths where certain facts need to be established to determine various unknown matters—be they the identity of the deceased, cause of death, when/where the person died, or elucidation of the circumstances of the person's death, in such cases as sudden and unexplained deaths, and deaths of persons in the care or control of the police, prison authorities or a mental health facility or under child welfare legislation. The purpose is to establish whether the death resulted from natural causes or from unlawful homicide. The Coroner generally has the power to order a postmortem, require information to be provided and conduct an inquest, usually in a public forum.

Certain deaths involving childbirth may well come under the definition of a death that must be notified.

Indeed, in New Zealand under the *Coroner's Act 2006*, there is mandatory reporting under s13 to a member of the police (who then reports to the Coroner) for cases that may involve midwifery including 'any death of a woman that occurred while the woman concerned was giving birth, or that appears to have been a result of that woman being pregnant or giving birth' or; of a death that was 'without known cause'; or may have resulted from 'a medical procedure and was medically unexpected' (s14(2)). Some jurisdictions in Australia provide for penalties for failure to inform the Coroner of a 'suspicious death'. A midwife is not under an obligation to report a death that has already been reported to the Coroner or the police (or, in New Zealand, will be reported).

Coroners do not have the power to investigate stillbirths. Somewhat controversially in Australia, coroners have shown a rising inclination toward challenging long-established parameters of stillbirth by expanding the definition of 'signs of life', particularly in relation to homebirth. In high-profile home birth coronial inquiries, including the Inquest into the deaths of Tate Spencer-Koch (baby), Jahli Hobbs (Baby), Tully Kavanagh (baby), Unnamed child from Western Australia, 2010, signs of life were considered to include those not associated with the infant's body or consciousness, such as whether the umbilical cord is still pink or there is some indication of a very low electronic pulse reading medically associated with dying or death. Such findings could have significant implications for organ donorship and women's fundamental right to bodily autonomy. Home birth midwives in particular should be cognisant of the requirements for reporting a death in the jurisdiction in which they practise.

RESEARCH ACTIVITY

A pre-term baby dies shortly after birth, which was not totally unexpected given the gestational age; however, babies of 800 g do survive. Consider the registration requirements of the birth and death, and whether a coronial inquest may be held, by consulting the legislation in your jurisdiction.

The number of deaths referred to coroners in New Zealand and Australia is growing and it is increasingly likely that a midwife, at some time in her career, will be involved in a coronial investigation or called to give evidence at an inquest. This can be a difficult and stressful experience. It is prudent for midwives to be aware of the procedures set out in the Coroner's legislation governing her practice and to seek legal advice as soon as possible. When the Coroner's office is notified of a death, the body should be left until such time as that office instructs that the body can be moved. All intravenous lines, catheters and drains are left in situ or capped as necessary, and the physical scene is left as undisturbed as possible. Any midwives involved in the care should make full retrospective notes regarding the case as soon as possible (Box 14.10), but should not disclose these to anyone except *their nominated* lawyer so that legal privilege is maintained.

Box 14.10   Advice regarding coronial inquests

Staunton & Chiarella (2016, p. 275) endorse the New South Wales Nurses and Midwives' Association Guidelines in relation to a potential Coronial inquiry. For the Association, simply read your relevant professional or industrial body.

1. Contact the Association for advice. To obtain the necessary advice you should find out details of the matter in which you are involved, the name and contact number of the investigator and the proposed date and time of the interview or the date for submission of the statement.

2. The Association will contact the investigator on your behalf and seek full particulars.

3. Following this, you should be given at least 24 hours' notice of the time, date and place of the proposed interview. You should not attend any interview until advised by the Association.

4. You have a right to access a health record of a client relating to a request for an interview or statement, before you provide a statement or attend an interview, to refresh your memory.

5. Members attending interviews may be accompanied by an Association representative who has knowledge of the issues and rights of the member.

6. Prior to attending any interview, you should be advised by the interviewer that:

    a. anything you may say and the transcript of the interview may be used in evidence in any subsequent legal or disciplinary proceedings

    b. you have the right to either allow or refuse audio or video taping of the interview, and

    c. you may be asked to provide a written statement subsequent to the interview. However, you cannot be made to provide this written statement.

7. If, in the course of any interview, matters are raised which go beyond those previously disclosed to you, the interview should be adjourned or concluded so that you can obtain full particulars of the new issue(s) and gain further advice.

8. You should be aware that the interviewer is not permitted to use intimidatory or accusatory terms. If this approach is adopted, the interview should be terminated immediately.

9. Persons conducting the interview should be totally impartial.

10. You should be provided with a copy of the tape and transcript of the interview as soon as practicable after its completion. You should not sign any transcript or record of interview unless you have read it and are satisfied that it is true and correct in every respect.

11. The Association maintains that its members are entitled to a fair, proper and prompt outcome of such investigations and attempts to assist its members to achieve this end.

Where a matter is referred to the Coroner, in Australia and New Zealand, uniformed police officers assist the Coroner in its inquiries. They gather evidence and interview or request reports and sworn statements from those involved. Sometimes the police will ask midwives to disclose medical information or clinical records. Poor records may suggest that the care given to the patient prior to death was also inadequate. If asked for an interview or a written statement, or for originals or copies of the notes, a midwife is well advised to seek independent legal advice. The provision of any information in relation to a coronial inquiry is not mandatory unless a statutory notice, subpoena or search warrant is issued. HCPs often believe (and are led to believe) that co-operation is an indication that no harm was intended or done. In addition to potentially violating a client's right to confidentiality, it is very damaging for a midwife to speak with or provide any documentation to the police before legal assistance is obtained, particularly as the police may also be assessing the situation in terms of a criminal investigation. In terms of legal advice, although an employed midwife may be offered the services of the hospital's lawyers, situations do arise where the midwife's and the institution's interests are in conflict.

The police are also authorised to receive the custody and care of a dead body immediately after a matter is notified. If the matter appears to involve homicide or manslaughter, the Coroner will usually pause its investigation pending resolution of the criminal investigation / prosecution through normal police processes.

REFLECTIVE THINKING EXERCISE

A policeman arrives at your door unannounced saying he is there on behalf of the Coroner in relation to the perinatal death of a baby of a woman you cared for. He demands the original notes immediately and wants you to attend the police station with him to give a statement.

1. Are you required to give the original notes or a statement to the police officer immediately?

2. What considerations are relevant when a midwife is confronted in such a manner?

3. Reflect and comment on how you can access your professional support systems in such a case.

The Coroner is concerned with causation, not fault. The Coronial inquiry is said to be inquisitorial, rather than adversarial, and it has been suggested that it plays a role in what is known as therapeutic jurisprudence (Freckleton, 2007). A Coroner's Court is generally more informal than an ordinary court and the rules of evidence do not apply. Nevertheless, the Coroner's Court has many of the trappings of an ordinary court. It is a public hearing where witnesses give sworn evidence and are questioned by the Coroner and may be cross-examined by lawyers representing the various parties. Witnesses can be summonsed to give evidence and the Coroner can impose penalties should a witness fail to appear. The highly emotive content of and sociopolitical interest in maternal and infant health often means that media is present and reputations are at stake. In the Australian context, where inter-professional collaboration problems remain unresolved, this leads to a tendency for medical professionals and midwives to seek to blame each other following an adverse event.

It is not the role of the Coroner to find a person or persons liable of negligence or guilty of a crime, but rather to establish how the person died. The Coroner cannot frame his or her findings in a way that indicates either the guilt or negligence of a person involved with the person prior to the death. In New Zealand, if a Coroner makes an 'adverse comment' about the acts or omissions of any provider, then he or she is required to give that person—or in the case of adverse comment about a dead person, to give the family—formal notice of the proposed comments and the opportunity to be heard in relation to the proposed comment (s58 *Coroner Act 2006*). This enables the person or their representative to make submissions to the Coroner in order to answer and defend the comments before the finding is released. If the Coroner believes that an indictable offence has been committed, the appropriate authority, in most cases the Director of Public Prosecutions, or in New Zealand, the Police will be notified. The findings at inquest may provide relatives of the deceased with information indicative of negligence. It is then up to the relatives to pursue the matter through the civil courts (Staunton & Chiarella, 2016). This does not mean that no consequences will follow for an HCP involved in the inquiry.

At the conclusion of an inquest, a Coroner may comment on any matter in relation to a death, including public safety or the administration of justice, and make recommendations. Although it is a recommendation, the appropriate departments have a responsibility to act on such a recommendation (Staunton & Chiarella, 2016). This includes a recommendation that the police or AHPRA investigate a practitioner based on the evidence collected during the inquest. The Coroner can send the recommendations to AHPRA for publication and distribution. Under New Zealand legislation, the Coroner is also charged with making recommendations to try to bring to the attention of the public the circumstances of the death, in the hope of avoiding future similar deaths. In Western Australia, a Coroner may refer the matter to the registering authority/disciplinary body if the Coroner believes that it may wish to inquire into the conduct of a member of that profession (s50 Coroner's Act 1996 [WA]). In New Zealand, the Coroner may inform the MCNZ of any competence concerns held by the Coroner.

It is important to note that, although other legislation may not have an express provision for informing a regulatory authority, related organisations, including the police and AHPRA, may choose to commence investigations on their own accord based on the findings of a Coroner.

CLINICAL POINT

A New South Wales midwife was struck off the register for 2 years in April 2009 after the Nurses and Midwives Tribunal found her guilty of professional misconduct. The Health Care Complaints Commission took action after a baby died in January 2006. The tribunal found that the midwife removed the fetal heart monitor and failed to consult a medical officer. The midwife told the tribunal she practised in the 'paradigm of the normal and natural childbirth and she allowed this to cloud her judgement'. The baby was placed on life support but later died. The midwife was eligible to reapply for registration in 2011.

(Source: *ABC News*, 2009)

REFLECTIVE CASE STUDY

Baby's tragic death

Baby Candice was born nearly 7 weeks premature with a birth weight of just over 2 kg, failed to thrive and died 10 days after birth. While the baby 'thrived' in hospital, there were problems with breastfeeding and weight gain.

The Coroner found that the early discharge of the baby did not in itself contribute to the death. However, she did find that the lack of discharge planning and the failure to communicate that to the various agencies did contribute to the death. Victorian Coroner Noreen Toohey commented that 'had adequate post-discharge follow-up arrangements been instituted, it is unlikely the baby would have died'. The Coroner found it remarkable that the documentation provided to the community nurse made no reference whatsoever to the feeding difficulties and weight loss. The day before the baby died, she was examined by a child health nurse who failed to recognise signs of serious illness and to arrange an urgent admission to hospital. This contributed to the baby's death. One of the doctors from the facility, the discharge coordinator and the child health nurse were all found to have contributed to the baby's death.

The Coroner recommended that babies be returned to the medical centre for weighing and a medical check a few days after discharge, and that adequate note taking be encouraged. The Coroner took the unusual step of sending a copy of her 57-page report to the Victorian Health Department for distribution to medical and nursing colleges and associations.

Questions

1. What signs in the baby prior to and after discharge should have alerted the nursing staff that a problem might exist?

2. What should have been done, and by whom, to avert these events?

(Adapted from *The Western Nurse*, 2002)

REFLECTIVE THINKING EXERCISE

A midwife may observe another midwife giving inappropriate advice to a woman and her partner or observe incorrect practice.

As a midwife, what should you do in this situation? Consider whether you would:

- interfere at the time
- take the midwife aside and point out 'best practice'

- notify the person in charge
- report the midwife to the midwives' registering authority.

It may be appropriate to do all of these, or it may be appropriate to do only one or some of them. What could be a determining factor in making your decision?

Conclusion

It may be surprising to find that so much law applies to midwifery practice, but midwives can be reassured that they are rarely the subject of criminal or civil proceedings. It is hoped that this chapter has provided a helpful guide to the key statutes that relate to midwifery practice in Australia and New Zealand.

Review questions

Australia

1. Name the legislation that governs the regulation of midwifery practice.
2. What is the definition of 'professional misconduct'?
3. What is the role of the Coroner?
4. What might happen following a coronial inquest where the standard of the midwife's care had been in question?
5. What privacy requirements govern practice?
6. What would a plaintiff need to prove in a case of negligence against a midwife?
7. What is the role and function of the nursing and midwifery registering authorities?
8. What options does an aggrieved patient and her family have available to make a complaint to seek redress following an adverse outcome?

New Zealand

1. Where, how and for how long should health information be stored?
2. Describe the circumstances under which a midwife may sign a death certificate following a stillbirth.
3. What should a midwife discuss with the woman when prescribing a medication?
4. What is the role of the Coroner, and what deaths must be reported in the maternity setting?
5. List five legislative powers of the Midwifery Council, and identify its primary role.
6. What are three steps that it is recommended a midwife take following receipt of a complaint regarding that midwife's practice?
7. When assessing what is a 'reasonable standard of care' in any given case, name three sources of practice standards that could be referred to.

NOTE

a. (Where definitions differ between Australia and New Zealand they are provided in the text.) *Common law:* originally defined as the ancient unwritten law of England, but it has come to mean the system of law based on old customs or court decisions, as distinct from statute law or the laws enacted by Parliament (Orsman & Wattie, 2001). *Regulation:* (for the purposes of this chapter) a rule or other order issued by a ministry or (government) department under authority delegated by Parliament. A regulation has the force of law in Australia and New Zealand. *Statute:* a law made by an Act of Parliament passed by a majority of elected representatives (Orsman & Wattie, 2001).

Acknowledgements

With acknowledgement to Mary Chiarella, who was one of the original authors of this chapter, and whose work has been updated for the current edition.

Online resources

Australasian Legal Information Institute: http://www.austlii.edu.au.
Australian College of Midwives: http://www.midwives.org.au/.
New Zealand Health and Disability Commissioner: http://www.hdc.org.nz.
Midwifery Council of New Zealand: https://midwiferycouncil.health.nz.
Ministry of Health, New Zealand: http://www.health.govt.nz.
New Zealand College of Midwives: http://www.midwife.org.nz.
Privacy Commissioner, Te Mana Matapono Matatapu: http://www.privacy.org.nz.
Public Access to Legislation Project: http://www.legislation.govt.nz.

References

ABC News. *Midwife banned over baby death (Article)*. 2009.
Australian College of Midwives (ACM). *National Midwifery Guidelines for Consultation and Referral*. 3rd ed. Issue 2. Canberra: ACM; 2013. Online: https://issuu.com/austcollegemidwives/docs/guidelines2013.
Australian Health Practitioner Registration Authority (AHPRA). *Glossary—definition of AHPRA*. 2015. Online: https://www.ahpra.gov.au/Support/Glossary.aspx.
Australian Health Practitioner Registration Authority (AHPRA). *What we do*. 2017a. Online: http://www.ahpra.gov.au/About-AHPRA/What-We-Do.aspx.
Australian Health Practitioner Registration Authority (AHPRA). *Find out about the complaints process*. 2017b. Online: http://www.ahpra.gov.au/Notifications/Find-out-about-the-complaints-process.aspx.
Australian Health Practitioner Registration Authority (AHPRA). *How are complaints and concerns managed?* 2017c. Online: http://www.ahpra.gov.au/Notifications/How-are-complaints-managed.aspx.
Bates PW. *An overview of professional liability in health care. Keynote lecture presented by invitation to the Annual Seminar of the Medico-Legal Society of Singapore, 14–15 October*. 1989.
Beaupert F, Carney T, Chiarella M, et al. Regulating healthcare complaints: a literature review. *Int J Health Care Qual Assur*. 2014;27(6):505-518.
Commonwealth of Australia. *Health Legislation Amendment (Midwives and Nurse Practitioners) Act 2010*. ParlInfoSearch; 2010. Online: http://www.aph.gov.au.
Council of Australian Governments (COAG). *Summary of the Draft Health Practitioner Regulation National Law Amendment Law 2017*. Barton, ACT: COAG; 2017:7. Online: https://www.anzcp.org.au/wp-content/uploads/2017/05/Summary-of-HPRNL-Amendment-Law_FINAL.pdf.
Department of Health and Ageing (DOHA). *Maternity Services Review: Overview*. 2008. Online: http://www.health.gov.au/internet/main/publishing.nsf/Content/maternityservicesreview.
Devereux J, Parker M. Competency issues for young persons and older persons. In: Freckleton I, Petersen K, eds. *Disputes and Dilemmas in Health Law*. Sydney: Federation Press; 2006:54.
Freckleton I. Death investigation, the Coroner and therapeutic jurisprudence. *J Law Med*. 2007;15(1):1-12.

Health and Disability Commissioner (HDC). *Code of Health and Disability Services Consumers' Rights*. Regulations 1996 [NZ]. Online: https://www.hdc.org.nz/your-rights/about-the-code/code-of-health-and-disability-services-consumers-rights/.
Health and Disability Commissioner (HDC). *Code of Health and Disability Services Consumers' Rights*. 1998. Online: https://www.hdc.org.nz/your-rights/about-the-code/code-of-health-and-disability-services-consumers-rights/.
Health and Disability Commissioner (HDC). *A Guide for Providers: HDC's Investigation Processes. 2013, under update in 2022*. Online: https://www.hdc.org.nz/news-resources/search-resources/leaflets/guide-for-providers-hdc-investigation-process/.
Health and Disability Commissioner (HDC). *Annual Report for the Year Ended June 2020*. Wellington: HDC; 2020. Online: https://www.hdc.org.nz/media/5696/hdc-annual-report-2020.pdf.
Health Professions Councils Authority (HPCA). *Complaints and concerns*. 2018. Online: https://www.hpca.nsw.gov.au/complaints.
House of Lords [UK]. Decision in *F v West Berkshire Health Authority* [1989] 2 All ER 545. 1989.
International Confederation of Midwives (ICM). *International Code of Ethics for Midwives*. 2008. Reviewed 2014. Online: https://www.internationalmidwives.org/assets/files/general-files/2019/10/eng-international-code-of-ethics-for-midwives.pdf.
Kennedy I. The patient on the Clapham Omnibus (1984) 47 MLR 454, 460.
Kerridge I, Lowe M, Stewart C. *Ethics and Law for the Health Professions*. 3rd ed. Sydney: Federation Press; 2013.
Levi-Faur D. *Handbook on the Politics of Regulation*. Cheltenham: Edward Elgar Publishing; 2012:459.
Midwifery Council of New Zealand (MCNZ). *Competencies for Entry to the Register of Midwives*. Wellington, NZ: MCNZ; 2007. Online: https://www.midwiferycouncil.health.nz/common/Uploaded%20files/Registration/Competencies%20for%20entry%20to%20the%20Register.pdf.
Midwifery Council of New Zealand (MCNZ). *Code of Conduct*. Wellington, NZ: MCNZ; 2010. Online: https://www.midwifery-council.health.nz/common/Uploaded%20files/Registration/Code%20of%20Conduct.pdf.
Midwifery Council of New Zealand (MCNZ). *Statement on Cultural Competence for Midwives*: MCNZ; 2011. Online: https://www.midwiferycouncil.health.nz/common/Uploaded%20files/About%20Us/Statement%20on%20cultural%20competence.pdf.
Midwifery Council of New Zealand (MCNZ). *MCNZ Annual Report for the Year Ended 31 March 2020*; 2021. Online: https://www.midwiferycouncil.health.nz/Public/Publications/Annual-reports/Public/03.-Publications/Publications-Type-A/Annual-Reports.aspx?hkey=ad216505-605a-44cd-93c8-922bebc33f67.
Ministry for Social Development (MSD). *White Paper for Vulnerable Children*. Vol. I. Wellington, NZ: MSD; 2012. Online: https://www.orangatamariki.govt.nz/assets/Uploads/white-paper-for-vulnerable-children-volume-1.pdf.
Ministry of Health (MOH). *Guidelines for Consultation With Obstetric and Related Services (Referral Guidelines)*. Wellington, NZ: MOH; 2012. (Under review 2022). Online: https://www.health.govt.nz/publication/guidelines-consultation-obstetric-and-related-medical-services-referral-guidelines.
Ministry of Health (MOH) *Sharing information safely, Guidance on sharing personal information under the Family Violence Act 2018*: MOH; 2019. Online: https://www.justice.govt.nz/justice-sector-policy/key-initiatives/addressing-family-violence-and-sexual-violence/a-new-family-violence-act/information-sharing-guidance/.

Ministry of Health (MOH) *New Zealand EPrescription Service.* MOH; 2021. Online: https://www.health.govt.nz/our-work/digital-health/other-digital-health-initiatives/emedicines/new-zealand-eprescription-service.

Ministry of Health (MOH). *Primary Maternity Services Notice 2021. New Zealand Gazette Notice number 2021-go2473 30 June 2021.* MOH; 2021a. Online: https://gazette.govt.nz/notice/id/2021-go2473.

Ministry of Health (MOH). *Access Agreement.* MOH; 2021b. Online: https://www.health.govt.nz/system/files/documents/publications/maternity_facility_access_agreement.docx.

National Health and Medical Research Council (NHMRC). *General Guidelines for Medical Practitioners on Providing Information to Patients.* 2004a. Online: https://www.nhmrc.gov.au/_files_nhmrc/publications/attachments/e57_guidelines_gps_information_to_patients_150722.pdf.

National Health and Medical Research Council (NHMRC). *Communicating With Patients: Advice for Medical Practitioners.* 2004b. Online: https://www.nhmrc.gov.au/_files_nhmrc/publications/attachments/e58_communicating_with_patients.pdf.

New Zealand College of Midwives (NZCOM). *Unexpected Outcome? (Booklet).* Christchurch, NZ: NZCOMa. Online purchase: https://www.midwife.org.nz/product/unexpected-outcome/.

New Zealand College of Midwives (NZCOM). *Consensus Statements* Christchurch, NZ: NZCOMb; Online: https://www.midwife.org.nz/midwives/professional-practice/consensus-statements/.

New Zealand College of Midwives (NZCOM). *Multi-disciplinary guidelines,* NZCOMc; Online: https://www.midwife.org.nz/midwives/professional-practice/multi-disciplinary-guidelines/.

New Zealand College of Midwives (NZCOM). *Philosophy and Code of Ethics.* Christchurch, NZ: NZCOM; 2015a. Online: https://www.midwife.org.nz/midwives/professional-practice/philosophy-and-code-of-ethics/.

New Zealand College of Midwives (NZCOM). *Midwives Handbook for Practice.* Christchurch, NZ: NZCOM; 2015b. Online purchase: https://www.midwife.org.nz/product/midwifery-standards-review-handbook/.

New Zealand College of Midwives (NZCOM). *Consensus Statement: Informed Consent and Decision Making.* Christchurch, NZ: NZCOM. 2016. Online: https://www.midwife.org.nz/wp-content/uploads/2019/05/Informed-Consent-and-Decision-Making.pdf.

New Zealand College of Midwives (NZCOM). *Health and Safety Policy.* Christchurch, NZ: NZCOM; 2017. Online: https://www.midwife.org.nz/wp-content/uploads/2019/06/Health-and-Safety-Policy-2017.pdf.

New Zealand College of Midwives (NZCOM). *Prescribing information Reminder and Medsafe Alert re Codeine and Tramadol.* Online: https://www.midwife.org.nz/wp-content/uploads/2019/06/Prescribing-Reminder-and-Medsafe-Alert.pdf.

New Zealand College of Midwives (NZCOM) *The effect on midwives of the changes to the information sharing legislation.* NZCOM; 2019. Online: https://www.midwife.org.nz/news/significant-changes-to-information-sharing-starting-the-1st-july-impact-for-midwives/.

New Zealand College of Midwives (NZCOM). *Child Protection Policy 2021.* NZCOM; 2021. Online: https://www.midwife.org.nz/.wp-content/uploads/2021/04/Child-Protection-Policy-2021.pdf

Nursing and Midwifery Board of Australia (NMBA). *Fact Sheet: Continuing Professional Development.* Melbourne: NMBA; 2017a. Online: http://www.nursingmidwiferyboard.gov.au/Codes-Guidelines-Statements/FAQ/CPD-FAQ-for-nurses-and-midwives.aspx.

Nursing and Midwifery Board of Australia (NMBA). *Registration Standard: Endorsement for Scheduled Medicines for Midwives.* Melbourne: NMBA; 2017b. Online: http://www.nursingmidwiferyboard.gov.au/Registration-Standards/Endorsement-for-scheduled-medicines-for-midwives.aspx.

Nursing and Midwifery Board of Australia (NMBA). *Safety and Quality Guidelines for Privately Practising Midwives.* Melbourne: NMBA; 2017c. Online: http://www.nursingmidwiferyboard.gov.au/Codes-Guidelines-Statements/Codes-Guidelines.aspx.

Nursing and Midwifery Board of Australia (NMBA). *Fact Sheet: Audit on Safety and Quality Guidelines for Privately Practising Midwives.* Melbourne: NMBA; 2017d. Online: http://www.nursingmidwiferyboard.gov.au/Codes-Guidelines-Statements/FAQ/Fact-sheet-Safety-and-quality-guidelines-for-privately-practising-midwives.aspx.

Primary Maternity Services Notice 2021 (NZ) – see MOH 2021a above.

Nursing and Midwifery Board of Australia (NMBA). *Code of Conduct for Midwives.* Melbourne: NMBA; 2018. Online: http://www.nursingmidwiferyboard.gov.au/Codes-Guidelines-Statements/Professional-standards.aspx.

Office of the Australian Information Commissioner. *National Privacy Principles.* 2017. Online: https://www.oaic.gov.au/privacy-law/privacy-act/.

Office of the Health Ombudsman (OHO). *About us.* 2017. Online: http://www.oho.qld.gov.au/about-us/office-of-the-health-ombudsman/.

Office of the Privacy Commissioner (NZ). *Health Information Privacy Code.* 1994. Online: https://www.privacy.org.nz/privacy-act-2020/codes-of-practice/hipc2020/.

Oranga Tamariki (Ministry for Children) (OT). *Working with Children Information Sharing.* OT; 2019. Online: https://www.orangatamariki.govt.nz/working-with-children/information-sharing/.

Orsman HW, Wattie N, eds. *The Reed Dictionary of New Zealand English.* 3rd ed. Auckland: Reed; 2001.

Re C. Adult: Refusal of Treatment. 1 WLR 290, [1994] 1 All ER 819. Online: https://www.independent.co.uk/sport/law-report-patient-can-refuse-treatment-re-c-family-division-mr-justice-thorpe-14-october-1993-1510908.html.

Reader T, Gillespie A, Roberts J. Patient complaints in healthcare systems: a systematic review and coding taxonomy. *BMJ Qual Saf.* 2014;23:8. Online: http://qualitysafety.bmj.com/content/qhc/23/8/678.full.pdf.

State of Queensland. *Health Practitioner Regulation National Law Act 2009.* 2018. Online: https://www.legislation.qld.gov.au/view/pdf/inforce/current/act-2009-045.

Staunton P, Chiarella M. *Nursing and the Law.* 8th ed. Sydney: Elsevier; 2016.

The Western Nurse. *Baby's tragic death (Article).* The Western Nurse; 2002.

World Health Organization (WHO) Europe. *European Union Standards for Nursing and Midwifery: Information for Accession Countries.* 2nd ed. Geneva: WHO; 2009. Online: http://www.euro.who.int/__data/assets/pdf_file/0005/102200/E92852.pdf.

Statutes and case law

Abortion Law Reform Act 2008 (Vic).

Accident Compensation Act 2001 [NZ].

Adoption Act 1955 [NZ].

Annesley v Earl of Anglesea 1743 16 State Tr 1139.

Attorney-General (UK) v Heinemann Publishers Australia Pty Ltd 1987 10 IPR 153 (NSW CofA).

B v Medical Council of New Zealand HC Auckland HC11/96, 8 July 1996.

Births Deaths and Marriages Registration Act 1995 (NSW).

Births Deaths and Marriages Registration Act 1995 [NZ].

Births Deaths and Marriages Registration Act 1996 (NT).

Births Deaths and Marriages Registration Act 1996 (SA).

Births Deaths and Marriages Registration Act 1996 (Vic).

Births Deaths and Marriages Registration Act 1997 (ACT).

Births Deaths and Marriages Registration Act 1998 (WA).
Births Deaths and Marriages Registration Act 1999 (Tas).
Births Deaths and Marriages Registration Act 2003 (Qld).
Births Deaths Marriages and Relationships Registration Amendment Act 2008 [NZ].
Burial and Cremation Act 1964 [NZ].
Child Young Persons and their Families Act 1989.
Children's and Young People's Well-being Act 1989 (also known as Tamariki Oranga Act 1989) [NZ].
Community Health Services Complaints Act 1993 (ACT).
Contraception, Sterilisation and Abortion Act 1977 [NZ].
Coroner's Act 1996 (WA).
Coroner's Act 2006 [NZ].
Crimes Act 1961 [NZ].
Criminal Code Act 1924 (Tas).
Criminal Code Act Compilation Act 1913 (WA).
Criminal Law Consolidation Act 1935 (SA).
Donoghue v Stevenson 1932 AC 562.
F v West Berkshire Health Authority 1989 2 All England Reports.
Family Violence Act 2018 [NZ]
Finch v Rogers 2004 NSWSC 89.
Hart v Herron [1984] Aust Torts Report 80-201.
Health Act 1911 (WA).
Health Act 1956 [NZ].
Health Act 1993 (ACT).
Health and Community Services Complaints Act 1988 (NT).
Health and Community Services Complaints Act 2004 (SA).
Health and Disability Commissioner Act 1994 [NZ].
Health and Disability Commissioner (Code of Health and Disability Services Consumers' Rights) Regulations 1996 [NZ].
Health and Disability Services (Safety) Act 2001 [NZ].
Health and Safety at Work Act 2015 [NZ].
Health and Safety at Work (General Risk and Workplace Management) Regulations 2016 [NZ].
Health Care Complaints Act 1993 (NSW).
Health Complaints Act 1995 (Tas).
Health Information Privacy Code 2020 [NZ].
Health Practitioner Regulation National Law Act 2009 (Qld).
Health Practitioner's Competence Assurance Act 2003 [NZ].
Health Quality and Complaints Commission Act 2006 (Qld).
Health (Retention of Health Information) Regulations 1996 [NZ].
Health Services (Conciliation and Review) Act 1987 (Vic).
Health Services (Conciliation and Review) Act 1995 (WA).
Human Rights Act 1993 [NZ].
Human Rights Act 2019 (Qld).
Human Rights Commission Act 2005 (ACT).
Human Tissue Act 2008 [NZ].
Inquest into the death of Joseph Thurgood-Yates (baby) 2013 Vic Coroner COR 2010 4851.
Inquest into the deaths of Tate Spencer-Koch (baby), Jahli Hobbs (Baby), Tully Kavanagh (baby), Unnamed child from Western Australia, 2010 SA Coroner 17/2010 (0984/0207).
Medical Services Act (NT).
Medicines Act 1981 [NZ].

Medicines Amendment Act 2013 [NZ].
Medicines Regulations 1984 [NZ].
Misuse of Drugs Act 1975 [NZ].
Misuse of Drugs Amendment Regulations 2014 [NZ].
Misuse of Drugs Regulations 1977 [NZ].
Montgomery v Lanarkshire Health Board[2015] UKSC 11
New Zealand Bill of Rights Act 1990 [NZ].
Nurses Act 1977 [NZ].
Nurses Amendment Act 1990 [NZ].
Privacy Act 1988 (Cth).
Privacy Act 2020 [NZ].
Privacy Amendment (Private Sector) Act 2000 (Cth).
Public Health and Disability Act 2000 [NZ].
Public Records Act 2005 [NZ].
Radiation Protection Act 1965 [NZ].
Rogers v Whitaker [1992] HCA 58.
Social Security Act 1964 [NZ].
Summary Proceedings Act 1957 [NZ].
Tamariki Oranga Act 1989 (also known as Children's and Young People's Well-being Act 1989) [NZ].
Trans-Tasman Mutual Recognition Act 1997 (Cth).
Vulnerable Children Act 2014 [NZ].
Z v Dental Complaints Assessment Committee 2008 NZSC 55.

Further reading

Balkin R, Davis J. *Law of Torts*. 4th ed. Sydney: Lexis Nexis Butterworth; 2008.
Chiarella M. *The Legal and Professional Status of Nursing*. Edinburgh: Churchill Livingstone; 2002.
Mellars C, Cronin L, Merry A. *Is nursing a crime?* Nurs N Z. 1995;26.
Newnham H. Fetus v mother: who wins? *Aust J Midwifery*. 2003; 16(1):23-26.
Newnham H. To assist or not to assist: the legal liability of midwives acting as Good Samaritans. *Women Birth*. 2006;19(3): 62-64.
NSW Health. *Consent to Medical Treatment—Patient Information*. Policy Directive PD2005_406. 2005. Online: http://www.health.nsw.gov.au/policies/pd/2005/PD2005_406.html.
Office of Safety and Quality in Healthcare, Western Australia Department of Health. *Consent to Treatment Policy for the Western Australian Health System 2011*. 2011:20-25. Online: http://health.wa.gov.au/circularsnew/pdfs/12789.pdf.
Office of the Australian Information Commissioner. *National Privacy Principles*. Canberra: Office of the Australian Information Commissioner; 2017. Full text of privacy principles. Online: https://www.oaic.gov.au/individuals/privacy-fact-sheets/general/privacy-fact-sheet-17-australian-privacy-principles.
Seymour J. *Childbirth and the Law*. Oxford: Oxford University Press; 2000.
Skene L. *Law and Medical Practice: Rights, Duties, Claims and Defences*. 3rd ed. Sydney: Lexis Nexis Butterworth; 2008.

CHAPTER 15

Ethical frameworks for practice

Emma Tumilty

CHAPTER OVERVIEW

In this chapter, you will learn about the difference between professional ethics and values and personal ethics and values. You will be introduced to some of the stated values of your profession and the ethical codes of conduct for practice. This is followed by an introduction to bioethics and a selection of ethical concepts and theories. These concepts and theories are useful for understanding ethical situations that occur when providing care. Bioethical explanation, argumentation and justification are explained, as well as their relationship to practice.

The second half of the chapter then explains how to engage in ethical decision making when ethical dilemmas (due to conflict or uncertainty) arise in providing care. The process of engaging in ethical reasoning, while drawing on things like codes of ethics and bioethical concepts, is set out. Ethical decision making includes identifying clearly and explicitly what is in conflict or at stake, thinking through what options for action are available, and then evaluating how these options align with various appeals or justifications while considering what constraints are relevant. The resolution is an ethically reasoned and justified solution that focuses on the needs and values of the person being cared for, while operating within the ethical, legal and other constraints of the situation.

Sometimes practitioners can feel that a situation was not resolved ethically. This can lead to what is called moral distress. In the final section of the chapter, I outline what is understood by the term moral distress, how it arises, and what can be done to ameliorate it.

KEY TERMS

autonomy
beneficence
bioethics
codes of ethics
codes of professional conduct

ethics
informed choice
informed consent
justice
moral distress

non-maleficence
professional ethics
reasoning
values

INTRODUCTION

Health professionals exist in a special relationship with society (Abbott & Meerabeau, 2020). In recognition of the knowledge and skill exercised, health professionals are afforded special status that is protected; in return they provide service to society and individuals in a manner that meets ethical and practice standards. Midwives play a vital role in supporting people and their babies through the journey of pregnancy, birth, and postnatal care. During this time, people need to be able to trust midwives to support them in their decision making and further their own and their baby's wellbeing.

As students, one of the first things we learn and then later have to navigate in the transition to practice is the ethical standards of the profession and how these are applied.

CODE OF ETHICS FOR MIDWIVES

Professional ethics guide practitioners specifically in their work and are distinct from personal ethics (Comartin, 2011). Professional ethics are a collectively agreed set of ethical norms for a profession. They dictate how professionals should act per their socially-approved role as a professional. Personal ethics are the set of ethical norms you abide by in your life, informed by your culture, religion, upbringing, education, experiences, and so on. Your personal **ethics** will in many ways influence how you practise, but you must agree to uphold the ethical norms of the profession as part of being recognised as a professional.

The midwifery professions in Australia and Aotearoa New Zealand both have a range of guiding documents on practice that include codes of conduct, descriptions of competencies and standards of practice, scope of practice, descriptions of the philosophy of care and the partnership model (see Online resources for links to these resources). The International Confederation of Midwives (ICM), as the global professional association for midwives, also has a code of ethics that describes the moral commitments the profession has made in delivering service to the community. The midwifery professional associations in New Zealand and Australia have similar ethical codes. These codes often describe the philosophy of midwifery and provide detailed descriptions of what it is that is expected of midwives in their engagement with women, other birthing people, babies and their families, colleagues, other health professionals and society. Below are excerpts (Fig. 15.1) from the ICM's International Code of Ethics for Midwives (2008) that drew on the New Zealand College of Midwives' 1993 Code of Ethics (Fig. 15.2) in its development. The Australian Board of Nursing and Midwifery replaced their own code with the International Confederation's Code in 2018 and provides a range of other guidance (Fig. 15.3). New Zealand maintains its own code, with the inclusion of explicit commitments to Māori. These codes set out at a high level what the standards are for the profession to practise ethically.

The full range of documents relevant to your setting should be read in their entirety and clearly understood as you begin to practise. Some overarching themes throughout the **codes of ethics** are commitments to shared decision making, empowerment, partnership and trust-building, equity and advocacy with the people midwives will serve, but the codes also reference important ethical mandates in terms of ongoing learning and training of others and research. A midwife in their practice should be considering how their actions align with these commitments and what actions that honour them look like.

BIOETHICS AND MIDWIFERY: THEORIES AND PRINCIPLES AND THEIR APPLICATION

While codes of ethics provide a framework that can indicate to professionals what the expectations of the profession are for behaviour, they do not always make clear what actions should be taken in a context of conflict or uncertainty.

Bioethics—a discipline centred on value identification, ethical theorisation, analysis and justification—has much to offer health professionals in explicitly working through what ethical practice might mean. Bioethics is an interdisciplinary area of scholarship that provides theories, principles, and processes for understanding and **reasoning** through ethical situations.

By using bioethical theories and principles, health professionals have the means of analysing and communicating ethical issues and decisions across disciplinary boundaries in the clinical setting.

Ethical theories

Ethical theories help us understand and articulate the way we[a] approach or evaluate a situation and figure out what we want to do. Theories can be grouped in a variety of ways but here we will look at their locus of value. That is, a theory can take agents, actions or outcomes as a focus in determining whether something is the ethical thing to do and can be used in different ways for different types of questions.

Using a theory, you can either figure out what would be the right thing to do or justify to others what you think the right thing to do is based on your explanation of a situation using a particular theory. See Table 15.1.

Aside from this traditional collection of theories, new approaches have developed over time. These include feminist, race / ethnicity and disability approaches to bioethics, where issues and actions are evaluated through a lens of justice for particularly marginalised groups, or ideas about **values** are broadened beyond Western[b] conceptions. Using these kinds of approaches we can further understand why the prioritisation of particular values or actions may lead to further disadvantage or fail to address the needs of different populations. These kinds

I. Midwifery Relationships

a) Midwives develop a partnership with individual women in which they share relevant information that leads to informed decision-making, consent to an evolving plan of care, and acceptance of responsibility for the outcomes of their choices.
b) Midwives support the right of women/families to participate actively in decisions about their care.
c) Midwives empower women/families to speak for themselves on issues affecting the health of women and families within their culture/society.
d) Midwives, together with women, work with policy and funding agencies to define women's needs for health services and to ensure that resources are fairly allocated considering priorities and availability.
e) Midwives support and sustain each other in their professional roles, and actively nurture their own and others' sense of self-worth.
f) Midwives respectfully work with other health professionals, consulting and referring as necessary when the woman's need for care exceeds the competencies of the midwife.
g) Midwives recognise the human interdependence within their field of practice and actively seek to resolve inherent conflicts.
h) Midwives have responsibilities to themselves as persons of moral worth, including duties of moral self-respect and the preservation of integrity.

II. Practice of Midwifery

a) Midwives provide care for women and childbearing families with respect for cultural diversity while also working to eliminate harmful practices within those same cultures.
b) Midwives encourage the minimum expectation that no woman or girl should be harmed by conception or childbearing.
c) Midwives use up-to-date, evidence-based professional knowledge to maintain competence in safe midwifery practices in all environments and cultures.
d) Midwives respond to the psychological, physical, emotional, and spiritual needs of women seeking health care, whatever their circumstances (non-discrimination).
e) Midwives act as effective role models of health promotion for women throughout their life cycle, for families, and for other health professionals.
f) Midwives actively seek personal, intellectual and professional growth throughout their midwifery career, integrating this growth into their practice.

III. The Professional Responsibilities of Midwives

a) Midwives hold in confidence client information in order to protect the right to privacy, and use judgment in sharing this information except when mandated by law.
b) Midwives are responsible for their decisions and actions, and are accountable for the related outcomes in their care of women.
c) Midwives may decide not to participate in activities for which they hold deep moral opposition; however, the emphasis on individual conscience should not deprive women of essential health services.

FIGURE 15.1 The International Code of Ethics for Midwives
(Source: International Confederation of Midwives, 2008)

of approaches can offer us new ideas and tools for analysing ethical situations. Feminist bioethics and philosophy, for example, have provided new ways of understanding concepts such as care and autonomy (Leach Scully et al., 2010), and concepts such as **moral distress** (Morley et al., 2021). Indigenous and race-related writing and research make clear how our systems and actors within them cause harm to people of colour through colonialist and white supremacist logics (Bardill & Garrison, 2016; McNeill et al., 2005; Russell, 2016) (see Chapters 10 and 11). Disability writing informs us of the myriad and insidious ways that we reinforce ableist thinking in the very settings that should be safe (Garland-Thomson, 2017; see also Further reading).

Ethical thinking and knowledge is an area of life-long learning, one that will extend beyond your time in training (much like clinical thinking and knowledge). Reading diverse authors on these topics throughout your career can help you to become a better ethical practitioner.

Principles

In addition to theories, bioethicists also work with ethical principles. Principles can be thought of as a set of guiding points or markers for factors that require attention in our normative evaluation (normative ethics is a name for deciding what is right and wrong). There are generally a set of four principles that are considered across all health professions as the core principles that underpin ethical decision making. These are autonomy, beneficence, non-maleficence and justice (Beauchamp & Childress, 2001). These principles are not exhaustive but can act as a set of tools to explore what matters in a particular situation. This does not mean that other concepts and ideas, such as dignity or solidarity, might not be important in a given situation, or that public health ethics concepts like necessity and proportionality might not apply (Barrett et al., 2016). The four principles function as a starting point for ethical analysis in healthcare.

Responsibilities to the woman
- Midwives work in partnership with the woman
- Midwives accept the right of each woman to control her pregnancy and birthing experience
- Midwives accept that the woman is responsible for decisions that affect herself, her baby and her family/whānau
- Midwives uphold each woman's right to free, informed choice and consent throughout her childbirth experience
- Midwives respond to the social, psychological, physical, emotional, spiritual and cultural needs of women seeking midwifery care, whatever their circumstances, and facilitate opportunities for their expression
- Midwives respect the importance of others in the woman's life
- Midwives hold information in confidence in order to protect the woman's right to privacy. Confidential information should be shared with others only with the informed consent of the woman, unless otherwise permitted or required by law
- Midwives are accountable to women for their midwifery practice
- Midwives have a responsibility not to interfere with the normal process of pregnancy and childbirth
- Midwives have a responsibility to ensure that no action or omission on their part places the woman at risk
- Midwives have a professional responsibility to refer to others when they have reached the limit of their expertise
- Midwives have a responsibility to be true to their own value system and professional judgments. However, midwives' personal beliefs should not deprive any woman of essential health care.

Responsibilities to the wider community
- Midwives recognise Māori as tangata whenua of Aotearoa and honour the principles of partnership, protection and participation as an affirmation of the Treaty of Waitangi
- Midwives encourage public participation in the shaping of social policies and institutions
- Midwives advocate policies and legislation that promote social justice, improved social conditions and a fairer sharing of the community's resources
- Midwives acknowledge the role and expertise of community groups in providing care and support for childbearing women
- Midwives act as effective role models in health promotion for women, families and other health professionals.

Responsiblities to the profession
- Midwives support and sustain each other in their professional roles and actively nurture their own and others' sense of self-worth
- Midwives actively seek personal, intellectual and professional growth throughout their career, integrating this into their practice
- Midwives are responsible for sharing their midwifery knowledge with others
- Midwives are autonomous practitioners regardless of the setting and are accountable to the woman and the midwifery profession for their midwifery practice
- Midwives have a responsibility to uphold their professional standards and avoid compromise just for reasons of personal or institutional expedience
- Midwives acknowledge the role and expertise of other health professionals providing care and support for childbearing women
- Midwives take appropriate action if an act by colleagues infringes accepted standards of care
- Midwives ensure that the advancement of midwifery knowledge is based on activities that protect the rights of women
- Midwives develop and share midwifery knowledge through a variety of processes such as midwifery standards review and research
- Midwives participate in education of midwifery students and other midwives
- Midwives adhere to professional rather than commercial standards in making known the availability of their services.

FIGURE 15.2 New Zealand College of Midwives Philosophy and Code of Ethics, 1993
(Source: NZCOM, 1993)

Autonomy and relational autonomy

The principle of **autonomy** states that a person has the right to make their own decisions about their life, body and health. It also encompasses the right of a person to control the information known about them, meaning our laws regarding privacy and confidentiality are grounded in the principle of autonomy.

In clinical practice, this is foundational to all other principles but has some caveats. A person's autonomy can only be directly respected when they are capable of exercising it (it is still respected when they cannot, but through other measures). We generally consider this to be the case when people have decision-making capacity and are provided informed consent (discussed later in this chapter). A person has decision-making capacity when they can understand information, weigh options and alternatives against their values and goals, and come to a decision and communicate it freely. Decision-making capacity is decision- and time-specific. That is, a person may demonstrate decision-making capacity for one type of decision but lack it for another, or they demonstrate decision-making capacity at one moment in time and then not in another.

For those who are in labour, this is particularly relevant, because a person's capacity to engage in decision making in labour has historically (and sometimes still today) been questioned solely on the basis of being in labour, which is wrong (Villarmea & Kelly, 2020). One

Code of professional conduct for midwives

Midwives practise competently in accordance with legislation, standards and professional practice

1. Midwives practise in a safe and competent manner.
2. Midwives practise in accordance with the standards of the profession and broader health system.
3. Midwives practise and conduct themselves in accordance with laws relevant to the profession and practice of midwifery.
4. Midwives respect the dignity, culture, values and beliefs of each woman and her infant(s) in their care and the woman's partner and family, and of colleagues.
5. Midwives treat personal information obtained in a professional capacity as private and confidential.
6. Midwives provide impartial, honest and accurate information in relation to midwifery care and health care products.

Midwives practise within a woman-centred framework
7. Midwives focus on a woman's health needs, her expectations and aspirations, supporting the informed decision making of each woman.
8. Midwives promote and preserve the trust and privilege inherent in the relationship between midwives and each woman and her infant(s).
9. Midwives maintain and build on the community's trust and confidence in the midwifery profession.

Midwives practise midwifery reflectively and ethically
10. Midwives practise midwifery reflectively and ethically.

FIGURE 15.3 Code of professional conduct for midwives in Australia, Nursing and Midwifery (2018)
(Source: Nursing and Midwifery Board of Australia, 2018)

Table 15.1 Ethical theories

	Agent-centred	Deontology	Utilitarianism
Focus	Agent	Action	Outcome
Key figure	Aristotle	Immanuel Kant	John Stuart Mill
Main concept	*Virtues*: Acquired habits, skills, or dispositions that make people effective in social or professional settings	*Duties*: Ethical rules or commands that constrain one's action or define obligations owed to others	*Results*: Good or bad outcomes of actions and policies or their beneficial or harmful effects on individuals and society
Examples	Honesty, courage, modesty, trustworthiness, transparency, reliability and perseverance	Ethical and religious commandments, obligations to seek justice or respect persons and their rights	Burdens, risks, harms, or costs versus the benefits, advantages, or savings resulting from interventions or policies
Ethical action	Doing what a virtuous person would do in a given situation	Fulfilling an obligation or duty owed to oneself or society	Maximising the net balance of benefits over harms
Uses	Assessing skills and capacities needed for success in midwifery practice	Establishing compliance rules and regulations, and setting standards for evaluating actions and behaviour	Conducting cost–benefit, risk–benefit, or cost–effectiveness analyses in a variety of situations (individual / community / population, etc.)

(Adapted from Barrett et al., 2016)

should always assume a person has decision-making capacity until demonstrable evidence to the contrary. But there are also situations when a person may not be able to demonstrate full decision-making capacity that can happen at any time during pregnancy or labour. Sometimes people can have impaired decision making based on already-existing conditions, accidents / injuries, pregnancy-related interventions and so on. Despite this, we can still do our best as health professionals to respect their autonomy. This can be done in multiple ways depending on the nature of their lack of capacity. It may involve abiding by their previously expressed wishes, engaging with surrogate decision makers they have nominated, and always continuing to communicate what is happening to them when they are aware of their surroundings, for example. Women may have impaired capacity during labour, although this should never be assumed as something inherent to labour. It is always the goal to have a person engage in their decision making as much as possible, so where time may allow capacity to return (and that time is available) or an intervention may improve a person's capacity, this should be attempted before alternatives to direct patient involvement in decision making are used.

One of the criticisms of autonomy has been the overly individualistic way that it has been interpreted and applied (Stirrat & Gill, 2005). To counter this, relational autonomy was described by feminist philosophers. Relational autonomy recognises that people are not isolated individuals living in a vacuum but are rather relational beings who make decisions under the influence (both positive and negative) of their various relationships where they depend on and are depended on by others and in the context of varied histories and cultures (Christman, 2004). This means when engaging in shared decision making with a person, being aware of what influences their decision making can help in supporting them to make choices that align with their values and goals.

Beneficence

The principle of **beneficence** relates to a health professional's fiduciary duty to the person they are caring for: to act in ways that put that person first and prioritise their wellbeing and interests. For midwives, this is at the core of the partnership model (Pairman, 2010). It can be complicated when the dyad that is the pregnant woman and baby have competing needs, known as maternal-fetal conflict (Fasouliotis & Schenker, 2000). This can occur in cases where either the pregnant woman or the baby have an illness or injury that requires intervention that is in some way harmful to the other party; examples include cancer treatment for pregnant women or surgery for babies. These are often tragic and challenging situations that require a midwife to support the person through very difficult decision making and experiences.

It should also be noted that the best thing to do in a given situation is not always clear. Sometimes a person's autonomous decision making may not align with what clinically would be considered in their best interests. A person has the freedom to make poor choices. This is of course complicated in the case of pregnant women by the fact that their choices affect both themselves and their babies. These are situations in which ethical analysis and deliberation will be required and a process for this is discussed fully in the section Ethical Decision-Making in Practice.

Non-maleficence

Non-maleficence is the equal and opposite principle to beneficence. It prescribes that health professionals should do no harm. The most obvious understanding of the principle is to avoid causing pain, injury (short- or long-term) and death. However, there are also other kinds of harms that health professionals can cause in their interactions with the people they care for, and these include causing stigma, psychological harm (from discrimination, for example), and breaches of privacy or trust. All health professionals—and, therefore, midwives—are obligated to treat everyone with respect. It is not acceptable to treat a person differently based on your personal beliefs or judgments about their identity, lifestyle/behaviours, religion, and so on. It is your responsibility to be as caring for a pregnant woman who might, for example, be incarcerated as you are for a pregnant woman who might be a charity worker. They both equally require your professional support in their birthing journey to bring their baby into the world and they have a human right to that support enshrined by law.[c]

Justice

The principle of not harming people (non-maleficence) through judgmental and discriminatory practices, language, and behaviours is also related to issues of justice. The principle of justice dictates that all people should receive fair and equal treatment. Justice can be considered at the client–practitioner level (in midwifery, the partnership) and the system–society level.

At the client–practitioner level justice is about equal and fair treatment. This is the idea that what resources and support you utilise in your care of a woman is not determined by your personal biases, but by your client's needs. This is fundamental to all healthcare. This is also sometimes referred to as equitable care. Health equity is:

> *... the absence of systematic disparities in health (or in the major social determinants of health) between social groups who have different levels of underlying social advantage / disadvantage—that is, different positions in a social hierarchy. Inequities in health systematically put groups of people who are already socially disadvantaged (for example, by virtue of being poor, female, and / or members of a disenfranchised racial, ethnic, or religious group) at further disadvantage with respect to their health; health is essential to wellbeing and to overcoming other effects of social disadvantage.*
>
> (Braveman & Gruskin, 2003)

This means that sometimes you will treat people differently to be just. One person may need more or different support to achieve the same outcome. They may need services tailored in different ways to account for their circumstances. Treating people in our care differently based on their needs is not unfair and, in fact, where treatment is responsive to a person's culture, socioeconomic standing or education, it is most just. Culturally unsafe care is clinically unsafe care.[d]

Midwives involved in policy making, planning or resource allocation issues may also be involved in systemic-level decision making. Systems can also provide more or less justice. Equity should always be a key measure of whether something is the right decision or not. This means ensuring that the resources you prioritise or the service you design account for the needs of the diversity of the people you serve in the fairest way possible using ethical analysis, reasoning and justification.

Justice is closely tied to ideas of human rights. For pregnant and birthing people, reproductive rights are central to their ability to live their lives. Reproductive justice, a concept coined by black feminists in the US context, encompasses the range of rights a person has concerning contraception, birthing, fertility and the ability to parent in safety (Hill, 2008). A midwife can support pregnant and birthing people to exercise these rights through providing information, shared decision making, and care.

Justice is as important as autonomy in the provision of care to people. Beneficence and non-maleficence are principles that help us to weigh what our duties are to prioritise wellbeing and avoid harm and balance the various risks and benefits actions may present for a person. Together these principles help us to unpack situations and pay attention to a variety of competing demands. By being able to explicitly identify these demands, we can be clearer in a path to a solution.

Applying theories and principles

One particular application for ethical analysis and reasoning that is often discussed in midwifery and obstetric care is informed consent and informed choice.

Informed consent

In clinical practice, one of the key ways we respect autonomy is to provide those we care for with **informed consent**. Informed consent in clinical settings is both a process and a legal / administrative step. Informed consent in healthcare is sought for any medical intervention, such as prescribing medications, surgical intervention or diagnostic testing. Informed consent requires a conversation and, for some tasks, documentation. Informed consent requires:
1. capacity (as previously discussed)
2. disclosure
3. understanding
4. voluntariness.

Disclosure and understanding are the content of shared decision making. Informed consent conversations include disclosure of all the relevant information to make a decision: the options available (including in some cases doing nothing), the various risks and benefits associated with the options, both short- and long-term, and the assessment of how these options align with a person's expressed needs, values or goals. Throughout this conversation, a practitioner should be assessing how well a person understands the information being provided, giving extra explanation and clarification as needed. These conversations may occur in a single encounter, but in some contexts will happen over the course of many encounters; this is especially the case for midwifery, where the woman's options and preferences may be discussed over many weeks or months before a decision is reached.

Voluntariness dictates that the person in our care is free from external coercion or pressures in making their decisions. These pressures can come from families, but can also come from health professionals, including midwives. Ensuring you are not pressuring or overly influencing a person you are caring for in their decision making in a way that undermines their autonomy is important. Equally important is advocating for that person when you are in situations where others may be trying to coerce or pressure them.

One of the areas where informed consent is often (somewhat falsely) questioned is during labour—are people in pain, who might be exhausted or distressed, capable of providing consent? Do they have the capacity to do so?

The assumption should always be that a person does have capacity to consent unless proven otherwise. It should also be clear that when good information sharing has happened early on and frequently during pregnancy, consent conversations during labour can be simpler and more justifiable.

Informed choice

Traditionally, women do not provide informed consent for vaginal birth. They will provide informed consent for surgical interventions, for analgesia, and for other delivery interventions dependent on the circumstances (in some situations, consent is not sought justified by the presence of an emergency). However, some obstetricians have argued for a formal informed consent process (both the conversational element and a legal / administrative step) for vaginal delivery, on the basis that it comes with significant risks with varying short- and long-term outcomes, and these should be properly discussed with each woman when they make their choices regarding their mode of delivery (Dietz & Callaghan, 2018). Research on birth trauma has shown that not knowing what will likely occur and what the outcomes of differing choices may be may contribute to women's negative experiences (Kitzinger & Kitzinger, 2007; Priddis et al., 2018).

Vaginal birth is a natural process and requires **informed choice** rather than informed consent. Informed choice involves many of the same conversations that occur in informed consent processes using shared decision-making approaches. Midwifery supports this process with women in partnership. It may sometimes be the case that a vaginal birth will require medical intervention; that does not mean that the vaginal birth requires informed consent. It does mean that women should be made aware of potential risks and interventions early and have full and helpful conversations about what these are, their risks and benefits (for baby and mother). Doing so respects a person's autonomy by ensuring that the decisions they make for themselves and their baby are in line with their needs, values and goals. Midwives are well-placed to have many of these discussions while creating birth plans. Being fully informed also allows women to be better placed to make decisions in the context of labour, further supporting their ability to exercise their autonomy in challenging circumstances. When midwives are in hospital settings with women they are caring for, they may also need to advocate for them to other healthcare professionals where they know a woman's preferences and the woman is unable to advocate for herself. This calls on a midwife to embody the values of the profession (also justified by virtue ethics) while protecting a woman's right to make decisions for herself (autonomy).

ETHICAL DECISION MAKING IN PRACTICE

The aim of ethical decision making is to reason through, decide upon and communicate the ethical justification for a clinically appropriate action(s) that meets the person's goals of care while ensuring respect for all parties' values in situations of conflict or uncertainty.

Some ethical decisions are simple and made quickly in everyday practice with the people we care for and our colleagues, but in some cases, an ethical dilemma emerges that requires a thorough and thoughtful process to reach a solution. This can be the case in midwifery where the care of a woman and her baby can come into conflict, or different health professionals come into conflict (amongst other complexities).

The previous theories and principles outlined in this chapter will feed into this process—they help us to analyse and understand what is at stake and what can be balanced. The following steps are described linearly, but in practice often occur in parallel and with some back-and-forth as more aspects of a particular situation become clear or raise more questions. While the reasoning process itself may be dynamic and iterative, an ethical justification provided to others for a recommendation (or recommendations) should be clear and comprehensive. It should succinctly identify what the issue was (*Identification*), what information decision making rested on (*Information gathering*), what the options were (*Options*), how these options aligned with various appeals (*Appeals*) and why a certain solution(s) was the best choice in the given circumstance (*Recommendation*) (Bruce et al., 2015).[e] A succinct summary of this reasoning and justification should be documented.

Identification

Some ethical dilemmas or decision-making points are obvious: there are two (or more) ethically justifiable courses of action that contradict each other.

Alternatively, in less obvious situations, a midwife may intuit that there is an ethical issue at stake, but they are not able to identify it specifically. Ethical intuitions are phenomena that combine emotions, knowledge and various cues from the social environment to spontaneously arrive at a judgment without explicit reasoning being available to the person who has the intuition (Allman & Woodward, 2008). Intuitions, therefore, are grounded in information, but because that information is not transparent to the person having the intuition it cannot be assessed as to its relevance or truth. The information intuitions rest on can be mistaken, biased or outdated (McMahan, 2013). Intuitions should be

considered starting points in identification but further investigation and analysis are necessary.[f]

Multiple ethical issues may also occur at the same time. It is important to identify all issues separately even though they will likely require parallel consideration in their resolution.

Appropriate identification is crucial in setting the parameters of information gathering.

Information gathering

Once a midwife or healthcare team identifies the ethical issue at stake, they should aim to collect all relevant information to understand the situation. Relevant information will vary by case and setting but will include a combination of:

- a woman's values and goals of care
- a woman's cultural, social and financial situation relevant to the clinical encounter (regarding support required, or access to services, etc.)
- birth plans or where appropriate advanced care-planning, or advanced psychiatric care planning documentation
- information regarding surrogate decision makers, medical power of attorneys (MPOAs) or guardians
- if a person lacks capacity, loved ones' and appropriate decision maker's opinions regarding the situation, noting that a substituted judgment (what would this person do if they could make the decision themselves) or best interest standard (what provides the best clinical outcome, where a person's preferences are not known) should guide the formal decision maker depending on what information is available
- clinical options available, including risks and benefits, short- and long-term outcomes, etc. (this should also include healthcare team differences of opinion regarding these aspects)
- professional and institutional guidelines relevant to the case
- legal constraints on action.

The sources of this information will be manifold and will vary case-by-case. Ideally, information about a person in your care should be collected directly from that person or, when they are unable to provide it, directly from their appointed representatives.

Information gathering is likely to continue throughout the process as new options and their viability are considered or the person's preferences inform the prioritisation of appeals, and require further information to evaluate.

Options

Options for action will sometimes be apparent early on, but new options may be explored in the process of trying to resolve the situation. Each option for action should be grounded in the information available and be supported or constrained by the appeals (see next step) relevant to it.

It is in this stage that *ethical imagination* (also called 'moral imagination') is engaged (Carson, 2003). Ethical imagination is a combination of empathy and creativity used to think through the position of others and the outcomes of various actions. While ethical decision making will sometimes be conducted by a midwife in isolation with a woman in their care or their decision maker, it can also involve bringing together a team of relevant people to discuss options and their appeals, or engaging a hospital's clinical ethics consultation service, if available. Diverse perspectives can help, broaden or add specifics to the reasoning process and therefore improve the responsiveness of recommendations. Potential people to include in these discussions might be members of woman's care team (for example, family, other midwives, obstetricians, general practitioner), professionals in the person's life related to their religion or culture, or other midwives or obstetric specialists who have not been involved in the particular person's care (being mindful of privacy requirements).

Appeals

Each option and its consequences arrived at in the previous step must be weighed against the *appeals* it addresses: those ethical, legal and professional principles, concepts, rules or standards that apply in a healthcare setting and provide either justification for or reasons against actions. Appeals will include:
- ethical principles and concepts such as those outlined earlier
- legal principles, concepts, and regulations, such as the best interest standard, privacy laws, human rights, etc.
- institutional policies (including those of the institution where a woman is receiving care, a place of discharge, health insurers, government agencies, etc.)
- professional codes of conduct, standards or guidelines
- cultural norms and considerations
- health practitioner values or virtues.

The midwife / team should then assess each option to understand which appeals justify or contradict a particular course of action. In working through the options and their potential appeals, a clear understanding of how these relate to a woman's values or goals is required. This may require ongoing conversation with the woman or may have to occur with their decision maker.

Consultation with further parties may also be necessary. Where a midwife is working in a hospital they may seek their institution's legal assistance to help explain relevant legislative or regulatory details that apply. Similarly, help from an institution's spiritual or cultural services may be helpful to gain a better understanding of these aspects of a situation. Seeking outside consultation on specific elements to ensure a full understanding is encouraged where practically feasible.

Through this process of aligning options with appeals, some options may easily become dismissible due to inflexible constraints (such as regulations or funding, etc.). Depending on the nature of the case, it is possible that only one option aligns with appropriate appeals satisfactorily. However, it is more likely that two or more options may align with appeals in a way that provides justification for them as a course of action. This is dealt with at the recommendations stage.

Recommendations

Shared decision making is central to midwifery practice. In some complex ethical situations, as described above, some of the discussions may also happen with other parties to assess what are ethically justifiable courses of action. Even for relatively simple ethical dilemmas managed in a one-on-one process between a midwife and the person they are caring for, being able to describe what is ethically justifiable is important. Given the steps described here, a midwife or team with the woman being cared for may arrive at one option for action that is justified by a set of appeals (with a list of other options that are not possible because of the constraints of certain appeals). The described process ensured that this course of action was informed by the various stakeholders' considerations, including the woman in care, which play a central role. This option is then the recommendation for action and the midwife should discuss this with the woman (or their decision maker) explaining the reasoning for this course of action and seek their consent (which may be declined) to proceed. Where the issue is not a consent-related action, the midwife should communicate this to relevant parties. This communication should use the work done throughout these steps to succinctly explain and provide justification for the option chosen.

More often in complex cases, deliberations result in several options with different justificatory appeals. The midwife or team presents these options as recommendations to either the person in their care or the relevant parties that have to take the action. As before, this should be done with the same degree of communication about what led to these recommendations and what justifies them. In those situations, where women and / or their loved ones should be involved in the final deliberation of recommendations, this should proceed as in any other shared decision-making scenario. Where the situation is not a matter of client consent, then discussion with the relevant parties who have to decide on an action should proceed similarly, with a more explicit discussion about the appeals relevant to those particular decision makers.

The key to deciding between a variety of options with differing appeals is understanding what justifications are given higher importance or priority and what things are more acceptably compromised in the particular setting, with the particular stakeholders (ideally through shared deliberation), in the particular context.

While the description provided here is thorough and may sound complex, what this looks like in practice will vary hugely depending on the nature of the ethical dilemma itself and time constraints. Sometimes gathering relevant information and balancing the options versus appeals to meet the woman's values may be done in a conversation or two, while in complex cases this might involve multiple meetings with various stakeholders or in multidisciplinary teams. This is dependent on the context and case. The process is set out here to make explicit what will often happen as a matter of course and somewhat implicitly by experienced practitioners.

The ethics of ethical decision making

Process alone will not ensure that decision making is *conducted* ethically. There is a difference between the steps someone might take to resolve an ethical issue and the manner in which they undertake those steps. Midwives should aim to pay attention to the following behaviours and attitudes in their approach:

1. *openness*—be open to new information and ideas, from a variety of sources
2. *reflexivity*—consider your position explicitly, what perspectives and potential biases might influence your view;
3. *impartiality*—treat like situations alike; this requires a balance between objectivity in your handling of information while being responsive to an individual person's situations and needs
4. *transparency*—communicate clearly the actions and reasons taken throughout the process to affected parties to ensure they feel informed and fairly dealt with
5. *cultural humility*—engage in interpersonal thinking and actions that are responsive to the aspects of a person's cultural identity that are important to them, where culture is broadly understood (Hook et al., 2013)
6. *integrity*—be honest and trustworthy in your actions.

Ethical decision making marred by miscommunication, deception or prejudices cannot lead to ethically justifiable courses of action.

MORAL DISTRESS

Moral distress, first defined by Jameton (1984) in the nursing literature, is a particular psychological response to situations in which health professionals identify what they believe to be the (ethically) right course of action in a given situation, but they feel unable to take the action because of institutional constraints. Morley (2018) later broadened this definition so that it also included situations of ambiguity or uncertainty. By Morley's definition, moral distress may occur whenever a health practitioner encounters 'a moral event, experiences psychological distress, and the two are causally linked' (Morley, 2018). This means that health practitioners may feel moral distress also in scenarios where constraints may not be institutional or systemic: the right thing to do may not be evident even after investigation, or what is determined as a course of action seems to be the choice between equally poor options.

Moral distress is being explored in midwifery practice. Researchers have found that midwives feel moral distress when there are issues of uncertainty and constraints on their ability to advocate for women in their care, themselves and their profession (Foster et al., 2021). Midwifery is inherently relational in its commitment to the empowerment of women in their care through shared decision making and relationships of trust, but it also operates within systems that have power imbalances at their core (Oelhafen, 2020) and this can lead to experiences that cause moral distress.

Moral distress may be linked to burnout and staff turnover (Fumis et al., 2017; Lamiani et al., 2017). It is therefore important for individuals and institutions to be aware of moral distress and consider ways in which to address it. Engaging in explicit moral deliberation with colleagues and peers throughout the process can help individual practitioners have a clearer understanding of why decisions were made and their role, as well as being able to voice and explain their views. Reflective practice and debriefing exercises after experiencing moral distress may be useful in working through difficult feelings. This may take the form of journalling, counselling or team debriefs, for example. Self-care practices generally recommended to relieve stress and remain healthy as a health practitioner are also likely to be helpful. Lastly, advocating for change in constraints that are amenable to change may help midwives experiencing moral distress regain a sense of moral agency in their work.

Conclusion

Midwifery provides a crucial service to childbearing women and babies who will experience it variably as one of the most challenging, vulnerable, exciting and beautiful times of their lives. In its philosophy of relational practice, trust and empowerment midwifery centres the women it serves. To understand the ethical standards of one's profession and to be able to apply them in practice is a core competency for any health professional. To do this well requires not only knowing the codes of ethics of the profession but also how to apply them and ethically reason through and communicate justifiable actions. Midwives along with other health professionals can do this best when they use the tools of bioethics to identify ethical issues and relevant values, apply theories and principles to relevant information to understand the situation, deliberate on various appeals and constraints, and describe and justify ethically sound recommendations. Ethical knowledge and reasoning are much like clinical reasoning and knowledge, something that is capable of ongoing development and improvement.

REFLECTIVE CASE STUDY

Lily is a 33-year-old woman who is 28 weeks pregnant. Lily has been living with medically managed schizophrenia for four years. Once she became pregnant she chose to forego her regular medication despite advice that continuation was safe for her and the baby, because she didn't want to take any risk. You have worked with Lily on creating a birth plan and she wants to ideally give birth at home as she has a distrust of hospitals based on some of her experiences around her mental health. She is supported by her partner, Vanessa, who lives with her and attends most appointments with her.

Lily calls you and says she is worried as she is having some dizziness and heart racing that she finds worrying, but she does not want to go to hospital.

What are important ethical considerations in deciding how best to care for Lily both in terms of her immediate need and considering her long-term needs?

Case discussion

Working through the steps described in this chapter, think through:

- What information do you know and what information do you need to know?

This will include the clinical information about Lily's symptoms and help determine the urgency of the situation, but will also include trying to gain an understanding of Lily's capacity at this point in time and her decision making (it shouldn't be assumed she lacks capacity because of her mental health diagnosis).

- Based on the information you have available, what are the options in this situation?

It's important when thinking about options to not fall back on a binary—do X or don't do X. Often there are a many compromises or workarounds that can be worked out to accommodate a variety of ethical appeals and constraints.

- Consider what are the ethical, legal, and professional appeals and constraints on action in this situation

A course of action needs to be found here that appropriately respects Lily's needs and expressed wishes (autonomy and beneficence), while taking into account the safety of herself and her baby (beneficence / non-maleficence) depending on the severity / urgency of her situation, her decision-making capacity and what can be done.

- What other people may be helpful here (that can be involved with Lily's consent)?

Her partner is an important person in this scenario and especially if Lily's capacity to make decisions is impaired. But it may also be the case that throughout your time caring for Lily you have established relationships with her mental healthcare professional or her GP, they may also be helpful partners in this situation depending on the direction it takes.

Ultimately this case may resolve in many different ways dependent on factors that are currently uncertain. What should be paramount is respect for Lily and her expressed wishes and the safety of Lily and her baby. These factors shouldn't be considered as immutable and in conflict (i.e. that only one can be achieved) but rather as twin goals that need to be achieved together through compromise.

Review questions

1. What are the three foci of traditional ethical theories?
2. What constitutes decision-making capacity?
3. What are the four core principles in healthcare ethics?
4. What is relational autonomy?
5. What is informed choice?
6. What are the elements of good ethical decision making?

NOTES

a. 'We' is used here to speak collectively of people working in healthcare settings. I speak from the position of a clinical ethicist, but readers will be (student) midwives or may have different roles.

b. 'Western' is the term used in the bioethics literature, though it is imperfect.

c. Laws vary by country but the basic right to healthcare and non-discrimination exists in both Australia and New Zealand.

d. Phrase often used by Assoc. Prof. Lilon Bandler in talks, teaching, etc.

e. The framework set out here draws on Bruce et al., 2015. It has been adapted for this particular context but the main elements Identification, Options, Appeals and Recommendations are set out in their original work.

f. It should also be noted that people may have an ethical intuition as to what the right thing to do is in a given scenario (i.e. not just identification of an ethical issue). However, this too, requires investigation in order to ensure that it can be justified and does not rest on biases, misjudgments or mistaken information.

Online resources

Australian College of Midwives: http://www.midwives.org.au/.
Australian Nursing and Midwifery Council: https://anmac.org.au/.
International Confederation of Midwives: https://www.internationalmidwives.org/.
Midwifery Council of New Zealand: https://www.midwiferycouncil.health.nz/.
New Zealand College of Midwives: https://www.midwife.org.nz/.
Nursing and Midwifery Council, UK: https://www.nmc.org.uk/.

References

Abbott P, Meerabeau L. Professionals, professionalization and the caring professions. In: *The Sociology of the Caring Professions*. London: Routledge; 2020:1–19.

Allman J, Woodward J. What are moral intuitions and why should we care about them? A neurobiological perspective. *Philos Issues*. 2008;18:164–85.

Bardill J, Garrison NA. New words and old stories: Indigenous teachings in health care and bioethics. *AJOB*. 2016;16(5):50–2.

Barrett DH, W Ortmann L, Dawson A, et al. *Public Health Ethics: Cases Spanning the Globe*. Springer Open; 2016. doi:10.1007/978-3-319-23847-0.

Beauchamp TL, Childress JF. *Principles of Biomedical Ethics*. New York: Oxford University Press; 2001.

Braveman P, Gruskin S. Defining equity in health. *J Epidemiology Community Health*. 2003;57(4):254–8. Online: https://jech.bmj.com/content/57/4/254.

Bruce CR. *A Practical Guide to Developing and Sustaining a Clinical Ethics Consultation Service*. Baylor College of Medicine, Center for Medical Ethics & Health Policy; 2015.

Carson, RA. Educating the moral imagination. In: *Practicing the Medical Humanities: Engaging Physicians and Patients*. Hagerstown, MD: University Publishing Group, 2003.

Christman J. Relational autonomy, liberal individualism, and the social constitution of selves. *Philos Stud*. 2004;117(1/2):143–64.

Comartin EB. Dissonance between personal and professional values: Resolution of an ethical dilemma. *J Soc Work Values Ethics*. 2011;8(2):1–14.

Dietz HP, Callaghan S. We need to treat pregnant women as adults: women should be consented for an attempt at normal vaginal birth as for operative delivery, with risks and potential complications explained. *ANZCOG*. 2018;58(6):701–3.

Fasouliotis SJ, Schenker JG. Maternal–fetal conflict. *Eur J Obstet Gynecol*. 2000;89(1):101–7.

Foster W, McKellar L, Fleet JA, et al. Exploring moral distress in Australian midwifery practice. *Women Birth*. 2021. doi:10.1016/j.wombi.2021.09.006.

Fumis RR, Amarante GA, de Fátima Nascimento A, et al. Moral distress and its contribution to the development of burnout syndrome among critical care providers. *Ann Intensive Care*. 2017; 7(1):1–8.

Garland-Thomson R. Disability bioethics: From theory to practice. *Kennedy Inst Ethics J*. 2017; 27(2):323–39.

Hill BJ. Reproductive rights as health care rights. *Colum J Gender & L*. 2008;18:501.

Hook JN, Davis DE, Owen J, et al. Cultural humility: Measuring openness to culturally diverse clients. *J Couns Psychol*. 2013; 60(3):353.

International Confederation of Midwives (ICM). *The International Code of Ethics for Midwives*. 2008. Online: https://www.internationalmidwives.org/assets/files/general-files/2019/10/eng-international-code-of-ethics-for-midwives.pdf.

Jameton A. *Nursing practice: The ethical issues*. Englewood Cliffs, NJ: Prentice Hall, 1984.

Kitzinger C, Kitzinger S. Birth trauma: Talking with women and the value of conversation analysis. *Br J Midwifery*. 2007;15(5):256–64.

Lamiani G, Borghi L, Argentero P. When healthcare professionals cannot do the right thing: A systematic review of moral distress and its correlates. *J Health Psychol*. 2017;22(1):51–67.

Leach Scully J, Baldwin-Ragaven LE, Fitzpatrick. *Feminist Bioethics: At the Center, on the Margins*. Baltimore, MD: The John Hopkins University Press; 2010.

McMahan J, Moral intuition. In: LaFollette H, Persson I, eds. *The Blackwell Guide to Ethical Theory*. West Sussex: John Wiley & Sons; 2013:103–121.

McNeill PM, Macklin R, Wasunna A, et al. An expanding vista: bioethics from public health, indigenous and feminist perspectives. *Med J Aust*. 2005;183:8–9.

Morley G: What is "moral distress" in nursing? How, can and should we respond to it? *J Clin Nurse*. 2018;27(19–20):3443.

Morley G, Field R, Horsburgh CC, et al. Interventions to mitigate moral distress: a systematic review of the literature. *Int J Nurs Stud*. 2021. doi:10.1016/j.ijnurstu.2021.103984.

Morley G, Bradbury-Jones C, Ives J. Reasons to redefine moral distress: A feminist empirical bioethics analysis. *Bioethics*. 2021; 35(1):61–71.

New Zealand College of Midwives. *Philosophy and Code of Ethics*. 1993 (updated 2002, 2005, 2008, 2015). Online: https://www.midwife.org.nz/midwives/professional-practice/philosophy-and-code-of-ethics/.

Nursing and Midwifery Board of Australia (NMBA). *Code of Conduct for Midwives*. Melbourne: NMBA; 2018.

Oelhafen S, Cignacco E. Moral distress and moral competences in midwifery: a latent variable approach. *J Health Psychol*. 2020;25(13–14):2340–51.

Pairman, S. Midwifery partnership: a professionalizing strategy for midwives. In: Kirkham M, ed. *The Midwife-Mother Relationship*. Macmillan International Higher Education; 2010.

Priddis HS, Keedle H, Dahlen H. The Perfect Storm of Trauma: The experiences of women who have experienced birth trauma and subsequently accessed residential parenting services in Australia. *Women Birth*. 2018;31(1):17–24.

Russell CA. Questions of race in bioethics: Deceit, disregard, disparity, and the work of decentering. *Philosophy Compass*. 2016;11(1):43–55.

Stirrat GM, Gill R. Autonomy in medical ethics after O'Neill. *J Med Ethics*. 2005;31(3):127–30.

Villarmea S, Kelly B. Barriers to establishing shared decision-making in childbirth: Unveiling epistemic stereotypes about women in labour. *J Eval Clin Pract*. 2020;26(2):515–9.

Further reading

McDougall R, Delany C, Spriggs M, et al. Collaboration in clinical ethics consultation: a method for achieving "balanced accountability". *Am J Bioeth*. 2014;14(6):47–48.

Rogers WA, Mills C, Scully JL, et al. *The Routledge Handbook of Feminist Bioethics*. Routledge; 2022.

Ross LJ, Solinger R. *Reproductive Justice: An Introduction*. Oakland: University of California Press; 2017.

Staunton PJ, Staunton P, Chiarella M. *Law for Nurses and Midwives*. Sydney: Elsevier Australia; 2012.

CHAPTER 16

Supporting midwives, supporting each other

Andrea Gilkison and Leonie Hewitt

LEARNING OUTCOMES

Learning outcomes for this chapter are:

1. To describe the benefits for women and for society of a sustainable midwifery profession
2. To explore the concepts of 'self-care' and 'work–life balance' in relation to sustaining midwifery practice
3. To reflect on how to be a sustainable midwife practitioner
4. To explore the midwife–midwife partnership relationship.

CHAPTER OVERVIEW

Midwifery is an incredibly rewarding profession, and midwives wherever they practise make a huge contribution to the health of mothers and babies, their families and communities. Midwives work in a diverse range of settings, contexts and models of care. Midwives may be self-employed, providing continuity of care, or be employed in a maternity facility; may work in urban, rural or remote rural settings; may practise in primary, secondary or tertiary maternity services; or may work in educational or research institutions. Whatever the role, each brings its own set of rewards, demands, issues and challenges.

In this chapter sustainable midwifery practice is explored, with discussion about the meaning of sustainable practice, and the importance of sustainability for midwives and midwifery. The practicalities of how midwives sustain and support each other in practice are explored separately for caseloading and employed midwives. Although there are similarities for midwives wherever they work, there are different considerations of what can help to sustain midwives during their career. Relationships and networks are identified as important to sustainability, with the partnership relationship explored to determine how it can work to promote sustainability, both between the woman and her midwife and also between midwives. Negotiating and developing respectful **professional relationships** can lead to improved support and sustainability for each individual midwife and the profession as a whole. Finally, two case studies are provided, one from Aotearoa New Zealand and the other from Australia, showing how midwifery models of practice can work to sustain each other.

KEY TERMS

boundaries
bullying
generosity of spirit
partnership

practice arrangements
professional relationships
resilience
self-care

sustainable midwifery
work–life balance

INTRODUCTION

Midwifery is a profession that brings a range of demands, issues and challenges that are experienced differently depending on each midwife's individual circumstances and her midwifery role. For example, some midwives working in a tertiary unit may find the intensity of continuously providing care to often highly complex women challenging. Alternatively, for caseloading midwives, the unpredictability of being easily accessible and frequently on call may be the challenge.

Whatever the role, the kinds of challenges and issues that arise for each individual midwife will be different, but there are frequently common threads which can support and sustain midwifery practice. It is important for each midwife to think about and discuss working in ways which are sustainable for her as an individual as well as the profession as a whole.

DEFINING SUSTAINABLE PRACTICE

This chapter focuses on midwifery sustainability rather than environmental sustainability, although both are equally important. Midwifery is an essential role and can influence the drive for social change that is necessary to promote environmentally sustainable strategies. In order to do that though, midwives need to be able to sustain themselves within their work.

Any discussion about **sustainable midwifery** needs to include a shared understanding of some of the key terms being used. The verb 'to sustain' means to:

Keep in existence; maintain, continue, or prolong, to keep up competently, to supply with necessities, to support spirits, vitality and to encourage.
(Farlex, 2020; http://www.thefreedictionary.com/)

'Sustainability' is a term often used in environmental science and means:

The ability to be maintained at a steady level without exhausting natural resources or causing severe ecological damage.
(Farlex, 2020; http://www.thefreedictionary.com/)

So the underlying principle of sustainability is that it 'continues to exist whilst maintaining the integrity of mental and physical wellbeing' (McAra-Couper et al., 2014, p. 29). This is what this chapter is all about: how midwives individually and as a profession continue to exist and maintain physical and mental health. Crowther et al. (2016) have said that 'sustainability is the capacity of systems or processes to maintain balance and endure' (p. 41). The word 'endure' when applied to midwives evokes the idea of continuing to practise in the face of the difficulties and adversities encountered in practice. Enduring in midwifery practice has been referred to as being resilient and is often related to the sustainability of the profession.

RESILIENCE AND SUSTAINABILITY IN MIDWIFERY

'Resilience' is a term that is frequently used during discussions on sustainability (and vice versa) and has come to the forefront of recent literature, with the suggestion that being resilient is an important feature of midwifery practice. Hunter & Warren (2014) define resilience as 'the ability of an individual to respond positively and consistently to adversity, using effective coping strategies' (p. 927). Resilience then can be interpreted as implying that the job is difficult, and midwives need to find ways to cope in a work setting that may be challenging and then bounce back and resume normal practice as soon as possible.

While an element of resilience is very important to sustain midwifery, it could also be argued that there should be a limit to what midwives should be expected to endure. For example, when there are staff shortages, should midwives individually continue to carry increasing responsibilities whatever the personal cost?

There are themes which traverse both sustainability and resilience, and which are important facets of sustainable midwifery practice. Table 16.1 identifies the different features of sustainability and resilience and how they differ in language and expectation.

CRITICAL THINKING EXERCISE

What are some of the ways that midwives can build their own resilience to support sustainable practice?

REFLECTIVE THINKING EXERCISE

With a friend, think about the terms 'sustainability' and 'resilience'.

- Can you think of times when a midwife may need to be resilient in her midwifery practice?
- What strategies could help midwives develop sustainability?
- How does the definition of resilience differ from that of sustainability?
- Many midwives enjoy midwifery because of the constantly changing nature of the work. What situations do you think would increase challenges for midwives? What would help you deal with a constantly changing and challenging work environment?

It appears that sustainability and resilience in midwifery practice are about maintaining a balance on the level of the individual midwife, maternity facilities, and the midwifery profession.

Table 16.1 Features of sustainability and resilience	
Sustainability	Resilience
Concerned with maintaining balance	Ability to withstand or recover quickly from difficult conditions and/or events
Avoidance of depletion and focus on conserving, ensuring something can continue to exist	Ability to hold steady or recover following difficult events
Ability to maintain integrity of mental, physical, emotional and environmental aspects of individual and organisation/institution	Individual resilience can contribute to the formation of resilient organisations/communities that lead to habitual protective mechanisms and strategies to deal with adverse and difficult events
Ensuring that practices and strategies are able to be maintained over time without harm to persons and environment	Resilient practices and strategies allows individuals and organisations/communities to continue despite circumstances
Working sustainably allows for practice to be nourishing and enable those involved to flourish and enjoy what they doing over time	Resilient working behaviours may or may not be nourishing and may or may not allow others to flourish over time
Sustainable practices/strategies lead to positive and effective long-term ability to work resiliently throughout times of adversity that acknowledges others as part of that process	Resilient responses can be consistently positive and effective in managing stress and adversity that may or may not acknowledge others as part of that process

(Adapted from Crowther et al., 2016, p. 44)

Midwifery as a socially sustainable profession

Midwifery is inherently a social model of care, which is unusual amongst healthcare services in that midwives do not work with sick people but with women who are generally well and healthy, and for whom pregnancy and birth are normal life events. Within recent history, in many countries around the world midwives and women have fought to regain or maintain autonomy for the midwifery profession; New Zealand is one such example. The **partnership** model of midwifery care developed in this country is a reflection of women and midwives working together to successfully achieve autonomy for the midwifery profession (Guilliland & Pairman, 2010).

Midwifery as a profession can add to the social sustainability of a population in a number of ways, by reducing maternal and neonatal mortality and morbidity (Nove et al., 2021), reducing interventions and supporting a positive experience for mothers and babies (Davis et al., 2011; United Nations Population Fund (UNFPA) et al., 2021). The report *The State of the World's Midwifery* (UNFPA et al., 2021) aims to ensure that all women will have available, accessible, acceptable and high-quality midwifery care. Access to high-quality, well-resourced midwifery care can reduce maternal and infant mortality (Nove et al., 2021).

In parts of the world which face rising intervention rates, again it is midwives who can help to keep birth normal (Sandall et al., 2016), which not only reduces the economic cost, but also improves satisfaction for both women and midwives (Downe et al., 2019; East et al., 2019). Midwifery therefore needs to be sustained so that all women have access to quality midwifery care.

Being a midwife requires many interpersonal skills such as empathy and compassion, effective communication, and an ability to work autonomously and take responsibility for decisions made. Being a midwife is a joyous, profound, energising, satisfying, life-affirming profession. It can also at times be stressful, tiring, challenging, demanding and hard work. As a midwife you regularly witness the birth of a baby, of a new mother, of a new father, of a new or enlarged family. In this, midwifery is at once both deeply sacred and profoundly practical, often at the same time (Crowther et al., 2015). Perhaps a midwife's strength is that ability to hold both aspects simultaneously.

For their own emotional health, midwives need to ensure that they are able to continue to do their work in a way that is sustainable for them. Each individual midwife should consider what they personally require to sustain themselves in their work, bearing in mind that this may change over time due to family or other life commitments. This involves understanding the nature and demands of midwifery work and identifying what part of the work provides them with the most satisfaction. They also need to identify what helps them to re-energise and relax so that they come to their work refreshed and prepared and able to work with passion and thoughtfulness. What then are the important elements of sustainability for midwives?

CLINICAL POINT

Sustainable midwifery is intertwined with sustainable birth, and the sustainability of midwifery operates on the level of the individual midwife, the maternity organisation, the midwifery profession and society as a whole.

MIDWIFERY SUSTAINABILITY—SOME KEY PRINCIPLES

There are four key principles of midwifery sustainability: enjoying the work being undertaken (getting a sense of satisfaction from your work); having a good work–life balance; having autonomy over your working life and having good working relationships. These key principles are important to maintain the integrity of the individual midwife's mental and physical wellbeing (McAra-Couper et al., 2014). Shown as the cogs in the wheel in Fig. 16.1, all of these principles work together to support and sustain midwives in their practice. The individual's ability to care for themselves and the practical working arrangements are both essential elements of sustainable practice. If one cog falters, the system will break down.

Work–life balance

Work–life balance is a contemporary concept which identifies the need to balance an individual's work and career with their lifestyle—the things they do outside of work and which bring them pleasure whilst also helping them to relax and re-energise (Table 16.2). This may be things like spending time with family and friends, being able to do sport or physical exercise, and having time to pursue hobbies and other lifestyle-related choices. When one or other element—work or lifestyle—is out of

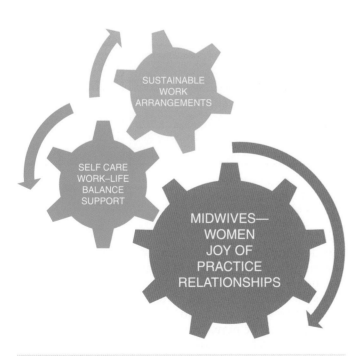

FIGURE 16.1 Key principles of sustainability cog diagram

Table 16.2 Self-awareness and work–life balance	
Self-awareness	Work–life balance
Knowing what sort of person you are	Physical, mental and emotional health
Knowing how you work best	Satisfying lifestyle choices (relaxation and leisure)
The stage of your life which you are at and which way of working fits you and your family best	Family and friends
	Cultural and spiritual dimension

balance there can be a negative effect on the emotional health of the individual.

Donald et al. (2014) undertook action research to support 16 caseloading midwives to improve their work–life balance. This involved focus group discussions to identify and reflect on how they worked and how they could make changes that would support an improved work–life balance. A tool was designed to help caseloading midwives identify whether they had an optimal balance between their work and lifestyle (Fig. 16.2). This tool provides elements to consider which can lead to poor or optimal lifestyle balance.

REFLECTIVE THINKING EXERCISE

Looking at Table 16.2, think about your own self-awareness. Think about the sort of person you are, and your stage of life.

- What kind of midwifery role would suit you the best?
- Can you envisage that this might change as your life circumstances change?
- Now look at the work–life balance side of the table.
- Write a list of things that sustain you in your life: things that you love to do, that bring you joy and pleasure, that make you smile or laugh.
- Reflect on how often you do those things that give you joy, pleasure or relaxation. What stops you from doing them? What supports you doing them?

Self-care

Midwives are dedicated and committed to caring for others, and although it is highly satisfying work, midwifery can also be a demanding profession. Long or irregular hours, shift work, a lot of time on call, irregular and/or insufficient sleep and a significant level of responsibility can all contribute to job-related stress

Work–life Balance (WLB) score for the LMC midwife

Name _____ Date _____

ARE YOU IN THE RED, YELLOW OR GREEN ZONE?			
select the closest description or add your own to fit your situation			

Points	0	1	2	Subtotal choose a point from each criteria
Personal relationships	Not enough time for family No social life Or _____	Difficult to plan activities with family and friends Or _____	Enjoy planned time to spend with family and friends Or _____	
Time off call	Difficult to get cover Or _____	Some cover but not as often as I need it Or _____	Regular cover for days off Or _____	
Group/team work	Work on my own but struggle Or _____	Tension between members Some conflict, difficult to resolve Or _____	Great team work and support Or Happy working on my own and have support if needed Or _____	
Physical wellbeing	Not enough sleep No recreation Poor eating habits Or _____	Struggle at times to catch up on sleep Irregular recreation Irregular eating pattern Or _____	Able to catch up on sleep Regular recreation Healthy eating Or _____	
Life satisfaction	Life is a constant struggle Or _____	Feel up and down Feel guilt if not available for women Or _____	Life feels great Or _____	

0 to 3: Red Zone	Life needs urgent attention! Intervene now before possible burnout.	Total Score
4 to 7: Yellow Zone	The work–life balance needs some attention. Life could be better. Continuing like this could make continuity of care difficult to sustain long term.	
8 to 10: Green Zone	Well done! A great work–life balance. There is enough time for work and enough time to have a personal life and to enjoy both.	

FIGURE 16.2 Work–life balance score for the LMC midwife
(Source: Donald, Smythe & McAra-Crouper, 2014)

(Arbour et al., 2020; Donald et al., 2014; Flo et al., 2012). Midwifery can be an unpredictable life as births follow their own timetable, and the work of a midwife does not finish when the baby is born. It is important that midwives are supported to look after their wellbeing and maintain their work–life balance by keeping physically and mentally healthy, taking regular time off to enjoy leisure and family activities, and having enough holidays each year to be able to rest and recover from the demands placed on them. Midwifery can be all-consuming, so a midwife will bring a more rounded and balanced perspective to practice when there is time to focus on other things, and an enjoyment in life outside of midwifery. There are two vital components to a midwife reducing or managing that potential stress: being self-aware and having work–life balance. (See Ch. 5 for a discussion of the need to use caution when using the term 'self-care'.)

Self-determination and autonomy

Equally important is the need to consider the midwife's autonomy within her midwifery working role. Midwifery autonomy is embedded in midwifery practice in New Zealand and relates to providing care under a midwife's own professional responsibility (Clemons et al., 2021). Midwives are able to work in a diverse array of settings from providing care to a caseload of women to working in small birthing units or large busy maternity hospitals. In addition, they can work in education or research. It is important that midwives are able to change roles during their working careers; a change will often bring new challenges and new learning experiences. When midwives feel that they 'have to' take on extra clients, take on extra shifts, work longer hours, stay in the same role—then there is the potential for the midwife to become overworked and dissatisfied.

Having control over the practice environment is also important to midwives' job satisfaction and sustainability (Clemons et al., 2021; Gilkison, 2014; Gilkison et al., 2017). For example, if core midwives have some control over their shift roster and are able to take annual leave when they request it they have better job satisfaction—these are important issues that contribute to work–life balance.

Despite the high satisfaction that working with women provides, it is also important that midwives are able to ensure their professional and personal lives are integrated and balanced, and therefore can be more easily sustained (McAra-Couper et al., 2014).

Relationships between midwives

Relationships with women provide midwives with high levels of joy and satisfaction from their work. In addition, the relationships that midwives have with their colleagues are equally important and provide the foundation for sustainable midwifery practice in any context.

Collegial relationships can affect how a midwife feels about going to work, can influence how a midwife provides woman-centred care, and can also affect their autonomy and sustainability of the practice or service (Clemons et al., 2021; Gilkison et al., 2015). Midwives work together in a variety of settings—it might be in hospitals, in other institutions or in communities. Collegial relationships are important to midwives no matter what services they work in because such relationships can influence engagement, job satisfaction and support retention within the profession (Catling et al., 2017).

When midwives work in cohesive groups where they enjoy each other's company, the practice or service they work in is more sustainable than those practices where they do not get on (Gilkison et al., 2015). The resource that comes from these social relationships is also known as 'social capital'. The key components of social capital are perceptions of trust, reciprocity and recognition both horizontally and vertically (Stromgren et al., 2016). The culture of an organisation can be one of the most important aspects of a workplace for those that work there and within health

may have an impact on patient outcomes (Braithwaite et al., 2017). Satisfaction with co-workers and interaction opportunities have been associated with work satisfaction and wanting to stay in a role (Jarosova et al., 2016).

Another essential component to midwifery partnerships is a shared philosophy. Catling et al. (2017) found that differing perspectives on risk and philosophies around childbirth can lead to communication breakdown and disrespect. Having a shared philosophy is therefore an essential component to a unified work environment and a key aspect to the midwifery partnership. Supportive midwifery partnerships that are philosophically aligned are a major factor in sustainability of a service or practice (McAra-Couper et al., 2014). Midwives that work in a positive culture have more job satisfaction and are more likely to stay, thereby encouraging sustainability and retention. Supportive midwifery partnerships between midwives enables midwives to work in partnership with women, whether they are providing continuity of care or not. A shared philosophy, trust and a '**generosity of spirit**' are essential to good midwifery partnerships, and in turn can help midwives recover from significant events. No matter what environment midwives choose to work in, their midwifery partnerships will affect the partnerships they have with women, and can affect the profession and the maternity service.

Support

Midwifery at times can be challenging, so it is important for midwives to build a strong support network around themselves. Support can come from midwifery colleagues in caseloading practices and from hospital midwives, from other health professionals and from family and friends. It is important for physical, mental, social and emotional health and personal sustainability to have professional and collegial support. Building support takes time and effort and often these support networks need nurturing too.

While all of these elements of sustainable midwifery are applicable to whatever context midwives are working in, there are some features of sustainable practice which are specific to the type of work and role undertaken—specifically caseloading or core hospital midwives. Table 16.3 summarises sustainable caseloading and core midwifery practice.

DIFFERING ROLES AND SUSTAINABILITY— CASELOADING PRACTICE

For midwives working in caseload practice together, it is important that **practice arrangements** are fair and equitable. This involves the following:

- having fair and regular time off for each team / practice member
- ensuring a manageable caseload for each practice partner

- ensuring fair and equitable ways of working together as a practice
- having regular practice/team meetings
- ensuring that practice arrangements are shared with women
- having a shared midwifery philosophy
- having clear financial arrangements (in self-employed practice).

Having regular and equitable time off is important for each midwife in a practice. This involves discussing how they manage time off and annual leave. Many midwifery practices will plan annual leave in advance so as to ensure they can stagger holidays, and that midwifery care is still available for women in the practice across the year. Also necessary to consider is how to ensure that when a practice member is on leave the others will not be overloaded with work. In New Zealand, midwives in practice together will often arrange to have blocks of 4 weeks leave at a time. They will often reduce bookings at this time so that their practice partners can more easily cover their caseload during their leave.

Most importantly, whatever arrangements for time off are made, they need to be described to the women prior to registration with the midwife so that the women are aware of the midwife's need for regular time off and have information about back-up arrangements—who to call, when and how. Ideally this would be provided to the woman in written format (Gilkison et al., 2015).

Table 16.3 Sustainable practice summarised	
Sustainable caseloading practice	**Sustainable core midwifery practice**
Passion for midwifery and joy of practice	
• The joy of midwifery practice • Pride and passion in the midwifery profession • Contributing to society • Upholding professional practice standards	• Love of variety and diversity of work options • Making a difference to women • Pride in the midwifery profession • Providing some continuity of care and seeing clients over a period of days • Enjoying caring for women with multiple challenges and complications
Self-care	
• Regular time off from being on call • Support of family and friends • Clear boundaries • Managing the unpredictability of being on call • Sustainable practice arrangements • Having the ability to say 'no' • Having support during critical practice events	• Punctuating work and home life • Physical activity • Other out-of-work activities • Talking and debriefing
Self-determination	
• Ability to control ebb and flow of practice, being self-directed • Ability to work/decide between caseloading or hospital midwifery practice in response to personal life • Providing continuity of care • Being an autonomous practitioner • Managing caseload size	• Having control over work: choosing to do shiftwork or not/annual leave/number of hours worked • Using the flexibility that midwifery offers • Fitting work around life
Relationships sustain	
• Partnership relationships with women and whānau/families • Good relationships with colleagues • Supportive friends and families • Generosity of spirit between midwifery colleagues • Working well together as a practice with partners with similar philosophical beliefs • Supporting/mentoring others (students and new graduates)	• Effective relationships with women, whānau, colleagues and managers • Valuing each other's skills and supporting each other • Feeling part of a team • Being mindful of what has been going on for other team members • Team is bigger than just midwifery • You have not hit rock bottom because you are all in it together and they catch you • Supporting each other through life's events • Supporting new people and new graduates

(Adapted from Gilkison et al., 2015, 2017)

Administration support

Midwives working in group practice will need to have well-organised administration systems that support them in their practice. This will cover issues such as accounts, taxes, equipment, consumables replacements, etc. In addition, midwives need to consider how they share information and ensure they have records of phone calls, clinical visits, filing systems, vehicle log, expense records, etc. It is important that midwives working in group practice together establish clear and equitable working arrangements. There are several electronic midwifery management and calendar systems that provide administrative and claiming support for caseloading midwives (e.g. Tiaki in New Zealand: https://mmpo.org.nz/how-we-help/).

Manageable caseload size

Having a manageable caseload size is important to sustaining caseloading practice and this is dependent on where the midwives work (urban/rural, etc.). It appears that, for many, four to six women per month for 10–11 months of the year is a sustainable caseload size although 30–40 women annually may be more sustainable when there is increased complexity within the woman's needs and therefore increased information sharing and care needs (Dixon, 2017); it is important that practice partners take a similar caseload, so that when one is off the other isn't left covering for a large number of women.

Financial arrangements

When working together in a practice it is important to negotiate and agree on financial arrangements. Midwives in New Zealand claim from the government for each woman they care for, whereas private midwives in Australia are usually paid by the woman.

For many midwifery practices there will be some shared costs such as clinic room rental, equipment, supplies and telephone services. The midwives in the practice will need to determine how the costs will be divided and who is responsible for paying bills, replenishing supplies, etc.

An issue to consider is payments for births when a midwife is having time off and care is provided by her practice partner. There are different ways of managing this situation, for some practices a 'give and take' reciprocal financial arrangement works, where the lead midwife for the woman keeps the birth payment knowing that there will be a time in the future when the role is reversed. For others, a specific percentage of the birth fee goes to the practice partner. Whatever the arrangement, it is important to be very clear from the beginning how this works, and to review regularly.

Boundaries

Another element of **self-care** is negotiating and creating clear professional **boundaries** with women. Midwives are involved in an intimate and special part of women's lives.

Women can feel safe and share personal issues during the midwifery relationship, but it is important that the relationship is based on partnership principles and avoids dependency. A co-dependent relationship is one where the woman feels dependent on the midwife for her emotional wellbeing. In addition it is important to set clear boundaries. This involves identifying optimal times for contact and when it is appropriate for the woman to contact a midwife outside of working hours. Midwives may also want to consider what is important for her to ensure that her work is sustainable, and allows her to achieve her desired work–life balance. If the midwife sets clear boundaries at the outset of a relationship, then her clients know how to contact her and her boundaries will be respected. While a midwife's role in providing maternity care includes being a source of information and support to women, it is not her role to fix her life for her. A midwife should know what agencies and community groups are available to meet some of the non-maternity needs of women, and refer as appropriate.

It can be hard providing maternity care for families that are experiencing stress, trauma or loss but it is important to share the families' feelings and provide support whilst ensuring that you are supported yourself. When midwives are unsupported or highly stressed they may fail to recognise the issue and can become distant and disconnected from their clients and their colleagues. Eventually this can lead to burnout and to midwives leaving the profession. Midwifery is a profession which has a high risk of burnout (Creedy et al, 2017; Dixon et al., 2017). Having good mentorship and self-reflection is essential to help especially the vulnerable students and early-career midwives to develop ways of caring that don't involve self-sacrifice (Gilkison & Cummins, 2021; Pedersen & Sivonen, 2012).

Relationships between caseload midwives

Midwives working in continuity-of-carer models find good relationships with their midwifery colleagues essential. When midwives are working in a way that they are dependent on a colleague to cover for them when they require time off-call, a 'generosity of spirit' within the group is vital (Hunter et al., 2016). Kupfer (1998) describes 'generosity of spirit' as benefiting the recipient out of concern for their welfare and forms a culture of reciprocity within the group. Examples in the midwifery context include concern for each other's wellbeing, offering to take over from someone when they need a break, and offering to take their phone if they are needing 'time off'. Midwives need to be able to balance their professional and personal lives, as otherwise the service they are providing will not be sustainable (Hunter et al., 2016).

One of the other ways midwives in all work environments can support each other is in the willingness to listen and share about the care of a woman, especially when she is in labour. This should never be viewed as the

Table 16.4 Guide to sustainable midwifery practice arrangements	
Regular time off	• As a practice, plan time off a year in advance where possible so that the holidays are staggered • Plan to have 1–2 months off each year • Plan regular time off during the year at weekends and/or weeknights off call
Caseload size	• 4–6 women per month for 10–11 months of the year as a full-time caseload is sustainable • Caseload needs to be similar size to that of practice partner/s
Financial arrangements	• Important that financial arrangements are discussed, agreed and clear to all from the beginning • Financial arrangements for back-up midwife who covers for the midwife on leave need to be agreed in advance • May be a 'give and take' arrangement • May have a specific percentage of birth fee going to the back-up midwife • Consider how rent, equipment, supplies are paid for
Meet regularly	• Regular practice meetings to build a team, support each other, plan time off, discuss practice issues, share learning
Have a shared midwifery philosophy	• Women chose their midwife according to her philosophy of birth, so it is important that practice partners who may be a back-up have the same shared philosophy
Share arrangements with women	• Describe the arrangements before women book in • Include information about time off and back-up arrangements, who to call, when and how
(Adapted from Gilkison et al., 2015, p. 16)	

midwife not knowing what she is doing. It should be encouraged between midwives, be part of the culture of the practice or service and be viewed as a quality assurance measure. By sharing concerns, midwives can organise their thoughts, formulate a plan of care, brainstorm and gain another midwife's opinion (Table 16.4).

SUSTAINABLE CORE HOSPITAL MIDWIFERY

The term 'core hospital midwife' has been used to refer to midwives who are employed (but not caseloading) and are based in hospitals, maternity units or other employed roles. These midwives staff the facilities and usually undertake shift work. The term 'core' midwife refers to the wide variety of midwifery roles that are performed by employed midwives, and that are pivotal—indeed a 'core' function to the provision of midwifery care and the continued day-to-day running of maternity facilities (Gilkison et al., 2017).

Australian midwives work mostly in either public or private hospitals as employees, and most midwives work in shift-based staffing models (Newton et al., 2016). Remote area maternity care is where a remote area midwife provides antenatal and postnatal care, with intrapartum care provided in regional and metropolitan hospitals.

In Australia, some hospitals provide models of care where midwives can work in groups providing continuity of carer (Newton et al., 2016); this may be in 'midwifery group practice', 'caseload care' or 'team midwifery care' (Donnolley et al., 2016). However, less than 10% of women in Australia have access to a publicly funded continuity-of-carer model (Cooper & King, 2020; Dawson et al., 2016).

Some midwives in Australia are self-employed and are known as privately practising midwives (PPMs). PPMs work in collaboration with doctors in the event of identified risks, and provide continuity of care to the women who employ them (Donnolley et al., 2016). However, only a small proportion of midwives work as PPMs. The barriers to working as a PPM include difficulties accessing indemnity insurance, collaborative agreements, lengthy registration processes and difficulty gaining access to hospital visiting rights (Catling & Homer, 2016).

Variety and diversity

Core hospital midwives have variety and diversity in their roles. The ability to move to a new area, for example, adds variety to a core midwife's working life, and enables her to develop new and different skills (Gilkison et al., 2017). The diversity of the women and the differing core midwifery roles mean that 'no two days are the same', which supports satisfaction for the midwife in her work. The ability to change roles according to life changes adds to the sustainability for core hospital midwives. Of importance, though, is that the variety and diversity is sustainable only if the midwife herself is in control of those changes. If the midwife is required to move to fill gaps in service by maternity service/manager requirements, midwives may become dissatisfied and feel overstretched, which is unsustainable long term.

Having enough resources

Sustaining core hospital midwifery relies on having enough midwifery staff and resources for midwives to provide high-quality care that meets women's needs. If a maternity unit is understaffed and poorly resourced, so that there are insufficient midwives to ensure women's needs are met, then the resulting care rationing can cause dissatisfaction. In New Zealand the Midwifery Employee Representation and Advisory Service (MERAS) have developed midwifery Staffing Standards for Maternity Facilities (2014) and a Recruitment, Retention and Responsiveness Strategy (2018) to identify optimal staffing arrangements and ways of achieving this for maternity facilities. Acute health care needs to be prioritised and when there are not enough midwives, other important midwifery care cannot be provided, resulting in frustration, which over time can result in midwives leaving the service and in retention/recruitment issues for that service.

Management

Managers of maternity units have a major influence on the culture of the unit. If managers work with a team of core midwives to build functional, supportive collegial relationships, the culture of the unit will greatly add to the sustainability of the midwives within it. Managers can ensure that the unit is well resourced so that midwives can practise in a way that is satisfying for them and for the woman who they care for.

In Australia publicly funded continuity of midwifery carer is provided through midwifery group practice (MGP). This model has been established within the hospital system so the midwives working in this service generally have a midwifery unit manager (MUM). The position of MUM can be challenging, requiring her to juggle 'outside forces' like funding and competing paradigms that threaten the sustainability of the practice (Hewitt et al., 2019). The MUM is the buffer between the midwives who are trying to provide a holistic model of care and the requirements of an institutional system designed to process sick people. The MUM, therefore, is required to be sensitive to the needs of the midwives in the practice while also meeting the demands of the institution. Studies have indicated that a transformational style of leadership works well for this role (Hewitt et al., 2019), and for the management of midwives in general (Byrom et al., 2011).

Relationships between employed midwives

Despite an inability to choose who they work with, hospital midwives still need positive, supportive relationships with their colleagues. Midwives who work with each other in employed situations still need to have a culture of trust, respect and collaboration to encourage a healthy work culture (Catling et al., 2017). This can take the form of warm and open communication, reciprocity and teamwork. Sometimes attending social occasions such as birthday celebrations or Christmas parties can also improve collegiality. Taking time to enquire about each other's wellbeing and connecting on a human level can help build relationships. Catling et al. (2017) found a positive work culture nurtures the midwives within it, enabling them to flourish in their careers and to provide quality care.

Midwives traversing caseloading and core

Moving between caseloading and core practice can really help to build relationships between midwives. In New Zealand, where caseloading midwifery has been integrated into the maternity system since 1990, midwives have had the opportunity to work in both models. Each has its advantages and disadvantages. For example, core hospital midwives know their working hours in advance, so for some midwives that is important to accommodate their family commitments. Self-employed caseloading midwives find that providing continuity of care for women gives them greatest satisfaction, and like being able to have control over things such as the number of women they care for and which days they have their clinics.

Midwives can change their roles throughout their careers to fit in with their own passions and life circumstances. Moving between caseloading and core practice improves the understanding of both roles, and adds to the sustainability of midwifery practice.

New graduates and students increase sustainability

To grow the next generation of midwives, and ensure the midwifery profession's sustainability, means that registered midwives have a commitment to supporting student midwives and new graduate midwives. Again, relationships are the key to growing new midwives. Students and new graduates can be either enabled or disabled in their learning based on the relationships and attitudes they encounter with other midwives. Relationships are always multifaceted and require work from those within the relationship to maintain optimal outcomes. Registered midwives speak of the joy of nurturing the next generation of midwives as something that sustains them in practice (Gilkison et al., 2017) and, so long as the relationships are respectful, learning is enabled on both sides.

A maternity unit or practice which models respectful behaviours and welcomes students and graduate midwives is critical for growing and sustaining the midwifery profession. If a culture is created which encourages questioning, and encourages all to ask if there is uncertainty, an environment is promoted which is safe for all who come into the unit, especially the woman.

While it is important to nurture the next generation and to share our knowledge, we also need to model respect for each other. This not only helps new midwives to stay in the profession but also encourages sustainability within the profession. It can also be of benefit for more experienced midwives, giving them the opportunity to learn about the latest research and evidence. Caring for the next generation of midwives is critical to meeting the workforce requirements of the future; encouraging and sharing our knowledge, teaching and educating our next generation of midwives is part of being a midwife (Gilkison & Cummins, 2021; Tuckett et al., 2015).

Challenges to sustainability

Midwifery belongs to those professions that can be physically, emotionally and mentally demanding, making midwives particularly prone to stress and burnout (Young et al., 2015).

Core midwives and midwives providing standard care may not always find their work satisfying, owing to high workloads and the inability to form relationships with women. Feeling unable to provide woman-centred care may lead to less job satisfaction and a higher rate of burnout (Newton et al., 2014). Fergusson et al. (2010) explored the pressures that the core midwives on the floor in New Zealand experienced, where being understaffed and feeling unable to provide adequate care was often a reality. Catling et al. (2017) described how midwives working in standard care believed that the system was seen as being more important than the midwives themselves. The same authors advised greater emphasis on positive cultures across all environments, suggesting that giving midwives more control over their workplace would go a long way to addressing these concerns (Box 16.1).

Burnout

There may come a period in a midwife's life when the work becomes overwhelming or seems unreasonably demanding. The midwife may feel exhausted, depleted, constantly stressed, overwhelmed, burdened by responsibility and unable to find time for herself, family and friends. She may be irritable and impatient with the women she provides care for, and feel little or no enjoyment in her work (Young, Smythe, & McAra Couper, 2015). This state is often referred to as 'burnout'.

If this occurs, the midwife needs to reflect on why and how this situation has arisen: 'What is going on in my life at the moment?', 'Is it the work?', 'Is it the way I'm doing my work?', 'Is it the place of work in the whole of my life?', or 'Has something happened that has triggered this event for me?' The midwife will need to work out whether what is occurring is about the pressures of the work, related to the person she is, or about the attitudes, skills and abilities she has or has not developed to assist her to manage her work.

The midwife will need support from her family, colleagues and managers, and may need professional psychological support from a counsellor, therapist or mental health services. She may need time off work to be able to work out what the issues are for her. If she is employed, her employer may have an Employee Assistance Programme (EAP) available, and if caseloading, then counselling is available in New Zealand through the New Zealand College of Midwives (NZCOM). A health check may be needed to exclude underlying physical causes such as anaemia or hypothyroidism, or whether clinical depression, anxiety disorder or another mental health issue is a contributing factor.

Midwives need to learn the necessity for self-care, to ensure that the midwifery role remains sustainable as midwives move through phases of their lives. Midwifery colleagues have a responsibility to be supportive and engaged with one another, and to let each other know if or when a colleague is beginning to become overburdened by working as a midwife.

CRITICAL THINKING EXERCISE

What are some of the ways that you can promote more self-care and care for your colleagues to support sustainable practice?

Horizontal violence or workplace bullying

Building midwifery relationships at work starts with kind and respectful communication and should include students and graduate midwives. Unfortunately, **bullying** remains a major issue within the workplace with bullying identified amongst peers, between management and staff and with students and new midwifery staff members (Catling & Rossiter, 2020; Catling et al., 2017). The practice experience of student midwives is deeply influenced by the workplace culture, with students often describing negative experiences (Arundell et al., 2018).

When midwives experience intimidation and bullying behaviour, it increases their emotional vulnerability and can lead to low morale and resignations within the workplace. Most workplaces have zero tolerance guidelines to reduce and remove the opportunity for individuals to be bullied. Supportive networks are important in reducing bullying behaviours. Midwives should not accept a culture where horizontal violence, bullying or incivility exist. Friendships formed at work can create a constructive

---

Box 16.1   Workplace culture

Workplace culture relates to the unwritten rules within a workplace which can often cause conflict for midwives (Davis et al., 2016). It can lead to expectations of being seen to be busy as a behavioural norm as opposed to 'being with' women during labour.

A survey of 322 Australian midwives found less than a third of midwives thought their workplace had a positive culture (Catling & Rossiter, 2020). Many identified limited resources, inadequate staffing levels, poor communication, time pressures and a lack of leadership. Those who identified a positive workplace culture found positive support from managers, and inspiring role models.

environment where learning, teaching and working can be enjoyable (Ambler et al., 2016).

Bullying behaviour needs to be addressed immediately, especially as some perpetrators are unaware of their harmful behaviour. The victim should express to the perpetrator how the bullying behaviour 'feels' to prevent the perpetrator feeling accused but helping them to self-reflect on the behaviour (Egues & Leinung, 2013). Participating in courses aimed at giving midwives strategies to resolve conflict and deal with bullying can be helpful. However, it is essential that midwives support each other to report and stand up to bullying behaviour. Encouraging each other to engage in self-care and self-reflection can be a good start towards curtailing horizontal violence. Caring and respect for ourselves and each other goes a long way toward a healthier workplace.

(See the Online resources for dealing with workplace bullying at the end of the chapter.)

CRITICAL THINKING EXERCISE

What would you do in a situation where a colleague asked your advice on a time they had been bullied?

Relationships between caseloading and core midwives

New models of care have the potential to create tensions and subcultures within the workforce with differing perceptions on risk and differences in philosophy leading to lack of respect and breakdown in communications (Catling et al., 2017). In Australia, Catling et al. (2017) found in a qualitative study looking at midwives' workplace culture that hostility towards midwives who were new to the service, student midwives and midwives providing continuity of care was often reported. The study linked this behaviour to an 'us and them' culture within a hierarchical structure. The trauma of introducing new models of care can be lessened by forward planning and inclusion of all stakeholders. Hartz et al. (2012) discovered that extensive multidisciplinary education to increase awareness of and to explore the concept of midwifery continuity of care helped to explore fears and concerns, to find possible solutions and to make transition into the new models less stressful when introducing a new model of care.

Fox et al. (2014) investigated women's experience of transfer into hospital from planned home birth, finding the home-birth midwives were sometimes met with open hostility from colleagues. This hostility, unfortunately, was often witnessed by the women, adding to their sense of vulnerability and fear (Fox et al., 2014). For women who have planned a home birth or birth in a birth centre, transfer to another facility can feel stressful and traumatic. Clear and respectful communication between midwives

not only helps make a difficult time for a woman less distressing, but ensures safe care for her.

Women choose different models of care, with some choosing to birth outside standard models. Midwives also choose to work in different settings providing different ways to care for women depending on their own personal needs, belief systems and values. Maternity care providers need to reflect on the reasons that women choose different models of care, reflecting on their own views around safety and risk. Creating a positive workplace culture is the responsibility of all healthcare workers; respectful communication between each other can be the catalyst to a safer and happier workplace for professionals and a better environment for women (Box 16.1).

REFLECTIVE THINKING EXERCISE

Think about times in your life you have been treated well and times you might have been treated poorly by your colleagues. How do you like to be treated? Is this how you treat your colleagues?

What can you do in your everyday work life to encourage a culture within your group or workplace that is respectful, has reciprocity and would make your colleagues want to work with you?

How can you as an individual help the culture within your group or workplace to be a better place to work?

Unexpected outcomes

Midwives may be involved in providing care to a woman or baby who becomes unwell and for whom there may be an unexpected outcome. These events can occur at any time during a midwife's career and may result in the midwife being required to account for her practice in a number of differing ways. Midwives in New Zealand who are members of the NZCOM are advised to contact the College legal advisor for advice when they have had an unexpected outcome. A booklet outlining what to do when an unexpected outcome occurs is also available for members through the College website. Being involved in an unexpected outcome is stressful and difficult, both professionally and personally. Often midwives will experience a range of differing responses including grief, fear, anger, shame and guilt. Support from colleagues as well as family and friends is important at this time. Any discussion about the case will need to be confidential. Further support can be accessed through the NZCOM legal advisor or through the hospital EAP. In Australia support can be found at: https://www.nmsupport.org.au/accessing-support/its-ok-to-ask-for-help, or the EAP. Sometimes a mentor midwife can help support the midwife; at other times colleagues can support the individual. Being 'midwifed' back into practice by supportive colleagues has been found to be of benefit in regaining confidence after a significant event (Hunter et al., 2016). Hunter & Warren (2014) found that in difficult circumstances peers could play a key role in promoting resilience and helping with recovery. Reflection and review of events is important but this needs to be undertaken in a non-judgmental manner with processes and systems included within any review. Midwives need to support each other through these difficult events.

The following two case studies, one from Australia and the other from New Zealand, demonstrate how midwifery models of practice can work to sustain each other.

CASE STUDY

Australia: my experience working in a cohesive group practice

I worked in a freestanding birth centre for 11 years; it was situated within a small hospital with no onsite obstetric services. The freestanding birth centre was run by a group of employed midwives who each cared for a caseload of women. Working in this practice taught me the importance of friendship, unity, a shared empathy and a sense of reciprocity or 'spirit of generosity' within the group. The midwife turnover was low, and we took every opportunity to bond as a group resulting in a practice where everyone knew each other very well. My time working with these midwives taught me that friendship, relationships and cohesiveness within the group has a direct correlation with midwife work–life happiness and service sustainability.

The 'spirit of generosity' within the group meant that midwives happily offered to take each other's phones so they could attend functions important to having a normal life outside of midwifery. The culture within the group encouraged each individual to take time off as needed. Things happen to us all and so it is important to be kind to each other to offer support, in the form of listening, offering to take the phone, or offering to take over the care of a woman when you know they need to go home. I have found time and time again that, although it might be a colleague needing help today, tomorrow it could just as easily be me.

There have been many times that I have taken help when it was offered; one such time was after a critical incident. It was a public holiday; the woman I was caring for was having her second baby with me. During the second stage of labour she collapsed and had a cardiac arrest. Working in a freestanding birth centre meant we could call an emergency response team, but we had no obstetric or paediatric doctors on hand. On this occasion we were able to call them in. I am so thankful that I had a colleague with me at the time; the whole ordeal would have been so much harder on my own.

In a wonderful show of unity all of my colleagues came in and supported us; one came up to the theatre where we were doing the caesarean section and helped with the resuscitation of the baby. My manager came in and gave us support and reminded us to do paperwork that we may have forgotten in the moment. My colleagues cleaned the birth centre, which resembled a 'bomb site' where the emergency had occurred, and restocked the unit. The doctor who had supported our service from the time the birth centre was established also came in to support all of us involved, and continued to support us through our many debriefing sessions.

The support and love my colleagues showed me was what got me through this incident, even though it could have ended my and my colleague's careers. This support came in the form of constantly touching base with us through text messages and phone calls, taking our phones to let us have time out for a few days and coming in to support us with the next birth. The midwife who was with me during the incident and I spent many hours on the phone going over what had happened and planning how to recover, which proved to be very therapeutic. Although supportive, my family had trouble understanding the gravity of the situation for me. They seemed to think I should be used to losing mothers and babies and were surprised it affected me so much. It meant a lot to know my colleagues understood how devastating it was for us.

The outcome of this incident was that, although the baby was relatively easy to resuscitate, he did not survive having been in his arrested mother's body. His life support was turned off several days after birth. The woman, however, did survive, although she needed many trips back to theatre to stop bleeding, and her recovery was slow, she went home to her husband and first child several weeks later. It was thought she had suffered an amniotic embolism; however, without an autopsy we can never be absolutely sure. She was too unwell to attend her baby's funeral, and unfortunately has only seen photos of the beautiful little boy she had got so close to having.

As a group, we prioritised our relationships by ensuring we attended the weekly meetings, and tried to spend time together as much as possible. The friendship, trust, shared philosophy and reciprocity helped me through some dark times in my career and gave me great joy in better times. Being on-call, responsible to the women in your care and working long hours can be hard at times, but the joy that comes from the woman–midwife relationship, and the support and friendship from a cohesive group practice, make this a wonderful way to work.

CASE STUDY

New Zealand Midwifery Practice by Juliet Thorpe

Since 1990 New Zealand (NZ) midwives have had legislated autonomy, allowing them to work with women and their families in a fully funded continuity model of care. For over a quarter of a century, NZ midwives have adopted a multitude of ways of working in an attempt to meet their professional and personal requirements as well as the needs of birthing women. The demands of providing a 24-hour on-call service is a constant challenge, but some midwifery group practices have managed to maintain their passion for midwifery despite the potential for burnout. I am fortunate enough to work in such a practice. I work with three other midwives and we provide midwifery care to women wanting to birth at home. We take two to four women per month depending on other midwifery work and family commitments and consider four women per month to be a full-time caseload. As we are self-employed we have been able to design our own practice model, without the constraints of an institution. This is our group's 25th year of providing an on-call midwifery service to the home-birthing women of our city and the rural surrounds. It is a job we adore and rarely tire of.

Essential to the sustainability of our group is the clarity we have with regard to our philosophical framework for practice. The luxury of working with home-birthing families is that they too share our belief that pregnancy and birth are normal life processes and that being in the familiar environment of their home maximises their potential for a normal healthy outcome. Women choose home birth for a variety of reasons but in the main it is due to the faith they have in their bodies and the impact of a positive birthing environment. We work in partnership with each family, combining our midwifery expertise with the knowledge each woman holds with regard to her own health and wellbeing. As colleagues we have a shared philosophy, which means that every birthing family receives the same care no matter who attends them. I rarely miss a birth but when I do, owing to time off/holidays/illness or just being tired, I know that my clients are in the best hands. It allows me to have a break, without feeling that I have let my clients down should they labour and birth without me. As a practice, we also attempt to keep our caseload to a number where we can earn a reasonable living yet not be too busy for our clients and our own families.

For effective collegial support to be possible we commit to a regular weekly meeting but will also often talk to each other daily. We don't have a communal work setting, so talking to each other on a regular basis creates its own setting and allows us to build professional and social support, which are possibly taken for granted by those working in an institution.

A typical day begins with a round of texts and phone calls with colleagues to find out who has been up all night at a birth, who needs appointments postponed or rescheduled and can one of us do some work for a tired colleague so they can sleep? We visit women in their homes but also have a clinic where women can come to us. It can be a bit of a juggle if we have been up during the night with a woman in labour. Normally we will call a back-up midwife to support us at the birth, meaning at least two in the practice have had a broken night's sleep. Generally we will triage the day so that women with very new babies and women with pregnancy or postnatal issues have priority and that at least one of us can sleep!

Our midwifery day then involves visiting women at various stages of their pregnancy and postnatal experience. We may be doing a pregnancy test or a first-trimester booking visit in one house and be weighing and assessing a 2-week-old baby at the next. We plan our visits but, even with the best-laid plans, all it can take is a woman with reduced fetal movements or a woman in early labour to turn the day pear shaped. Never a dull moment! The days are often full and when we finally get home there is the paperwork to catch up on. This may involve following up on ultrasound and blood results, writing referral letters to obstetricians and GPs, accounting for tax purposes or emailing clients' information they have requested on various subjects. Then it is time to check in with colleagues again so that we can organise who will have the energy to provide support if there is another birth in the night.

Not every day is 9 to 5 and we will try to diary an appointment-free day if we can. I don't plan any visits before 10 a.m. most days, in anticipation of sometimes needing a sleep-in. Over the last few years I have started swimming for an hour twice a week during which time I am unavailable. My clients and colleagues know this and respect it. Sustainability is so important for our profession and it can be achieved so easily if we prioritise time to breathe and enjoy some midwifery-free time.

One of the highlights of our week is the practice meeting. It is a precious time where we all get to hear how each of our weeks has been. We bring food to share and then settle in with our diaries and we each tell the story of our week with all of its highs and lows. The putting aside of 4 hours a week to devote to talk may seem to some to be indulgent and even excessive but illustrates the most beneficial tool used by the practice in ensuring its sustainability. Rarely do people in their working lives get that chance to totally debrief to others in a forum where they know they will be heard and cared for. It is a luxurious process, which is not difficult to maintain, and its benefits are considerable. By hearing about each other's clients we get to know more about the clients but also about each other.

Our midwifery practice is alive and well after 25 years and we put it down to daily communication with like-minded supportive colleagues, regular time off, a manageable caseload and a strong belief in birthing women.

Conclusion

Midwives, wherever they work, are sustained by their passion for the profession and the joy and satisfaction they experience when working alongside women and their families in a partnership relationship (Kirkham, 2011; Leap et al., 2011; McAra-Couper et al., 2014). Being with women and their families when they go through pregnancy, labour and birth, and as they become mothers, fathers and families, is a positive experience for the woman and the midwife, and provides the midwife with a sense of her work being valued and important.

This chapter has explored sustainable midwifery practice. Whatever the midwife's role, the most satisfying part of her work is the meaningful relationships she develops—relationships with the women and families she is caring for, positive working relationships with colleagues, practice partners, students and new graduates, and supportive relationships at home. It is the quality of these relationships with women and families and with colleagues that gives the midwife fulfilment in her work, and strengthens the sustainability of midwifery.

Underpinning supportive and sustaining relationships, the midwife needs to work in an environment where she is able to provide quality care for women and families. An environment which fosters supportive relationships needs to be well resourced, with colleagues and practice partners who communicate well and are supportive. Midwives are sustained when work and life outside work are balanced. Ultimately when the midwifery profession is sustained then the care that women and their families receive will be enriched, which in turn sustains the profession.

Review questions

1. How are resilience and sustainability important for a midwife? How can a midwife develop resilience and sustainability in her practice?
2. If you were thinking about joining a caseloading practice, what would you want to consider and discuss with the practice before deciding to join?
3. If you were setting up your ideal working environment, what would that look like?
4. How does the culture of a practice or service influence the midwives and does this have any impact on the women?
5. Who is responsible for the culture of a practice, or workplace?
6. What can you do as a midwife or student midwife to help change the workplace culture?
7. Does the workplace culture influence the sustainability of that practice or service? If so, how does it?

Online resources

Dealing with workplace bullying (Australia)

In Australia, fact sheets such as 'Workplace bullying: violence, harassment and bullying' and 'What you can do to stop bullies—Be a supportive bystander: violence, harassment and bullying', as well as hotline phone numbers for help with bullying in each state or territory, are found on the Australian Human Rights Commission website: http://www.humanrights.gov.au/employers/good-practice-good-business-factsheets/workplace-discrimination-harassment-and-bullying.

The Australian College of Midwives and the Australian Nursing and Midwifery Federation can offer information and support: http://www.midwives.org.au/; http://anmf.org.au/documents/policies/P_Bullying.pdf.

Links to helpful resources to develop resilience: http://www.apa.org/helpcenter/road-resilience.aspx; https://www.mindtools.com/pages/article/resilience.htm.

New Zealand

Midwifery Representation and Advisory Services (MERAS): http://www.midwife.org.nz/meras.

Work Safe New Zealand has fact sheets available about workplace bullying: http://www.worksafe.govt.nz/worksafe/toolshed/bullying-prevention-toolbox?searchterm=guide+to+bullying+in+the+workplace.

References

Ambler T, Harvey M, Cahir J. University academics' experiences of learning through mentoring. *Aust Educ Researcher*. 2016;3(5): 609–627. doi:10.1007/s13384-016-0214-7.

Arbour MW, Gordon IK, Saftner M. et al. The experience of sleep deprivation for midwives practicing in the United States. *Midwifery* 2020, 89: 102782. doi.org/10.1016/j.midw.2020.102782

Arundell F. Mannix J, Sheehan A. et al. Workplace culture and the practice experience of midwifery students: A meta-synthesis. *J Nurs Manag*. 2018;26(3), 302–313. doi:10.1111/jonm.12548.

Braithwaite J, Herkes J, Ludlow K, et al. Association between organizational and workplace cultures, and patient outcomes: systematic review. *BMJ Open*. 2017;7(11), e017708–e017708. doi:10.1136/bmjopen-2017-017708.

Byrom S, Byrom A, Downe S. Transformational leadership and midwifery: a nested narrative review. In: Downe S, Byrom S, Simpson L, eds. *Essential Midwifery Practice: Leadership, Expertise and Collaborative Working*. Oxford: Blackwell; 2011:23–24.

Catling C, Homer C. Twenty-five years since the Shearman Report: how far have we come? Are we there yet? *Women Birth*. 2016;29:93–99.

Catling C, Reid F, Hunter B. Australian midwives' experiences of their workplace culture. *Women Birth*. 2017;30(2):137–145. doi:10.1016/j.wombi.2016.10.001.

Catling C, Rossiter C. Midwifery workplace culture in Australia: A national survey of midwives. *Women Birth*. 2020;33(5), 464–472. Doi:10.1016/j.wombi.2019.09.008.

Clemons JH, Gilkison A, Mharapara TL, et al. Midwifery Job Autonomy in New Zealand: I do it all the time. *Women and Birth: journal of the Australian College of Midwives*. 2021;34(1), 30–37. doi:10.1016/j.wombi.2020.09.004.

Cooper M, King R. *Women's experiences of maternity care during the height of the COVID-19 pandemic in Australia*; 2021. Online: www.midwives.org.au.

Creedy DK, Sidebotham M, Gamble J, et al. Prevalence of burnout, depression, anxiety and stress in Australian midwives: a cross-sectional survey. *BMC Pregnancy and Childbirth*. 2017;17(1), 13–13. doi:10.1186/s12884-016-1212-5.

Crowther S, Smythe E, Spence D. Kairos time at the moment of birth. *Midwifery*. 2015;31(4):451–457.

Crowther S, Hunter B, McAra-Couper J, et al. Sustainability and resilience in midwifery; a discussion paper. *Midwifery*. 2016;40:40–48. doi:10.1016/j.midw.2016.06.005.

Davis D, Baddock S, Pairman S, et al. Planned place of birth in New Zealand: does it affect mode of birth and intervention rates among low-risk women? *Birth*. 2011;38(2):111–119. doi:10.1111/j.1523-536X.2010.00458.x.

Dawson K, McLachlan H, Newton M, et al. Implementing caseload midwifery: Exploring the views of maternity managers in Australia—a national cross-sectional survey. *Women Birth*. 2016;29:214–222. doi:10.1016/j.wombi.2015.10.010.

Dixon L. Looking for ways to improve maternity care? It's time to listen to midwives. *Midwifery News*. 2017;84(March):9–11.

Dixon L, Guilliland K, Pallant JF, et al. The emotional wellbeing of New Zealand midwives: comparing responses for midwives in case loading and shift work settings. *NZCOM J*. 2017;53:5–15.

Donald H, Smythe L, McAra-Couper J. Creating a better work–life balance. *NZCOM J*. 2014;49:5–10.

Donnolley N, Butler-Henderson K, Chapman M, et al. The development of a classification system for maternity models of care. *Health Inf Manag*. 2016;45(2):64–70. doi:10.1177/183338316639454.

Downe S, Finlayson K, Tunçalp Ö, Gülmezoglu AM. Provision and uptake of routine antenatal services: a qualitative evidence synthesis. *Cochrane Database of Systematic Reviews* 2019, Issue 6. Art. No.: CD012392. DOI: 10.1002/14651858.CD012392.pub2.

East CE, Biro MA, Fredericks S, et al. Support during pregnancy for women at increased risk of low birthweight babies. *Cochrane Database of Sys Rev*. 2019(4). doi:10.1002/14651858.CD000198.pub3.

Egues AL, Leinung EZ. The bully within and without: strategies to address horizontal violence in nursing. *Nurs Forum*. 2013;48(3):185–190.

Farlex, ed. *The Free Dictionary*. Boston, MA: Houghton Mifflin Harcourt; 2020. Online: http://www.thefreedictionary.com/.

Fergusson L, Smythe L, McAra-Couper J. Being a delivery suite coordinator. *NZCOM J*. 2010;42:7–11.

Flo E, Pallesseen S, Mageroy N, et al. Shift work disorder in nurse-assessment, prevalence and related health problems. *PLoS ONE*. 2012;7(4):e33981. doi:10.1371/journal.pone.0033981.

Fox D, Sheehan A, Homer C. Experiences of women planning a home birth who require transfer to hospital: a metasynthesis of the qualitative literature. *Int J Childbirth*. 2014;4(2):103–119.

Gilkison A. Sustainable midwifery practice. *NZCOM J*. 2014;49:2.

Gilkison A, McAra-Couper J, Gunn J, et al. Midwifery practice arrangements which sustain caseloading Lead Maternity Carer midwives in New Zealand. *NZCOM J*. 2015;51:11–16. doi:10.12784/nzcomjnl51.2015.2.11-16.

Gilkison A, McAra-Couper J, Fielder A, et al. The core of the core: what is at the heart of core hospital midwifery practice in New Zealand? *NZCOM J*. 2017;53:30–37.

Gilkison A, Cummins A. Sustainable midwifery: Supporting new graduates' transition to practice. *Women Birth*. 2021;34(2), 111–112. doi:https://doi.org/10.1016/j.wombi.2020.09.019.

Guilliland K, Pairman S. *Womens business: The story of the New Zealand College of Midwives 1986–2010*. 2010 Christchurch: New Zealand College of Midwives.

Hartz D, White J, Lainchbury K, et al. Australian maternity reform through clinical redesign. *Aust Health Rev*. 2012;36:169–175. doi:10.1071/AH11012.

Hewitt L, Priddis H, Dahlen HG. What attributes do Australian midwifery leaders identify as essential to effectively manage a Midwifery Group Practice? *Women and Birth*. 2019;*32*, 168–177. doi:https://doi.org/10.1016/j.wombi.2018.06.017.

Hunter B, Warren L. Midwives' experiences of workplace resilience. *Midwifery*. 2014;30:926–934. doi:10.1016/j.midw.2014.03.010.

Hunter M, Crowther S, McAra-Couper J, et al. Generosity of spirit sustains caseloading Lead Maternity Carer midwives in New Zealand. *NZCOM J*. 2016;52:50–55.

Jarosova D, Gurkova E, Palese A, et al. Job satisfaction and leaving intentions of midwives: analysis of a multinational cross-sectional survey. *J Nurs Manag*. 2016;24:70–79. doi:10.1111/jonm.12273.

Kirkham M. The potential of flow experience for midwives and mothers. In: Davies L, Daellenbach R, Kensington M, eds. *Sustainability, Midwifery and Birth*. London: Routledge; 2011:87–100.

Kupfer J. Generosity of spirit. *J Value Inq*. 1998;32:357–368.

Leap N, Dahlen H, Brodie P, et al. Relationships: the glue that holds it all together. In: Davies L, Daellenbach R, Kensington M, eds. *Sustainability, Midwifery, and Birth*. Abingdon, Oxon: Routledge; 2011:61–74.

McAra-Couper J, Gilkison A, Crowther S, et al. Partnership and reciprocity with women sustain Lead Maternity Carer midwives in practice. *NZCOM J*. 2014;(49):23–33.

Newton M, McLachlan H, Willis K, et al. Comparing satisfaction and burnout between caseload and standard care midwives: findings from two cross-sectional surveys conducted in Victoria, Australia. *BMC Pregnancy Childbirth*. 2014;14(426):1–16. doi:10.1186/s12884-014-0426-7.

Newton M, McLachlan H, Forster D, et al. Understanding the 'work' of caseload midwives: A mixed-methods exploration of two caseload midwifery models in Victoria, Australia. *Women Birth*. 2016;29:223–233. doi:10.1016/j.wombi.2015.10011.

Nove A, Friberg I, Bernis L et al. Potential impact of midwives in preventing and reducing maternal and neonatal mortality and stillbirths: a Lives Saved Tool modelling study. *Lancet Glo Health*. 2021 9(1) e24–e32 doi: 10.1016/S2214-109X(20)30397-1.

Pedersen B, Sivonen K. The impact of clinical encounters on student nurses' ethical caring. *Nurs Ethics*. 2012;19(6):838–848. doi:10.1177/0969733012447017.

Sandall J, Soltani H, Gates S, et al. Midwife-led continuity models versus other models of care for childbearing women. *Cochrane Database Syst Rev*. 2016;(8):CD004667, doi:10.1002/14651858.CD004667.pub5.

Stromgren A, Eriksson A, Bergman D, et al. Social capital among healthcare professionals: A prospective study of its importance for job satisfaction, work engagement and engagement in clinical inprovements. *Int J Nurs Stud*. 2016;53:116–125.

Tuckett A, Eley R, Ng L. Transition to practice programs: what Australian and New Zealand nursing and midwifery graduates said. A graduate eCohort sub-study. *Collegian*. 2015;347:8.

United Nations Population Fund (UNFPA), ICM, WHO. *The State of the World's Midwifery 2021*. Online: http://www.unfpa.org/sowmy.

Young CM, Smythe L, McAra-Couper J. Burnout: lessons from the lived experience of case loading midwives. *Int J Childbirth*. 2015;5(3):154–165.

Further reading

Davies L, Daellenbach R, Kensington M, eds. *Sustainability, Midwifery and Birth*. Oxon, United States: Routledge; 2011.

Practising partnership

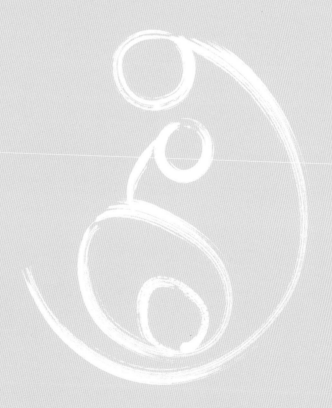

CHAPTER 17

Midwifery partnership

Suzanne Miller and Rebecca Jane Bear

LEARNING OUTCOMES

Learning outcomes for this chapter are:

1. To explore the nature of partnership between women and midwives
2. To describe the difference between caring for a woman as the midwifery 'expert' and working with a woman as an equal partner
3. To describe the key theoretical frameworks for culturally competent midwifery practice: midwifery partnership, cultural safety and, in Aotearoa New Zealand, Tūranga Kaupapa
4. To discuss the implications of midwifery partnership, cultural safety and cultural competence for midwifery professionalism.

CHAPTER OVERVIEW

This chapter encompasses midwifery partnership and the frameworks with which relationships with wahine and whānau may be supported. Firstly, there is exploration of what it means to work in partnership with wāhine, their partners and whānau during their childbearing experience. The next section focuses on the three major frameworks for midwifery practice—cultural safety, midwifery partnership and, in Aotearoa New Zealand, Tūranga Kaupapa—and identifies their practice as components of cultural competence.

Midwives and women can both benefit from mutually negotiated relationships, and care practices that support partnership are shown to improve outcomes for women and babies. In order for midwives to work in partnership with women, they need to be open, self-aware, reflexive and mature, with a strong commitment to honouring the woman's ways of knowing about herself, her body and her baby. Midwives also partner each other in a diverse array of practice settings and enable sustainable midwifery practice as a result.

This chapter examines the relationship and partner roles of midwives, including the ways that midwives partner with women, each other and their communities to enhance the development of socially sustaining communities. It also examines cultural competence and the requirement of midwives and other health professionals to understand and apply it, in both Aotearoa New Zealand and Australia.

The frameworks of cultural safety, midwifery partnership and Tūranga Kaupapa were developed in New Zealand and arose out of that country's unique historical, social and cultural context. Tūranga Kaupapa is one set of principles to describe the cultural values of Māori in pregnancy and childbirth which may be relevant to midwives working with Māori women anywhere, including Australia. These theoretical frameworks can be applied with caution by indigenous and non-indigenous people for midwifery practice in Australia and other countries, as the principles articulated in each theory describe values, beliefs, understandings and behaviours that any midwife and midwifery partnership may choose to embrace.

KEY TERMS

continuity of care
cultural safety and cultural
  competence

informed choice and consent
midwifery partnership
theoretical frameworks

Te Tiriti o Waitangi
Tūranga Kaupapa

INTRODUCTION

Working in partnership with wāhine, their partners and whānau is the touchstone of midwifery practice. The relationship between an individual wahine and her midwife is centred on mutual trust and respect, power sharing and recognition of the impact this can have on whole communities. The concurrent aims of midwifery care encompass the protection of physiological birth and the enabling of women to embrace fully their role as confident mothers. The power of these aims, when enacted, cannot be underestimated in their potential to transform society. To enable the highest potential of partnership, a range of relationships and value-based frameworks lend structure to a shared understanding and form the foundations of healthy partnership. The Midwifery Council of New Zealand (MCNZ) identifies the integrated practice of cultural safety, midwifery partnership and Tūranga Kaupapa as strategies to demonstrate cultural competence (MCNZ, 2012). A culturally competent midwife is able to interact respectfully and effectively with people from backgrounds different to the midwife's own (MCNZ, 2012). A culturally competent midwife will be able to work effectively with women with different cultural beliefs through the development of skills to better understand others' cultures and through recognition of the impact that one's own culture has on one's interactions. Better health outcomes occur when culturally competent midwives partner with women and their families.

This chapter will explore the nature of working in partnership, and midwifery's varied relationships and theoretical frameworks for practice. An examination of the relationships themselves, the role of midwives in different working contexts, and the frameworks for how midwives may work in partnerships with each other and with their communities is undertaken. In doing so, we help to reveal the dimensions of the importance both of midwifery to women and their families, and of midwifery as a public health strategy.

PARTNERING WITH WOMEN

The relationship

Partnering women throughout the pregnancy: the first phone call to the discharge visit at 4–6 weeks

Women in Aotearoa New Zealand and Australia can access maternity **continuity of care** from the same midwife during their childbearing journey. Continuity of midwifery care is described in various ways, but the relationship between a woman and her midwife has been described as that of a 'professional friend' (Pairman, 1998, 2000a; Wilkins, 2000). This relationship is the basis of what is termed the 'partnership model'. This unique relationship between the woman and midwife was first described by New Zealanders Sally Pairman and Karen

Guilliland in their 1995 monograph, *The Midwifery Partnership: A Model for Practice*, updated in 2010 (Guilliland & Pairman, 1995, 2010a). Strongly embedded in this model is the notion of 'being with' as opposed to 'doing to', which is associated with rites of passage such as birth and death (Kennedy et al., 2003). Partnership includes an emotional engagement, with each party placing the other within a personal and biographical context (Wilkins, 2000). The needs of the woman will vary with her personal context but will also vary due to the midwife and the midwife's context. The **midwifery partnership** will typically begin when the woman first contacts the midwife, usually early in pregnancy, though first contact may be initiated during the pre-conceptual period for discussion about creating an optimal environment for a planned pregnancy. The partnership continues until the new baby is integrated into the family and the woman perceives she is ready to be discharged to the relevant ongoing care provider in each country, which occurs between 4 and 6 weeks postnatally.

Partnership in midwifery can take many forms. The partnership model (Guilliland & Pairman, 1995, 2010a) as a framework for practice describes the potential for developing relationships that are mutually satisfying and that optimise care for women and their families. This model is perhaps most visibly manifested in the continuity-of-care context where self-employed practice is situated. Outcomes of this model of care have consistently demonstrated both increased satisfaction for women and midwives and reduced intervention rates in childbirth (Sandall et al., 2016). Midwives who are employed in maternity facilities (called 'core midwives' in Aotearoa New Zealand) are also highly skilled at developing shorter-term partnerships with women and their families that are no less mutually beneficial and satisfying. These occur in a time frame that may be limited to episodic antenatal care, labour care provision, or care during a postnatal stay in a facility or in the community following discharge.

Whatever a midwife's practice context, practising partnership requires her[a] to respect and support the woman's beliefs, knowledge and decision-making processes. Partnership asks that she meet the woman where she is at, assess her health and education needs in relation to her care, and create a safe and trusting environment in which they can, together, plan the woman's ongoing care. This may involve members of the woman's whānau/family as well, as determined by her. Like any partnership, in order for a trusting relationship to form, time may be needed to get to know one another, and the midwife may need to share something of herself as a person to allow this relationship to flourish. This need not extend to sharing intimate details about her own life or family, or about her own decision making in relation to healthcare but should be enough to enable the woman to gain a sense of shared experience as people journeying together towards a common goal.

Carolan & Hodnett (2007) suggest the midwife–woman relationship has been 'portrayed as going beyond more usual professional relationships in terms of importance, intimacy and intensity' (p. 146) and requires considerable emotional investment on the part of the midwife. They argue that there is little suggestion that creating partnership relationships is 'ever other than seamless' (p. 147) and question whether this close relationship is as important to women as it appears to be for midwives. Expression of how the midwifery relationship is valued by women can be seen both in the numbers of women choosing this model of care and in consumer satisfaction surveys conducted at intervals by the Ministry of Health. In Aotearoa New Zealand, over 90% of women select a midwife lead maternity carer (LMC) from among the choices on offer to them, which include obstetrician or GP provision of maternity care (Ministry of Health (MOH), n.d.). In 2014 (the latest consumer satisfaction survey available), 87% of women were 'very satisfied' or 'quite satisfied' with their overall care from an LMC midwife, which represented the highest satisfaction rating among caregiver types (MOH, 2015a).

Of course, working in partnership with women can sometimes be challenging, especially in situations where the relationship does not feel *equal*—for example when the behaviour of either the woman (and perhaps her family) or the midwife is not mutually supportive, or shows no recognition of each other's day-to-day 'busy-ness'. The provision of continuity of care and its challenge for midwives has increasingly been a topic of research and debate within the profession over the last decade or so. Some studies have focused on 'burnout' or how midwives are supported following sentinel events (Calvert, 2011; Sandall, 1997; Young, 2011). Others have explored why midwives cease caseloading practice (Ball et al., 2002; McLardy, 2003; Wakelin & Skinner, 2007). Salutary aspects of midwifery caseloading—exploring what enables midwives to stay in practice (Kirkham & Stapleton, 2000; McAra-Couper et al., 2012) and the satisfaction midwives feel in relation to their work (Page et al., 2006)—have also been documented. What is clear from these studies is that being a midwife is demanding and can occasionally feel overwhelming. Midwifery frameworks support midwives to work in sustainable ways, and the choices individual midwives make about how they work (caseload size, practice arrangements for time off and cover for holidays, etc.) can positively impact sustainability and longevity in practice (Gilkison et al., 2015; Hewitt et al., 2021; Hunter, 2016).

○ CLINICAL POINT

Tips for demonstrating partnership in practice

Initiating your relationship: the first phone call is often the point at which the pregnant person will form powerful first impressions of you as their chosen midwife. If a message has been left, it is important to respond in a timely manner, so they feel valued and knows that they are important to you. If you are unable to accept them for booking, make sure you contact them to let them know, and ensure they have some alternative options. If you are able to book them, remember to offer your congratulations! It could be

that if they are very young and newly pregnant, you may be the *first* person they have that congratulates them, and this will set the scene well for your ongoing relationship. Even people who find themselves unexpectedly pregnant enjoy the feeling that someone cares about their pregnancy. Arrange to meet with them by asking when they would like to connect with you, and where. Depending on their situation, they may need to be seen quickly, in order to facilitate discussions about managing early-pregnancy symptoms or to talk about screening options. If they will be coming to your midwifery clinic, ensure they have clear instructions about where to come; if late for the appointment, they may feel nervous about how they will be received. If you are going to them, being on time is important too; if you know you are going to be late, let them know in advance so they aren't left wondering if you have forgotten their visit.

As your relationship develops, and trust begins to form, it becomes easier to address those aspects of care which require particular sensitivity—for example discussions about screening for STIs, or family violence. These topics for discussion need not necessarily be part of your booking visit unless disclosure is spontaneous, and having developed a warm relationship in advance will enhance the likelihood that the pregnant person will trust you enough to be honest with you about their relevant history. At the end of each antenatal visit, ask them when they would like to see you next. The decision points (New Zealand College of Midwives (NZCOM), 2015) give some guidance about the spacing of antenatal visits, but it is useful to empower them to articulate their own preferred pattern of visits.

If the person contacts you outside of a planned antenatal visit to discuss a concern (e.g. an episode of diarrhoea and vomiting), it is helpful if you follow up this call the next day to ensure they are feeling better. This is a simple way of demonstrating that their wellbeing is important to you, and will give them confidence that their needs and concerns will be taken seriously. Feeling *cared for* is a really important contributor to a person's sense of overall wellbeing in pregnancy.

As birth approaches, ensure you tell the pregnant person and their family positive stories about birth, to enhance their confidence and decrease their anxiety (Dahlen et al., 2008). This will support them to explore other physically or emotionally challenging events in their life so that they can identify coping strategies which have previously been successful for them. When they phone to say they are in labour, be as excited as they are (!) because if they feel that you are too busy, or don't want to get out of bed, they may feel deflated by your lack of enthusiasm. Ensure they know that when they feel the need for your continuous presence this will be at *their* discretion, not as predetermined by a particular pattern of length, strength and frequency of contractions.

Concluding your partnership in a way that supports the person's transition out of your care is every bit as important as how you supported their introduction into it. It is valuable to begin to negotiate the completion of care early in the postpartum period by assisting the person to identify their ongoing support systems, and discussing their options for well child healthcare. As their discharge date approaches, it is vital that the person knows *in advance* which visit will be their last, as finding out on the day that this visit is the last may be disempowering and potentially distressing. Your goal as a midwife is to leave the person feeling strong and independent as they embark on their parenting role. Spending time together to reflect on your mutual experience of care is an important way to stimulate ongoing learning for you as their midwife, and beginning resolution of the experience for them (Baxter et al., 2014; Fryer & Weaver, 2014; Sheen & Slade, 2015). Midwives can do this with each and every partnership they form (Leap & Pairman, 2010) even in the context where a more formal process of feedback provision is in place, for example midwifery standards review consumer feedback forms.

Specific aspects of working in partnership during pregnancy, labour and birth, and the postpartum period are covered in Chapters 23, 25 and 30 so please make sure you read these closely.

What do women want from their midwife?

Like any human relationship, the development of partnership between a midwife and a childbearing woman is a complex process requiring self-knowledge, well developed communication skills, willingness, honesty, trust, generosity and time.

(Pairman, 2006, p. 74)

Women want a partnership with a midwife who has a strong clinical background with current knowledge and experience, and with a clear understanding of the evidence around childbirth (Homer et al., 2008). Women's needs of their midwives include professional and personal characteristics such as having confidence in women's abilities, skills to ensure normality is maintained, expertise in communication, the ability to collaborate with other care providers and the ability to provide continuity of care and carer (Homer et al., 2008). Women have also identified that being engaged in continuous learning (Nicholls et al., 2011), being 'an immediately available presence', supporting 'embodied limbo' and 'helping to go with the flow' (Borelli et al., 2016, p. 103) were characteristics of the 'good' midwife. From their interviews with fourteen first-time mothers Borelli et al. (2016) described the 'kaleidoscope midwife' who is 'ever-changing in the light of women's individual needs', who can 'create an environment that enables her to move forward despite uncertainty and the expectations / experiences gap' (p. 103).

The notion of 'advocacy' is complex in a relationship that is mutual and 'two-way' (Leap et al., 2010). It is important that the midwife and woman identify the women's individual characteristics and knowledge within the context of the partnership. The midwife then works with the woman to develop the woman's skills and confidence so that she is able to advocate for herself effectively and has faith in her own abilities to mother. In situations where women feel less able to advocate for themselves, often in the face of illness or extreme dominance of

medicalisation in birth, the significant and long-lasting relationship between the midwife and woman enables the midwife to honestly and actively reflect the woman's wishes, alongside other people that the woman has chosen to support her.

Ross-Davie & Cheyne's (2014) structured literature review reported on themes from 91 studies examining what women find most helpful about professional support during the intrapartum period. Their main finding, 'high-quality continuous support', was characterised by the following behaviours:

. . . supportive presence; enabling the woman to have a sense of control, asking the woman and her birth partner what kind of care they would like; presenting a positive, calm and friendly attitude; providing reassurance and praise; coaching the woman and her partner in ways to cope, such as breathing and relaxation, when needed; ensuring the woman feels respected and cared for as an individual; keeping the couple informed about progress; ensuring the partner feels involved and supported and providing physical support, such as touch and assisting with position changes, when wanted.

(Ross-Davie & Cheyne, 2014, p. 57)

The authors concluded that provision of intrapartum care that included these measures resulted in high satisfaction for women and fewer medical interventions. Feeling in control of their own experience was highly valued by women, and they reported improved postnatal wellbeing when they had received highly supportive care, regardless of the outcomes of their births.

In order to promote confidence in women, the midwife needs to be secure and confident in herself, both as a woman and as a midwife (Kirkham, 2010). This often entails a mature approach to resisting the temptation to 'make things better', 'sort everything out' and take control as the 'expert' (Leap & Pairman, 2010). The relationship needs to ensure independence of both parties and recognition of potential co-dependencies. It is also important that, whilst midwives have confidence in their own expertise, they do not see themselves as superior or 'experts' who need to 'instruct' and 'educate' women; midwives need to conceptualise the relationship as one based on mutual learning and reciprocity (Guilliland & Pairman, 2010a; Pairman, 1998). Women want midwives with excellent communication skills (Homer et al., 2008, p. 676) and the midwife's ability to listen and communicate openly is the first step in developing a meaningful relationship.

If a relationship is such that the practitioner does not listen, does not come to know the hopes and fears of the woman, does not respond to her anxieties, then the mode of care can only ... be based on the semblance of what the practitioner thinks should be happening. It lacks attention to the things that are 'mattering'. It traps the woman into a passive role of accepting inappropriate, unsafe care, rather than freeing her to involve herself in the accomplishment of personalised care that promotes all that is safe.

(Smythe, 1998, p. 202)

Partnering women in decision making: informed choice and consent

Decision making in pregnancy, birth and post birth is a complex process and it is not only the decisions but also the process of decision making that some women may find challenging. This period may be the first time women feel and respond to the full responsibility of decision making. Women's confidence and mental wellbeing is often affected by how well they are supported whilst exploring evidence and making decisions. Within the partnership model, the midwife can enable situations in which women have a chance to develop their confidence in this area, with acknowledgement that the midwife also grapples with the uncertainty and complexity that surrounds much decision making (Downe & McCourt, 2008; Page & Mander, 2014).

The partnership model provides for mutual information exchange between the woman and midwife in an egalitarian process. It is not possible to completely eliminate restrictions in a woman's life circumstances that impact on choice. Choices are influenced by intersections of ideology, resources, ethnicity, and other factors, such as obstetric regimens and value systems, over which women have little control (Leap & Edwards, 2006; Quigley, 2014). However, it is strongly suggested that partnership provides women with the greatest opportunity to obtain evidenced-based information and to seek all options and alternatives in her care. A decision can be made, in the absence of coercion by any party, that reflects self-determination, autonomy and control (Health and Disability Commission (HDC), 1996; National Health and Medical Research Council (NHMRC), 2010). Often there is little recognition of the complex nature of 'informed choice' and the fact that the person who does the 'informing' will play a major role in determining the 'choice' that is made (Leap, 2010; Menage, 2016). In the Australian context, Stevens et al. (2014) noted the seeming paradox between women feeling a high level of 'decisional autonomy' over their choices regarding the model of care they wish to engage with and having insufficient information on which to base these decisions. In their Queensland-based study, although 83% of the over 5000 women responding to a survey reported active involvement in deciding the model of care that would best meet their needs, only 8.2% of these women were given information about the option of having a home birth with a private midwife. Midwifery partnership is by definition non-coercive so recognition of the intricacies of the relationship in sharing information and allowing open discussion in relation to decision making is essential for midwives working in the partnership model. The New Zealand College of Midwives has developed a *Consensus Statement on Informed Consent and Decision Making* (NZCOM, 2016) outlining midwives' responsibilities in relation to **informed choice and consent**, which affirms the dynamic process of decision making and the centrality of the woman to this process.

Midwives are challenged regularly around the 'advice' provided to women, particularly in situations where the woman is facing a decision that is not straightforward. The attitude of the midwife is important not only in the decision, but additionally in how the woman reflects on the decision she has made. This is especially important in circumstances where midwives are challenged by the decisions that women make and find it hard to support their choices (Holten & de Miranda, 2016). In New Zealand, the *Referral Guidelines* (MOH, 2012) protect both the informed choice of the woman who makes an 'unorthodox' choice *and* the LMC midwife who may find herself practising outside her scope by the explication of a clear pathway which can be followed in this event. Midwives are directed to *advise* the woman about recommended care, including the evidence supporting that recommendation, *explain* the LMC's potential need to discuss the case with another practitioner, ensuring the woman's right to privacy, *share* the outcomes of this discussion with the woman, and *document* these discussions and any decisions the woman has made clearly in the clinical record (MOH, 2012, p. 18). Similarly, in Australia, the Australian College of Midwives' *National Midwifery Guidelines for Consultation and Referral* (2017) contain Appendix A and B, which outline steps that midwives can take when a woman chooses a course of action which sits outside the guidelines. Appendix B is a 'Record of Understanding' template which can be used to document the discussions, decisions made and ongoing management plan in this circumstance. The midwife's ability to share messages which demonstrate to the woman that the midwife trusts in her, and her ability to consider all elements and make appropriate decisions may go a long way to building up women's confidence in their ability to cope with the challenges of new motherhood.

Partnering women in communication—written and verbal

If we conceptualise midwifery care as a blend of art and science, then communication falls squarely into the midwifery 'arts'. The nature of the communication between women and midwives is a powerful indicator of the way the relationship is progressing. In a social landscape where communication is becoming increasingly 'clipped' by technology (Twitter is a prime example of saying as much as possible in as few words as possible) the conversations between women and midwives remain an important tool for information sharing, exploring hopes and fears, settling nerves and expressing joy and triumph. Effective communication is a two-way process which involves 'giving and receiving information, which requires efficient use of language, effective listening, observation, accurate interpretation, and appropriate responses to verbal and non-verbal clues' (England & Morgan, 2012, p. 1). Listening is an especially important part of communication in midwifery, as it involves using the mind, senses and emotions to understand what is being communicated, not just the words that are being spoken (Deane-Gray, 2008). From the first phone call to the discharge visit, being supportive and showing genuine interest in, and care for, the woman are vital to developing a partnership that will be mutually satisfying.

The *Midwives Handbook for Practice* (NZCOM, 2015) outlines midwives' responsibilities around both written and verbal communication, with both the *Standards for Practice* and the *Competencies for Entry to the Register of Midwives* containing statements requiring that a midwife 'communicates effectively with the woman/wahine and her family/whānau, as defined by the woman/wahine' (p. 6), that she 'facilitates open interactive communication and negotiates shared decision-making' (p. 18), and that she 'documents her assessments and uses them as a basis for ongoing midwifery actions in consultation with the woman' (p. 20). Midwives need to remain mindful at all times that the language used in both their verbal encounters and their written documentation supports and affirms the woman. In particular, words and phrases that imply poor bodily function ('failure to progress', 'incompetent cervix', 'irritable uterus') or that are patronising ('aren't you clever', 'good girl') should be avoided at all costs.

Partnering women in written communication is an important contributor to a woman's sense of ownership of her experience. Women-held notes enable both the woman and her midwife to contribute their individual expertise, by developing a record that reflects each person's input to decision making and the development of care planning. It is a requirement in New Zealand (under Section 88) that LMCs arrange for the woman to hold her clinical record unless she prefers to be given a copy at the completion of each module (MOH, 2009). Fleming (1998) suggested the possibility that the joint construction of the written clinical record by both midwives and women might enable the explication of a body of midwifery knowledge by using language that is woman centred and thus different from objective medically focused language commonly found. She argued that midwifery knowledge is in part derived from an oral culture shared through story and reflective practice, but that documentation has not traditionally reflected those aspects of the woman's experience that remain meaningful for her over time—her emotional or intuitive context. Documentation which is an artful blend of both the objective findings and the social/emotional context may articulate additional dimensions of midwifery knowledge as effectively as empirical knowledge derived from research and deserves to be as highly valued by health professionals as it is by women. Shared construction of knowledge also reflects a commitment to partnership by surfacing women's voices and the aspects of care most valued by them—that is, those things that are *mattering* (Smythe, 1998).

Women-held notes create an opportunity to promote women's active participation in their care (Kerkin, et al., 2017). They enable excellent communication between practitioners in the event that a woman's experience becomes complex and additional input is required from other health professionals.

Documentation in the clinical record should contain sufficient information to demonstrate the midwife's decision-making processes, especially in the labour context. Clinical records that find their way to a review process (for example, in the event of an unexpected poor outcome) are closely scrutinised to discern why the practitioner acted in the way they did, and well-constructed documentation can be highly protective where clinical decision making has been reasonable. Notes need to reflect not just *what* was done, but *why* a decision was made to intervene, or to continue without intervention. Davies (2010) suggests that a guide to the effectiveness of your documentation is to ask yourself 'if I was relieving this midwife, would I easily grasp the progress or current concerns of this woman/whānau and/or baby?' (p. 553). A recently published literature review concluded that the purpose of midwifery documentation is multidimensional and extends beyond the mere reportage of clinical and legal details about the woman's care (Kerkin et al., 2017). The authors note the potential for enhancement of the woman's experience through co-construction of the record and support for the role of the midwife by 'making visible' the extent of what midwives do. They suggest a positive contribution to collaborative relationships with other healthcare practitioners can be achieved via the woman's written records. Organisational processes and research are other areas where documentation can play a key role to increase our understanding of midwifery practice and women's experience of maternity care (Kerkin et al., 2017).

With the advent of electronic health records now a reality in most clinical settings, midwives are coming to understand both the benefits and the limitations of this technology. Whilst some studies have reported improved completion of perinatal data collection once e-health records have been implemented (Craswell et al., 2013), others have described qualitatively how the inclusion of yet more technology in the woman's birthspace can be intimidating for women (Brooke-Read et al., 2012). The student midwives in this study could articulate some benefits of e-health records such as improved availability of information, the lack of legibility problems associated with hand-written records and ease of referral to another clinical area. Balancing this, they also described feeling nervous about the 'instantaneousness' of the records being 'in the system' when as a student they were used to negotiating handwritten documentation with their preceptor or mentor midwife before committing to paper. One student midwife described disruption to her care (and therefore her partnership with the women) saying 'We also need to think about the perception of the woman, because you're standing there, banging away at the computer, and you feel like you're on the checkout at a supermarket and she feels like she's a tin of beans or something!' (Brooke-Read et al., 2012, p. 444).

If one purpose of documentation is to provide a record for a wahine and her whānau of their childbearing journey, it will be important for midwives to think about how they document their care so that it still reflects the narrative of the episode of care in a meaningful way for whānau.

For a closer examination of the legal requirements relating to documentation, please refer to Chapter 14.

Communication—a word about texting

Although fairly ubiquitous as a communication medium in our social world, texting as a means of communication between a midwife and her client can be potentially risky and is discouraged when a clinical issue is the subject of the communication (Fig. 17.1). Inappropriate text communication has been highlighted in at least one case brought to the attention of the Health and Disability Commission, following the death of a baby (Barker et al., 2012). Whilst it may be an easy and efficient method for making or changing an appointment, in the event that a clinical issue is being communicated it is important that the midwife responds with a phone call, rather than texting a reply. Coverage issues and occasional network glitches can see messages delivered sometimes several hours after they were sent, and this can potentially compromise safety for the woman and/or her baby. The Midwifery Council of New Zealand *Code of Conduct* (2010) gives some specific guidance in this area:

> *Text messaging can be an unreliable method of communication, with message transmission delayed at times or messages open to misinterpretation. While women may use texting to contact a midwife, midwives must consider the appropriateness of using text communications and ensure that their communication with women occurs through reliable methods such as telephone. All communication with women should be appropriately documented.*

(MCNZ, 2010, p. 7)

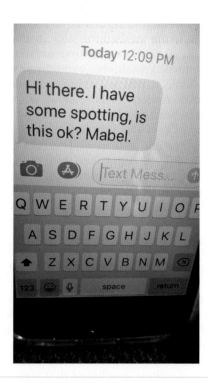

FIGURE 17.1 Example of text message received by a midwife
(Image courtesy the author (SM))

Barker et al. (2012) describe the potential for misinterpretation of text messages, noting that in most circumstances other than appointment-related messages the midwife needs to communicate more directly with the woman, in order to make an appropriate assessment about the woman's concern. A message regarding ruptured membranes, for example, requires an in-depth conversation as a number of considerations will impact the woman's decision making in this instance.

REFLECTIVE THINKING EXERCISE

Communication

Words are extremely powerful. Take these six, for example:

For sale: Baby shoes. Never worn. (Anon)

This could be a classified ad, or the saddest poem ever written. So when you are communicating with a woman, the words you choose can have a lasting effect. Think of what words you might choose in the following situations:

- You are learning to use a Pinard to auscultate the baby's heartrate. You carefully palpate the woman's abdomen and place your Pinard where you think you will be most likely to hear the heartbeat. You hear nothing.

- You have been with Saele, who is in labour, for most of the night. Her contractions are regular, and she has been finding them really challenging, and feels exhausted. She requests a vaginal examination. She is 2 cm dilated.

- Manu is supporting his partner Jasmin in labour. She is in the bath, and Manu is reading the emergency management posters on the wall of the birthing suite room. He asks you 'what does "remove the posterior arm" mean?'

- You are meeting with Kiriana and Alex for a booking visit and are discussing the options for first trimester screening. They ask what will happen if they have a combined first trimester result which indicates increased chance of having a baby with one of the conditions tested for.

- You have received an hCG result for Amanda and the level is not as high as you would expect for her 8-week-gestation pregnancy. You ring Amanda to discuss this result with her.

THE ROLE OF THE MIDWIFE
The changing landscape of midwifery practice in Australia

Until recent years working in partnership with women has been seriously restricted in Australia owing to the lack of continuity-of-care models. In 2008, consumer demand for midwifery continuity of care was demonstrated within a national review of maternity services in Australia receiving unprecedented submissions asking for improved access for women to midwives (Australian

Government Department of Health, 2009, p. 60). Subsequently, a number of legislative and regulatory changes for midwives have enabled women to access directly Commonwealth-rebated care from self-employed midwives for most elements of their care including birth care in hospital. This review led to the development of a *National Maternity Services Plan* (Australian Government Department of Health, 2011), which works to implement greater access to Commonwealth funding (Medicare) for midwives and for expanded options for state-employed midwives to work in continuity-of-care models (see Ch. 1). The landscape in Australia continues to evolve and greater access to continuity of care also means greater demand for midwives, including graduates, to work in these models. Midwives working in partnership have a greater level of occupational autonomy and flexibility, therefore organising and prioritising their workload becomes a valued skill for midwives who are working in continuity-of-care models (Hewitt et al., 2021).

The transition requires midwives to make changes in the way that they work, including potentially where they work (hospital or community based), the hours they work (shiftwork or a flexibility-responsive pattern to deal with the needs of women) and, as indicated above, responsibility (all clients admitted 'under' a medical officer and a line of reporting through the midwife 'in charge' of the shift instead of the woman being admitted as a client of the midwife with the responsibility to seek consultation and referral as required resting with the midwife). It is important that midwives making this transition are supported by other midwives who are already working this way (Queensland Government, 2012, p. 17).

There are a variety of models within Australia that are now designed to provide, or increase, access to midwifery continuity of care, most of which are for midwives employed by hospitals and state-based facilities. These include: models where midwives work in groups (midwifery group practice or caseload practice (McLachlan et al., 2012; Tracy et al., 2013) and are on call for labour and birth care (Homer et al., 2008, p. 17); and a range of team models that are variously defined in terms of whether they are on call for women in birth or work in a rostered arrangement to provide birth care. Many models also provide antenatal care in groups based in the Centring Pregnancy model of antenatal care (Homer et al., 2008, p. 14).

Midwives working in self-employed practice in increasing numbers are able to provide continuity of care to women in all contexts. The ability for self-employed midwives to provide care to women who are admitted to hospital at any time, including for labour and birth, has not been possible in Australia since the indemnity insurance crisis, and prior to this most midwives did not work this way. Midwives may now apply to the Australian Health Practitioner Regulation Agency (AHPRA) for registration as an 'endorsed midwife', which qualifies the midwife to prescribe certain scheduled medicines (see Ch. 13). The endorsement also enables midwives to apply and receive a Medicare provider number, which may enable more midwives to make the step into self-employed practice as a financially viable option. A Medicare rebate is available for a range of services including provision of antenatal care, postnatal care and birth care in hospital but not at home. For a rebate for private birth services to be available the midwife must be credentialed and have visiting or admitting rights to the hospital where the woman gives birth to her baby. Midwives providing care as endorsed midwives with admitting rights to a hospital provide that care in collaboration with private practitioners and the hospital team. This way of working is limited to a small number of areas in Australia. A number of evaluation studies are emerging in the Australian midwifery literature about these evolving models of care, which are showing favourable outcomes including for young and Aboriginal women (see, for example, Allen et al., 2015; Scherman et al., 2008; Wilkes et al., 2015).

Aotearoa New Zealand—LMC and core midwifery roles

Since 1990, midwives have worked under contract to the Ministry of Health to provide primary maternity services (since 1996 as 'lead maternity carer' (LMC) midwives). Women who seek continuity of care in this context will sign a registration form, which renders the LMC responsible for coordinating the woman's care across the spectrum of her childbearing experience, and accountable for the care that she provides. The woman is free to change LMC at any time in her pregnancy. With the exception of non-resident women, and a few other selected circumstances, this care provision is free of charge to the woman. Currently 32% of the midwifery workforce provides care to women in this model. A further 49% of the workforce is employed as core midwifery staff in District Health Boards (MCNZ, 2020). Core midwives are the backbone of the maternity facility workforce, providing care to women who have no LMC, or who have chosen an obstetrician as their LMC, as discussed further below. Wherever a midwife chooses to practise, she works autonomously across the full scope of midwifery practice and is accountable for the care that she provides. The remainder of the midwifery workforce comprises midwives working in research, education, administrative roles, etc., and those who hold an Annual Practising Certificate, but who are not currently practising due to maternity leave, etc.

Provision of continuity of care— outcomes of one-to-one care

Midwifery continuity of care demonstrates significant benefits to women. In their Cochrane review, Sandall et al. (2016) compared midwife-led care in a community and hospital setting with medical-led models—excluding homebirth and women with complex medical and obstetric needs. The findings concluded that women choosing midwife-led care were less likely to have surgical interventions such as episiotomy, forceps and ventouse extraction, and had less analgesia and anaesthesia during the intrapartum period (Sandall et al., 2016). The study also found a reduction in the rate of pre-term births under 37 weeks, and an increase in spontaneous vaginal birth compared with other models of care. Interestingly, the caesarean section rates were comparable across models (Sandall et al., 2016). However, the CoSMos trial has demonstrated that caseload care for women of low obstetric risk at the onset of pregnancy demonstrated promise for decreasing caesarean section rates, whilst also demonstrating increased vaginal birth rates in primiparous women, decreased likelihood of epidural anaesthesia, and lower episiotomy rates (McLachlan et al., 2012). The study by Wax et al. (2010) demonstrated that birth-centre and home births, related to midwifery-led care, were associated with improved maternal and perinatal outcomes compared with hospital births in healthy women. In Australia, research regarding continuity models has demonstrated improved outcomes for young women. Significantly fewer pre-term births and admissions to neonatal intensive care facilities were shown for newborns of women under 21 who received caseload care, compared with standard care (Allen et al., 2015). Wilkes et al. (2015) described reduced rates for induction of labour, less use of pharmacological pain medications, lower caesarean section rates and fewer admissions to neonatal intensive care facilities in their cohort of 323 women who received caseload care from a privately practising eligible midwife compared with national rates for these outcomes for women receiving standard care. The overarching view of most research is that there is a reduction in intervention, an increase in safety, improved satisfaction for recipients of care and increased access to care for indigenous people in midwifery continuity-of-care models (Fernandez Turienzo et al., 2019; Forster et al., 2016; Sandall et al., 2016; Turnbull et al., 2009).

The feeling of safety and the associated reduction of uncertainty that partnership with a known midwife in a continuity-of-care model during pregnancy, birth and the postnatal period confers is of paramount importance in terms of aiding a mother's sense of wellbeing. Matthias (2009) observed in her study comparing the way obstetricians and midwives manage uncertainty that the midwife–woman relationship revolved around education and informing the mother of ideas and choices relating to birth care. Where uncertainty arose, the midwife helped the mother reframe her fears to find new ways to cope with vulnerability. In contrast, the obstetrician–woman relationship was more formal, with less conversation around social and emotional issues and more focused on medical aspects of care. The relationship of women and their midwives is based in a completely different context to that of women and obstetricians, which has a more demonstrated power imbalance (Matthias, 2009).

In Aotearoa New Zealand, where the one-to-one (LMC) model of care has been embedded for many years, it is possible to discern measurable benefits for women and their babies, including those of so-called 'hard-to-reach' populations (young mothers, Māori and Pacific women).

In 2018, the latest year for which statistics are available, approximately 92.9% of women chose an LMC as their caregiver; within this number, 94.5% chose a midwife LMC, with 0.2% choosing a GP and 5.3% an obstetrician (MOH, n.d.). The online Maternity Report Webtool (MOH) outlines outcome data on a range of parameters associated with pregnancy, birth and postpartum care. The increasing complexity of the maternity cohort has seen recent increases in intervention rates (2018 data) such as induction of labour (26.4%), caesarean section (28.4%) and episiotomy rates (16%), but, in an international context of more pronounced increases, Aotearoa is holding its rates at lower levels than comparable countries (MOH, n.d). Two-thirds of women are now booking with an LMC in the first trimester of pregnancy, compared with just 50% less than a decade ago, and the statistically significant reduction in the stillbirth rate reported in the *Tenth Annual Report of the Perinatal and Maternal Mortality Review Committee* (PMMRC, 2016) has continued since 2007.

Enabling midwives to work in partnership with women

Australia

The frameworks for midwives in Australia have moved towards articulating the partnership model, but still reflect the history of midwifery as a specialty of nursing. The AHPRA is the overarching regulatory body within Australia, with the Nursing and Midwifery Board of Australia (NMBA) being the board responsible for both nurses and midwives. Several documents contribute to the framework for midwives including *A Midwife's Guide to Professional Boundaries* (NMBA, 2010) and refer to partnership, but also talk about a 'zone of helpfulness, under and over involvement' (NMBA, 2010) within midwifery care. There is a recommendation that midwives not have a dual role—that is, friendship with women for whom they care, which may be difficult in situations where women are cared for over more than one pregnancy and where the professional friendship develops. In Australia, midwives who are working in continuity-of-care models, and in longer-term partnerships with women, are seen as the minority of the workforce. Most policy documents and guidelines reflect a nursing-based culture of fragmented care; however, this is changing. Effective from March 2018, the *Code of Conduct for Midwives* (NMBA, 2018) articulates an expectation of the provision of safe, woman-centred and evidence-based midwifery care that reflects partnership and promotes shared decision making with women.

Birthing on Country represents a further crucial understanding of partnership with Aboriginal and Torres Strait Islander women and their families, and its principles can be applied regardless of the setting for birth. The integration of these principles into midwifery practice is supported by the Joint Birthing on Country Position Statement developed collaboratively by the Australian College of Midwives, CATSINaM and CRANAplus (2015).

The Birthing on Country (BoC) project seeks to improve outcomes for indigenous women and babies by bringing community members and health services together, supported by State and National Governments to establish models of maternity care that embed Birthing on Country principles (see https://anmj.org.au/birthing-on-country-improving-indigenous-health/). Please also see Chapter 10 for further discussion about Birthing on Country.

The opportunity for Australian midwives to reflect on all elements of midwifery care in relation to the regulatory framework is possible within the Australian College of Midwives (ACM) midwifery practice review (MPR). The MPR is based on New Zealand midwifery standards review (MSR) and occurs every 3 years. Reflection is the central tenet of the review process and women working in continuity-of-care models must provide their statistics, satisfaction surveys, and reflection on the way they work with women (see ACM website). MPR can be accessed as an online video review process in the wake of the COVID-19 pandemic.

Aotearoa New Zealand

The frameworks that enable midwives in Aotearoa New Zealand to work in partnership with women are well established and embedded from the first moment in a student midwife's educational journey. The *Midwives Handbook for Practice* (NZCOM, 2015) articulates the philosophy and scope of midwifery practice, the code of ethics, competencies for entry to the Register of Midwives, standards for practice, **Tūranga Kaupapa** statements, and decision points for the provision of care. Partnership is a foundational principle in each of these frameworks, and is underpinned by an expectation of cultural competence, which among other things involves a midwife's responsibility to reflect on her own background and attitudes, so that she can provide care that focuses on power shifting/sharing, even when a woman's views are at odds with her own.

Other frameworks that highlight the reciprocal nature of midwifery partnership provide service users (consumers) with opportunities to contribute their expertise, by way of engagement with the Midwifery Standards Review process, the Resolution Committee process, and by participation in all aspects of the structure and decision making of both the professional (New Zealand College of Midwives/Te Kāreti o Nga Kaiwhakawhanau ki Aotearoa) and the regulatory (Te Tatau o te Whare Kahu/Midwifery Council) bodies of the profession. These frameworks are discussed in detail in Chapter 13.

Partnerships with consumer organisations

In both Australia and Aotearoa New Zealand, consumer groups are actively engaged in partnerships with the midwifery profession. The Maternity Coalition and Homebirth Australia have been working alongside the Australian College of Midwives in political activity directed towards ensuring women's options for place of birth and access to continuity-of-care models continue to be on the political radar. Representatives from Homebirth Aotearoa, the Royal New Zealand Plunket Society, Parents Centre New Zealand and La Leche League all hold positions in the New Zealand College of Midwives National Committee, where they actively engage in policy debate and ensure the voices of women are heard. In both countries, maternity consumers have taken to the streets alongside midwives in recent years to protest about the erosion of services, be it closures of small primary maternity facilities or threats to the option of homebirth. Women and midwives working together politically was the genesis of the sweeping maternity reforms of the late 1980s and 1990s in Aotearoa New Zealand (Guilliland & Pairman, 2010b), and this effort has been mirrored in Australia in recent years where momentum is gathering with the extension of Medicare access to midwives.

Partnerships with other midwives — group practice

Midwives working in continuity of care are challenged working on their own and therefore there is a tendency towards midwifery group practice to increase sustainability. There are some midwives who prefer to essentially work alone, but this model presents significant challenges including fatigue and burnout. The attributes of individual midwives and midwifery group practices that contribute to effective and sustainable care provision are discussed in more detail in Chapter 16. Midwives in continuity-of-care models usually work in partnership either consistently (i.e. with the same partner all the time) or with a back-up midwife from within a wider midwifery group usually chosen for the care of each woman. The group practice model relies on more than just a partnership to provide cover for holidays, other leave and unexpected events. However, the relationships that midwives have with each other offer more than a practical back-up. These relationships also have the potential to provide:

- friendship, support, laughter and fun
- reflection in and on practice
- debriefing
- the sharing of ideas, information and evidence
- a safe place to express uncertainty and fear
- mentoring and peer review
- support for students and new graduates
- opportunities to locate individual experiences in the wider political context
- strategising and action to enable political and policy change
- the breaking down of hierarchical barriers
- a sense of 'belonging' and professional identity (Leap & Pairman, 2010).

The partnership between midwives cannot be forced; it is important that—like the partnership between a woman and her midwife—there is common ground that brings the midwives together. This may be a shared or similar philosophy. There are also important considerations such as the way the midwives approach work (Leap & Pairman, 2010) and additionally the stage of life of the midwife. For example, midwives with small children may work well together having a shared understanding of the commitments that this requires; however, midwives at different points having different commitments (no children, children left home or other carer commitments) may prefer to work together (Queensland Government, 2012). The personal relationship between midwives working together relies on trust and communication. Sustainability of midwifery practice is covered substantially in Chapter 16.

There are a range of decisions to be made when working in a midwifery group practice. These include how the midwives organise on- and off-call time, the mechanisms for ensuring that women know both/all midwives who may be involved in her care, and how communication occurs both between midwives and between women and midwives (Queensland Government, 2012).

In Australia, most midwives working in caseload practice—particularly in employed settings—are employed on a specific caseload award. The scheduling of on- and off-call time in these models varies, with some having significant flexibility and some looking more like a roster of on- and off-call time. These ways of working have been described in four ways (Queensland Government, 2012):

- caseload—care of allocated women
- caseload—rostered time off call
- caseload—rostered time on call
- team.

The care of allocated women is the mechanism employed by most self-employed midwives so that they provide care to their primary clients for the majority of time. There may be some decision about off-call time, say every second weekend or similar, but the midwives primarily remain available for birth care.

Where midwives in Australia are employed on an award system, they are primarily required to roster some time off call. In most models, this requires an allocation that midwives have two days per week off duty. Some models work this very flexibly—rarely providing this care when births do not occur—and therefore would be referred to as providing care for allocated women. However, some models these days are more rigidly allocated and women will know that the back-up midwife will attend them if they require assistance or birth on their midwife's 'days off'.

A model that appears to be developing throughout Australia is a more rigid model of having midwives on call only for small periods of time. This model is referred to as 'caseload—rostered on call' (Queensland Government, 2012, p. 67). The midwife may still be allocated women for whom they provide primary care; however, they are 'on call' (typically overnight) for only short periods—for instance, they may have on call periods of one or two nights at a time or may have two nights on call per week.

The team model means generally that the woman is not allocated a primary midwife but is cared for within the team. The midwives are typically rostered on- and off-call time.

The differences between these four ways of working are not well articulated and therefore do not appear to be well evaluated; however, it is clear that continuity of midwifery care is impacted. It is fundamental that as more models evolve in Australia the recognition of the need for continuity of midwifery care, which is the driver for development, is also balanced with the midwives' needs.

Community-based midwives also work alongside hospital-based midwives. In Aotearoa New Zealand there are 'core' midwives who are rostered on shifts. The role of these midwives has changed in response to the development of midwifery caseload practice. The majority of women—around 95% (MOH, n.d.)—continue to birth in a maternity facility and most of these women (90%) come into it under the care of their midwife LMC. Employed midwives may be involved directly in the care of women with serious complications who have been admitted under the care of the hospital obstetric team, or women whose clinical responsibility has been 'transferred' under the *Referral Guidelines* (MOH, 2012). In this circumstance, it is common for the LMC to remain involved in the provision of the woman's midwifery care, alongside a core midwife who may provide clinical support for more complex areas of care (e.g. insulin infusions). A few women who choose a general practitioner (GP) or private obstetrician for their LMC, or who arrive at a facility without a named caregiver, will also be cared for by core midwives. Therefore, a role has been articulated for the 'core' midwife: one that is based on supporting the primary woman–midwife partnership (Campbell, 2000; Guilliland & Pairman, 2010a; Pairman, 2000b). The core midwife can be viewed as the 'wise woman' of the maternity facility:

her skills in facilitating and negotiating the interface between primary services and secondary/tertiary services have a major impact on each woman's experience of birth and each midwife's ability to continue to provide the woman's midwifery care, even when obstetric interventions may be required. In order for this to happen, both LMC midwives and core midwives have to develop clear understandings of each other's roles and the need to work in partnership in the interests of woman-centred care.

(Leap & Pairman, 2010, p. 346)

The recognition and valuing of each other's roles contributes positively to women's experience, as each strives to maintain normality in the context of complexity. Earl (unpublished thesis) has described a number of ways in which core midwives work to retain a 'normal birth' focus in a facility setting. These include holding on to a firm belief that birth is a normal life event, developing 'little rules of thumb' to prevent further intervention, and utilising the knowledge of more experienced midwives. She concludes her thesis thus (p. 164):

[core midwives] demonstrate a quiet yet determined courage to constantly question the decisions that might take away from the 'normal' experience. They do not say that intervention is not necessary, but rather, they raise questions about their automatic use, and ask, 'Do we really need to do this? Does it feel right? Is there another way?' Such questions keep normal birth a possibility.

365

Gilkison et al. (2017) similarly reported the unique and specific skill set of core midwives as contributing to the sustainability of core midwifery work. These skills include developing quick rapport with families, being prepared to deal with anything including critical incidents, managing complexity, being flexible and adaptable. They noted also that what might threaten the sustainability of this type of work was feeling invisible and undervalued at times (p. 36). As midwives traverse their life's path, it is increasingly common for them to move both into and out of self-employed and employed practice, as family responsibilities and other opportunities (e.g. postgraduate study, becoming a midwifery educator, or working in developing countries) place different demands on their time, and the need for flexibility/structure around their working world ebbs and flows.

REFLECTIVE THINKING EXERCISE

Working within a midwifery group practice (MGP) is a rewarding but challenging experience. Consider the following issues:

1. Mary, Jenny, Kate and Tahnee are working together in a group practice. The workload appears to be being unevenly shared, with Mary having many additional days where she has been unable to work due to commitments to a research project. Jenny, Kate and Tahnee are unsure about how to resolve this issue.

2. Saskia and Clare work in partnership. Clare has a noticeably reduced number of satisfaction surveys completed. When Saskia speaks to a client of Clare's about this, the client indicates that she thinks it is probably because Clare is lovely, but her approach to care feels really disorganised so no one wants to say anything.

3. An MGP within Somewhere Hospital is having trouble communicating with a new medical officer. Some of the MGP midwives favour approaching the medical officer directly and inviting him to lunch to discuss matters, whilst others favour going to the medical director to discuss this potential risk to client safety.

4. Aleta is concerned about one of the midwives in her group practice. She regularly advises women to use a variety of complementary therapies without consulting relevant complementary therapists, which Aleta believes is outside her colleagues' scope of practice. Additionally, she becomes agitated if previous clients choose another midwife and tries to make contact with her previous clients to convince them to change care provider. There are clearly serious practice issues, but Aleta is new to the group practice and wonders how to deal with this issue.

5. Kerri is joining a new group practice where she will be the only midwife without children at home. Her colleagues are jokingly discussing how they like to roster off-call time regularly to spend time with their kids. Kerri prefers to organise time off around births.

Student midwives—partnering midwives and women

Student midwives also work in partnership relationships alongside midwives and pregnant women as they gain knowledge, insight and clinical experience in their journey to becoming midwives. As a midwife, sharing one's expertise is not only a professional and ethical responsibility (NZCOM, 2015); it is described by many midwives as also a joy, a wonderful opportunity to maintain currency via robust discussion and critique of practice, and a further opportunity to engage in reflective practice for the midwife. James (2012) described the 'excitement' midwives felt when students began integrating theory and practice well, the 'bringing it all together' (p. 15). Precepting and mentorship of students and midwives is discussed further elsewhere in the text.

Women also appear to value highly the relationships they develop with student midwives, describing a sense of 'solidarity' in their 'mutual newness' (Snows, 2010). Snows discusses how this fosters 'a unique bond, strengthened through a shared transition and negotiation of complex obstacles' and contends that 'students who offer themselves as companions to women in a medicalised birth culture deserve recognition, and should perhaps be timely reminders to all midwives of what it truly means to be with woman' (p. 40).

REFLECTIVE CASE STUDY

Thoughts on partnership from 'Kelly'—student midwife

Guilliland & Pairman (2010a) define the many aspects underpinning the partnership that enables midwives and women to work together throughout the maternity journey and into motherhood. Alongside a steadfast woman-centred approach, I see one of the most important aspects as being mutual trust. Developing relationships of trust with women as a student of midwifery has been one of the most challenging aspects of the degree. As is their right, women want to know they are receiving the best care available and the term 'student' implies one's skill level is below this standard. Nevertheless, we are students, requiring hands-on learning opportunities with women, babies and families to gain and develop skills, which will in turn facilitate trust. I have lost count of the moments where I silently straightened my spine when introduced to women and their families, trying to feign an aura of confidence that would allow them to see my competence. Usually we as students have not had much time to develop a relationship which can traverse times of heightened fear or emotion, and I wonder if this leaves women feeling their experience of continuity was lacking when it was most needed/anticipated. Initially I felt enormous pressure to practise building 'midwifery partnerships' with women to combat this; however, what resulted was never fully a midwifery partnership, but rather a student/woman relationship. I can see now that this is because the midwifery partnership, in its fullness, requires a framework which I am unable to offer women as a student. I think developing a sort of student/midwife partnership with the midwives I work alongside facilitates learning experiences which are more woman centred, as the midwife often knows the woman's hopes and expectations, and she can help ensure the student's involvement is appropriate. I have also noticed that when the midwives I work with trust me then this flows on to the woman through the way I am introduced, and the confidence the midwife shows in my skills. Hence, I would say lately that I have been focusing on developing partnerships with the midwives, and then if the woman is consenting I am brought into the midwifery partnership with the woman via the midwife. From that point, it is a three-way, collaborative experience, within which I can establish a relationship of trust and participate in some aspects of a partnership that already exists. In this way, I have been able to develop and better understand the concept and realities of establishing partnerships with women, and with midwives.

Other partnerships—the midwife and her community

As primary healthcare practitioners who cross the interface between hospital and community services, the majority of a midwife's work takes place in the community. This means that midwives need to have a sophisticated understanding of the importance of networking and establishing partnerships with other agencies and practitioners in their local communities in initiatives that employ the principles of primary healthcare and community development.

Effective partnerships underpin the role of midwifery as a woman-centred, public health strategy (Kaufmann, 2000, 2002). Midwives who are community based, providing continuity of care that 'follows the woman' across the interface of community and hospital services, are ideally placed to engage with women around strategies for health promotion, including addressing social exclusion and isolation (Leap, 2004). They therefore need to understand the social determinants of health and the complex politics of how inequalities affect women's lives.

In particular, there are opportunities for midwives to 'dovetail' their services and liaise with child health nurses, Well Child services and community-based organisations. Because the midwife is alongside the woman on her journey through pregnancy, birth and the initial weeks of new motherhood, she is ideally placed to keep an overview of all the interacting needs of the woman in terms of accessing appropriate services and support structures. This is about physical, emotional and cultural safety. Midwives can engage with women in ways that avoid dependency and maximise the potential for women to learn from each other and build supportive networks in the community.

The midwife maintains the 'midwifery overview' ensuring that all the interwoven elements of a woman's life are kept in relief, whatever the events that unfold. The midwife works with the woman and her community, collaborating with other health professionals if necessary, to ensure that everything is done to ensure a safe and supported transition to new motherhood, taking into consideration the woman's individual circumstances and wishes (Leap, 2010).

 Midwifery Practice Scenario

I was working on the Assessment, Labour and Birthing Unit when I had the privilege of working with Aroha, a 16-year-old Māori primigravida woman in established labour. Aroha was of term gestation and had a well pregnancy where she enjoyed attending her antenatal appointments. In labour her parents and multiple whānau and friends, eight in total, supported her. On discreet communication with Aroha it was determined that having her whānau and friends present was important to her. She reported that their presence distracted her from the discomfort of labour and made her feel safe and strong.

I advised her that if her feelings changed at any time she could advise me and I would ask for her visitors to allow us space. I communicated the situation in our suite to the charge midwife, which is of great importance for ensuring that a woman-centred approach to care is negotiated. Advocating for flexibility of the visitor policy to respond to Aroha's cultural needs, both Māori and teenage, was required in this situation, alongside being mindful of other women using the facility and ensuring that Aroha's whānau and friends knew that if we required space they would be asked to wait outside the suite.

I later received a phone call from the ward clerk who questioned how many visitors we had in our suite as there was 'another' visitor at reception. Knowing that Aroha valued her whānau and friends' presence I spoke to Aroha again informing her of who was at reception. She was excited that this person had arrived and asked that they come to support her, stating 'baby can come now that Auntie is here'. I advocated for Aroha's request and advised the ward clerk that it was appropriate to allow this visitor entry to the unit.

Aroha requested that we play music so she could relax and move around the room. This enabled us to utilise the art of pelvic rocking and lumbar massage to the rhythm of her music to aid descent of the fetus through the pelvis, which was a beautiful experience to be a part of. Aroha burst into laughter throughout her labour with her whānau and friends verbally and physically supporting her through her birth experience, where her non-pharmacological pain relief plan resulted in a normal vaginal birth. Surrounded by her whānau and friends we welcomed her new baby boy into the world as all in attendance spoke, 'Tihei Mauri Ora'. Aroha's Auntie thanked me for acknowledging that Aroha's birth experience was a special event.

I believe that the woman is 'Te Whare Tangata' (the house of the people) and is the most important determinant of a well pregnancy, birth and parenthood. Advocating for the woman, respecting her 'knowing' and life experience, supporting her choice to birth her way, believing in her mana (power), and having faith in her natural potential and instinctive knowledge of how to birth when in a comfortable, supportive environment without fear is of great importance to the midwifery partnership, recognising that when the opportunity for normal birth is maximised then positive outcomes occur.

CRITICAL THINKING EXERCISE

1. Tūranga Kaupapa is a set of statements about the cultural values of Māori in relation to childbirth. What cultural values are present in this story?
2. What are the issues that need to be considered when a midwife is navigating and balancing the policies of an institution with needs and wishes of the woman and her whānau?
3. This midwife talks about 'a woman-centred approach to care' being negotiated. What skills do you need to carry out such negotiation?

THEORETICAL FRAMEWORKS FOR PRACTICE

Two **theoretical frameworks** have been developed in New Zealand that can provide some guidance for midwives engaging in these types of relationships with women. *Midwifery partnership* describes and explores how midwives can work in partnership with women. *Cultural safety* supports partnership relationships through focusing on invisible structures of power that exist between any two partners and in wider contexts within healthcare service institutions and society. Cultural safety, like midwifery partnership, seeks to make these power differentials visible so that both partners can negotiate how they work together and ensure that the woman, as the recipient of care, receives care that meets her needs and leaves her individuality intact and strengthened.

Cultural safety and midwifery partnership both also have a political imperative. Cultural safety challenges any personal, professional, institutional, social issues or structure that 'diminishes, demeans or disempowers the cultural identity and wellbeing of an individual' (NZCOM, 2015, p. 53). Midwifery partnership challenges professional power structures and medical dominance over childbirth, through recognising childbearing women as active partners of equal status in the shared experience of maternity care (Guilliland & Pairman, 1995, 2010a).

What is a theoretical framework?

Theoretical frameworks are tools for making sense of and explaining reality, and for thinking about practice. They provide ways in which midwifery care may be examined, understood, tested and developed (Forster et al., 2011).

In her seminal work Rosamund Bryar (1995) contends that the essence of the art of midwifery is intuition and empathy that is informed by theory, knowledge and reflective thinking. Exercising the art of midwifery requires combining the personal qualities of the midwife with reflective thinking about how theory and knowledge can best be used in the care of individual women. Theory is an integrated set of defined concepts and statements that present a view of a phenomenon and can be used to describe, explain, predict and/or control that phenomenon (Burn & Grove, 1995). Also, 'theory provides a structure within which midwives can compare the present experiences of the woman they are caring for with the responses identified in the theory' (Bryar, 1995, p. 5).

Theory arises from midwifery practice and a range of other disciplines and provides a broad framework for practice and articulates the goals and core values of a profession (Halldorsdottir & Karlsdottir, 2011). The thinking of midwives about this theory in relation to their daily practice with women will lead to further development of practice theories, which are '… intended to be tested, modified or abandoned in the light of new evidence' (Bryar, 1995, p. 40).

The two theoretical frameworks presented in this chapter—midwifery partnership and cultural safety—arose from practice and describe and explain living processes (relationships) that are always engaging, challenging and changing. 'Partnership' and 'cultural safety' exist only in encounters between individuals, groups or cultures, and have a moral and ethical imperative as well as a theoretical one. Both theoretical frameworks identify a number of concepts and values, and these are described below as tools for helping midwives to think about themselves and explore how they engage with others in their professional roles as midwives.

THE ORIGINS OF CULTURAL SAFETY AND MIDWIFERY PARTNERSHIP

Cultural safety and midwifery partnership were both developed in Aotearoa New Zealand and both arose out of its unique historical, cultural and social context. Aotearoa New Zealand's constitutional and legislative structure is founded on **Te Tiriti o Waitangi**/The Treaty of Waitangi, signed in 1840 between Māori (New Zealand's indigenous peoples) and the British Crown. Te Tiriti o Waitangi articulates a particular relationship between Māori and generations of settlers who have come to New Zealand since the early 1800s. This relationship is a bicultural partnership between Māori and the Crown that recognises the unique place and status of the indigenous people and assures the place of both Māori and the colonists in New Zealand (Ramsden, 1990, 2002).

Rapid British colonial expansion in the 19th century meant that immigrants from Britain and the four continents as well as the Pacific rapidly outnumbered Māori. There has been ongoing debate and dispute about the meaning of te Tiriti and biculturalism in a society made up of a variety of ethnicities, languages and religions. These debates have been compounded by a long-standing struggle by Māori to have the Crown recognise and meet its partnership obligations under te Tiriti. The 1980s and 1990s saw increased efforts by Māori and government to address te Tiriti claims and construct a bicultural relationship based on the principles of partnership, protection, participation and equity. One result of this work has been that the notion of 'partnership' is culturally embedded in New Zealand society.

New Zealand women drew on this cultural understanding of partnership when they actively sought changes to the way in which maternity services were delivered, and in particular demanded the choice of a midwife as their caregiver for childbirth (Dobbie, 1990; Strid, 1987). In the mid 1980s, maternity consumer organisations joined with midwifery's professional organisation (at that time the Midwives Section of the New Zealand Nurses Association, now the New Zealand College of Midwives) in an organised political campaign to reinstate midwifery autonomy and enable women to have a choice of caregiver for childbirth (Donley, 1989; Guilliland, 1989; Guilliland & Pairman, 2010b). The campaign took place in a context in which women's issues were high on the political agenda and the Cartwright Inquiry[b] had raised awareness of patients' rights and issues of informed consent (Guilliland & Pairman, 1995, 2010b). Together, women and midwives succeeded in bringing about legislative change, and the resulting 1990 amendment to the *Nurses Act 1977* reinstated midwives as autonomous practitioners and gave women the choice of a doctor or a midwife, or both, as their lead caregiver for childbirth.

Another result of this political campaign was midwifery's recognition of its political partnership with women and its determination to enact this partnership by establishing representation for women (as maternity service consumers) at every level of midwifery's professional structure through the NZCOM. It was then only a short step for midwives to understand that their individual relationships with women were also partnerships, or could be. Exploration of the political and professional relationships between midwives and women has led the NZCOM to identify partnership as a philosophical stance, a standard for practice and an ethical principle (NZCOM, 2015).

New Zealand midwifery has redefined midwifery professionalism to mean midwifery partnership. In doing so, it seeks to replace traditional hierarchical professional relationships with negotiated ones, where power differentials are acknowledged and actively shifted from the midwife to the childbearing woman so that she can control her own birthing experience (Guilliland & Pairman, 1995, 2010a; Pairman, 2005).

All healthcare professionals in New Zealand and Australia are required by their respective regulatory frameworks to be culturally competent (see Chs 13 and 14), but cultural competence is not specifically defined in the *Health Practitioners Competence Assurance Act*, which regulates midwifery practice in Aotearoa New Zealand. The Midwifery Council of New Zealand considers that a culturally competent midwife integrates midwifery partnership, cultural safety and Tūranga Kaupapa into her practice (MCNZ, 2012). We will explore Tūranga Kaupapa and the concept of cultural competence later in this chapter.

CULTURAL SAFETY AND MIDWIFERY PARTNERSHIP IN OTHER CONTEXTS

The theoretical frameworks of cultural safety and midwifery partnership both explore relationships and therefore, although both arose out of the New Zealand context, are applicable in other countries, cultures or contexts (Phiri et al., 2010). Indeed, the Nursing and Midwifery Board of Australia (NMBA) *National Competency Standards for the Midwife* require midwives to provide culturally safe midwifery practice and to plan and evaluate midwifery care in partnership with the woman (NMBA, 2006). The NMBA Midwife Standards for Practice articulate a clear vision for the application of cultural safety in the context of Australian midwifery practice.

In all contexts, midwifery must be concerned with relationships because, unlike any other healthcare professional, midwives are privileged to have the opportunity to be 'with' women throughout the life experiences of pregnancy, birth and new motherhood. In their professional roles, midwives are able to develop relationships with women that last up to 10 months (sometimes longer) and they have the opportunity to work with women in their own homes and communities, away from the influence and control of institutions. In such settings the traditional practitioner/patient relationship, where the practitioner is the 'expert' and has the authority to make decisions, is clearly inappropriate (see Ch. 13). Midwives who work within continuity-of-care models work in contexts in which relationships are valued and where midwifery attributes such as support, caring and enabling are recognised as skilled midwifery practice. Midwives and childbearing women in these settings need to develop relationships of equity, trust and mutual understanding. So too do midwives and women working within the constraints of hospital services with fragmented care, insufficient staffing numbers, hierarchies and organisational control. Such settings can undermine midwifery knowledge and midwifery confidence and trust, making it difficult for midwives to support women in taking control of their own birthing experiences (Hunter, 2006; Kirkham, 2000a, 2010). Both midwives and women need to take hold of their power in order to begin to change the culture of these institutions. The political partnership experienced by women and midwives in New Zealand offers some guidance (Guilliland & Pairman, 1995, 2010b; Kirkham, 2000b). Listening to women is at the heart of understanding women's needs. In Western Australia, women clearly articulated their views about choosing their caregiver in research by Davison et al. (2015) examining 14 women's experience of private midwifery care. These women 'knew exactly what they wanted' from their caregivers (p. 772). Davison et al. concluded that 'the relationship is everything' (p. 776); these women valued the shared vision for normal birth that was achieved in their relationships with their midwives and suggested that no care would be preferable to medical-led care if they could not find their way to a caregiver that met their needs.

No matter what the context, midwives should examine their relationships with childbearing women because these relationships are at the heart of midwifery practice. When New Zealand women fought for midwifery autonomy they did so because they believed that midwives would provide an alternative model to medicine—a model of care in which women would be in control as the decision makers (Strid, 1987). These same arguments were made by Australian women and midwives to bring about legislative and practice changes that strengthened midwifery autonomy with the new role of 'eligible midwife', now termed 'endorsed midwife' (Australian Government Department of Health, 2013; Maternity Choices Australia, n.d.).

Midwifery autonomy in New Zealand brought with it a social mandate for midwives to practise across the Midwifery Scope of Practice and on their own responsibility. This social mandate carries with it a moral obligation for midwifery to provide the service that women have called for. There is also a moral obligation to recognise and respect individual differences in those we work with as midwives, no matter what other structures encourage us to do.

Midwives in any country and from any cultural context will work with childbearing women who are different from them. Midwives need to examine their relationships with the women they care for if women are to become active agents in their own care (Kirkham, 2000b). Cultural safety and midwifery partnership provide frameworks for achieving meaningful relationships between midwives and childbearing women and for practising in a culturally competent manner.

Embracing the challenge of gender-inclusive midwifery

Midwifery models of care, including Aotearoa's foundational partnership model for midwifery practice, have been premised and articulated with the assumption of pregnant women as the centre of care (Guilliland & Pairman, 1995, 2010a). However, globally, and within Australasia, assumptions about the gender of pregnant and birthing people are being challenged (see for example: Botelle et al., 2021; Moseson et al., 2020). This is leading to calls for greater recognition of, and responsiveness to, gender diversity in midwifery care including attention to the specific experiences and realities of transgender, non-binary, and indigenous gender diverse pregnant people and families (see for example: Charter et al., 2018; Hoffkling, Obedin-Maliver & Sevelius, 2017).

The challenge to embrace gender inclusion in midwifery, and specifically to ensure the provision of culturally safe and responsive midwifery care to gender diverse pregnant people, is increasingly being recognised by midwifery professional bodies. The International Confederation of Midwives in its position statement 'Human rights of Lesbian, Gay, Bisexual, Transgender and Intersex (LGBTI) people' has recognised the right of all people to receive humanised and inclusive midwifery care regardless of gender identity or expression and the importance of care that respects self-determination and the right to receive care that is free of discrimination including transphobia and prejudice (International Confederation of Midwives, 2017).

The principles of gender-inclusive midwifery care are being identified and articulated in research evidence and in maternity service statements and resources (see for example: Brighton & Sussex University Hospitals, 2021). These principles include the importance of capturing gender identity in maternity data collection systems, the use of gender-inclusive or gender-additive language in midwifery at a service and practice level, gender-inclusive cultural safety education for midwives and other maternity providers, gender-inclusive facilities and resources, and explicit policies and statements in maternity services and within midwifery professional bodies that affirm non-discrimination and inclusion for gender diverse pregnant people and families (Brighton & Sussex University Hospitals, 2021). The importance of research which addresses the specific midwifery care needs of gender diverse pregnant people and whānau has also been affirmed.

Gender-inclusive midwifery can be understood as part of the challenge to extend midwifery care beyond models of care that privilege Western understandings and heteronormative family units in order to ensure midwifery partnership is responsive and sustainable in a twenty-first century world.

CULTURAL SAFETY

Cultural safety was initially defined as:

The effective nursing or midwifery practice of a person or family from another culture, and is determined by that person or family. Culture includes, but is not restricted to, age or generation; gender; sexual orientation; occupation and socio-economic status; ethnic origin or migrant experience; religious or spiritual belief; and disability.

The nurse or midwife delivering the nursing or midwifery service will have undertaken a process of reflection on his or her own cultural identity and will recognise the impact that his or her personal culture has on his or her professional practice. Unsafe cultural practice comprises any action which diminishes, demeans or disempowers the cultural identity and well-being of an individual.

(Nursing Council of New Zealand (NCNZ), 2002, p. 7)

Intrinsic to the concept and practice of cultural safety is the notion of 'right relationship'. Whether that relationship is between two persons, two groups, two cultures or two countries, right relationship recognises and honours the rights and responsibilities of each (McAra-Couper, unpublished paper, 2005). Cultural safety seeks to establish the practice of right relationship at a personal, professional and institutional level.

What is meant by 'culture'?

… we learn from the experiences of the past to correct the understanding of the present and create a future which can be justly shared.

(Ramsden, 2002, p. 182)

The understandings of culture expressed in nursing and midwifery today have evolved over a long period. It is important to be familiar with this evolution of understandings in order to appreciate the significance and place of cultural safety.

Historically culture was invisible in nursing and midwifery curricula. In part this reflected a context in which assimilation was prevalent. For example, in Aotearoa New Zealand, despite the existence of Te Tiriti o Waitangi, assimilation policy influenced the social thinking of the 19th and early 20th centuries, and led to the establishment of structures and processes that denied differences between Māori and Pākehā (non-Māori) in an attempt to make Māori more like Pākehā and absorb them into Pākehā-dominated culture and society (Walker, 1987).

In this context, nurses and midwives were encouraged to give care to patients 'irrespective of differences such as nationality, culture, creed, colour, age, sex, political or religious belief or social status' (Ramsden, 1990, p. 79). This understanding of culture informed the practice of nurses in New Zealand and elsewhere until the early 1970s. It was well intentioned but served only to reinforce assimilation (Spence, 2001). The long-term consequences of assimilation are suppression and destruction of the culture of indigenous people, which results in mental, physical and spiritual stress (NCNZ, 1992). This stress is seen only too readily in the present-day health statistics of indigenous peoples in New Zealand and Australia and throughout the world (Australian Institute of Health and Welfare, 2018; Health Quality and Safety Commission [HQSC], 2019).

In the 1970s a new understanding of culture developed. Anthropological understandings of culture emerged that led to greater cultural awareness and cultural sensitivity. Transcultural nursing theory, developed by nurse theorist Madeline Leininger in the early 1970s, influenced nursing education. Transcultural nursing was based on nurses having knowledge about a range of different cultures from which they could respond therapeutically to their clients' needs (Campinha-Bacote, 2011; Papps, 2005). Nurses and midwives were taught to gather information about the beliefs, patterns and behaviours of other cultures, so that they would be able to identify 'specific cultural patterns that occurred' and provide culturally sensitive care (Richardson, 2000, p. 32; Spence, 1999).

Nurses and midwives were taught about the concepts of *cultural awareness* (becoming aware of difference) and *cultural sensitivity* (sensitivity to the legitimacy of difference and the impact the midwife's own culture may have on others) (NCNZ, 2002). Nursing and midwifery knowledge considered culture and ethnicity from the perspective of the nurse or midwife, as an observer, exploring and understanding what makes the other person different from themselves (Ramsden, 2000; Richardson, 2000). Such approaches allowed the nurse or midwife to be patronising and powerful as they identified the needs of people from other ethnic groups and did not require any self-knowledge or change in attitude (Ramsden, 2000). In New Zealand, the dominance of transcultural nursing in nursing education and practice was challenged by the alternative theory of cultural safety.

Developed in the 1980s by Māori nurse educator, Irihāpeti Ramsden, cultural safety or *kawa whakaruruhau* provided another theoretical framework for understanding culture. This sociopolitical definition of culture had Te Tiriti o Waitangi as its starting point, and involved recognition that power needed to be shared and racism deinstitutionalised (Spence, 1999). Cultural safety focused on the sociopolitical factors that affected healthcare (Richardson, 2000).

By contrast, notions of cultural sensitivity and cultural awareness avoided the more difficult recognition of power relationships that existed in the delivery of healthcare and led to cultural stereotypes and simplistic notions such as cultural checklists (Ramsden, 2000). Cultural safety focused not on the 'other' but on the nurse and midwife. The process of cultural safety began with self-reflection and attitude change (see Fig. 17.2). This process required the nurse or midwife to recognise themselves as 'powerful bearers of their own life experience and realities and the impact this may have on others' (Ramsden, 2000, p. 117).

The notion of power is inherent in the concept of and processes associated with cultural safety. The nurse or

Cultural safety
Is an outcome of nursing and midwifery education that enables safe service to be defined by those who receive the service.

Cultural sensitivity
Alerts students to the legitimacy of differences and begins a process of self-exploration as the powerful bearers of their own life experience and realities and the impact these may have on others.

Cultural awareness
Is a beginning step towards understanding that there is a difference. Many people undergo courses designed to sensitise them to formal ritual and practice rather than to emotional, social, economic and political context in which people exist.

FIGURE 17.2 Developing understanding of cultural safety
(Source: Ramsden I. *Kawa Whakaruruhau: Guidelines for Nursing and Midwifery Education.* Wellington, NZ: Nursing Council of NZ; 1992)

midwife is challenged to recognise her personal power and the power of the institutions and society in which they work and live (Richardson, 2000). Cultural safety is primarily about establishing trust, gaining a shared meaning of vulnerability and power, and carefully working through the legitimacy of difference (Ramsden, 2000). Cultural safety makes visible the invisible structures of power (including our own) and attempts to transform anything that creates inequality and inequities in the healthcare services. In the Aotearoa New Zealand context this also includes actions that do not uphold Te Tiriti ō Waitangi in the delivery of healthcare services. In Australia, the Congress of Aboriginal and Torres Strait Islander Nurses and Midwives (CATSINaM) has produced a range of position statements that identify current priorities for working meaningfully as, and for, Aboriginal maternity workers and consumers of maternity care. Student midwives are encouraged to engage with the following two position statements: Cultural Safety (CATSINaM, 2014) and the Position Statement: Embedding Cultural Safety Across Australian Nursing and Midwifery (CATSINaM, 2017a). These documents provide excellent guidance towards facilitating cultural safety within midwifery practice.

Fig. 17.2 describes the progression of students towards understanding cultural safety and the differences in meaning of the commonly used terms 'cultural safety', 'cultural sensitivity' and 'cultural awareness'.

Thus cultural safety and transcultural nursing present different theoretical understandings of culture. Transcultural nursing exists in a multicultural context and focuses primarily on defining culture as race and ethnicity (Ramsden, 2002). Transcultural nursing places the nurse or midwife in the position of 'external observer' for the purpose of providing culture-specific care. On the other hand, cultural safety addresses the issue of power between the client (woman) and the nurse (midwife) and interprets 'culture' in the broadest possible sense (Ramsden, 2002). Contemporary understandings preclude the use of terms such as 'race' which are socially constructed and contested, preferring 'ethnicity' as a descriptor.

Leininger's culturally congruent care model is different from Cultural Safety in that nurses and midwives need to move from treating people regardless of colour or creed towards a model of treatment that was regardful of all those things that make them unique.

(Ramsden, 1993, p. 5)

This movement from 'regardless to regardful' is one of the most important contributions cultural safety makes in ensuring the safety of the care that midwives give. Midwives and student midwives who are interested in understanding more about the development of cultural safety theory through the 1990s and early 2000s are encouraged to read *Cultural Safety in Aotearoa New Zealand* (Wepa, 2015).

It was Ramsden's view that future evolution and direction for cultural safety would not focus on the customs, habits and cultural practices of any group, but rather would continue to be about an analysis of power and relationships of power (Ramsden, 2002). Cultural safety is simply an instrument that allows the woman and her family to judge whether the health service and delivery of healthcare are safe for them (Kruske et al., 2006; Ramsden, 2002). Therefore, the next step in this journey of cultural safety will need to be centred on the facilitation of a process whereby women and their families can tell midwives about the safety of the care they receive (Ramsden, 2002). This next step will facilitate the focusing of cultural safety not just on 'ethnicity', but rather will increasingly 'promote the uniqueness of each person resulting from multiple intersecting cultural layers' (Clear, 2008, p. 4).

Student Midwifery Practice Scenario

I was working as a student with my independent midwife when a young Filipina woman came in to book with her mother. She looked very embarrassed and would not speak to us or even look at us. It was really difficult to understand what the young woman wanted for her pregnancy, labour, birth and postnatal. Any advances made by the midwife regarding information or options available were met by the mother with, 'You decide what is best.' At delivery time the young woman lay in the bed with a flannel over her face and really appeared to be in a lot of pain. The midwife was very anxious about the young woman being in so much pain and not really coping with it. The midwife suggested pain relief to the family in terms of an epidural. She suggested this because the young woman had been in labour for 10 hours, the baby was in an occipitoposterior position, and there was little progress being made; the midwife thought that Syntocinon augmentation was indicated.

The family took the midwife outside and said that the pain was the young woman's punishment and she and they would cope with it. I felt so angry and upset with this, I had to excuse myself and go and have a cup of coffee. One hour later the midwife decided that she would try another approach, as it was clear that the young woman needed pain relief if the labour was to progress. The midwife rang the consultant on call and told him about the situation and asked if he would come and assess the situation and talk to the family regarding the epidural. The doctor did this and the family agreed to an epidural after listening to the doctor who said exactly the same things as the midwife. Six hours later the baby was born by ventouse delivery. I was very impressed that the midwife could step aside and involve someone else, hoping that the perceived 'status' of the doctor would be the thing that would get the family to agree to the much-needed epidural.

Questions

1. Describe the culturally unsafe issues in this story.
2. Identify the principle/s of cultural safety that inform the midwife's practice.

3. Describe how the midwife facilitated cultural safety in this difficult situation.

4. The student midwife states, 'I felt so angry and upset with this I had to excuse myself and go and have a cup of coffee.' What made the student midwife angry?

5. Discuss other ways you could navigate this situation in order to promote the cultural safety of the woman and her family.

6. Describe how you would have handled this situation, in order to facilitate the cultural safety of the woman and her family.

Principles of cultural safety

Cultural safety is facilitated by communication, understanding the diversity in worldviews, and understanding the impact of colonisation (NCNZ, 2002).

There are four principles of cultural safety (NCNZ, 2002):

• Cultural safety seeks to improve the health status of all people.
• Cultural safety seeks to enhance the delivery of healthcare and disability services through a culturally safe workforce.
• Cultural safety is broad based and broad in its application.
• Cultural safety focuses closely on 'understanding of self, the rights of others and the legitimacy of difference' (Ramsden, 2002, p. 200).

Implications for midwifery practice

Learning about cultural safety and thinking about its implications for practice can be challenging. Students who are part of the dominant culture (such as being a white Australian or New Zealander with a European background) can be challenged by issues such as history, Te Tiriti o Waitangi, partnerships between Tangata Whenua and Tangata Tiriti and cultural safety. It is important that a framework that is working towards the transformation of everything that diminishes, demeans and disempowers does not do precisely this in working towards awareness. In the Australian context, preregistration health professional education is guided by the Aboriginal and Torres Strait Islander Health Curriculum Framework, released in 2015 by the Australian Government Department of Health (Commonwealth of Australia, Department of Health, 2014). The Framework seeks to promote consistency across the health professions in terms of the development of cultural capability during health professional education programs. This document has been adapted further to focus specifically on the education of midwives and nurses and is called The Nursing and Midwifery Aboriginal and Torres Strait Islander Health Curriculum Framework: an adaptation of and complementary document to the 2014 Aboriginal and Torres Strait Islander Health Curriculum Framework (CATSINaM, 2017b).

 Reflection from a non-indigenous midwife on providing care to indigenous families by Kate Nicholl

As a Pākehā midwife who has had the privilege of attending at the continuation of whakapapa Māori, as pēpi Māori are being born into their whānau, I have grappled with what it means to be in partnership inside a health system that is Eurocentric in its creation and delivery. It is a system that invariably upholds the power imbalance created by ongoing colonisation and discrimination, leading to large inequities in health outcomes for whānau Māori.

The term Tangata Tiriti helps me identify my place and responsibilities within Aotearoa. It reminds me that I have benefited from the signing of Te Tiriti O Waitangi and that this enables me to live on this beautiful land with a wide range of privileges. Benefits however inherently require accountability and it is through my mahi (work) as a midwife that I work to realise these, for a future that truly embodies partnership for my own mokopuna.

Working with whānau there are some key elements that underpin the midwifery relationship I offer to whānau. I enter the relationship with honesty and openness, this means offering information, including challenges, to both the systems ways of doing, as well as to commonly held views on health and haputanga. I have a strong belief that the midwifery partnership is with whānau and not only an individual person. I am only one person who comes briefly in and out of their lives. Mostly they have a wide range of other important relationships that form their support networks, their social structures and who influence and impact on their lives. The knowledge that is held within whānau has strength beyond my clinical view as the midwife and is their expression of tino rangatiratanga, self-determination. I come with a curiosity around what those strengths are for whānau, who they are, where do they come from and what has and is happening for them, how do they experience and understand the world? As a midwife I intentionally ensure manaakitanga and whanaungatanga occurs with the whānau. I am open in sharing who I am, where I come from and who my people are and how this has influenced what I do. I recognise the inadequacies of a workforce that is not diverse enough to reflect the community it sits within. I ensure that I educate myself around the political-socio-cultural context of whānau, and what services, particularly Kaupapa Māori, are available in the community to support their haputanga journey. The beauty of all of this is that I have been embraced into a community far wider than my midwifery space.

The ultimate measure of partnership can only be assessed by the recipients of care and there are few opportunities to formally engage with whānau around this. As a midwife I will ask whānau to complete the feedback form that informs part of my Midwifery Standards Review, however this is limited in its ability to reveal how the partnership was understood and experienced by the whānau. A truer gauge for me is the whānau who return over many years and different connections—cousins, sisters, Aunties—looking for the same midwife to provide the care to them during their haputanga. This speaks of a trust in the relationships that we have created over time.

Glossary for the reflection

- Aotearoa—New Zealand
- hapūtanga—pregnancy
- Kaupapa Māori—Māori ways of thinking, philosophy, Māori approach
- Manaakitanga—behaviours that enhance and acknowledge the equal, if not greater importance, of another person, through hospitality, generosity, kindness and nurturing relationships
- Māori—normal, the indigenous peoples of Aotearoa, a term applied as an identifier after the colonisers arrived
- mokopuna—grandchildren, ancestors to come
- Pākehā New Zealander of European descent, usually those whose ancestors came to New Zealand as settler colonisers
- pēpi—baby
- Te Tiriti (o Waitangi)—the founding document of Aotearoa signed between some Māori and the colonising government
- tino rangatiratanga—the right to exercise self-determination and authority, sovereignty
- whakapapa—geneaology, lines of descent
- whānau—family unit, as defined by the person and may include those not related via kinship ties
- whanaungatanga—ways in which the relationship to each other is discovered and upheld

Spence (2004) suggests that the process of engaging with people who differ from the nurse and midwife is unlikely to ever be free of tension. She argues that nurses (and midwives) need to learn to live with the uncertainty and paradox that difference constantly presents to them. The process of becoming culturally safe and learning to live with uncertainty and paradox takes courage, patience and kindness: courage to enter into the process, patience to stay with the process, and kindness towards self and others in the struggle with what the process requires. As Ramsden reminds us, the process of cultural safety calls for 'excellence in the service to other human beings' (Ramsden, 2000, p. 12).

We finish this section by acknowledging that cultural safety was 'designed as an educational process by Māori and it is given as koha [gift] to all people who are different from the service providers, whether by gender, sexual orientation, economic or educational status, age or ethnicity' (Ramsden, 2002, p. 181).

CRITICAL THINKING EXERCISE

Cultural safety is not about extraordinary events but about the everyday situations midwives find themselves in. It is the handling of these ordinary situations that requires a midwife to be culturally safe.

MIDWIFERY PARTNERSHIP

Midwifery partnership was first articulated as a theoretical model in 1994 when Guilliland and Pairman wrote *The Midwifery Partnership: A Model for Practice* (Guilliland & Pairman, 1995). Midwifery autonomy had been re-established four years earlier with the passing of the *Nurses Amendment Act 1990* and the time was right to capture the profession's growing understanding about what it meant for women and midwives to work together *in relationship* with one another. The model continued to evolve over the following two decades, in response to further research by Pairman, and support from local and international studies. These studies examined relationships between women and midwives, and noted similar concepts, thus lending weight to the theoretical underpinnings of the model (Hatem et al., 2008; Hunter, 2006; McCourt et al., 2006; Powell Kennedy, 1995, 2002, 2004; Sandall et al., 2006; Walsh, 1999). In 2010 the model underwent further revision and refinement by the original co-authors (Guilliland & Pairman, 2010a) who wished to emphasise midwifery relationships as 'existing within the context of pregnancy and childbirth and influenced by the scope of practice and the competence and qualities of each midwife' (Pairman & McAra-Couper, 2015). The model reflects a relationship that is equal, reciprocal and positive, and which recognises the professional role that the midwife occupies within it—bringing her knowledge and skill to active decision making when required with the priority of contributing to the wellbeing of the woman and her baby. As well as being the framework for a professional relationship between women and midwives, it serves as a model for midwife-to-midwife partnerships as well, such as between members of a group practice, or between community- and hospital-based midwives.

Overview of midwifery partnership: a model for practice

The midwifery partnership model (Fig. 17.3) presents the partners, their shared experiences, the philosophies that underpin their relationships, and the context that relationships exist within. Some deconstruction of the component parts of the model allows further reflection on the concepts and the research which led to the model's refinement over time. It is acknowledged that critique of the model from indigenous perspectives challenges the assumption of an individualistic framing of the partners

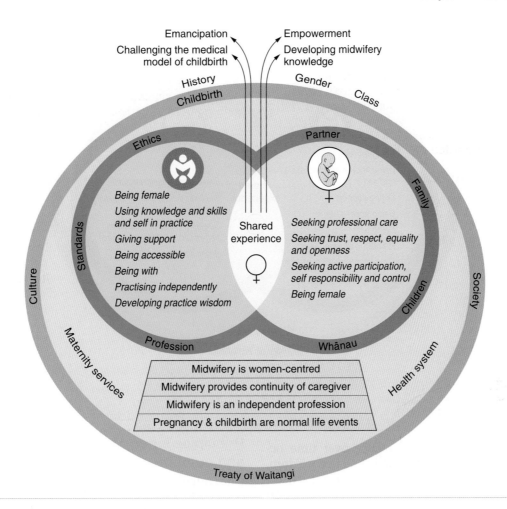

FIGURE 17.3 Midwifery partnership model
(Source: Based on Pairman, 1998)

as being a woman and a midwife (Kenney, 2011) and that people who are pregnant do not always identify as women. The following description honours the original explication of the model as proposed by Guilliland and Pairman (1995, 2010a). It was always envisaged by the authors that the model would 'continue to evolve further' (Pairman, 1999, p. 7).

The partners

The two partners in a midwifery relationship are a woman and a midwife. They come together at a time that is specific to the woman's childbirth experience, in a relationship that may last for up to a year and may include ongoing episodes of care within this relationship in future pregnancies. The woman brings her knowledge and expertise about her 'self' in the context she is situated in, along with her experiences, expectations, hopes and fears. She is within a context that includes whoever she wishes to acknowledge as part of her experience—her partner and family—and will be influenced by the beliefs and culture of these people. The midwife brings her self, her knowledge and midwifery expertise, which is in turn shaped by her professional ethics, standards for practice, and her

own cultural context. The area where these people meet is their shared experience, and the environment that wraps around this shared experience is tempered by wider societal and cultural influences such as gender, class and history including, in Aotearoa, Te Tiriti o Waitangi.

Pairman's (1998) research examined the nature of the relationships between women and midwives—*their shared experience*—by qualitative exploration of the experience of six woman-and-midwife pairs, including reflection by these participants on the 1995 model as part of the research process. This led to the addition of some further concepts to each circle, which more explicitly described what women seek from midwives in their relationships with them, and what qualities midwives can bring to the partnership. For the woman, 'seeking professional care', 'seeking active participation, self-responsibility and control', 'seeking trust, respect, quality and openness' and 'being female' were added. For midwives, 'being female', 'using knowledge, skill and self in practice', 'giving support', 'being accessible' and 'being with' were added. As well as 'being with women', midwives wished to acknowledge how their independent midwifery practice was embedded in their identities beyond their working world,

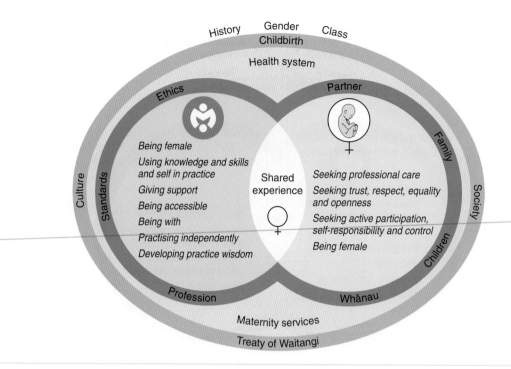

FIGURE 17.4 The partners
(Source: Based on Pairman, 1998)

and that development of their practice over time occurred via reflection and trust in their practice wisdom, and so these two concepts were added also (Fig. 17.4).

A full description of the research can be accessed at: https://viewer.waireto.victoria.ac.nz/client/viewer/IE937751/rep/REP937787/FL937788?dps_dvs=1518135702398,221.

The shared experience

The partnership relationship is far from being just about what each partner brings to it—indeed what happens *within* their shared experience reflects the strength and political potential to change society. What happens when women and midwives 'be together in relationship' encompasses inherent principles which are necessary for the successful functioning of the partnership. These principles—theoretical concepts—as defined in the earlier model, are individual negotiation, equality, shared responsibility and empowerment, and informed choice and consent. Pairman's (1998) study resulted in a more specific articulation of how women and midwives actually work together and brought the *outcomes* of the relationship into sharper focus. 'Being equal', 'sharing common interests', 'involving the family', 'building trust', 'reciprocity', 'taking time' and 'sharing power and control' were thus identified in the refined model.

When the shared experience functions optimally in this way, the whole is greater than the sum of its parts. The relationship itself can become an incubator of wider societal enhancement, by enabling the development of new midwifery knowledge, mutual empowerment, emancipation and ultimately providing the evidence for challenging the medical model of childbirth.

Principles inherent in the partnership model and outcomes of midwifery partnership

Once integrated into practice, the following key principles (Fig. 17.5) demonstrate midwifery partnership in action. These principles are important touchstones regardless of whether the relationship is between a woman and her LMC, or between a woman and a core midwife who is supporting her relationship with her LMC.

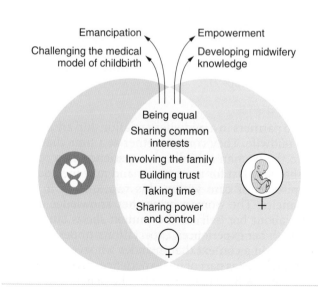

FIGURE 17.5 Principles inherent in the partnership model and outcomes of midwifery partnership
(Source: Based on Pairman, 1998)

376

Equality and reciprocity

Both the woman and the midwife bring to their relationship a sense of being equal—which does not negate or diminish their differences, or mean they are the same. They have equal rights in this relationship (Guilliland & Pairman, 2010a). They reciprocate by sharing their individual knowledge, which becomes beneficial to both. Power in the relationship is shared by the mutual exchange of expertise, and how the partnership will progress is negotiated.

Negotiation

The uniqueness of each partnership is assured because each person contributes their own 'self'—and power is shared through decision making which is based on honouring the woman as the decider, following a process of informed choice and consent. The expectation of equal contribution from both partners requires effective communication to arrive at mutually satisfying outcomes—working things out together.

Trust and time

As with any relationship, time is an important consideration in the development of trust. Some midwifery relationships are brief, in the context of an episode of care in a birthing facility, and midwives working with women in this space are highly skilled at developing respectful and trust-promoting relationships very quickly. For most women though, their relationship with their midwife will develop over several months, and as they grow to know more about each other the sense of mutual trust in the relationship is enhanced. A woman will usually feel freer to disclose her hopes and fears within a relationship that feels safe to her, and her chosen circle of support may extend to her partner and whānau as well as her midwife. Time spent with women at appointments, time to make important decisions during labour and time taken encouraging the woman as she grows into her mothering role all contribute to her feeling of trust, safety and support.

Sharing power and responsibility

In a mutually negotiated relationship, where both partners have equal rights, it follows that power sharing underpins all aspects of the relationship. This includes not only decision making based on informed choice and consent, but also acceptance that each partner shares accountability and responsibility for the choices that are made. In practice this is sometimes challenging; often expressed when third parties become involved in decision making as well, as in the situation of a proposed transfer of clinical responsibility when a complex situation arises. For the woman to be able to exercise her power, she needs to have all options (including the 'do nothing' option) explained to her fully, so that she can choose what will be best for her.

Acknowledging that the woman is accepting the responsibility for her choices does not absolve the midwife from her responsibilities to act professionally and in accordance with her scope of practice and professional standards and codes of ethics and conduct (Guilliland & Pairman, 2010a). Midwives always remain accountable for the midwifery actions they take and have sound frameworks available to them to guide their practice when a woman declines a recommended treatment or course of action.

Empowerment and emancipation

The women in Pairman's (1998) study (five of whom identified as Pākehā or European, the ethnicity of the sixth is not reported) were clear that taking responsibility for their decisions was empowering for them. But working with women in this way proved equally empowering for midwives, with one midwife describing how much it had meant to her seeing a woman apply her newly acquired sense of control to other areas of her life outside her pregnancy. Women who experience this kind of empowerment can encourage others to also seek relationships of equality with midwives, or even other health professionals, and this can lead to emancipation for birthing women as a wider community. Support networks that midwives encourage women to form around themselves have the power to transform women's lives so, by believing in women and inspiring confidence in their abilities as mothers, midwives can play a key facilitation role that will last well beyond the scope of their individual relationships with women.

Professional friendship

An important new concept surfaced during Pairman's research—the notion of the midwife as a 'professional friend'. The women described the relationship between themselves and midwives as being akin to friendship, but also acknowledged the 'time-boundedness' of the relationship and the professional focus of the midwife. Further research exploring this notion of professional friendship could further illuminate these ideas.

> *I think we had a really good relationship, actually. It was more of a friend relationship, but a friend you could trust in—a professional friend you could rely on.*
>
> (BF, in Pairman, 1998, p. 163)

REFLECTIVE CASE STUDY

Reflection on partnership from 'Helen'—a mother

I was pregnant with my third baby and was surprised when the expected due date came and went. I had the same midwife during all of my pregnancies, and it really helped that she knew my family and our pregnancy/birth philosophy and history so well. My midwife reassured me that I was not 'overdue' for another 2 weeks; however, it felt that every person I spoke to asked if I was going to be induced, simply because I had hit the 40-week mark! I also had the added pressure of my mum visiting from overseas and so I really wanted our baby to be born whilst she was here to support me. I was relieved that my midwife was happy to discuss my options and talk about the process of 'being induced' even though I knew I still had lots of time before I had to make those types of decisions. Just being able to talk about the processes, gave me, my husband and mum reassurance that our 'let's wait and see' attitude was best for us at that time.

I wanted to have regular telephone calls and check-ups with my midwife during this time, especially as I always felt better when I could discuss my thoughts and worries, and hear the baby's heartbeat, check their position and that we were both healthy. In addition, I was having regular (and sometimes strong) Braxton-Hicks from about 38 weeks of the pregnancy and this was becoming draining and disheartening, since it felt like labour was never going to start! Empathy was shown every time I had a 'false start' and I always felt that my midwife was so patient with me, my questions, and with trusting in the process of labour and birth.

When I was over 41 weeks pregnant I noticed that the baby's movements had reduced. My midwife discussed our options and alongside the normal checks she asked if my husband and I wanted to go into hospital and have fetal monitoring done. We agreed to have this, as it felt like it could provide a lot of reassurance that our baby was well, or give more information if things were not as they should be. Whilst we were there, I asked if there was any benefit to having a vaginal examination to help establish if I was close to going into labour. My midwife discussed the pros and cons of doing this, and me and my husband were given time to talk through how we felt about it. Overall, I decided not to have an examination as I felt it wouldn't have changed anything at that present time.

The next day I woke at 5 a.m. and knew our baby was going to be born on this day! Since so much time had been spent discussing the labour and birth of our baby with our midwife, it felt that very little needed to be said during those crucial few hours. I felt so much trust, respect and support from my midwife during the entire labour and birth, and interestingly the only time I remember her assisting me was to listen to the baby's heartbeat. In addition, when my baby's head was being born he 'got stuck at his nose', some gentle encouragement for me to bear down was all that was needed. As I held onto my mum's body, our third son was breathed gently into the world, in our living room at midday, into the arms of his dad and big brothers.

Through having a partnership between my midwife and myself, alongside my husband and whānau it allowed me to be given all the facts needed for informed consent to be carried out at all times. It always felt that the care and information was individualised, research based and given with respect but tenderness and feeling.

Quote from Heider's adaptation of Lao Tsu (Chinese philosopher 604–531 BC)—on being a midwife

Remember that you are facilitating another person's process. It is not your process. Do not intrude. Do not control. Do not force your own needs and insights into the foreground. If you do

not trust a person's process, that person will not trust you.

Imagine that you are a midwife. You are assisting at someone else's birth. Do good without show or fuss. Facilitate what is happening rather than what you think ought to be happening.

If you must take the lead, lead so that the Mother is helped yet still free and in charge. When the baby is born, the mother will rightly say: 'We did it ourselves'.

(Heider, 1997)

Reflection on partnership from 'Michael'—a father

In 2009, my wife and I were expecting our first baby. During our midwife appointments we talked about our thoughts for the pregnancy, labour and birth. One of the poignant discussions was about where we would like to birth our baby. Our initial reaction was that we would have a hospital birth, as that was our perception of where all babies were born.

Because of our philosophy of wanting a gentle, natural birth, without medical intervention, our midwife asked us whether we would be open to considering a home birth? We said we could be, but wanted more information in order to make a fully informed decision. Our midwife did a fantastic job of providing current facts and research about home birth, including highlighting the benefits and potential risks. Over time, and after regular discussion with our midwife, we felt home birth was the safest and best option for us. It made complete sense that if we were in our own relaxed, calm, comfortable environment, with the best possible care available to us, we were much more likely to achieve the birth experience we wanted. Birth isn't meant to be medicalised, and we quickly realised that by going to hospital it would likely lead to a cascade of intervention.

As the due date in May 2010 approached, we started to look forward to the impending birth, but we did have some apprehension. Two days after the expected due date, we woke up with my wife reporting that she was having a few twinges. During the morning, the sensations continued and my wife went for acupuncture to support the labour process. Throughout the afternoon, the contractions were more regular, and by 5 pm we were calling our midwife. As soon as she arrived at our home, her presence calmed our nerves.

As the labour progressed, our midwife reminded us of the pain relief techniques we had learned in our antenatal classes, and had included in our birth plan (such as breathing techniques, acupressure and getting in a warm bath). Other than our baby's heart rate being monitored and dilation checked (at my wife's request), there was no other intervention from our midwife. Before our baby was born, the second midwife was called to attend the birth (as with all home births in New Zealand) as a precautionary measure. My wife and I were able to successfully birth our first son calmly together, with the support of the midwives. It brought me to tears when I looked directly into my son's eyes for the first time.

Post birth, because we were at home, we were already in our own comfortable environment and able to snuggle up in bed with our son to establish early skin-to-skin contact and breastfeeding.

Since this time, we have had two further home births, in 2013 and 2016. We wanted to have even more control of these birth experiences than with our first, and my wife laboured for longer each time before we called our midwife. Again, during each labour our midwife provided the reassurance we needed, while allowing the process of labour and birth to take place naturally. On both occasions, I had the absolute privilege of delivering my sons. In 2016, we went full circle with our third boy being caught by both my eldest son and I together. This was without any doubt the most special moment of my life, and one which would not have been possible without being at home under the outstanding care and supervision of our experienced midwife.

Theoretical underpinnings

Supporting the shared experience of the partners are the philosophical underpinnings which shape the partnership relationship between women and midwives, and direct midwifery practice. The beliefs inherent in these philosophical statements are universal in midwifery and are articulated in the International Confederation of Midwifery (ICM) definition of a midwife, and the philosophies of a range of international professional organisations for midwives (ACM, n.d.; Midwives Alliance of North America (MANA), 1991).

Supporting structure for the midwifery partnership (Fig. 17.6)

Midwifery is women centred

The basic premise of midwifery care is 'to facilitate the optimal experience of birth for pregnant women and

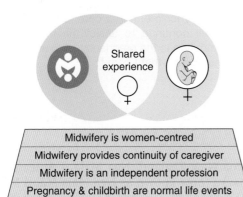

FIGURE 17.6 Supporting structures for midwifery partnership
(Source: Based on Guilliland & Pairman, 1995)

their babies' (Guilliland & Pairman, 1995, p. 41). It is the woman who defines her own needs, and the midwife's focus is on her. It should be remembered that at all times the term 'woman' is not exclusive—others she may define as being important to her may be included in this concept. The woman has a primary relationship with her baby, and midwifery sees the needs of both the woman and baby as intertwined—meeting the woman's needs will meet the baby's needs, and vice versa. Similarly, the woman has a relationship with her family, so the midwife recognises their needs through her relationship with the woman. Each woman is unique so her needs will also be unique, and midwifery recognises each woman's context, beliefs and values accordingly. 'Woman-centredness just means working with a woman in whatever way she wants' (Pairman & McAra-Couper, 2015, p. 399).

Midwifery provides continuity of caregiver

Working together through pregnancy, birth and the postpartum period strengthens the relationship between the woman and her midwife by allowing time for trust to develop. Continuity of caregiver 'means one midwife (and her back-up colleague) providing midwifery care throughout the entire childbirth experience' (Guilliland & Pairman, 1995, p. 39). The midwife can practise across her scope within this relationship, and she is the only maternity caregiver who can provide all aspects of necessary care where the woman's experience remains uncomplicated. Getting to know the woman's dreams for her birth, along with her anxieties, positions the midwife well for providing support that will address her concerns, and assist with manifesting her dreams. Evidence increasingly supports continuity of care as the model of maternity care which produces excellent outcomes for women in terms of their satisfaction (Hatem et al., 2008; Sandall, 2004; Sandall et al., 2016), but also in relation to outcomes such as a reduction in the rate of pre-term fetal loss, reductions in use of technology and some birth interventions, and cost savings from decreased use of technology, pharmacology and personnel associated with highly medicalised birth. No adverse outcomes have been associated with this model of care (Sandall et al., 2016).

Midwifery is an independent profession

Independence, in this context, is about *practice autonomy*, not about where/how the midwife is employed or the birth place the woman chooses. Accepting accountability for practice and being able to provide the full scope of midwifery care on her own account without oversight from another health discipline, exemplifies autonomous practice. Practice colleagues assist midwives to meet these responsibilities by providing support and back-up when required. The Code of Ethics (NZCOM, 2015, p. 13) outlines a midwife's accountabilities to the woman, her profession and the wider community. When other practitioners become involved in the woman's care owing to additional complexity, the midwife ensures that the woman remains at the centre of care, supported to make decisions that will best meet her needs. Clear role definitions about the woman's ongoing care provision

379

are negotiated and understood by all, and the midwife remains accountable for midwifery care she provides alongside her medical colleagues.

Pregnancy and childbirth are normal life events

For millennia women have been giving birth; a physiological process that results in the birth of a baby human. In the 21st-century context, both in resource-rich countries and increasingly in resource-poor countries, technology and the rise of biomedicine has placed birth into a category of human endeavour that has been 'risk-managed' to the extent it is barely recognisable as a physiological life event. Scammell & Alaszewski (2012) use the phrase 'the ever-narrowing window of normality' (p. 207) to describe how health professionals are taking a more and more precautionary approach to the uncertainties that are part and parcel of maternity care. With most births now taking place in highly medicalised settings, women are less and less likely to achieve spontaneous physiological birth experiences despite midwifery's commitment to being the guardians of normal birth. So it behoves women and midwives to strongly resist the notion that birth is unsafe unless under the surveillance of biotechnology. A huge body of evidence has established that birth at home and in primary birth spaces produces optimal outcomes for well women who are experiencing uncomplicated pregnancies (see for example Birthplace in England Collaborative Group, 2011; Cheyney et al., 2014; Davis et al., 2011, Janssen et al., 2009). Belief that birth is normal is a fundamental position for midwives and women to take. Because each woman's experience is unique to her, the term 'unique normality' has been coined and is the most fitting for ongoing understanding of women's experience. Maternity systems that embrace each woman's unique normality will be best placed to 'engage with complexity and uncertainty, and to maximise holistic wellbeing, while ensuring appropriate responses to pathology when it arises' (Downe & McCourt, 2004, p. 174).

REFLECTIVE CASE STUDY

Thoughts on partnership from 'Keesie'—a new graduate midwife

Partnership is the first key principle of midwifery that as students we are immediately encouraged to learn, understand and embrace. The theory that to work with women and provide the best midwifery care possible we first need to develop an honest, trusting and reciprocal relationship in which to share information and enable a woman to make the decisions that are best for her.

As a midwifery student walking alongside and learning from both women and midwives, I had a unique opportunity to forge strong partnerships with women without the substantial clinical responsibility that goes along with the relationship of being the 'actual midwife'. As a relatively new midwifery student I was intently focused on developing strong partnerships with women because

that is what I was learning about and it is what a number of our assessments and exams were based on. As I gained clinical knowledge and practical experience walking alongside women in midwifery relationships, I developed a deeper understanding and appreciation of partnership as a core foundation for midwifery. I believe our intent and ability to forge partnerships with women are what sets midwives apart from other healthcare professionals.

Over time I have realised that good communication, honesty, openness and the ability to remain non-judgmental are key aspects in the ability to develop a midwifery partnership. Awareness of self, of cultural differences and cultural safety are also imperative in developing partnerships, as without this it is impossible to understand the individual needs of the women I care for. I am now in my first year of practice and have found it hard at times to balance my desire to forge partnerships with the often-overwhelming clinical responsibility that comes with the transition from student to midwife. My path to midwifery and the student to midwife transition has cemented one thing very clearly—the tools that enable every other aspect of developing midwifery partnerships are time and the ability to listen.

Every woman is different. In order to develop a partnership with women there first needs to be understanding. Understanding of who they are and where they come from, and this only comes from allowing women the time to talk, to tell you what they want or need to—understanding of what your role in their journey is, how you communicate, when you will meet and what their expectations of you are and equally your expectations of them. When we give women the time they need and actually listen to them we are better equipped to share information in a way that suits them, to openly talk about risks, benefits and alternatives, to provide evidence-based information and to assist them to make the decisions that feel safe and feel right for them—to empower them with informed choice.

As I move forward in my midwifery career I hope to maintain this clarity of what partnership is, what it means to me and the tools that ensure it has ample opportunity to develop. The principle of partnership is not merely theory for me, it is a core foundation for my practice. It will continue to assist me in providing a positive contribution to the pregnancy, birth and postnatal journey of the women that I care for.

TŪRANGA KAUPAPA

In Aotearoa New Zealand, Nga Maia o Aotearoa me te Waipounamu (now known as Nga Maia Māori Midwives Aotearoa) developed Tūranga Kaupapa, a set of philosophical principles that express the cultural values of Māori in relation to childbirth (Fig. 17.7, Box 17.1). The statements provide insight into how Tangata Whenua

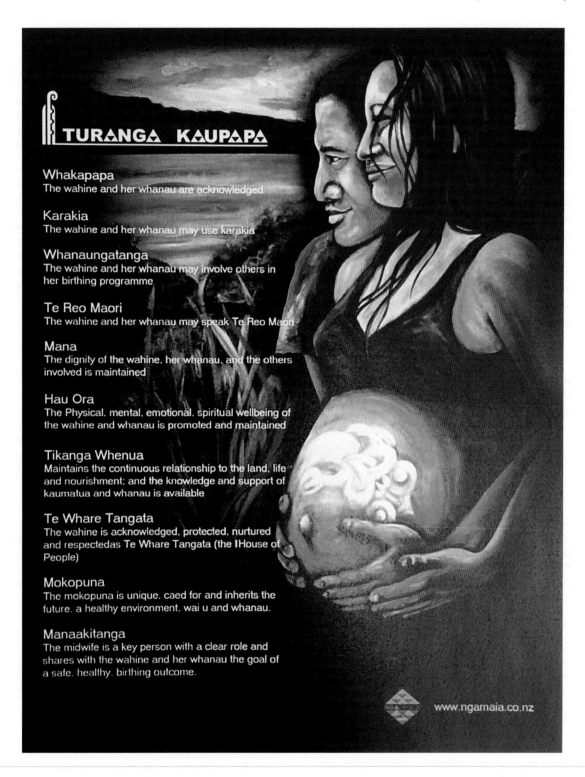

Whakapapa
The wahine and her whanau are acknowledged

Karakia
The wahine and her whanau may use karakia

Whanaungatanga
The wahine and her whanau may involve others in her birthing programme

Te Reo Maori
The wahine and her whanau may speak Te Reo Maori

Mana
The dignity of the wahine, her whanau, and the others involved is maintained

Hau Ora
The Physical, mental, emotional, spiritual wellbeing of the wahine and whanau is promoted and maintained

Tikanga Whenua
Maintains the continuous relationship to the land, life and nourishment; and the knowledge and support of kaumatua and whanau is available

Te Whare Tangata
The wahine is acknowledged, protected, nurtured and respected as Te Whare Tangata (the lHouse of People)

Mokopuna
The mokopuna is unique, caed for and inherits the future, a healthy environment, wai u and whanau.

Manaakitanga
The midwife is a key person with a clear role and shares with the wahine and her whanau the goal of a safe, healthy, birthing outcome.

www.ngamaia.co.nz

FIGURE 17.7 Tūranga Kaupapa poster (© Ngā Maia)

(indigenous people of the land) value aspects of the childbearing experience, and as a framework for midwifery practice provide clear guidance about working with wāhine Māori and their whānau.

Nga Maia gifted this framework to the New Zealand College of Midwives and the Midwifery Council of New Zealand, and Tūranga Kaupapa now sit alongside the Standards of Practice (NZCOM, 2015) and Competencies for Entry to the Register of Midwives (MCNZ, 2007). Tūranga Kaupapa are a fundamental aspect to preregistration midwifery education in Aotearoa New Zealand and registered midwives have ongoing opportunities available to them to learn about Tūranga Kaupapa through workshops, and by reflecting on how they apply

Box 17.1   Tūranga Kaupapa glossary

- wahine—woman
- whānau—family
- whakapapa—genealogy
- karakia—incantation, prayer
- whanaungatanga—relationships
- Te Reo Māori—Māori language
- mana—prestige, standing
- hauora—wellbeing (holistic)
- tikanga Māori—Māori traditions
- whenua—placenta, land
- Te Whare Tangata—mother, woman, the House of the People (womb)
- Mokopuna—child, grandchild, face of ancestor
- Wai ū—breast milk
- Manaakitanga—actions of respect and caring

the statements to their own midwifery practice during their Midwifery Standards Review process. Please also see Chapter 11 for further discussion of this topic.

REFLECTIVE CASE STUDY

Reflection on Tūranga Kaupapa from Tungane—an MSR reviewer

For a majority of wāhine Māori, the relationship with their midwife will be the first encounter with a health professional. Tūranga Kaupapa has given midwives a resource that when actioned can enrich this partnership. For over a decade Tūranga Kaupapa has existed in New Zealand midwifery culture, sitting alongside the Standards, as a framework which midwives can use to reflect on their practice—defining how they work and walk alongside women.

As a Midwifery Standards Reviewer during these years I have to say that the potential has barely been tapped by the vast majority of midwives, who are influenced by the attitudes and leadership of our profession. Tūranga Kaupapa educational workshops were relegated as elective education for midwives. The Midwifery Council has denied the opportunity in this term to make cultural competence a compulsory requirement for recertification and has radically reduced ongoing education to one study day per year. Māori birth is on the rise and makes up a significant percentage of many caseloading around the country. Where is the accountability for ensuring that professional development is culturally appropriate? That outcomes for whānau Māori improve with quality care? I guess the old adage still rings true, 'you can lead a horse to water but you can't make it drink!' This comment from a current consumer reviewer colleague was her response when discussing the limited uptake of Tūranga Kaupapa:

'... as a reviewer I'm sick of hearing midwives go on about bad stats for Māori ... as I'm sitting straight opposite them ... I want to hear from them what the solutions might be, to answer their own complaints instead ... My disappointment is that she isn't able to talk to what or how to make the changes, and the positive influences a midwife has on a hapū mama ... using Tūranga Kaupapa as "the" resource.'

On a more hopeful note it has been heartening reviewing new graduate midwives who have had Tūranga Kaupapa as a natural part of their midwifery landscape. These midwives have no problem in acknowledging that in Aotearoa New Zealand there can be no true partnership model without acknowledging Tangata Whenua values, and freely and confidently are using Tūranga Kaupapa and the Standards as a framework to demonstrate how they work in partnership with women—whether they be Māori or tauiwi.

As a reviewer I extend an invitation to my sister midwives, dip your toe in, take a refreshing drink! Read the Tūranga Kaupapa statements. So you are passionate about breastfeeding for example, have you read the Mokopuna statement? The Mokopuna is unique, cared for and inherits the future, a healthy environment, wai ū and whānau. Do you agree? Let's make that a goal for your next review to give an example from your practice that demonstrates how you have achieved this whainga.

Tūranga Kaupapa belong to the midwifery profession, he taonga tuku iho!

While Tūranga Kaupapa gives guidance specific to the values of Māori, the principles inherent in the statements can be effectively applied to women of all cultures. As with all mahi involving recognition of Te Ao Māori, what is of benefit to Māori is of benefit to all.

PERSPECTIVES ON BICULTURALISM AND MIDWIFERY FROM A CONSUMER

Rebecca Bear

I feel deeply humbled by the opportunity to comment on biculturalism in midwifery today and I will begin by making explicit my status as a non-Māori New Zealander from outside of the midwifery profession. My life has brought me close to both midwifery and biculturalism over the last two decades, particularly as they relate to health and education in this land. As a consumer of midwifery services, I take my responsibility to both midwifery partnership and the women I represent very seriously and I appreciate the political and legislative gains for autonomy that midwives and women won together in partnership. I do not proclaim expertise on this topic and yet I am deeply moved to share my perspective as a person who was born into the dominant Eurocentric culture that was Aotearoa New Zealand in the 1970s—an influence I have been working to raise my own awareness of through an understanding of our colonisation history ever since.

Firstly, it seems appropriate to voice my beliefs about biculturalism, including a definition and principles that I connect to in daily life. Accentuating that contemporary Aotearoa/NZ was founded on Te Tiriti o Waitangi and therefore bicultural, rather than multicultural, is important to me. In my experience, discussions about culture in this country are often dominated by the word 'multiculturalism', bypassing the fact that our foundational culture consists of the indigenous people, Māori, and non-Māori (Pākehā and tau iwi, or other non-Māori). I believe this undermines the status of Tangata Whenua and hinders the development of true partnership between Māori and non-Māori, recorded in our founding document, Te Tiriti o Waitangi. This personal definition of biculturalism in Aotearoa/NZ informs me:

> Aotearoa is a bicultural society whose founding agreement between Māori and non-indigenous peoples was Te Tiriti o Waitangi. Its principles of partnership, participation and protection guide the inclusion of many different cultures into its social fabric, whilst acknowledging that biculturalism remains firmly at centre-stage of any dialogue regarding best outcomes for all New Zealanders. To this end, bicultural dialogue, system creation and strategic planning, particularly where there is inequity for Māori people, must be ensured. Visible, measurable and accountable frameworks in pursuit of bicultural parity, most notably in healthcare, are of utmost importance.

I acknowledge the status of Māori as Tangata Whenua of Aotearoa, an equal partner with the Crown as stated in Te Tiriti o Waitangi, maintaining tino rangatiratanga (chiefly autonomy). I deeply respect Māori values and connection to their reo (language), tikanga (cultural practices), whenua (land), taonga (treasures), mātauranga Māori (indigenous knowledge) and their whakapapa (genealogy). I attempt to remain reflexive with my thoughts and behaviours in all interactions, aware that my experience has been dominated by a Eurocentric worldview and the privilege associated with that. Embedding these principles into my understanding, I endeavour to work in partnership with other New Zealanders for equity in healthcare, education and social justice issues, and one role where I have been particularly active is as a consumer reviewer of the Midwifery Standards Review (MSR) process.

In my endeavours to remain current with issues facing midwives, wāhine and whānau, I have been particularly interested in the commentary on biculturalism as it relates to this group. Specifically, I have focused on the efforts to bring forth and embed a Māori worldview and framework, Tūranga Kaupapa, to support the development of cultural competence and the midwifery partnership model in service of those who identify with Māori culture. I have learnt much about this framework through the NZ College of Midwives and a Tūranga Kaupapa workshop held by Nga Maia's

Henare Kani, and yet have found it almost invisible in the reflections of women in their Midwifery Standards Reviews over the last 6 years. I therefore share some of the concerns written about by Kenney in her 2011 paper, 'Midwives, women and their families: a Māori gaze', questioning whether true partnership was attained with Māori when creating the foundations of midwifery practice; the partnership model (Kenney, 2011). This, in turn, may be reflected in ongoing difficulty in retaining Māori midwifery students and building the Māori midwifery workforce, stated by McEldowney as central to the improvement of Māori health outcomes (O'Connor, 2012).

It seems important to continue to acknowledge the 'spiritual wounds of colonisation' (Farry & Crowther, 2014, p. 33) with regards to their prolonged and negative effect on traditional Māori childbirth practices. Inclusion of Māori ways of knowing and being in the world, including the use of language and concepts relevant to those who hold the Māori worldview, would go a long way to raising the awareness of all New Zealanders and avoiding the trap of cultural tokenism (Farry & Crowther, 2014). One example of differences between Māori and non-Māori perspectives is found when comparing words for childbirth assistants in each culture. 'Kaiwhakawhānau' means to 'facilitate the creation and development of whānau' (Kenney, 2011, p. 126), whereas the Eurocentric word 'midwifery' means 'with women'. Some feel that the Māori perspective is diminished when appropriate language is absent and suggest that cultural safety can be achieved only through truly bicultural frameworks which are highly visible throughout the profession (Kenney, 2011).

I feel privileged to be a part of the profession of midwifery as a consumer. I acknowledge the huge work and efforts of midwives and women to assert their autonomy as practitioners and individuals who work in partnership, which enables the sharing of my perspective. After the efforts of the 80s and 90s in developing the relationships and frameworks that they have, I would like to be part of a renewed momentum for developing partnership between the midwifery profession and the public. Especially, that there is no 'slippage' in the energy applied to ensuring that the indigenous people of this land enjoy health, educational and social policy which reflect the principles of partnership, participation and protection detailed in Te Tiriti o Waitangi, as determined by their own worldview. An active and developing foundation of biculturalism in Aotearoa will serve as a prominent model for true partnership with people of all cultures, enhancing the childbearing experience of all women and families.

Student Midwifery Practice Scenario

I was caring for a woman who was in early labour. As part of the gathering of support around her at this important time, her grandmother and six other elders visited for prayers. This was very important for the woman and her family, both to give strength and to make safe the important event about to take place. During this time the charge midwife came into the room to introduce herself. I could see her looking around with some dismay and I knew she was about to say that there were too many visitors in the room. I quickly and politely interjected to introduce the people in the room and to let her know that the elders had come for prayers. This was a very uncomfortable situation for myself as the midwife, as I knew how important these elders were to the woman. Even though I felt I had pre-empted the situation regarding the charge midwife, the woman over the next 2 hours made excuses for the religious needs of herself and her family. There was no doubt she had picked up what had been about to happen. I, of course, felt most uncomfortable with her obvious discomfort and did all I could to reassure her that the elders were welcome and that her needs and the family's needs were important. I really had a deep sense of unease at how institutions and their policies can negate a woman's right to her family's cultural and spiritual needs. As a culturally competent midwife I am very aware of the need to ensure that the imbalance of power that can exist in these situations is addressed, and I work to protect and provide a safe environment for the woman and her family.

Questions

1. Identify and explore the principles of cultural safety and midwifery partnership that promote culturally safe practice.
2. Describe your own culture and identify five things that are really important to you.
3. Describe how the assumptions, beliefs and values that you hold may affect your practice as a midwife.
4. Describe how the protocols and policies of institutions may impact on culturally competent care.
5. Identify three ways in which you can promote cultural safety within your midwifery practice.
6. Explore how you would address this situation if it arose with a colleague.

CULTURAL COMPETENCE

The concept of 'cultural competence' was initiated by the work of Madeleine Leininger on Transcultural Nursing. Leininger's work had its roots in anthropology and was focused initially on the need for health professionals to understand cultures other than their own (Andrews, 2012). In New Zealand, the *Health Practitioners' Competence Assurance Act (2003)* (HPCAA) requires the Midwifery Council, along with all the other regulatory authorities, to set standards not only of clinical competence but also of cultural competence (MCNZ, 2012). This requirement by the HPCAA has led to a growing acceptance of the notion of cultural competence in New

Zealand (De Souza, 2008). Cultural competence is viewed by some as being more comprehensive than cultural safety, as it includes an understanding of systems, organisations and institutions (Adams, 2010). However, others see it as being 'neutral' about the social, economic and political structures, which lead to health inequities and power imbalances (De Souza, 2008).

The Midwifery Council of New Zealand's *Statement of Cultural Competence* sets out the frameworks for cultural competence (MCNZ, 2012). These frameworks are: midwifery partnership, cultural safety and Tūranga Kaupapa. Cultural competence involves an ongoing process whereby there is an integration of knowledge, awareness and cultural encounters (Campinha-Bacote, 2011). The midwife is required to apply these frameworks to her practice, to ensure that the woman and her family feel safe and have the optimal experience and outcome.

The Australian Nursing and Midwifery Accreditation Council (ANMAC, 2014) has determined the national accreditation standards for programs of midwifery education (Midwife Accreditation Standards, 2014, https://www.anmac.org.au/sites/default/files/documents/ANMAC_Midwife_Accreditation_Standards_2014.pdf). These include Standard 2.4(i) 'to promote emotional intelligence, communication, collaboration and teamwork, cultural safety, ethical practice and leadership skills' (p. 14). In regard to curriculum development, Standard 4.6 requires 'inclusion of content giving students an appreciation of the diversity of Australian cultures to develop and engender their knowledge of cultural safety and respect' (p. 18). The Nurses and Midwives Board of Australia states in its National Competency Standards for Midwives what is expected of a midwife in relation to cultural competence in that country. Competency 10 states what is required for a midwife in Australia to be culturally safe. From 2018, the International Confederation of Midwives *Code of Ethics for Midwives* is in effect for all Australian midwives. Section II Practice of Midwifery requires that 'Midwives provide care for women and childbearing families with respect for cultural diversity while also working to eliminate harmful practices within those same cultures' (ICM, n. d., p. 2).

Research into cultural competence and its implications for midwifery practice is limited. In Western Australia a study researched antenatal services for Aboriginal women because of significantly poorer Aboriginal perinatal outcomes. This research found that 75% of the services delivered to Aboriginal women did not deliver care in line with culturally responsive values (Reibel & Walker, 2010). Research in Aotearoa New Zealand has examined the engagement of Pasifika women with antenatal care, as these women continue to have significantly poorer outcomes than other sectors of the population (Perinatal Maternal Mortality Review Committee (PMMRC), 2021). This research showed that two of the main barriers to engaging with care were women's lack of information about the services available and the fact that access to and delivery of the services was not culturally safe or appropriate for these women (Corbett & Okesene-Gafa,

2013; Priday, 2011). Also from Aotearoa New Zealand, the experiences of Japanese women giving birth within the New Zealand maternity context was explored, and researchers found that some women faced cultural differences and language challenges that result in 'an inability to genuinely express their aspirations and concerns' (Doering et al., 2015, p. 9).

Chapters 10 and 11 of this text identify and discuss the health disparities that still exist for Māori, Aboriginal and Torres Strait Islanders in Aotearoa New Zealand and Australia. The provision of culturally competent health services is one strategy to reduce these disparities and improved clinical outcomes are being reported from such services (Kildea et al., 2021).

It is clear that one strategy to enhance indigenous women's experience during childbirth is the option to be cared for by a midwife of their own culture. In both Australia and Aotearoa New Zealand, low numbers of indigenous midwives in the workforce means this option is not fully recognisable. Providers of midwifery education strive to increase recruitment and retention of indigenous students in their programs, and clear benefits to Aboriginal women in Australia have been described, including the importance of 'knowing how we feel', when Aboriginal student midwives work alongside Aboriginal and Torres Strait Islander women during their Bachelor of Midwifery education (Kelly et al., 2014). However, several studies have highlighted the difficulty experienced by some indigenous students of health programs in successfully completing their education (Hall et al., 2013; Milne et al., 2015; Oliver et al., 2013; Rigby et al., 2011; West et al., 2014). Some recent research in Australia has led to the development of a tool for assessing the cultural safety of academics who are involved in midwifery and nursing education (Milne et al., 2016). The Awareness of Cultural Safety Scale (ACSS) shows promise as a means to 'foster purposeful consideration by nursing and midwifery academics about their perceptions and approaches to teaching in order to improve indigenous student success' (Milne et al., 2016, p. 20). Similarly, a midwifery education provider in Aotearoa undertook a Kaupapa Māori (indigenous research methodology) research project to understand the experiences of indigenous students in its Bachelor of Midwifery program, resulting in several recommendations from students about how the program could strengthen its support of indigenous learners (Patterson et al., 2017). During 2021, the Te Ara ō Hine—Tapu Ora project in Aotearoa New Zealand was funded by the Ministry of Health (MOH, 2021). This project aims to improve recruitment and retention of Māori and Pasifika midwifery students by providing financial and pastoral assistance to support successful degree completion. In Australia, the Australian Catholic University is now offering a Bachelor of Midwifery (Indigenous) for Aboriginal and Torres Strait Islander students (Australian Catholic University (ACU), n.d.).

There is a rapidly growing awareness of the issue of cultural competence among midwives, and their role in creating birthing environments that promote culturally safe care. The following example comes from a new graduate midwife, describing something of her journey in ensuring holistic and culturally responsive care when she was involved in the postnatal care of a woman whose pre-term baby died.

Student Midwifery Practice Scenario

Lelei, a 20-year-old Pasifika woman, G 4, P 0 presented at 21 weeks and 3 days, obviously unwell with abdominal pain and pyrexia. Lelei was found to have prelabour premature rupture of membranes and, following consultant review, a plan was made to commence induction of labour. Approximately 5 hours later Lelei gave birth to a live female infant. I became involved in Lelei's care postnatally; she had minimal support, with only the neighbour who brought her in waiting outside. Lelei was aware that Agelu was unable to survive extrauterine at such early gestation, and was prepared for her to pass away without resuscitation. On entering the room I found that Agelu was not showing any signs of life. I was unable to palpate a heart rate, and required a neonatal stethoscope to make a further assessment; however, there was not one available in the room. Therefore I needed to retrieve one from another room, and on examination I was unable to auscultate a heart rate. I appropriately informed Lelei of my findings, indicating that Agelu had passed away. I expressed my condolences and supported Lelei emotionally, as well as providing ongoing postnatal care and completing required procedures and processes in the event of a neonatal death. This included the weighing of Agelu and the placenta on a communal set of scales. I handed over Lelei's care to another staff member and on return to work the following day found that the room had not yet had spiritual follow-up or 'blessing', which I was advised by a senior staff member occurs to maintain holistic care and cultural responsiveness with regard to the room and equipment that was being transferred for use between well and deceased neonates.

I discussed my experience with a small group of midwife colleagues who agreed that a holistic and culturally responsive process in such events is required, and that they would support the implementation of a documented process which responded to the holistic and cultural wellbeing of staff, women and whānau (family) in relation to facility and equipment use in the event of perinatal death.

As a result of this experience and investigation I proposed to Maternity Service management that a Holistic and Culturally Responsive Care Process be implemented into practice within the service for use when perinatal death occurs. This process includes steps to ensure that in the event of perinatal death women, whānau, staff and lead maternity carers (LMCs) are provided with appropriate support that responds to their cultural needs and maintains holistic wellbeing.

Having this process in place enables staff to arrange appropriate cultural support for women and their whānau throughout maternity care, and provides guidance on how to manage equipment for use when perinatal death occurs and how to arrange a spiritual response on discharge of the woman and their whānau.

As a consequence, the Holistic and Culturally Responsive Care Process is in place. Designated equipment has been purchased to furnish an equipment room for use in the event of perinatal death, to ensure that equipment used for care and assessment of the deceased is kept separate from equipment used to care for and assess well neonates; the resuscitaire in the designated room to care for women and whānau who are expecting a perinatal death has been modified so it can fold away; a Holistic and Culturally Responsive Care Team is to be formed, as a resource for supporting women, whānau, staff and LMCs, completing the care process by being available to give support and perform prayer. A closer working relationship with the Chaplaincy Service has allowed for an improved referral process to be devised. Furthermore a *Tikanga Best Practice in Women's Health Guideline* has been written, and is endorsed by Māori Health Services.

This is an encouraging example of cultural competence in action. The provision of such important resources will positively affect the way midwives in this maternity service provide holistic maternity care to women and whānau in the event of perinatal death. It will assist midwives to navigate encounters with individual women and whānau in a manner that acknowledges and respects different worldviews and perspectives, while providing care with competence and cultural humility.

It is important to acknowledge, however, that there remains a philosophical tension between the concepts of **cultural safety and cultural competence** (De Souza, 2011). While cultural competence focuses on the culture of the consumer, cultural safety focuses on the worldview and culture of the health professional. Cultural safety has always acknowledged and critiqued the political, social and economic milieu in which healthcare is delivered, whereas cultural competence is more neutral in these matters (De Souza, 2008). Cultural safety in effect seeks the transformation of social and economic structures and addresses inequities and power imbalances, whereas cultural competence does not. De Souza (2008) claims that further discussion and research is required to understand fully the application and relevance of these two approaches to midwifery practice. Vernon & Papps (2015) suggest the following: 'Cultural safety and cultural competence are different discourses. Both however are appropriate and neither is necessarily right or wrong. Cultural safety is about the client feeling comfortable or safe with healthcare, while cultural competence is about the ability of health practitioners to demonstrate what is needed to achieve that' (p. 60).

A culturally competent midwife recognises that many different elements of culture exist side by side and that at any time one aspect may be more important than another. Through the development of skills to understand others' cultures better, the culturally competent midwife will be able to work effectively with women with different cultural beliefs. As cultural safety theory shows us, the acquisition of skills to understand others' cultures better cannot be through checklists or a standardised approach based on assumptions about the beliefs and values of specific cultures. Rather, midwives need well-developed personal and communication skills so as to talk with women about their cultural needs and to enable each woman to define what is important for *her*. Guidance for working towards achieving culturally competent care when working with Aboriginal women has been provided by the Australian Government Department of Health (2012).

'Cultural fluency' as a concept has surfaced more recently. It has been described as going beyond cultural awareness, sensitivity *and* safety, by including an understanding of 'how or by whom decision-making is made in a whānau, and considerations of how Māori values, beliefs and experiences might impact on the establishment and maintenance of a therapeutic relationship' (Best Practice Advocacy Centre (BPAC), 2010, p. 19). Ramos (2010) in his description of cultural fluency, describes putting 'culture at the core of creating a better health experience' (p. 58) by incorporating more-inclusive wellness practices that are meaningful to different communities—in Australasia this would include *rongoā* and 'bush medicine', smoking rituals and other Aboriginal practices to maintain health. The notion of cultural fluency suggests it is not possible to say one *is* culturally competent, as this suggests a state of 'arrival', whereas cultural fluency suggests a dynamic and ongoing learning about other cultures and reflection on one's own.

Curtis et al. (2019) undertook a literature review of 59 international articles which described definitions of cultural competence and cultural safety. They concluded that a move towards cultural safety from cultural competence would more directly improve health equity, and proposed a new definition of cultural safety:

Cultural safety requires healthcare professionals and their associated healthcare organisations to examine themselves and the potential impact of their own culture on clinical interactions and healthcare service delivery. This requires individual healthcare professionals and healthcare organisations to acknowledge and address their own biases, attitudes, assumptions, stereotypes, prejudices, structures and characteristics that may affect the quality of care provided. In doing so, cultural safety encompasses a critical consciousness where healthcare professionals and healthcare organisations engage in ongoing self-reflection and self-awareness and hold themselves accountable for providing culturally safe care, as defined by the patient and their communities, and as measured through progress towards achieving health equity. Cultural safety requires healthcare professionals and their associated healthcare organisations to influence healthcare to reduce bias and achieve equity within the workforce and working environment.

(Curtis et al., 2019, p. 14)

Conclusion

This chapter has explored how midwives partner with women, each other and their communities to enhance and optimise care. Key to working in partnership is the ability to engage in open, reflective relationships that honour and value the expertise that each person brings to the relationship. For the woman, it is her own knowing about her body, her baby and her family and social context. For the midwife it is these things too, but also her skills and knowledge derived from multiple 'ways of knowing' in midwifery. A critical skill for midwives in this partnership is that of balancing the art and science of supporting a physiological process of pregnancy, birth and the postpartum period with the sensitivity to acknowledge its complexity and uncertainty, Also, to engage meaningfully with women as they journey together along this woman's childbirth path, intervening where necessary, but always with the woman's active participation in informed decision making—in essence, being truly 'with women'.

Midwifery partnership provides a framework for a negotiated and reciprocal relationship of equity and power sharing between a midwife and a woman. Cultural safety provides a framework for recognising cultural 'difference' between a midwife and a woman, the power inherent in the professional role of a midwife and the impact that the culture of the midwife may have on her professional practice. A key aspect of cultural safety in relation to midwifery practice is that it is the childbearing woman and her family, not the midwife, who determine that the midwifery care is effective and 'safe'. Tūranga Kaupapa provide guidance on specific Māori values in relation to pregnancy and childbirth. A culturally competent midwife draws on midwifery partnership, cultural safety and Tūranga Kaupapa in the development of skills that will help her to understand each woman's needs and values better, how her own culture impacts on her professional practice and how to provide midwifery care that will meet each woman's needs and improve her health outcomes and those of her baby.

Review questions

1. What is meant by 'midwifery partnership'?
2. What do women want from their midwife?
3. How would you describe the terms 'informed consent' and 'informed choice'?
4. What are the benefits for women who receive one-to-one midwifery care?
5. In your birth documentation, what are the key things you will need to demonstrate?
6. How would you decide whether a colleague would make a good midwifery partner?
7. Describe the differences between cultural awareness, cultural sensitivity and cultural safety.
8. Identify three ways you experience the world and explore how that may differ for someone different from yourself (in age, gender, sexual orientation, socioeconomic status, ethnicity, religious or spiritual belief and disability).
9. Identify and discuss the concepts of empowerment, negotiation, reciprocity and trust in relation to midwifery partnership.
10. Describe how the frameworks of midwifery partnership, cultural safety and Tūranga Kaupapa can influence midwifery practice.

Acknowledgements

The authors wish to particularly acknowledge Sally Pairman, Judith McAra-Couper and Liz Wilkes as authors of previous iterations of some of this chapter content. In places their writing remains largely unchanged, apart from updating of references where applicable.

NOTES

a. The word 'she' is used primarily because the vast majority of midwives in Aotearoa New Zealand and Australia at the present time are women. The Midwifery Council of New Zealand's workforce survey in 2020 noted that there are six practising male midwives (0.18% of the workforce) currently holding Annual Practising Certificates (Midwifery Council of New Zealand (MCNZ), 2020) and the Australian Government Department of Health reports that 1.3% of its midwifery workforce in 2019 was male (*Midwives NHWDS Fact Sheet 2019*). To date data capture mechanisms have only provided an opportunity to identify as female or male.

b. In 1987 a Committee of Inquiry was established to investigate allegations concerning the treatment of cervical cancer at National Women's Hospital in Auckland New Zealand. Known as the Cartwright Inquiry, the Committee looked into the treatment of a group of women who had precancerous conditions of the cervix, yet who were not treated for the disease but 'monitored' over a 20-year period. In that time 26 of the women died. The Inquiry highlighted many problems with the treatment of cervical cancer and provided recommendations for healthcare system reform based on four principles of accountability, patients' rights, self-determination and cultural sensitivity.

Online resources

Australian College of Midwives: http://www.midwives.org.au.

Australian Government Department of Health: http://www.health.gov.au.

Australian National Health and Medical Research Council: http://www.nhmrc.gov.au.

Midwifery Council of New Zealand: http://www.midwifery-council.health.nz.

New Zealand College of Midwives: http://www.midwife.org.nz.

New Zealand Health & Disability Commissioner: http://www.hdc.org.nz.

New Zealand Ministry of Health: http://www.health.govt.nz.

Nursing and Midwifery Board of Australia: http://www.nursingmidwiferyboard.gov.au.

References

Adams K. Indigenous cultural competence in nursing and midwifery practice. *Aust Nurs J.* 2010;17(11):35–38.

Allen J, Gibbons K, Beckmann M, et al. Does model of maternity care make a difference to birth outcomes for young women? A retrospective cohort study. *Int J Nurs Studies.* 2015;52(8):1332–1342.

Andrews MM. Editorial—Dr Madeleine M. Leininger. *OJCCNH.* 2012;2(4):1–2. doi:10.9730/ojccnh.org/v2n4e1.

Australian Catholic University. *Bachelor of Midwifery (Indigenous).* n.d. Online: https://www.acu.edu.au/course/bachelor-of-midwifery-indigenous

Australian College of Midwives (ACM). *Midwifery Philosophy.* n.d. Online: https://www.midwives.org.au/midwifery-philosophy.

Australian College of Midwives (ACM). *National Midwifery Guidelines for Consultation and Referral.* 3rd ed. Canberra: ACM; 2017. https://1-midwives.cdn.aspedia.net/sites/default/files/uploaded-content/field_f_content_file/with_covers_guidelines_3rd_edition_issue_2_final_2017.pdf. Online.

Australian College of Midwives, CATSINaM, CRANAplus (2015). *Joint Birthing on Country Position Statement.* Online: https://8-midwives.cdn.aspedia.net/sites/default/files/uploaded-content/field_f_content_file/birthing_on_country_position_statement.pdf.

Australian Government Department of Health. *Improving Maternity Services—Report of the National Maternity Services Review.* 2009. Online:http://www.health.gov.au/internet/main/publishing.nsf/content/maternityservicesreview-report.

Australian Government Department of Health. *National Maternity Services Plan 2010.* 2011. Online: http://www.health.gov.au/internet/main/publishing.nsf/Content/maternityservicesplan.

Australian Government Department of Health. *The Characteristics of Culturally Competent Maternity Care for Aboriginal and Torres Strait Islander Women.* 2012. Online: http://www.health.gov.au/internet/main/publishing.nsf/Content/maternity-pubs-cultur.

Australian Government Department of Health. *Eligible Midwives Questions and Answers.* 2013. Online: http://www.health.gov.au/internet/main/publishing.nsf/Content/midwives-nurse-pract-qanda.

Australian Nursing & Midwifery Accreditation Council (2014) *Midwife Accreditation Standards.* 2014. https://www.anmac.org.au/sites/default/files/documents/ANMAC_Midwife_Accreditation_Standards_2014.pdf

Ball I, Curtis P, Kirkham M. *Why Do Midwives Leave?* London: Royal College of Midwives; 2002.

Barker R, Hiskemuller Y, Kyle M. Do you text? *Midwifery News.* 2012;December:28.

Baxter JD, McCourt C, Jarrett P. What is current practice in offering debriefing services to post partum women and what are the perceptions of women in accessing these services: A critical review of the literature. *Midwifery.* 2014;30(2):194–219.

Best Practice Advocacy Centre (BPAC). Substance abuse and addiction in Māori. *Best Pract J.* 2010;28:18–35.

Birthplace in England Collaborative Group. Perinatal and maternal outcomes by planned place of birth for healthy women with low risk pregnancies: the Birthplace in England national prospective cohort study. *BMJ.* 2011;343:d7400. doi:10.1136/bmj.d7400.

Borelli S, Spiby H. Walsh D. The kaleidoscopic midwife: A conceptual metaphor illustrating first-time mothers' perspectives of a good midwife during childbirth. A grounded theory study. *Midwifery.* 2016;39: 103–111. http://dx.doi.org/10.1016/j.midw.2016.05.008

Botelle R, Connolly D, Walker S, et al. Contemporary and future transmasculine pregnancy and postnatal care in the UK. *Prac Midwife.* 2021;24(5), 8–13.

Brighton and Sussex University Hospitals. *Gender inclusive language in perinatal services: Mission rationale.* 2021. Online: https://www.bsuh.nhs.uk/maternity/wp-content/uploads/sites/7/2021/01/Gender-inclusive-language-in-perinatal-services.pdf

Brooke-Read M, Baillie L, Mann R, et al. Electronic health records in maternity: the student experience. *Br J Midwifery.* 2012; 206:440–445.

Bryar R. *Theory for Midwifery Practice.* London: Macmillan; 1995:5–40.

Burn N, Grove SK. *Understanding Nursing Research.* Philadelphia: WB Saunders; 1995.

Calvert I. *Trauma, Relational Trust and the Effects on the Midwife* (Unpublished thesis). Palmerston North, New Zealand: Massey University; 2011.

Campbell N. Core midwives—the challenge. *Proceedings of the New Zealand College of Midwives Sixth National Conference,* Cambridge 28–30 September. Christchurch: NZCOM; 2000:187–193.

Campinha-Bacote J. Coming to know cultural competence: an evolutionary process. *Int J Hum Caring.* 2011;15(3):42–48.

Carolan M, Hodnett E. 'With woman' philosophy: examining the evidence, answering the questions. *Nurs Inq.* 2007;14(2):140–152.

Charter R, Ussher JM, Perz J, et al. The transgender parent: Experiences and constructions of pregnancy and parenthood for transgender men in Australia. *Int J Trans.* 2018;19(1), 64–77.

Cheyney M, Bovbjerg M, Everson C, et al. Outcomes of care for 16,924 planned homebirths in the United States: The Midwives Alliance of North America statistics project, 2004 to 2009. *J Midwifery Womens Health.* 2014;59(1):17–27. doi:10.1111/jmwh.12172.

Clear G. A re-examination of cultural safety: a national imperative. *Nurs Praxis N Z.* 2008;24(2):2–4.

Commonwealth of Australia, Department of Health. *Aboriginal and Torres Strait Islander Health Curriculum Framework.* 2014. Online: http://www.health.gov.au/internet/main/publishing.nsf/Content/aboriginal-torres-strait-islander-health-curriculum-framework.

Congress of Aboriginal and Torres Strait Islander Nurse and Midwives (CATSINaM). CATSINaM. *Cultural Safety Position Statement.* 2014. Online: https://www.catsinam.org.au/static/uploads/files/cultural-safety-endorsed-march-2014-wfginz phsxbz.pdf.

Congress of Aboriginal and Torres Strait Islander Nurses and Midwives (CATSINaM). *Position statement: Embedding cultural safety across Australian nursing and midwifery.* 2017a. Online: https://www.catsinam.org.au/static/uploads/files/embedding-cultural-safety-accross-australian-nursing-and-midwifery-may-2017-wfca.pdf.

Congress of Aboriginal and Torres Strait Islander Nurses and Midwives (CATSINaM). *The Nursing and Midwifery Aboriginal and Torres Strait Islander Health Curriculum Framework*. 2017b. Online: https://www.catsinam.org.au/static/uploads/files/nursing-midwifery-health-curriculum-framework-final-version-1-0-wfffegyedblq.pdf.

Corbett S, Okesene-Gafa K. Pasifika women and barriers to the initiation of antenatal care at CMDHB; July 2013. Conference Presentation at the Pacific Society for Reproductive Health.

Craswell A, Moxham L, Broadbent M. Perinatal data collection: current practice in the Australian nursing and midwifery healthcare context. *Health Inf Man J*. 2013;42(1):11–17.

Curtis E, Jones R, Tipene-Leach D, et al. Why cultural safety rather than cultural competency is required to achieve health equity: A literature review and recommended definition. *Int J Equity in Health*. 2019;18:174. https://doi.org/10.1186/s12939-019-1082-3

Dahlen HG, Barclay LM, Homer C. Preparing for first birth: mothers' experiences at home and in hospital in Australia. *J Perinat Educ*. 2008;17(4):21–32.

Davies R. Completing the midwife–woman partnership. In: Pairman S, Tracy SK, Thorogood C, et al, eds. *Midwifery: Preparation for Practice*. 2nd ed. Chatswood. NSW: Elsevier; 2010:677–693.

Davis D, Baddock S, Pairman S, et al. Planned place of birth in New Zealand: does it affect mode of birth and intervention rates among low-risk women? *Birth*. 2011;38(2):111–119.

Davison C, Hauck Y, Bayes S, et al. The relationship is everything: women's reasons for choosing a privately practicing midwife in Western Australia. *Midwifery*. 2015;31(8):772–778.

De Souza R. Wellness for all the possibilities of cultural safety and cultural competence in New Zealand. *J Res Nurs*. 2008;13:125–135. doi:10.1177/1744987108088637.

De Souza R. *Migrant Maternity* (Doctoral thesis). Auckland: Auckland University of Technology; 2011. Online: http://hdl.handle.net/10292/4249.

Deane-Gray T. Effective communication. In: Peate I, Hamilton C, eds. *Becoming a Midwife in the 21st Century*. Chichester, UK: John Wiley; 2008:10–29.

Dobbie M. *The Trouble With Women. The Story of Parents Centre New Zealand*. Whatamango Bay, NZ: Cape Catley; 1990.

Doering K, Patterson J, Griffiths C. Experience of the New Zealand maternity care system by a group of Japanese women in one centre. *NZCOM J*. 2015;51:5–10.

Donley J. Professionalism. The importance of consumer control over childbirth. *NZCOM J*. 1989;Sept:6–7.

Downe S, McCourt C. From being to becoming: reconstructing childbirth knowledges. In: Downe S, eds. *Normal Childbirth: Evidence and Debate*. London: Churchill Livingstone; 2004:174.

Downe S, McCourt C. From being to becoming: reconstructing childbirth knowledges. In: Downe S, eds. *Normal Childbirth: Evidence and Debate*. 2nd ed. Edinburgh: Elsevier; 2008:3–28.

England C, Morgan R. *Communication Skills for Midwives: Challenges in Everyday Practice*. Milton Keynes, UK: Open University Press; 2012.

Farry A, Crowther S. Cultural safety in New Zealand midwifery practice: Part 2. *Pract Midwife*. 2014;17(7):30–33.

Fernandez Turienzo C, Roe Y, Rayment-Jones H, et al. Implementation of midwifery continuity of care models for Indigenous women in Australia: Perspectives and reflections for the United Kingdom. *Midwifery*. 2019;69:110–112 https://doi.org/10.1016/j.midw.2018.11.005

Fleming V. Women and midwives in partnership: a problematic relationship? *J Adv Nurs*. 1998;27(1):8–14.

Forster D, McLachlan H, Davey MA, et al. Continuity of care by a primary midwife (caseload midwifery) increases woman's satisfaction with antenatal, intrapartum and postpartum care: results from the COSMOS randomised controlled trial. *BMC Pregnancy and Childbirth*. 2016;16:28. doi 10.1186/s12884-016-0798-y

Forster D, Newton M, McLachlan H, et al. Exploring implementation and sustainability of models of care: can theory help? *BMC Public Health*. 2011;11(suppl 5):S8.

Fryer J, Weaver JJ. Should a postnatal birth discussion be part of routine midwifery care? *Br J Midwifery*. 2014;22(2):118–123.

Gilkison A, McAra-Couper J, Gunn J, et al. Midwifery practice arrangements which sustain caseloading Lead Maternity Carer midwives in New Zealand. *NZCOM J*. 2015;51:11–16. http://dx.doi.org/10.12784/nzcomjnl51.2015.2.11-16

Gilkison A, McAra-Couper J, Fielder A, et al. The core of the core: What is at the heart of hospital core midwifery practice in New Zealand? *NZCOM J*. 2017;53:30–37 http://dx.doi.org/10.12784/nzcomjnl53.2017.4.30-37

Guilliland K. Maintaining the links—a history of the formation of the NZCOM. *NZCOM J*. 1989;Sept:14–15.

Guilliland K, Pairman S. The Midwifery Partnership: a Model for Practice. Monograph Series: 95/1. Wellington: Department of Nursing and Midwifery, Victoria University of Wellington; 1995.

Guilliland K, Pairman S. *The Midwifery Partnership: A Model for Practice*. 2nd ed. Christchurch: New Zealand College of Midwives; 2010a.

Guilliland K, Pairman S. *Women's Business: The Story of the New Zealand College of Midwives 1986–2010*. Christchurch: New Zealand: NZCOM; 2010b.

Hall M, Rata A, Adds P. He Manu Hou: the transition of Māori students into Māori studies. *Int Indigenous Policy J*. 2013;4(4):1–19.

Halldorsdottir S, Karlsdottir S. The primacy of the good midwife in midwifery services: an evolving theory of professionalism in midwifery. *Scand J Caring Sci*. 2011;25(4):806–817.

Hatem M, Sandall J, Devane D, et al. Midwife-led versus other models of care for childbearing women. *Cochrane Database Syst Rev*. 2008;(4):CD004667, doi:10.1002/14651858.CD004667.pub2.

Health and Disability Commissioner (HDC). *The HDC Code of Health and Disability Services Consumers' Rights Regulation*. 1996. Online: http://www.hdc.org.nz/the-act—code/the-code-of-rights.

Heider J. *The Tao of Leadership: Lao Tsu's Tao Te Ching Adapted for a New Age*. Georgia, USA: Humanics New Age; 1997.

Hewitt, L, Dadich A, Hartz D, et al. management and sustainability of midwfiry group practice: Thematic and lexical analyses of midwife interviews. *Women Birth*. 2021;(in press). https://doi.org/10.1016/j.wombi.2021.05.002

Hoffkling A, Obedin-Maliver J, Sevelius J. From erasure to opportunity: a qualitative study of the experiences of transgender men around pregnancy and recommendations for providers. *BMC Pregnancy Childbirth*. 2017;17(2), 1–14.

Holten L, de Miranda E. Women's motivations for having unassisted childbirth or high-risk homebirth: An exploration of the literature on 'birthing outside the system'. *Midwifery*. 2016;38:55–62. http://dx.doi.org/10.1016/j.midw.2016.03.010

Homer C, Brodie P, Leap N, eds. *Midwifery Continuity of Care: A Practical Guide*. Chatswood, NSW: Elsevier; 2008.

Hunter B. The importance of reciprocity in relationships between community-based midwives and mothers. *Midwifery*. 2006;22:308–322.

Hunter M, Crowther S, McAra-Couper J, et al. Generosity of spirit sustains caseloading Lead Maternity Carer midwives in New Zealand. *NZCOM J*. 2016;52:50–55. http://dx.doi.org/10.12784/nzcomjnl52.2016.8.50-55

International Confederation of Midwives (ICM). *Code of Ethics for Midwives*; n.d. Online: http://internationalmidwives.org/assets/uploads/documents/CoreDocuments/CD2008_001%20V2014%20ENG%20International%20Code%20of%20Ethics%20for%20Midwives.pdf.

International Confederation of Midwives. (2017). *Position Statement: Human Rights of Lesbian, Gay, Bisexual, Transgender and Intersex (LGBTI) People*. https://www.internationalmidwives.org/assets/files/statement-files/2018/04/eng-lgtbi.pdf

James L. Nurturing the next generation: midwives' experiences when working with third year midwifery students in New Zealand. *NZCOM J*. 2012;47:14–17.

Janssen P, Saxell L, Page LA, et al. Outcomes of planned home birth with registered midwife versus planned hospital birth with midwife or physician. *CMAJ*. 2009;181(6–7):377–383.

Kaufmann T. Public health: the next step in woman-centred care. *RCM Midwives J*. 2000;3(1):26–28.

Kaufmann T. Midwifery and public health. *MIDIRS Midwifery Digest*. 2002;12(S1):S23–S26.

Kelly J, West R, Gamble J, et al. 'She knows how we feel': Australian Aboriginal and Torres Strait Islander childbearing women's experience of Continuity of Care with an Australian Aboriginal and Torres Strait Islander midwifery student. *Women Birth*. 2014;27(3):157–162.

Kennedy HP, Rousseau A, Kane Low LK. An exploratory metasynthesis of midwifery practice in the United States. *Midwifery*. 2003;19(3):203–214.

Kenney CM. Midwives, women and their families: a Māori gaze. *AlterNative (Nga Pae o te Maramatanga)*. 2011;7(2):123–137.

Kerkin B, Lennox S, Patterson J. Making midwifery work visible: the multiple purposes of documentation. *Women Birth*. 2017;(17):doi:10.1016/j.wombi.2017.09.012. [Epub ahead of print]; pii:S1871–5192, 30123–3.

Kildea S, Gao Y, Hickey S, et al. Effect of Birthing on Country service redesign on maternal and neonatal health outcomes for First Nations Australians: a prospective, non-randomised, interventional trial. *Lancet Glob Health*. 2021;9:e51–59. https://doi.org/10.1016/S2214-109X(21)00061-9

Kirkham M, ed. *The Midwife–Mother Relationship*. London: Macmillan; 2000a.

Kirkham M. How can we relate? In: Kirkham M, eds. The *Midwife–Mother Relationship*. London: Macmillan; 2000b:227–254.

Kirkham M. *The Midwife–Mother Relationship*. 2nd ed. London: Macmillan; 2010.

Kirkham M, Stapleton H. Midwives' support needs as childbirth changes. *J Adv Nurs*. 2000;32(2):465–472.

Kruske S, Kildea S, Barclay L. Cultural safety and maternity care of Aboriginal and Torres Strait Islander Australians. *Women Birth*. 2006;19(3):73–77.

Leap N. Journey to midwifery through feminism: a personal account. In: Stewart M, eds. *Pregnancy, Birth and Maternity Care: Feminist Perspectives*. London: Books for Midwives; 2004:185–200.

Leap N. The less we do, the more we give. In: Kirkham M, eds. *The Midwife–Mother Relationship*. 2nd ed. London: Macmillan; 2010:1–18.

Leap N, Edwards N. The politics of involving women in decision making. In: Page L, Campbell R, eds. *The New Midwifery: Science and Sensitivity in Practice*. 2nd ed. London: Elsevier; 2006:97–124.

Leap N, Pairman S. Working in partnership. In: Pairman S, Tracy SK, Thorogood C, et al, eds. *Midwifery: Preparation for Practice*. 2nd ed. Chatswood. NSW: Elsevier; 2010:337–350.

Leap N, Sandall J, Buckland S, et al. Journey to confidence: women's experiences of pain in labour and relational continuity of care. *J Midwifery Womens Health*. 2010;55(3):234–242.

McAra-Couper J. Right relationship and cultural safety. Unpublished paper. Auckland University of technology. 2005

McAra-Couper J, Gilkison A, Gunn J, et al. Sustainable Lead Maternity Care (LMC) midwifery practice: what sustains LMC midwives in practice in New Zealand; 2012. Conference Proceedings, New Zealand College of Midwives 12th Biennial National Conference, Wellington 24–26 August.

McCourt C, Stevens T, Sandall J, et al. Working with women: developing continuity of care in practice. In: Page L, McCandlish R, eds. *The New Midwifery: Science and Sensitivity in Midwifery*. 2nd ed. Churchill Livingstone, Elsevier; 2006:141–165.

McLachlan HL, Forster DA, Davey MA, et al. Effects of continuity of care by a primary midwife (caseload midwifery) on caesarean section rates in women of low obstetric risk: the COSMOS randomised controlled trial. *BJOG*. 2012;119(12):1483–1492.

McLardy E. *On-Call 24/7 Midwives Negotiating Home and Work Boundaries* (Master's thesis). Victoria: University of Wellington; 2003.

Maternity Choices Australia. n.d. Online http://www.maternity-choices.org.au/about-us.html.

Matthias MS. Problematic integration in pregnancy and childbirth: contrasting approaches to uncertainty and desire in obstetric and midwifery care. *Health Commun*. 2009;24(1):60–70.

Menage D. Part 2: A model for evidence-based decision-making in midwifery care. *Br J Mid*. 2016;24(2):137–143.

Midwifery Council of New Zealand (MCNZ). *Standards for Approval and Accreditation of Pre-Registration Midwifery Education Programmes*. Wellington: MCNZ; 2007.

Midwifery Council of New Zealand (MCNZ). *Code of Conduct*. 2010. Online: https://www.midwiferycouncil.health.nz/sites/default/files/documents/midwifery%20code%20of%20conduct%20feb%202011.pdf.

Midwifery Council of New Zealand (MCNZ). *Statement of Cultural Competence for Midwives*. Wellington: MCNZ; 2012.

Midwifery Council of New Zealand (MCNZ). *Midwifery Workforce Survey*. Wellington: MCNZ; 2020. Online: https://www.midwiferycouncil.health.nz/sites/default/files/site-downloads/Workforce%20Survey%202020.pdf.

Midwives Alliance of North America (MANA). *MANA Core Competencies for Basic Midwifery Practice*. Bristol, VA: MANA; 1991.

Milne T, Creedy DK, West R. Integrated systematic review on educational strategies that promote academic success and resilience in undergraduate indigenous students. *Nurs Educ Today*. 2015;36:387–394.

Milne T, Creedy DK, West R. Development of the awareness of cultural safety scale: a pilot study with midwifery and nursing academics. *Nurs Educ Today*. 2016;44:20–25.

Ministry of Health (MOH). *Notice Pursuant to Section 88 of the New Zealand Public Health and Disability Act 2000*. Wellington: Ministry of Health; 2009. Online: http://www.health.govt.nz/publication/section-88-primary-maternity-services-notice-2007.

Ministry of Health (MOH). *Guidelines for Consultation With Obstetric and Related Medical Services (Referral Guidelines)*. Wellington: Ministry of Health; 2012. Online: http://www.health.govt.nz/publication/guidelines-consultation-obstetric-and-related-medical-services-referral-guidelines.

Ministry of Health (MOH). *Maternity Consumer Survey 2014*. Wellington: Ministry of Health; 2015a. Online: http://www.health.govt.nz/publication/maternity-consumer-survey-2014.

Ministry of Health (MOH). *Maternity Report Webtool*. Wellington: Ministry of Health; n.d. Online: https://minhealthnz.shinyapps.io/Maternity_report_webtool/

Ministry of Health (MOH). *Te ara ō Hine – Tapu ora*. 2021. Online: https://www.health.govt.nz/our-work/life-stages/maternity-services/midwifery.

Moseson H, Zazanis N, Goldberg E, et al. The imperative for transgender and gender nonbinary inclusion: beyond women's health. *Obstet Gynecol*. 2020;135(5), 1059

National Health and Medical Research Council. *National Guidance on Collaborative Maternity Care*. Canberra: NHMRC; 2010. Online: http://www.nhmrc.gov.au/_files_nhmrc/publications/attachments/CP124.pdf.

New Zealand College of Midwives (NZCOM). *Midwives Handbook for Practice*. Christchurch: NZCOM; 2015.

New Zealand College of Midwives (NZCOM). *Consensus Statement: Informed Consent and Decision Making.* Christchurch: NZCOM; 2016. Online: https://www.midwife.org.nz/quality-practice/practice-guidance/nzcom-consensus-statements/.

New Zealand Government. *Health Practitioners Competence Assurance Act.* 2003. Online: http://www.legislation.govt.nz/act/public/2003/0048/latest/DLM203312.html.

Nicholls L, Skirton H. Webb C. Establishing perceptions of a good midwife: A Delphi study. *Br J Midwifery.* 2011;19(4): 230–236.

Nursing and Midwifery Board of Australia (NMBA). Midwifery Competency Standards; 2006. Online: http://www.nursingmidwiferyboard.gov.au/Codes-Guidelines-Statements/Professional-standards.aspx.

Nursing and Midwifery Board of Australia (NMBA). *Professional Boundaries for Midwives.* 2010. Online: http://www.nursingmidwiferyboard.gov.au/Codes-Guidelines-Statements/Professional-standards.aspx.

Nursing and Midwifery Board of Australia (NMBA). *Code of Conduct for Midwives.* 2018. Online: http://www.nursingmidwiferyboard.gov.au/Codes-Guidelines-Statements/Professional-standards.aspx.

Nursing Council of New Zealand (NCNZ). *Guidelines for the Cultural Safety Component in Nursing and Midwifery Education.* Wellington: NCNZ; 1992.

Nursing Council of New Zealand (NCNZ). *Guidelines for Cultural Safety, the Treaty of Waitangi, and Māori Health in Nursing and Midwifery Education and Practice.* Wellington: NCNZ; 2002.

O'Connor T. 'A powerful and disruptive position'—a cultural safety pioneer reflects. *Kai Tiaki Nurs N Z.* 2012;18(4):16–17.

Oliver R, Rochecouste J, Anderson R, et al. Understanding Australian Aboriginal tertiary student needs. *Int J High Educ.* 2013; 2(4):52–64.

Page LA, Cooke P, Percival P. Providing one-to-one care and enjoying it. In: Page LA, Campbell R, eds. *The New Midwifery: Science and Sensitivity in Practice.* 2nd ed. Edinburgh: Elsevier; 2006:123–140.

Page M, Mander R. Intrapartum uncertainty: A feature of normal birth, as experienced by midwives in Scotland. *Midwifery.* 2014;30:28–35. http://dx.doi.org/10.1016/j.midw.2013.01.012

Pairman S. *The Midwifery Partnership: An Exploration of the Midwife/Woman Relationship* (Master's thesis). Wellington: Victoria University of Wellington; 1998.

Pairman, S. (1999). Partnership revisited: Toward midwifery theory. *J N Z Coll Midwives, 21,* 6–1

Pairman S. Woman-centred midwifery: partnerships or professional friendships? In: Kirkham M, eds. *The Midwife–Mother Relationship.* London: Macmillan; 2000a:207–226.

Pairman S. Revitalising partnership; 2000b. Panel presentation, New Zealand College of Midwives Sixth National Conference, Cambridge, September (unpublished).

Pairman S. *Workforce to Profession; An Exploration of New Zealand Midwifery's Professionalisation Strategies From1986 to 2005* (Doctoral thesis). Sydney: University of Technology; 2005.

Pairman S. Midwifery partnership: working 'with' women. In: Page LA, Campbell R, eds. *The New Midwifery: Science and Sensitivity in Practice.* 2nd ed. Edinburgh: Elsevier; 2006:73–96.

Pairman S, McAra-Couper J. Theoretical frameworks for midwifery practice. In: Pairman S, Pincombe J, Thorogood C, et al, eds. *Midwifery Preparation for Practice.* 3rd ed. Sydney: Elsevier; 2015:383–411.

Papps E. Cultural safety: daring to be different. In: Wepa D, eds. *Cultural Safety in Aotearoa New Zealand.* Auckland: Pearson Education; 2005:20–28.

Patterson J, Newman E, Baddock S, et al. Strategies for improving the experiences of Māori students in a blended Bachelor of Midwifery programme. *NZCOM J.* 2017;53:45–52.

Perinatal and Maternal Mortality Review (PMMRC). *Tenth Annual Report of the Perinatal and Maternal Mortality Review Committee. Reporting Mortality 2014.* Wellington: Health Quality and Safety Commission; 2016. Online: https://www.hqsc.govt.nz/assets/PMMRC/Publications/tenth-annual-report-FINAL-NS-Jun-2016.pdf.

Perinatal and Maternal Mortality Review Committee (PMMRC). *Fourteenth Annual report of the Perinatal and Maternal Mortality Review Committee ☐ Te Pūrongo ā-Tau tekau mā Whā o te Komiti Arotake Mate Pēpi, Mate Whaea Hoki.* 2021. Online: https://www.hqsc.govt.nz/our-programmes/mrc/pmmrc/publications-and-resources/publication/4210/

Phiri J, Dietsch E, Bonner A. Cultural safety and its importance for Australian midwifery practice. *Collegian.* 2010;17(3):105–111.

Powell Kennedy H. The essence of nurse-midwifery care: the woman's story. *J Nurse Midwifery.* 1995;40(5):410–417.

Powell Kennedy H. The midwife as an 'instrument' of care. *Am J Public Health.* 2002;92(11):1759–1760.

Powell Kennedy H. The landscape of caring for women: a narrative study of midwifery practice. *J Midwifery Womens Health.* 2004;49(91):4–19.

Priday A. *A Successful Lead Maternity Care Practice in Counties Manukau. Ministry of Health Report.* Wellington, NZ: Ministry of Health; 2011.

Queensland Government. *Delivering Continuity of Care to Queensland Women an Implementation Guide.* Brisbane: Queensland Government; 2012.

Quigley M. Risk and choice in childbirth: Problems of evidence and ethics? *BMJ.* 2014;40(12): 791. doi:10.1136/medethics-2014-102558

Ramos R. The vital signs of culture. *Med Marketing Media.* 2010; 45(12):58(1). Online: http://www.mmm-online.com/features/the-vital-signs-of-culture/article/192273/.

Ramsden I. *Kawa Whakaruruhau: Cultural Safety in Nursing Education in Aotearoa.* Wellington, NZ: Nursing Council of NZ; 1990.

Ramsden I. *Kawa Whakaruruhau: Guidelines for Nursing and Midwifery Education.* Wellington, NZ: Nursing Council of NZ; 1992.

Ramsden I. Cultural safety in nursing education in Aotearoa (New Zealand). *Nurs Prax N Z.* 1993;8(3):4–10.

Ramsden I. Cultural safety/Kawa whakaruruhau ten years on: a personal overview. *Nurs Prax N Z.* 2000;15(1):4–12.

Ramsden I. *Cultural Safety and Nursing Education in Aotearoa and Te Waipounamu* (Doctoral thesis). Wellington: Victoria University of Wellington; 2002.

Reibel T, Walker R. Antenatal services for Aboriginal women: the relevance of cultural competence. *Qual Prim Care.* 2010;18: 65–74.

Richardson F. What is it Like to Teach Cultural Safety in a New Zealand Nursing Education Programme? (Master's thesis). Palmerston North: Massey University; 2000.

Rigby W, Duffy E, Manners J, et al. Closing the gap: cultural safety in indigenous health education. *Contemp Nurs.* 2011;37(1): 21–30.

Ross-Davie M, Cheyne H. Intrapartum support: what do women want? A literature review. *Evid Based Midwifery.* 2014;12(2): 52–58.

Sandall J. Midwives' burnout and continuity of care. *Br J Midwifery.* 1997;5(1997):106–111.

Sandall J. Promoting normal birth: weighing the evidence. In: Downe S, eds. *Normal Childbirth: Evidence and Debate.* London: Churchill Livingstone; 2004:161–171.

Sandall J, Page L, Homer C, et al. Midwifery continuity of care: What is the evidence? In: Homer C, Brodie P, Leap N, eds. *Midwifery Continuity of Care: A Practical Guide.* Sydney: Churchill Livingstone; 2006:25–43.

Sandall J, Soltani H, Gates S, et al. Midwife-led versus other models of care for childbearing women. *Cochrane Database Syst Rev.* 2016;(4):CD004667, doi:10.1002/14651858. CD004667.pub.5.

Scammell M, Alaszewski A. Fateful moments and categorization of risk: midwifery practice and the ever-narrowing window of normality during childbirth. *Health Risk Soc.* 2012;14(2):207–221.

Scherman S, Smith J, Davidson M. The first year of a midwifery-led model of care in Far North Queensland. *Med J Aust.* 2008;188(2):85–88.

Sheen K, Slade P. The efficacy of 'debriefing' after childbirth: is there a case for targeted intervention? *J Repr Infant Psychol.* 2015;33(3):308–320.

Smythe E. 'Being Safe' in Childbirth. *A Hermeneutic Interpretation of the Narratives of Women and Practitioners* (Doctoral thesis). Palmerston North: Massey University; 1998.

Snows S. 'Mutual newness'; mothers' experiences of student midwives. *Br J Midwifery.* 2010;18(1):38–41.

Spence D. The evolving meaning of 'culture' in New Zealand nursing. *Nurs Praxis N Z.* 2001;17(3):51–61.

Spence D. Prejudice, paradox and possibility: the experience of nursing people from cultures other than one's own. In: Kavanagh K, Knowlden V, eds. *Many Voices, Toward Caring Culture in Healthcare and Healing.* Wisconsin: University of Wisconsin Press; 2004:140–180.

Spence DG. *Prejudice, Paradox and Possibility: Nursing People From Cultures Other Than One's Own* (Doctoral thesis). Palmerston North: Massey University; 1999.

Stevens G, Thompson R, Kruske S, et al. What are pregnant women told about models of maternity care in Australia? A retrospective study of women's reports. *Pat Ed Counsel.* 2014; 97(1):114–121.

Strid J. Maternity in revolt. *Broadsheet.* 1987;153:14–17.

Tracy SK, Hartz DL, Tracy MB, et al. Caseload midwifery care versus standard maternity care for women of any risk: M@NGO, a randomised controlled trial. *Lancet.* 2013;382:1723–1732.

Turnbull D, Baghurst P, Collins C, et al. An evaluation of midwifery group practice. Part I: Clinical effectiveness. *Women Birth.* 2009;22(1).

Vernon R, Papps E. Cultural safety and continuing competence. In: Wepa D, eds. *Cultural Safety in Aotearoa New Zealand.* 2nd ed. 2015:51–62.

Wakelin K, Skinner J. Staying or leaving: a telephone survey of midwives, exploring the sustainability of practice as Lead Maternity Carers in one urban region of New Zealand. *NZCOM J.* 2007;37:10–14.

Walker R. *Nga Tau Tohetohe, Years Of Anger.* Auckland: Penguin; 1987.

Walsh D. An ethnographic study of women's experiences of partnership caseload midwifery practice: the professional as friend. *Midwifery.* 1999;15:165–176.

Wax JR, Pinette MG, Cartin A, et al. Maternal and newborn morbidity by birth facility among selected United States 2006 low-risk births. *Am J Obstet Gynaecol.* 2010;202(2):152.e151–152. e155.

Wepa D, ed. *Cultural Safety in Aotearoa New Zealand.* 2nd ed. Cambridge, UK: Cambridge University Press; 2015.

West R, Usher K, Foster K, et al. Academic staff perceptions of factors underlying program completion by Australian Indigenous nursing students. *Qual Rep.* 2014;19(24):1–19.

Wilkes E, Gamble J, Adam G, et al. Reforming maternity services in Australia: outcomes of a private practice midwifery service. *Midwifery.* 2015;31(10):935–940.

Wilkins R. Poor relations: the paucity of the professional paradigm. In: Kirkham M, eds. *The Midwife–Mother Relationship.* London: Macmillan; 2000:28–54.

Young C. *The Experience of Burnout in Case Loading Midwives: An Interpretive Phenomenological Study* (Doctoral thesis). Auckland, New Zealand: Auckland University of Technology; 2011.

Further reading

Downe S, Simpson L, Trafford K. Expert intrapartum maternity care: a meta-synthesis. *J Adv Nurs.* 2007;57(2):127–140.

Hodnett ED, Gates S, Hofmeyr GJ, et al. Continuous support for women during childbirth. *Cochrane Database Syst Rev.* 2007;(3):CD003766, doi:10.1002/14651858.CD003766.pub2.

Kennedy HP, Shannon MT, Chuahorm U, et al. The landscape of caring for women: a narrative study of midwifery practice. *J Midwifery Womens Health.* 2004;49(1):14–23.

Sandall J. Promoting normal birth: weighing the evidence. In: Downe S, eds. *Normal Childbirth: Evidence and Debate.* Edinburgh: Elsevier; 2004:161–171.

Sandall J, Page LA, Homer CSE, et al. Midwifery continuity of care: what is the evidence? In: Homer C, Brodie P, Leap N, eds. *Midwifery Continuity of Care: A Practical Guide.* Chatswood, NSW: Elsevier; 2008:25–46.

Wepa D, ed. *Cultural Safety in Aotearoa New Zealand.* 2nd ed. Cambridge, UK: Cambridge University Press; 2015.

World Health Organization (Technical Working Group). Postpartum care of the mother and newborn: a practical guide. *Birth.* 1999;26(4):255–258.

CHAPTER 18

Working in collaboration

Suzanne Miller and Hannah G Dahlen

LEARNING OUTCOMES

Learning outcomes for this chapter are:

1. To describe the frameworks that relate to collaborative practice within which midwives practise
2. To discuss the nature of collaboration, consultation and referral
3. To articulate the professional requirements relating to collaboration, consultation and referral.

CHAPTER OVERVIEW

Collaborative practice is integral to the safety of midwifery practice. Midwives, as primary caregivers, need to negotiate evidence-based decisions with individual women in their care when the woman's circumstances suggest a need for referral or consultation with another caregiver during pregnancy, labour, birth, or the postnatal period. This chapter outlines the means of collaboration between midwives, the women they care for, and the other healthcare professionals with whom they may need to collaborate.

KEY TERMS

collaboration
consultation

referral
referral guidelines

transfer

INTRODUCTION

Engagement in collaborative effort is the midwife's *raison d'être*. 'Working together' is the thread that runs through every aspect of midwifery practice. The most fundamental understandings of the midwifery partnership model involve women and midwives working together to achieve positive experiences for all (see Ch. 17). Collaboration between women and midwives has resulted in widespread political change over the last 30 years, and has brought about the establishment of a truly women-centred maternity service in Aotearoa New Zealand and a movement towards this in Australia (see Ch. 1). At every level, from the individual woman and midwife to the professional and regulatory bodies, it is women and midwives working collaboratively who determine the vision and direction for the future of maternity services (Department of Health (DOH), 1993; Maternity Coalition, n.d.; New Zealand College of Midwives (NZCOM), 2015).

Midwifery care is centred on promoting and protecting birth as a normal physiological process. For many birthing women, the totality of their care falls within the scope of midwifery practice. There are occasions, however, when the complexity of a woman's experience may require that she also have some input from other midwifery colleagues or other healthcare professionals. Maternity care is dynamic, there can be expected or sudden complexities which require input from professionals from different disciplines who need to work together to ensure that the woman and her baby are offered appropriate, evidence-based care. Midwives must be skilled at assessing whether referral for **consultation** or **transfer** of clinical responsibility is necessary. To assist midwives with their decision making, in both New Zealand and Australia referral guidelines have been developed that outline a range of circumstances where referral may be warranted.

Collaborative practice is integral to the safety of midwifery practice and enshrined in midwifery policy. The New Zealand College of Midwives Code of Ethics states that: 'Midwives have a professional responsibility to refer to others when they have reached the limit of their expertise' (NZCOM, 2015, p. 13). Similarly, the Midwifery Scope of Practice, which legally defines midwifery in New Zealand, requires that: 'When women require referral, midwives provide midwifery care in collaboration with other health professionals' (Midwifery Council of New Zealand (MCNZ), 2004). In Australia, the National Midwifery Guidelines for Consultation and Referral (2021) aims to provide individual midwives with an evidence-informed national framework for consultation and referral of care between midwives, medical practitioners and other healthcare providers with the woman receiving care (Australian College of Midwives (ACM), 2021). These guidelines have now been endorsed by the Royal Australian and New Zealand College of Obstetricians and Gynaecologists (RANZCOG).

The Competencies for Entry to the Register of Midwives provide further clarification of what generally and specifically constitutes midwifery practice, in terms of the profession's and the public's expectations of woman-centred care. The Scope of Practice provides the broad boundaries of midwifery practice, whereas Competencies provide the detail of how midwives are expected to practise and what they are expected to be capable of doing; there is a set of minimum competencies required of all midwives who register in New Zealand and Australia (MCNZ, 2004, 2007; Nursing and Midwives Board of Australia (NMBA), 2018). It is expected that all midwives will demonstrate that they are able to meet the competencies relevant to the position they hold (Homer et al., 2005, p. 5). Specific competencies relating to **collaboration** are reproduced in Box 18.1.

Systems that enable midwives to work collaboratively are valued. The components of supportive systems include effective communication, consultation and referral between professionals. A collaborative relationship with medical colleagues is an important aspect of midwifery practice. Collaboration also includes working with others when the care of women falls outside the midwives' scope of practice. For example, the care of women with mental health conditions is seen as one area where collaboration is particularly needed (Homer et al., 2005).

THE NATURE OF COLLABORATION

Successful collaborative practice requires several conditions. First, and most importantly, the woman must remain at the centre of the process. In order that she may participate in informed decision making, information must be shared in a context where the woman's values and philosophical beliefs are respected and upheld. Midwives can assist women to examine critically the evidence presented to them, and help them make sense of those aspects that appear conflicting or inconclusive. When the woman is central to the collaborative process, her ability to tease out the important elements—to her—of both midwifery and obstetric (or other) practice will mean that she can negotiate a plan of care that will best meet her needs.

Theory continues to develop about the 'preconditions' for successful collaborative practice. Tracing the development of literature around collaboration, it can be seen that a number of scholars have examined the features most closely associated with successful collaboration, and the commonest thread running through the literature is that effective communication is a crucial prerequisite for working together. This requires that those involved in the collaborative effort are able to assert their point of view constructively, and at the same time are open to listening to the views of others.

Dorne's seminal work offered some useful insights into what she described as the Ten Major Tenets of Collaboration (Dorne, 2002, p. 17). They are as follows:

- provision of a non-competitive/non-hierarchical environment
- partnership between parties based on shared power and authority

Box 18.1 Competencies for Entry to the Register of Midwives, relating to collaboration

New Zealand competency 2

The midwife applies comprehensive theoretical and scientific knowledge with the affective and technical skills needed to provide effective and safe midwifery care.

Selected performance criteria:

The midwife:

2.3. assesses the health and wellbeing of the woman/wahine and her baby/tamaiti throughout pregnancy, recognising any condition which necessitates consultation with or referral to another midwife, medical practitioner or other health professional;

2.6. identifies factors in the woman/wahine or her baby/tamaiti during labour and birth which indicate the necessity for consultation with, or referral to, another midwife or a specialist medical practitioner;

2.7. provides and is responsible for midwifery care when a woman's/wahine pregnancy, labour, birth or postnatal care necessitates clinical management by a medical practitioner;

2.12. assesses the health and well-being of the woman/wahine and baby/tamaiti throughout the postnatal period and identifies factors which indicate the necessity for consultation with or referral to another midwife, medical practitioner, or other health practitioner;

2.18. collaborates and co-operates with other health professionals, community groups and agencies when necessary.

(Sources: NMBA, 2018; NZCOM, 2015)

Australian standard 2

Engages in professional relationships and respectful partnerships.

The midwife establishes and maintains professional relationships with the woman by engaging purposefully in kind, compassionate and respectful partnerships. The midwife will also engage in professional relationships with other health practitioners, colleagues and/or members of the public. These relationships are conducted within a context of collaboration, mutual trust, respect and cultural safety.

The midwife:

1.1 supports the choices of the woman, with respect for families and communities in relation to maternity care

1.2 partners with women to strengthen women's capabilities and confidence to care for themselves and their families

1.3 practises ethically, with respect for dignity, privacy, confidentiality, equity and justice

1.4 practises without the discrimination that may be associated with race, age, disability, sexuality, gender identity, relationship status, power relations and/or social disadvantage

1.5 practises cultural safety that is holistic, free of bias and exposes racism

1.6 practises in a way that respects that family and community underpin the health of Aboriginal and/or Torres Strait Islander Peoples

1.7 develops, maintains and concludes professional relationships in a way that differentiates the boundaries between professional and personal relationships, and

1.8 participates in and/or leads collaborative practice.

- the ability to jointly define work processes, relationships, mutual objectives and goals
- joint responsibility / accountability for decision making
- secure self-identity enabling clearly defined roles, with an emphasis on the function of each party
- power based on knowledge / expertise as opposed to power based on role and role function
- mutual trust, respect, cooperation and commitment
- time and space for open and effective communication and conflict resolution
- recognition / valuing of how differing perspectives inform decision making
- interdependence of work with dependent / independent functions within the collaborative practice.

In 2010, the National Health and Medical Research Council in Australia produced the National Guidance on

Collaborative Maternity Care (National Health and Medical Research Council (NHMRC), 2010). The purpose of this document was to provide a resource to support collaborative maternity care in Australia. It was part of the significant maternity reforms in 2010 and the definition given in this document was:

In maternity care, collaboration is a dynamic process of facilitating communication, trust and pathways that enable health professionals to provide safe, woman-centred care. Collaborative maternity care enables women to be active participants in their care. Collaboration includes clearly defined roles and responsibilities for everyone involved in the woman's care, especially for the person the woman sees as her maternity care coordinator.

(NHMRC, 2010, p. 1)

This document identifies the principles and key elements of maternity collaboration including: (NHMRC, 2010, p. 13):

- woman-centred care and communication
- communication among professionals
- awareness of disciplines and autonomy
- responsibility and accountability
- cooperation and coordination
- mutual trust and respect
- policy, procedures and protocols
- interprofessional learning
- organisational support systems.

Scholarship about collaboration has evolved to include theories around boundary work, communities of practice and emotional intelligence. Collaboration can be seen as being 'about what happens when effective working takes place at boundary junctions between distinctly different groups' (Downe & Finlayson, 2011, p. 157). Acknowledging that our understanding about collaboration has been partly shaped by exploring why collaboration can be difficult to achieve, Downe and Finlayson propose that using salutogenetic thinking (i.e. what works well) can be equally instructive at improving our understanding about how to achieve good collaborative practice. Schmied et al., (2010) identified that professional cultures can act as barriers to successful collaborative effort, as each culture has its respective values, worldviews, behaviours and attitudes which may not be mutually understood or respected. Scott (2005, cited in Schmied et al., 2010) argued that conflict should be a 'normal and expected part of collaboration', best managed by 'acknowledging it, normalizing it and identifying its source' (p. 3522), suggesting that the tensions inherent in making professional boundaries visible can thus be addressed.

In her qualitative study focused on exploring communication between community-based midwives (Lead Maternity Care) and obstetricians, Cassie (2019) interviewed eight midwives, three obstetricians and two obstetric registrars. She found mostly positive inter-professional interactions. Themes that emerged were the need to negotiate the differing professional philosophies, the need to clarify boundaries that were sometimes blurred to ensure clear lines of responsibility and the importance of the three-way conversation. The three-way conversation was helpful in negotiating the professional philosophical differences and clarifying blurred boundaries and supported optimal communication.

A significant challenge for midwives is that of 'working a "birth is normal" paradigm in an increasingly "birth is risky" social and political context' (Skinner, 2011, p. 17). Skinner (2011) argues that the referral practices of midwives are an expression of their risk management, which may be unique to the New Zealand context. In her mixed-methods study, Skinner (2011) examined the referral practices of 311 Lead Maternity Care (LMC) midwives who had provided care for 4271 women. She found that 35% of the women had been referred for obstetric consultation at some point in the childbearing continuum,

with 43% of *those* women having clinical responsibility for their care transferred, but overall 96% of the women continued to receive some of their midwifery care from their LMC despite their changed risk status and transfer of clinical responsibility (Skinner, 2011). This finding highlights the centrality of the woman to the midwife's practice, alongside her deep commitment to protecting those aspects of the woman's experience that remain normal in the presence of complexity. It presents a tension between research which concludes that having clear role boundaries around care provision is crucial to successful collaboration (Hall, 2005; Rushmer, 2004)—which in our context suggests that midwives should work only with 'low-risk' women, leaving 'high-risk' women to obstetrics—and that which focuses on the partnership relationship and continuity of care as pivotal to improving outcomes. The midwives in Skinner's study clearly saw their role as being 'with women' regardless of their risk profile, placing high value on continuity of care, and negotiating relationships with other care providers while keeping the woman's needs uppermost (Skinner, 2011). It must be remembered also that midwives are accountable for their midwifery actions, regardless of who accepts 'clinical responsibility'.

The concept of 'exnovation' has more recently been applied to our understanding of how successful collaboration occurs. Exnovation is a salutogenic approach which identifies and enhances already-existing competency in care practice by focusing on the 'invisible but necessary aspects of care work that promote quality' (van Helmond et al., 2015, p. 211). This approach recognises that different groups involved in maternity care may have different perspectives about what 'best practice' looks like; the scoping study by van Helmond et al., (2015) revealed 14 articles that explored good collaboration and communication between health professionals in maternity care. The authors concluded that there are explicit and implicit prerequisites of working together collaboratively. Explicit prerequisties for good collaboration included things linked to 'doing things together'— often enshrined in documents or topics for discussion such as the distribution of workload. Implicit prerequisites included ways of 'being together' emotionally rather than physically. Also noted was the important influence of the built environment on people's mood, emotional wellbeing and overall work experience (p. 218).

PARTNERING WOMEN WHEN COLLABORATION OCCURS

Midwives participating in a reflective midwifery partnership are in a position to have a positive impact on women's experiences in situations where **referral** is required. In addition to honouring the woman's own knowing about herself and her body, midwives can assist the woman to educate herself well, so that the consultation is not one in which the 'specialist' is the only 'expert'. Thus, a woman will ask the questions that will *meaningfully* aid her decision making, rather than following a predetermined protocol that may not reflect her values or beliefs. Midwives need to remain mindful of the fact that *within* midwifery there is an enormous resource and body of knowledge, and that sometimes it is to our colleagues that we should turn for discussion and advice. A study by one of the authors (SM) uncovered how collaboration between midwives can be protective of women's experiences in a labour context. This study explored labour and birth outcomes of first-time mothers in different birth settings. It revealed that when a woman's labour became complex and required additional input from the obstetric service, in situations where a second midwife was also involved in the woman's care she was more likely to achieve a spontaneous birth (68%) than when only an obstetrician was consulted (51%) (Miller, 2008).

Experienced midwives know well how judicious one needs to be about some indications for referral—the 'large-for-dates' baby, for example. Midwives can work to ensure that the experience of consultation will not negatively affect the woman's confidence in her ability to birth normally when the obstetrician has told her she has a high likelihood of needing a caesarean section. Midwives are obliged to discuss the recommendation for referral with the woman, and support her decision to consult or not, as the case may be. But they also need to balance the content of the obstetric consultation with midwifery knowledge about moulding, pelvic mapping, optimal baby positioning, working with labour pain, and mobility in labour to enhance the likelihood of the woman achieving a normal birth.

Sometimes the woman may request referral, or may self-refer, to healthcare professionals other than obstetricians/paediatricians/anaesthetists. This may involve referral to an acupuncturist, an osteopath, a homeopath or a naturopath to assist with the particular issue the woman faces. A respectful collaborative process can be achieved here also. Indeed, because of a greater appreciation for holism displayed by complementary therapists, many midwives find working alongside these practitioners a supportive and satisfying experience for all involved.

To conclude, it seems that communication, trust, mutual respect, power sharing, strategies for conflict resolution and accountability are all essential to good collaborative practice, and that firmly centring the woman in any process of decision making is the prime consideration for caregivers.

CRITICAL THINKING EXERCISE

Bella had gestational diabetes during her last pregnancy but was distressed by the way her pregnancy became medicalised and she felt pressured to have an induction of labour when she did not want one. She is pregnant again and has decided not to be tested, but to really watch her diet and do the occasional blood sugar test to check on herself. She also wants a home birth. How will you counsel her and support her choice while fulfilling your professional responsibilities?

COLLABORATION IN THE CONTEXT OF THE AUSTRALIAN MATERNITY REFORMS 2010

In Australia, following the introduction of the Health Legislation Amendment (Midwives and Nurse Practitioners) Bill 2009 on 24 June 2009, the Minister for Health Nicola Roxon proclaimed that midwives wishing to provide treatment under Medicare and prescribe certain medicines under the Pharmaceutical Benefits Scheme (PBS) would need to demonstrate that they met the eligibility requirements and that they had collaborative arrangements in place, including appropriate referral pathways with hospitals and doctors to ensure that women receive coordinated care and the appropriate expertise and treatment as the clinical need arose. The requirement for 'eligible midwives' to have a collaborative arrangement with an obstetrician (known as the *Determination*) was met with dismay by midwives across Australia, but eventually accepted with promises from the then Health Minister that if there was evidence that this led to medical veto over midwifery practice the legislation would be changed. Some years on, it is now clear that this requirement has not worked. While some states now have clinical-privileging arrangements allowing midwives access to hospitals, apart from Queensland there has been little uptake of this option. Midwives still find it hard to get obstetricians to collaborate if they are required to sign on the dotted line, so to speak. In September 2012, the Standing Council on Health (SCOH) agreed to vary the *Determination* on collaborative arrangements to enable agreements between midwives and hospitals and health services. This was signed into legislation in September 2013. Many midwives in Australia continue to lobby for formal 'clinical privileging', enabling them to engage with hospitals and benefit from the legislative changes.

Collaboration in healthcare occurs when experts from different disciplines work together in a combined effort to improve patients' needs (San Martín-Rodríguez et al., 2005; Saxell et al., 2009). Although the proposed maternity reforms intend to make interprofessional collaboration mandatory, it is usually by its very nature a negotiated process founded on all of the following key components: interprofessional willingness to collaborate, trust, mutual respect and good communication. Successful collaborative practice in midwifery is based on two broad categories of collaboration: interprofessional collaboration and patient-centred (or more specifically 'woman-centred') partnership. Both aspects are integral to the safety of midwifery practice.

Interprofessional collaboration occurs when two or more experts from different disciplines take joint ownership of decisions and collective responsibility for outcomes when working across professional and functional boundaries, for example within the hospital setting (Liedtka &

Whitten, 1998). A collaboration of healthcare professionals share responsibility for outcomes, see themselves playing a crucial role within a larger social system (healthcare service) and manage their relationships across organisational boundaries (Cohen & Bailey, 1997). Successful collaboration in healthcare teams can be attributed to several key elements, including interpersonal relationships within the team and favourable conditions within the organisation and the system within which collaboration takes place (San Martín-Rodríguez et al., 2005).

Despite the difficulties in keeping birth normal in large maternity units (Tracy et al., 2006), it is also quite clear that where there is a healthy collaborative culture in big maternity units continuity of midwifery care can bring extraordinary results in terms of safety and quality (Beasley et al., 2012; Homer et al., 2001; McLachlan et al., 2012). It also appears that, when working in continuity of care where collaboration is strong, midwives do not feel a sense of subordination or feel undervalued by their medical colleagues (Moore, 2009).

RESEARCH ACTIVITY

Complete a simple database search using keywords 'collaboration' AND 'maternity' AND 'interprofessional'. Have a brief look through the first 20 or so titles and journal names. Which profession is generating most of the research in this field? What does this tell us about the commitment to 'getting it right' for women? How visible *are* women in the studies about collaborative practice?

Few studies have investigated the influence of all these determinants of collaboration on interprofessional collaboration. However, an Australian randomised controlled trial of collaboration in the maternity services published by Homer et al., (2001) demonstrated that a community-based model of continuity of care provided by midwives and obstetricians improved maternal clinical outcomes, in particular a reduced caesarean section rate. Collaboration with medical colleagues in that study demonstrated how working together strengthened the ability of midwives to work to their full scope of practice, providing safe, high-quality care.

A study undertaken in Australia of the efficacy of a collaborative partnership between obstetric doctors and midwives providing Midwifery Group Practice (MGP) found that, of the 337 women booked with MGP, 50% were discussed at least once (Beasley et al., 2012). Of these, 35% were referred for consultation with an obstetrician. Women's clinical cases were most commonly discussed in these meetings, followed by educational discussions and anecdotes with equal verbal contributions from midwives and doctors. Plans for each case were recorded 97% of the time, and adhered to 90% of the time. A high level of consistency of care between similar cases (75% of the time) and with the ACM consultation and **referral guidelines** (85% of the time) was achieved. Professional satisfaction with this model of care rated highly for both groups. The authors concluded that interprofessional collaboration between midwifery and obstetric staff is attainable within this model of care and collaboration in the MGP model of care for women of all risk levels is effective and other maternity care providers should consider adopting this collaborative model.

Research published in 2003 and funded by the Australian Research Council and four state Departments of Health as industry partners found that in Australia one of the major barriers to collaborative practice is the competitive approach that exists both between professionals and between healthcare institutions (Barclay et al., 2003). Traditional structures for medical and nursing services have tended to concentrate and optimise the provision of care within their 'silos' from a provider perspective, rather than optimising the larger system from the patient's perspective.

In contrast, *women-centred (patient-centred) partnerships* support collaboration. In the midwifery model of care, women are at the centre of their pregnancy and birth care and from that point all decisions are made. In this way, collaboration plays a central role in coordinating care across the continuum of sites and services. In a woman-centred model of care healthcare resources are organised around the needs of women and their families rather than around the needs of service providers. In women-centred services each woman's values and philosophical beliefs are respected and upheld, thereby enabling each woman to participate in informed decision making and collaborate in her care. Midwives, doctors and other health professionals collaborate to ensure that each woman's maternity experience is seamless across all services that she requires.

REFLECTIVE THINKING EXERCISE

Following a primary postpartum haemorrhage of 1200 mL, Natalie has been offered a blood transfusion. She decides instead to take some organic iron tablets, which she took during pregnancy and which she feels her body tolerated really well. As her midwife LMC, how will you assess Natalie's ongoing wellbeing throughout the postnatal period?

PROFESSIONAL COLLABORATIONS

The midwifery profession in both New Zealand and Australia is involved in building relationships with the professional bodies of other healthcare disciplines. This is to ensure that those involved in the production of clinical guidelines for practice and in policy discussions are aware of the full scope of midwifery practice. This approach also ensures that the voice of women service users is heard at the highest levels, as their involvement is a requisite component of guideline development.

Recent examples in New Zealand include government-led initiatives resulting in national multidisciplinary guidelines relating to observation of neonates in the immediate postpartum period, management of postpartum haemorrhage, and screening for gestational diabetes mellitus (MOH, 2012, 2022c, 2014), and professional group-led guidelines such as the national induction of labour guideline (MOH, 2021) and prevention of early-onset group B *Streptococcus* (GBS) disease in neonates (GBS Working Group, 2014). The College (NZCOM) meets regularly with RANZCOG to discuss issues of mutual interest and they often agree to work collaboratively to progress issues of mutual concern.

REFLECTIVE THINKING EXERCISE

Jacinta comes into the birth unit in labour and has a positive swab for GBS, which she did not want to be screened for in the first place. She had had an unusual vaginal discharge during pregnancy and GBS was picked up when she had a swab for this. She tells you she had GBS in her first pregnancy and declined antibiotics and she does not want them this time either. It is your hospital's policy to give antibiotics in labour when women are GBS positive. How are you going to manage this and what are your ongoing responsibilities here?

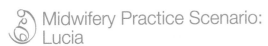

Midwifery Practice Scenario: Lucia

Lucia has approached you to provide midwifery care for her fifth pregnancy. She has a history of three spontaneous vaginal births, at term and with normal weight babies. Her fourth baby was born by caesarean section for breech presentation at 38 weeks. Lucia wishes to have a repeat elective caesarean section because her husband can have only limited time off owing to his new employment situation, and the ability to plan the birth date will be easier for their family.

What are your ethical, professional and legal responsibilities in this scenario? What frameworks for practice will assist you to negotiate care with Lucia? Write a referral letter to an obstetrician requesting a consultation to discuss Lucia's proposed birth plan. What information will you need to include in your letter?

THE NEW ZEALAND REFERRAL GUIDELINES

In New Zealand, the Guidelines for Consultation with Obstetric and Related Medical Services (Referral Guidelines) (MOH, 2022a) provide LMCs with clear guidance on referral and consultation procedures. They are used in conjunction with the Primary Maternity Services Notice 2021 (MOH, 2022a). This notice is pursuant to Section 88 of the New Zealand Public Health and Disability Act 2000 (MOH, 2000). The guidelines are well used and embedded in practice for LMC midwives; they provide guidance, support for appropriate management and optimal communication between the midwife, the specialist and the birthing person.

The Guidelines bring together the expertise of a working group of service users, midwives, obstetricians, paediatricians, anaesthetists and general practitioners who examine new clinical evidence and any relevant changes in policy or legislation that may affect the recommendations for practice in a referral context. These guidelines are reviewed at 5-yearly intervals.

The stated purpose of the Guidelines is an intention to:
1. improve maternity care safety and quality
2. improve the consistency of consultation, transfer and transport services
3. give confidence to women, their families and whānau, and other practitioners if a primary healthcare or specialist consultation, or a transfer of clinical responsibility, is required
4. promote and support coordination of care across providers.

Midwives also need to consider their responsibility to work with Te Tiriti principles when working with the woman and her whānau. They should have the capability to engage with Māori in ways that uphold Māori cultural identity and do not detract from it (MOH, 2022a). The Referral Guidelines (MOH, 2022b) define four categories of referral and consequent action. These categories are primary, consultation, transfer and emergency. Process maps have been provided to assist LMCs with their decision making around referral by showing critical steps that should be followed in each circumstance. Conditions and referral categories that might prompt a discussion about referral are listed in the document. There is a clear explication of the process an LMC can follow in the event that a woman declines any of the options offered to her, thus upholding the woman's right to informed consent and providing support to the LMC who may be left practising outside her scope of practice. Midwives are directed to *advise* the woman about recommended care, including the evidence supporting that recommendation, *explain* the LMC's potential need to discuss the case with another practitioner, ensuring the woman's right to privacy, *share* the outcomes of this discussion with the woman, and *document* these discussions and any decisions the woman has made clearly in the clinical record (MOH, 2022b, p. 18).

Student midwives are strongly encouraged to familiarise themselves with the Referral Guidelines.

THE PROCESS OF REFERRAL

In general, the booking interview is often the time when the woman will disclose a situation that may require referral. If this is because of something in her medical or maternity history, the midwife can discuss the recommendation for referral and, with the woman's informed consent, initiate the process immediately. For some conditions, the referral guidelines indicate the optimal timing for the referral to support decision making and care planning. Other indications for referral may arise later in the pregnancy—for example, the discovery of a twin pregnancy, or breech presentation that persists near term. Referral will occur in such instances as the particular issue arises. In some circumstance the referral condition may be identified as 'acute' and the guidelines may indicate the need for an immediate discussion and management plan.

CRITICAL THINKING EXERCISE

Jana discloses to you at her booking visit that she has epilepsy. She tells you that she has decided to discontinue her medication now that she is pregnant. How will you respond to this information?

If after discussion of the recommendation for referral the woman consents to being referred to a specialist, the midwife is responsible for undertaking the referral request. With the advent of integrated IT systems, there may be systems in place to support the midwife when referring. The referral form/letter should have sufficient information to enable the obstetrician to adequately assess the woman's situation. At the very least, it should contain:

- the woman's name, address, date of birth, National Health Index, gravidity/parity and contact details
- the reason that referral is sought, which may include the Referral Guidelines category code
- a brief statement outlining her medical and/or maternity history
- any relevant supporting documentation (e.g. blood test, customised growth chart or ultrasound reports)
- her midwife's name and contact details.

Whether or not the midwife accompanies the woman to the appointment is negotiated between the midwife and the woman. Skinner (2011) reported that in her study 40% of the antenatal 'first consultations' saw the midwife attending alongside the woman. She noted this was more likely to occur when the woman was seeing a member of a public hospital obstetric team, and least likely when the woman was seeing a private obstetrician. Some advantages of having the midwife present are that it can facilitate the process of 'three-way discussion' more easily, and some women find that the presence and support of the midwife can make the encounter less stressful. The midwife will be able to interpret the content of the discussion after the appointment if any issues need clarification. On the other hand, some women feel that the presence of the midwife might cause the obstetrician to withhold certain information, or to consider that the woman is incapable of understanding complex information or that she is needing her 'hand held' in some way.

The main outcome of the consultant review will be the formation of an ongoing plan of care that reflects the woman's informed choices regarding who will have clinical responsibility, who will provide her primary (midwifery) care if transfer occurs, and if not, then whether and when further consultation should occur. All these decisions should be clearly documented in the clinical record so that there is no confusion as to roles and responsibilities. Referral for consultation does not imply that the clinical responsibility for the woman's care will be assumed by the secondary service.

Box 18.2 summarises the process for immediate referral in the acute clinical situation.

Box 18.2   Referral in the acute clinical situation

There are times during childbirth when immediate referral for acute care is necessary. Referral may be through the sharing of information by telephone or face to face. At these times it is important to communicate the right information clearly and concisely. This involves the following principles:

Identify who you are—and who they are.

State why you are calling—what is the situation or issue.

State what you need from them—for example—I need your advice as to ....

Agree an action plan—next steps.

There are a range of tools that support practitioners to ensure they are able to provide the appropriate information clearly in urgent/emergent situations.

1. Identify whether communication tools are used in your region/hospital—what are they?
2. Undertake a literature review to identify other tools.
3. Consider which tools would be most supportive.

THE AUSTRALIAN NATIONAL MIDWIFERY GUIDELINES FOR CONSULTATION AND REFERRAL

The collaborative process

The 4th edition of the National Midwifery Guidelines for Consultation and Referral have been developed following rigorous review and extensive consultation (ACM, 2021). The original Guidelines (ACM, 2004) were developed based on comparable guidelines in use in other OECD countries as well as on a thorough review of current evidence-based practice in maternity care. This fourth edition is supported and informed by the Council of Australian Government's 'Women-centred care: strategic directions for Australian Maternity Service' (COAG, 2019).

Since their publication in 2004, the Guidelines have been well received. They are now in use in most maternity services across Australia; midwives working in all models of care and geographical locations have used/are using/will use them to inform clinical decision making. The Guidelines are designed to be relevant in all midwifery practice situations. They have been cited in major maternity service documents on collaborative practice (NHMRC, 2010) and by the Nurses and Midwives Board of Australia. Amongst the initiatives produced by state and territory governments and complementing the National Maternity Services Framework, the Guidelines have been endorsed in New South Wales, Queensland, Western Australia, Victoria and South Australia and are referenced in the National Consensus Framework for Rural Maternity Services.

The aim of the Guidelines is to promote a system of care based upon the principle of close mutual cooperation between primary, secondary or tertiary level maternity caregivers and the woman involved.

The Guidelines

(The information in this section is from the Australian College of Midwives (2021) National Midwifery Guidelines for Consultation and Referral, 4th edition.)

The National Midwifery Guidelines for Consultation and Referral (ACM, 2021) are intended to assist midwives in their provision of care but also to inform policies, clinical practice standards and guidelines across Australian jurisdictions. They provide an evidence-based structured decision-making framework for midwives caring for women. This fourth edition also includes guidance about the social indications that may warrant consultation with and/or referral to medical practitioners or other relevant healthcare providers. The Guidelines are not designed to be prescriptive but to support the midwife to integrate evidence with experience (clinical judgment) in providing midwifery care, and to assist midwives in their discussions with women. They should in no way be interpreted and/or be used as a substitute for an individual midwife's decision making and judgment in situations where care has been negotiated within the context of informed decision making by the individual woman.

The Guidelines have been organised into five sections to assist midwives to quickly identify situations that require the input of other healthcare professionals. These are:

1. Indications at commencement of care
2. Clinical indications developed or identified during pregnancy
3. Clinical indications during labour and birth
4. Clinical indications during the postnatal period
5. Social indications.

The Guidelines reflect the following guiding principles (the information in this section is taken directly from the Australian College of Midwives (2021) National Midwifery Guidelines for Consultation and Referral, 4th edition):

1. *Midwives, medical practitioners and all other health care professionals involved in a woman's childbearing experience, are responsible for their own professional decision-making. The Guidelines assist maternity health care providers in making decisions about the care of a woman and her baby.*

2. *Midwives, medical practitioners and other health care providers respect the conditions under which information about the woman and her infant(s) may or may not be shared with others.*

3. *If problems occur during pregnancy, birth or the postnatal period, the midwife may decide to discuss with peers in the first instance; or consult directly with a medical practitioner or other health care provider. A referral should occur where indicated.*

4. *At all times, the woman must be included in discussions that relate to both her and her baby such that she is able to make an informed decision and provide informed consent, with this including the recommendation for referral.*

5. *The midwife, medical practitioner and other health care providers involved in providing care to a woman and her baby will collaborate and cooperate in accordance with the Guidelines.*

6. *The level of consultation and/or referral that may be required will be influenced by the midwife's endorsement to prescribe scheduled medicines.*

7. *Where indicated, a medical practitioner may assume ongoing clinical responsibility of the woman's care. However, this does not preclude the midwife from providing midwifery care. As such, the ongoing role of the midwife in providing care will be agreed between the woman, the midwife, and the medical practitioner. This discussion will also include the possibility of and/or timing of transfer back to the midwife once the woman's condition permits.*

8. *The severity of the woman's condition will influence these decisions.*

(ACM, 2021)

Three main steps in consultation and referral

When a variance from normal arises during a woman's care, it is recommended the midwife undertake one or more of three steps:

A/A*. Discuss. Care is provided by the midwife who may discuss the situation with a colleague (midwife), and/or with a medical practitioner, and/or another healthcare provider. A* is the category for midwives endorsed to prescribe scheduled medicines.

B. Consult with a relevant medical practitioner or other healthcare provider.

C. Refer a woman and/or her infant to a relevant medical practitioner or other healthcare provider.

Where there are variations in the severity of a condition there may be more than one level recommended (e.g. B/C; A/B/C).

For more detail on these categories please visit the ACM website (https://www.midwives.org.au/Web/About-ACM/Midwifery-Guidelines-and-Standards/Web/About-ACM/Guideline-Statements.aspx?hkey51ac129e0-1241-4894-9efe-4edb089f31ec).

Fig. 18.1 summarises decision making by midwives, and Table 18.1 is a summary of the codes used for the healthcare providers.

Appendix A: when a woman chooses care outside the guidelines

The ACM Guidelines have final parts in the document, called Appendix A and Appendix B. These aim to assist midwives in continuing to provide midwifery care when a woman chooses a course of action against advice or outside the Guidelines. The ACM respects and supports a woman's legal right to make decisions regarding her care following a discussion of the risks and benefits of any aspect of care, including procedures.

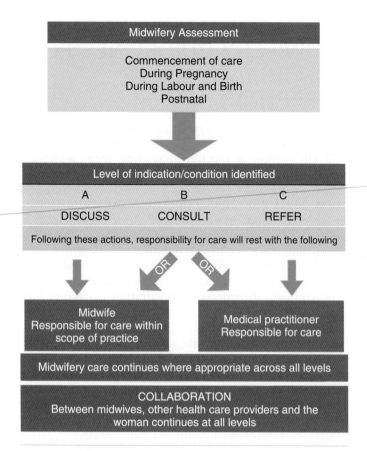

FIGURE 18.1 Decision making by midwives

This document can assist midwives to continue to provide midwifery care when a woman chooses a course of action against advice or outside the Guidelines. It should be read in conjunction with the ACM position statement about caring for women who make choices outside professional advice.

Table 18.1 Summary of codes used for the healthcare providers		
Code	Description	Care provider
A. DISCUSS	The responsibility for maternity care in the situation described is with the midwife.	Midwife and/or medical practitioner or other healthcare provider
B. CONSULT	Evaluation involving both primary and secondary care needs. The individual situation of the woman will be evaluated and agreements will be made about the responsibility for maternity care.	Midwife and/or medical practitioner or other healthcare provider
C. REFER	This is a situation requiring medical care at a secondary or tertiary level for as long as the situation exists. The request for referral will be made in writing. Alterations in care will be communicated in writing to the midwife.	Medical practitioner (for secondary or tertiary care); where appropriate the midwife continues to provide *midwifery* care

Midwifery Practice Scenario:
Sabina

Sabina and Anthony were migrants to Australia and proud parents of 2-year-old Joseph. During Joseph's birth Sabina had experienced a 2-hour second stage and a forceps delivery, which she had regrets about and wanted to avoid with a subsequent birth. She came to book into our group practice and really wanted a home birth this time. Sabina had a very straightforward pregnancy and it was lovely getting to know her and her beautiful family. At 36 weeks Sabina's little baby was settled comfortably into a breech position and seemed reluctant to change. At this point she started to get worried that her dream of an intervention-free home birth was slipping away. We had long discussions about what she could do to help turn the baby and what we could offer her to assist her in turning the baby. We had long conversations about the 'what ifs'. Sabina tried moxibustion, postural exercises and acupuncture. She indicated that if the baby had not turned by 37 weeks she wanted an external cephalic version (ECV) and if the baby did not turn she wanted a vaginal breech birth. We discussed the benefits of being in hospital should the baby remain breech and were able to let Sabina know that she was lucky to live near one of the best hospitals in Australia when it came to breech birth. Building her confidence in the wonderful obstetrician we collaborated with and staff of the hospital meant she came to terms with the possibility that she may give birth in hospital and we would all work together to make it a positive experience. Being a very organised person who liked to think through all the various scenarios, Sabina developed two birth plans: one for a breech birth in

hospital and another for a home birth should the baby turn. We worked through the birth plans together and felt we were all clear about Sabina's wishes and were able to get her to consider other possible scenarios as well, such as caesarean section and what we could do for her in that circumstance. Meeting the wonderful obstetrician we had spoken so highly of encouraged her further and she booked in for an ECV at 37 weeks. I had a conversation with the obstetrician beforehand about her background and her wishes and told him I thought this would be an easy ECV as the baby was very mobile and felt like a frank breech on palpation. Sure enough the baby was in a frank breech presentation and turned easily. Even better he stayed in a lovely, reassuring, head-down position. The long labour Sabina had been prepared for after her first birth was not to be her reality. After a fast 2-hour labour that took her by storm her little boy Rupert was born into Anthony's hands, healing both parents' trauma over Joseph's birth and giving them that wonderful 'I did it' sense of achievement that midwives love to witness. After the birth, I texted the obstetrician and told him the good news. His response needs to be quoted exactly: 'Whoo haa! Very pleased for her. Thanks for the message.' Now that's not the typical message you might expect from an obstetrician, but I have it in my phone and look at it every so often when I feel despair over obstetric attitudes. Yes, collaboration is possible and yes we can all work together to use the best of our complementary skills, to keep women at the centre of our care. Watching a mother glow after her achievement, or watching a proud father walk a little taller and a curious brother discover his protective big brother spirit, is why we do what we do. When we work together, we can do it even better.

 Midwifery Practice Scenario:
Jennifer

Jennifer and Angus phoned to ask if I could provide midwifery care for their unexpected, but welcome third pregnancy. I had cared for them twice previously. Jennifer had a history of endometriosis, which had contributed to some difficulty for her and Angus conceiving, and her two previous pregnancies were both IVF assisted. This time, 20 months following the birth of their second son, they had conceived spontaneously.

Their first baby had been born normally following a straightforward spontaneous labour at term. He had a gentle water birth and weighed 4005 g. In her second pregnancy, Jennifer experienced ongoing severe abdominal discomfort related to her endometriosis. At 37 weeks she developed hypertension and moderate generalised oedema, and she was referred to the secondary care service when she developed mild proteinuria. She continued in my care with episodic visits to the hospital for

monitoring, and at 39+ weeks the decision was made to induce her as her blood picture indicated preeclamptic changes. Despite 2 days of prostins, Jennifer's cervix remained unchanged and she did not establish in labour. On the third day, under some pressure from the medical staff, she 'chose' to undergo an elective caesarean section.

During the surgery, it was noted that Jennifer had three very tortuous large blood vessels running up the anterior surface of her uterus, which made it inadvisable to complete a low transverse incision. The consultant instead made a low vertical incision, resulting in an L-shaped scar on her uterus. Jennifer and Angus's second son weighed 3575 g. Jennifer made a good recovery, with no wound problems, but the surgeon advised no further pregnancies.

Jennifer's GP, who confirmed her pregnancy, referred her to the secondary team very early in her third pregnancy, because Jennifer understandably had some concerns

Continued

after being told not to contemplate another pregnancy. The specialist she saw at 8 weeks told her that there was no room for negotiation; she would be having an elective caesarean section at 38 weeks because there was a chance that even in pregnancy her uterus could rupture, let alone what might happen in labour!

Jennifer and Angus felt quite disappointed about this. They had experienced such a lovely water birth the first time, but were now faced with very limited or, as they saw it, no choice this time. We resolved to gather information about whether a low vertical incision posed risk over and above that of a low transverse incision, and to have another consultation later in the pregnancy to review the plan.

As the months went by, we collected together a file of studies reporting outcomes for subsequent pregnancy in women with previous low-vertical-incision caesarean section. These studies concluded that there was no apparent increased risk with the vertical incision when compared with transverse incision. Jennifer's confidence grew with her baby, and she enjoyed a pain-free and positive pregnancy. She thought some compromise was in order so, although not ruling out an 'elective' caesarean, she and Angus wanted to at least wait until she had reached her due date, and then make a decision about how to proceed. She was leaning towards wanting to request a VBAC (vaginal birth after caesarean section) by now; we all worried about the surgical risk involved because we knew from ultrasound scanning that the vascular anomalies were still present.

At 37 weeks, we organised another consultation, this time with the same specialist who had performed Jennifer's caesarean. We felt that his knowledge of the previous surgery would lead us to a better decision. We went 'armed' with our studies to discuss their findings if necessary. The specialist was very welcoming, and his first question to Jennifer and Angus was to ask them what they would like to do. Jennifer replied that they had looked at the evidence and were satisfied that an attempted VBAC would be a safe option, explaining that they were happy for early labour admission and intensive monitoring in labour to detect any deviation from normal. The specialist agreed with us that the surgery would be complex and potentially risky, and he felt on balance that a VBAC was not an unreasonable request, but that he would prefer not to 'let' Jennifer's pregnancy go much beyond 40 weeks and 3 or 4 days. Induction of labour was not an option.

We left feeling very buoyant and hopeful for a successful VBAC experience. Jennifer and Angus felt pleased that their wishes had been respected, and felt very optimistic about their approaching labour. In the event, despite membrane sweeps after 40 weeks and high hopes, Jennifer's baby was very comfortable in her space, and declined to participate. At 40 + 6, Jennifer underwent an elective caesarean section. The surgery was very complex as the vascularity of her uterus had proliferated, now including her bladder also. Her 4740 g baby girl was born through a diagonal incision in the body of her uterus.

Jennifer had a significant postpartum haemorrhage and required a blood transfusion.

Again Jennifer made a speedy recovery. She and Angus were mildly disappointed not to have had a normal birth experience, but were resolved about the situation, chiefly because of the respect that was shown to their autonomy around the decision making about their plan of care. A successful collaborative process was achieved at the second consultation, where information was exchanged rather than flowing in one direction. Each party to the decision making had the opportunity to express their opinions, and these were respected even where they differed.

Sample referral letter

Midwife's address

Date

Obstetric clinic or hospital address

Dear consultant

Re Jennifer X

d.o.b. xx/xx/xx

Address

National Health Number #

Phone number

Thank you for seeing Jennifer who is now coming up to 37 weeks pregnant. She requires review because of her previous caesarean section. Her history is as follows:

2004 39 weeks. Spontaneous onset of labour, 6 hours duration, normal birth of 4005 g boy

2007 40 weeks. IOL for preeclampsia. Failed IOL after 3 days, caesarean section performed. 3575 g boy.

Both of these pregnancies were IVF conceptions. This time Jennifer spontaneously conceived and her due date is xx/xx/xx. She has been keen to pursue VBAC for this birth, but was told at a consultation very early in this pregnancy that she should have elective LSCS at 38 weeks. This is because during her caesarean, once her uterus was visualised, she had some very prominent blood vessels lying anterior to her uterus, which precluded a full lower segment transverse incision. Dr Y completed a low transverse incision for a short distance, then modified it to a low vertical incision so as not to incise the blood vessels in front of the uterus.

Jennifer and Angus have researched the evidence regarding low vertical incisions in relation to trial of labour, and these studies have concluded that in an otherwise uncomplicated pregnancy the risks associated with trial of labour are not greater than for women with one prior low transverse incision. Jennifer does understand the increased risk from scar dehiscence/rupture generally associated with previous caesarean surgery. She made a good recovery with no wound infection present last time, and it has been more than 2 years since her surgery.

In view of this, she would like to at least wait until her due date to decide whether to proceed to elective caesarean section, or if labour ensues will be happy to have all the recommended observations usual for women undergoing trial of labour. We wonder whether the surgical risk posed to Jennifer from inadvertent incision of these blood vessels, which can be easily seen on scan, might perhaps outweigh the risk posed by her low vertical incision?

We look forward to discussing this with you at the clinic appointment. Jennifer's pregnancy has been straightforward this time; notably her blood pressure has remained stable and normal, and she has had no proteinuria or oedema. She is currently taking some iron to boost her stores. This baby is growing well and movements are reassuring.

I have included a copy of her blood and scan results for your information.

Kind regards (midwife's name, signature, registration number and contact details)

Conclusion

Collaboration in maternity care involves the incorporation of the woman as partner in all decision-making processes, in addition to working with others to implement the most appropriate and effective care. The challenge of collaborative practice is always to find a balance between midwifery skills, the notion of intensive 'presence' and minimal intervention, and the practice of medicine, in particular obstetrics, with its emphasis on technological expediency. Achieving collaboration and cooperation between the professional groups involved in maternity care involves recognising and acknowledging each other's particular expertise. Birth is a disorderly business. The multiple strategies of midwifery practice are negotiated through the intensity and immediacy of each birth experience, rather than defined in advance (Maher & Torney Souter, 2002). The way midwives work with each other, with women and with their professional colleagues shapes the experience of birth for both women and their families.

Review questions

1. What is the central principle to consider in the process of collaboration? Who is the most important person?
2. Can you describe at least five important tenets of collaboration?
3. How do the Competencies referring to collaboration relate to you as a student midwife?
4. What are the 'domains' of midwifery competency?
5. Describe, in your own words, what you understand as the Competencies that relate to legal and professional responsibilities.
6. 'Midwifery is a public health strategy'—what do you understand this statement to mean, and how does the need for collaboration 'fit' into this strategy?
7. How legally binding are the Referral Guidelines that guide your practice?
8. How would you describe the complementary roles of midwives and obstetricians?
9. What strategies might you employ in a situation where you are feeling that the person you are collaborating with does not understand your perspective?
10. What are your responsibilities when a woman declines your recommendation for referral?

Online resources

Australian College of Midwives, for midwives section: http://www.midwives.org.au.
Australian Nursing and Midwifery Council: http://www.anmc.org.au.
Midwifery Council of New Zealand: http://www.midwiferycouncil.health.nz.
New Zealand College of Midwives: http://www.midwife.org.nz.

References

Australian College of Midwives (ACM). National Midwifery Guidelines for Consultation and Referral. Canberra: ACM; 2004.

Australian College of Midwives (ACM). National Midwifery Guidelines for Consultation and Referral. 4th ed. Canberra: ACM; 2021. Online: https://www.midwives.org.au/shop/new-national-midwifery-guidelines-consultation-and-referral.

Barclay L, Brodie P, Lane K, et al. The Final Report of the Australian Midwifery Action Project. Sydney: The Centre for Family Health and Midwifery. University of Technology Sydney; 2003.

Beasley S, Ford N, Tracy SK, et al. Collaboration in maternity care is achievable and practical. *Aust N Z J Obstet Gynaecol.* 2012;52(6):576–581. doi:10.1111/ajo.12003.

Cassie R. How do midwives and obstetricians communicate at the primary/secondary interface? Unpublished Theses submitted in partial fulfillment of degree of Master of Midwifery; 2019.

Otago Polytechnic https://www.op.ac.nz/assets/OPRES/MID-Cassie-2019-thesis.pdf.

Cohen SG, Bailey DE. What makes teams work: group effectiveness research from the shop floor to the executive suite. *J Manag.* 1997;23(3):239–290.

Council of Australian Government (COAG). Woman-centred care: Strategic directions for Australian maternity services. 2019. Department of Health. Online: https://www.health.gov.au/resources/publications/woman-centred-care-strategic-directions-for-australian-maternity-services.

Department of Health (DOH) [UK]. The Cumberledge Report: Changing Childbirth: the Report of the Expert Maternity Group. London: HMSO; 1993.

Dorne A. Collaboration between healthcare professionals, what does it mean? The rhetoric and the reality (research paper). Wellington: Victoria University of Wellington; 2002.

Downe S, Finlayson K. Collaboration: theories, models and maternity care. In: Downe S, Byrom S, Simpson L, eds. *Essential Midwifery Practice: Leadership, Expertise and Collaborative Working.* Chichester: Blackwell Publishing; 2011:155–179.

GBS Working Group. The Prevention of Early-Onset Neonatal Group B Streptococcus Infection Consensus Guideline. NZCOM, The Paediatric Society of New Zealand, RANZCOG (NZ Committee), Australasian Society for of Infectious Diseases (NZ Sub-Committee). Christchurch: GBS Working Group; 2014. Online: https://www.midwife.org.nz/quality-practice/multidisciplinary-guidelines.

Hall P. Interprofessional teamwork. Professional cultures as barriers. *J Interprof Care.* 2005;19(S1):188–196.

Homer CS, Davis GK, Brodie PM, et al. Collaboration in maternity care: a randomised controlled trial comparing community-based continuity of care with standard care. *Br J Obstet Gynaecol.* 2001;108(1):16–22.

Homer C, Pincombe J, Thorogood C, et al. An Examination of the Role and Scope of Practice of Australian Midwives and the Development of Competency Standards for Midwifery. Final Report. Canberra: University of Technology Sydney, Sydney and Australian Nursing and Midwifery Council; 2005.

Liedtka JM, Whitten E. Enhancing care delivery through cross-disciplinary collaboration: a case study. *J Healthc Manag.* 1998;43(2):185.

McLachlan HL, Forster DA, Davey MA, et al. Effects of continuity of care by a primary midwife (caseload midwifery) on caesarean section rates in women of low obstetric risk: the COSMOS randomised controlled trial. *BJOG.* 2012;119(12):1483–1492. doi:10.1111/j.1471-0528.2012.03446.x.

Maher JM, Torney Souter KT. Midwifery work and the making of narrative. *Nurs Inq.* 2002;9(1):37–42.

Maternity Coalition. National maternity action plan. n.d. Online: http://www.maternitycoalition.org.au/uploads/1/5/1/4/15149676/the_final_nmap.pdf.

Midwifery Council of New Zealand (MCNZ). Midwifery Scope of Practice. Wellington: MCNZ; 2004. Online: https://www.midwiferycouncil.health.nz/midwives/midwifery-scope-practice.

Midwifery Council of New Zealand (MCNZ). Competencies for Entry to the Register of Midwives. Wellington: MCNZ; 2007. Online: http://www.midwiferycouncil.health.nz/main/Competencies.

Miller S. *First Birth at Home or in Hospital in Aotearoa/New Zealand: Intrapartum Midwifery Care and Related Outcomes.* Wellington: Victoria University of Wellington; 2008. Online: http://research archive.vuw.ac.nz/handle//10063/851.

Ministry of Health (MOH). *Public Health and Disability Act 2000.* Wellington: New Zealand Government; 2000.

Ministry of Health (MOH). Observation of the Mother and Baby in the Immediate Postpartum Period: Consensus Statements Guiding Practice. Wellington: Ministry of Health; 2012.

Ministry of Health (MOH). Screening, Diagnosis and Management of Gestational Diabetes in New Zealand. Wellington: Ministry of Health; 2014. Online: https://www.health.govt.nz/publication/screening-diagnosis-and-management-gestational-diabetes-new-zealand-clinical-practice-guideline.

Ministry of Health (MOH). Induction of Labour in Aotearoa New Zealand: A Clinical Practice Guideline. Wellington: Ministry of Health; 2021. Online: https://www.health.govt.nz/publication/induction-labour-aotearoa-new-zealand-clinical-practice-guideline-2019.

Ministry of Health (MOH). Maternity Services Notice Pursuant to Section 88 of the New Zealand Public Health & Disability Act 2000. Wellington: New Zealand Government; 2022a. Online: https://www.health.govt.nz/publication/primary-maternity-services-notice-2021.

Ministry of Health (MOH). Guidelines for Consultation with Obstetric and Related Medical Services (Referral Guidelines). Wellington: Ministry of Health; 2022b. Online: https://www.health.govt.nz/our-work/life-stages/maternity-services/national-maternity-clinical-guidance.

Ministry of Health (MOH). National Consensus Guideline for Treatment of Postpartum Haemorrhage. Wellington: Ministry of Health; 2022c. Online: https://www.health.govt.nz/our-work/life-stages/maternity-services/national-maternity-clinical-guidance.

Moore A. *Pioneering a New Model of Midwifery Care: A Phenomenological Study of a Midwifery Group Practice.* Melbourne: Australian Catholic University; 2009.

National Health and Medical Research Council (NHMRC). National Guidance on Collaborative Maternity Care. Canberra: NHMRC; 2010.

New Zealand College of Midwives (NZCOM). *Midwives Handbook for Practice.* Christchurch: New Zealand College of Midwives; 2015.

Nursing and Midwifery Board of Australia (NMBA). Midwifery Standards for Practice. Melbourne: NMBA; 2018. Online: http://www.nursingmidwiferyboard.gov.au/Codes-Guidelines-Statements/Professional-standards.aspx.

RANZCOG. Intrapartum Fetal Surveillance Guideline. 3rd ed. Victoria, Australia: RANZCOG; 2014. Online: https://www.midwife.org.nz/quality-practice/multidisciplinary-guidelines.

Rushmer R. Blurred boundaries damage interprofessional working. *Nurse Res.* 2004;12(3):74-85.

San Martin-Rodriguez L, Beaulieu MD, D'Amour D, et al. The determinants of successful collaboration: a review of theoretical and empirical studies. *J Interprof Care.* 2005;19(S1):132–147.

Saxell L, Harris S, Elarar L. The collaboration for maternal and newborn health: interprofessional maternity care education for medical, midwifery, and nursing students. *J Midwifery Womens Health.* 2009;54(4):314-320.

Schmied V, Mills A, Kruske S, et al. The nature and impact of collaboration and integrated service delivery for pregnant women, children and families. J Clin Nurs. 2010;19(23–24):3516–3526.

Skinner J. Being with women with risk. The referral and consultation practices and attitudes of New Zealand midwives. *J N Z Coll Midwives.* 2011;45:17-20.

Tracy SK, Sullivan E, Dahlen H, et al. Does size matter? The safety of giving birth in smaller maternity hospitals. *BJOG.* 2006;113:86–96.

van Helmond I, Korstjens I, Mesman J, et al. What makes for good collaboration and communication in maternity care? A scoping study. *Int J Childbirth.* 2015;5(4):210–223.

Further reading

Australian Health Ministers' Advisory Council. Clinical Practice Guidelines: Antenatal Care—Module 1. Canberra: Australian Government Department of Health and Ageing; 2012. Online: http://www.health.gov.au/antenatal.

CHAPTER 19

Promoting physiological birth

Nicky Leap

LEARNING OUTCOMES

Learning outcomes for this chapter are:

1. To explore the practicalities, sensitivities and systems that promote physiological birth
2. To highlight the factors and organisational culture that can inhibit this approach in midwifery practice
3. To explore the evidence concerning midwifery continuity of care
4. To provide information about midwifery practices that enhance physiological birth.

CHAPTER OVERVIEW

The focus of this chapter is the promotion of physiological birth by midwives. Strategies are suggested, including the need to develop systems and an organisational culture that nurtures the potential of birth to transform lives and strengthen women, their families and societies.

The imaginary story of the birth of Jack Taylor, presented in this chapter in a sequence of Midwifery Practice Scenarios, can be used for discussion and analysis in small groups as Critical Thinking and Reflective Thinking Exercises. As a similar group activity, practitioners and students can present 'real-life' stories from practice in order to analyse the factors that can promote or inhibit physiological birth in any given situation. Such an activity can be incorporated in continuing professional development activities, such as peer review, interdisciplinary learning, case review and workshops.

KEY TERMS

antenatal groups	midwifery continuity of care	physiological birth
empowerment	normal birth	place of birth
midwifery caseload practice	pain in labour	36-week home visit

INTRODUCTION

Birth is not only about making babies. Birth is also about making mothers—strong, competent, capable mothers who trust themselves and know their inner strength.

(Katz Rothman, 1996, pp. 253–4)

This oft-quoted statement by Barbara Katz-Rothman links the challenges women face during labour with the potential of birth to be transformative and empowering (Kurz et al., 2019, 2021). Studies suggest that healthcare professionals need to understand the importance of this potential and the relevance of not disturbing physiology unless it is necessary (Olza et al., 2018; Van der Gucht & Lewis, 2015). There is now robust international evidence that most women hope for a physiological labour and birth but acknowledge that birth is unpredictable. What is important to them is to have practical and emotional support from birth companions and reassurance from competent, kind midwives (Downe et al., 2018). All too often, however, women report feeling disempowered, emotionally fragile, and traumatised as a result of an experience of childbirth that rendered them passive in the face of intervention and poor communication from care providers (de Graaff et al., 2018; Kitzinger, 2006).

This chapter explores some of these issues, relating them to the practicalities of midwifery practice and initiatives that optimise women's potential to feel good about their experiences of pregnancy, giving birth and nurturing a new baby. Some strategies are suggested that might help to promote physiology, even in situations where midwives are 'swimming against the tide' of 'technocratic' thinking and practices. The word 'technocratic' (Davis-Floyd, 2001) rather than 'medicalised' is used in an attempt to acknowledge that it is not only doctors who can hinder physiological birth.

The phrase 'promoting physiological birth' is used in this chapter whilst recognising that women and most maternity care providers are likely to use the term 'normal birth' rather than physiological birth'. Efforts to conceptualise or describe 'normal' birth are fraught with difficulty (Darra, 2009; NCT/RCM/RCOG, 2007) and are dominated by a medical model that focuses on measurable parameters of labour progress. Within such definitions there is little room for articulating the midwifery skill of tolerating intrapartum uncertainty (Page & Mander, 2014) or for encompassing psychosocial and emotional factors for women (Gould, 2000). Furthermore, as Holly Kennedy (2009) has suggested, the notion of 'normal' is hardly in keeping with the midwifery philosophy of embracing the concept of each woman's birth being viewed by her as essentially 'special'.

Undoubtedly, however, the words 'normal birth' are embedded in the documentation and discourses that shape and reflect contemporary maternity service provision. Importantly, the term 'normal' is used to identify the primary domain of the midwife, a sphere of practice that is clearly defined as separate from the technological or medical interventions associated with complications. As identified on the website of the International Confederation of Midwives, the *International Definition of a Midwife* states that midwifery care includes 'the promotion of normal birth' (ICM, 2017).

Fulfilling this role is not as straightforward as it might seem in a Western maternity service culture of mounting intervention and caesarean section rates (Carolan-Olah et al., 2015; Davis, 2013; Delbaere et al., 2012), particularly where women have private obstetric care, do not know their midwives and where continuous fetal monitoring is the norm (Prosser et al., 2018).

In suggesting strategies to promote **physiological birth**, this author is mindful of the fact that the majority of midwives are working in institutions where 'normal' birth is not the most common experience for women. A recent study in Queensland, for example, identified that only 28.7% of 5840 respondents had a normal birth without: induction of labour, epidural, spinal and / or general anaesthesia, vaginal birth assisted with forceps or ventouse, caesarean section or episiotomy (Prosser et al., 2018).

Midwives in Western countries often work in hospitals where computerised summaries identifying 'normal birth' do not necessarily reflect physiological processes or the efforts of practitioners to promote physiological birth. There are mounting concerns about the limited learning opportunities for practitioners where the promotion of physiological birth is limited by 'technocratic' approaches and a culture of increasing intervention and epidural rates (Newnham et al., 2016). Concerns have also been raised about ethical issues associated with the promotion of 'normalcy' in situations where the majority of women have some form of intervention, particularly regarding the potential for these women to feel marginalised if birth is seen as a socially meaningful event only if it is 'normal' (Lyerly, 2013).

The concept of promoting normal birth is under threat in Western countries. In the UK, for instance, controversies abound concerning the public statements from the Royal College of Midwives of their intentions to disband the promotion of normal birth and focus instead on promoting 'positive' birth experiences. (These statements can be accessed online and can be used to promote conversations about the implications of removing the term 'normal birth' from nomenclature and how 'evidence' is being cited in a backlash against the promotion of physiological birth by midwives.)

Underlying power dynamics can subvert the efforts of midwives to promote physiological birth and practise according to their full role and scope of practice (Mander & Murphy-Lawless, 2013). Reflecting on how these dynamics have evolved over recent centuries may be useful in conversations about interdisciplinary working and how contemporary and future maternity care in Western countries is both enacted and experienced (Kurz, 2022).

THE MIDWIFE AS 'GUARDIAN OF THE NORMAL'

A long history of interprofessional rivalry lies behind the contemporary rhetorical notion of the midwife as 'guardian of the normal' as documented in several significant texts exploring the history of midwifery and childbirth. Before men entered the birthing arena, most women in European countries were attended at home by women they knew, one of whom might well be referred to as 'the midwife' owing to her acknowledged role and expertise (Donnison, 1977; Wilson, 1995). If problems occurred, it was not unusual for a more experienced midwife to be called to help out. As described in the diaries of Catharina Schrader, a 17th-century midwife who was called to complicated births in Holland, this often involved internal podalic version and bringing the baby out by its feet (Marland, 1987).

A core professionalising strategy used by midwives in Western countries in the 18th and 19th centuries was the relinquishing of complicated (and lucrative) birth practice to the medical profession in return for the domain of 'normal childbirth' (Donnison, 1977; Leap & Hunter, 2013). This strategy responded to, and set up, a dynamic that has had far-reaching consequences in terms of gender and class inequalities and the collective psychological effects of subordination (Witz, 1992). Pathology was the pivotal factor for role division, and doctors were presented as the superior professionals, educated at a higher level than midwives in order to carry out rescuing manoeuvres associated with the complications of childbirth. In comparison, the midwife's role was shrunk to that of 'caring' for women who did not need interventions, and to recognising problems and calling for a doctor to 'correct' the situation and intervene in a timely fashion.

The fraught negotiations that led to the role delineation between midwives and doctors have given way to a situation with its own set of interprofessional tensions (Sandall, 2012). While fulfilling the imperative to adopt good collaborative relationships with obstetricians in the interests of women and safe practice, the midwife often defines the boundaries of 'normal' in situations that are intricate and unclear. She engages with women and makes decisions in a culture dominated by the ideologies of authoritative medical science and its quest for certainty. Evidence-based protocols and policies often do not 'fit' with the complexity of individual women's psychological and social situations and the impact of the environment. This has led to a childbirth culture in which it is increasingly difficult to find consensus on what constitutes '**normal birth**' other than an absence of technical intervention (Downe & McCourt, 2019). The complex process of an interdisciplinary attempt to arrive at a consensus definition for normal labour and birth, one that involves women and measures the process of labour rather than outcomes, is discussed in *Making Normal Birth a Reality* (NCT/RCM/RCOG, 2007).

THE RATIONALE FOR PROMOTING PHYSIOLOGICAL BIRTH

The boundaries of what is considered 'normal' are at the heart of the passionate discussions that happen whenever midwives get together. In recent years, midwives have been addressing these issues by identifying the complexity of their role in being 'with woman' and promoting physiological birth. This is often explained in terms of the potentially self-transformative nature of birth and the profound long-term consequences of **empowerment** for women, their families and society (Kurz et al., 2019, 2021; Leap, 2004; Leap & Anderson, 2008). The promotion of physiology begins in early pregnancy and is about far more than aiming for an uncomplicated birth. It is concerned with a journey to motherhood that will have consequences for each individual woman in terms of how she feels about herself, her body and her capabilities (Thompson, 2004). Whether or not she eventually gives birth without intervention, a woman who feels powerful is in a good situation to take on becoming a new mother.

In this chapter, the telling and re-telling of the imaginary story of the birth of Jack Taylor teases out some of these issues, starting with Midwifery Practice Scenario One.

 Midwifery Practice Scenario One

The birth of Jack Taylor at St Average Hospital

This is an everyday story about the birth of a baby at St Average Hospital, in Australia. It's the story of the birth of Jack Taylor, first child of Michelle and Daniel Taylor. Michelle is a receptionist in a hotel and continued working up until she was 34 weeks pregnant. She has not had any problems in her pregnancy and has been coming to the antenatal clinic regularly, where, after waiting for over an hour, she has seen a different person at each visit for a 15-minute check-up. She attended antenatal classes at the hospital but could not persuade Daniel to come with her to these.

Daniel is a motor mechanic. He's a shy man who doesn't like hospitals. Secretly he's very worried about being with Michelle when she's in labour. He's scared that he'll faint, and is worried about seeing Michelle in pain. He didn't want to go to the classes in case they showed a video that might make him pass out or want to vomit. He has heard stories from his mates at work that make him shudder.

Michelle found the classes useful. They reinforced her idea that she would 'try for a normal birth', but it is

---

comforting to know that the epidural is there if she can't cope.

One Sunday evening, a week past her due date, Michelle starts having some low, period-type pains. She thinks her waters may have broken. She is very scared, and so is Daniel, who rings the hospital. The midwife on the phone asks him a lot of questions: 'How often are the contractions?', 'How long do they last?', 'What colour is the water?', and 'Is the baby moving?' The midwife suggests that it might be early days yet but to come in if they're worried. They are worried. They go in to St Average.

When Michelle and Daniel get to the 'delivery suite' at St Average, they are assigned to the care of midwife Sally, in Room 11. Sally is friendly and efficient, asks Michelle lots of questions, including whether she has been to classes and what her choices are for pain relief. Michelle says she's not sure how she'll cope, as she has a low pain threshold and already these pains are severe. The midwife says, 'We'll take it one step at a time, shall we? You're coping well at the moment.' She talks Michelle and Daniel through all the 'natural' methods of pain relief, and then explains that if Michelle can't cope with the pain, there are other things to help—she explains the pros and cons of gas, pethidine and epidurals.

Sally the midwife gives Michelle a hospital gown and carries out a series of tests: she takes Michelle's temperature, pulse and blood pressure, tests her urine and palpates her abdomen. She places Michelle on the monitor and explains the trace to Daniel, who is fascinated and remains glued to every variation in the lines. Sally reassures Michelle that the baby's heartbeat looks really good. She explains that she is looking after someone in the room next door, and that she'll come back in 10 minutes. She shows them a buzzer to press if they need her.

It will be a while before Sally can get back to Michelle. Next door, Sophie's contractions are suddenly very strong. She is having her second baby, and in order to have continuity of care with someone she trusts Sophie has booked with a private obstetrician, Edward Richman. Sally helps her get down onto all fours on a mattress on the floor. Sophie is bellowing. Sally asks someone to phone Dr Richman to come. He arrives 10 minutes later as the baby's head is crowning. Edward insists that Sophie get up onto the bed, cuts an episiotomy and hands her a healthy baby girl, who will be called Anna. Sophie and her partner thank Edward profusely. There is much jubilation all round.

Meanwhile, back in Room 11, Michelle and Daniel are still anxiously watching their baby's heartbeat on the monitor. Eventually Sally asks Rita, another midwife, to go and check on Michelle. They all look at the trace and admire its reassuring variations. According to the machine, Michelle is having what Rita interprets as 'irregular tightenings'. Michelle says that they are quite painful and Rita responds gently by telling Michelle that she's doing really well and that 'Bub's happy' but it looks as though it's early days yet. She asks Michelle what she has decided she'd like for pain relief if she needs it later. She reiterates what is on offer and tells Michelle that, as her waters may have broken, the doctor will come and examine her and have a look at her cervix using a sterile speculum.

Alexandria, the new resident, examines Michelle. She is kind and gentle but Michelle finds the examination painful. Alexandria asks Michelle what choices she has made for pain relief. She reassures her by saying, 'It's great if you can manage the pain but you don't have to be a martyr. If you're going to have an epidural don't wait until it's really bad before getting it inserted.'

It seems that Michelle's waters have broken but her cervix is still long and firm. She is offered the choice of going home and waiting for the contractions to establish, with daily review at the hospital, or having a 'bit of help to get things going'. She is too scared to contemplate going home and the thought of 'getting things going' is appealing. Michelle has some prostaglandins to help soften her cervix. She is given some sedatives to help her get some sleep, and Daniel goes home to get some rest.

The ensuing chain of events over the next day is familiar to all who have worked in large maternity units. For Michelle these events will remain embedded in her memory until the day she dies. She was very grateful to have an epidural to help her cope with the fierce contractions induced by a Syntocinon infusion. The pethidine she had had earlier hadn't touched the pain. She had a kind midwife called Sandra with her for most of the labour. Sandra was a mature woman whom Daniel would later describe as 'really knowing her stuff'.

Little Jack Taylor is pulled into the world with the aid of a ventouse after the monitor showed signs that he really would be 'better off out than in'. He is a fine, healthy baby, albeit a little confused about how to find his way around Michelle's breast. He is taken to the nursery for a few hours to be observed because he is 'breathing up a bit'.

Daniel didn't faint. He is in awe of Michelle and thanks God for the 'life-saving wonders of modern medicine'. Michelle and Daniel are very grateful to the staff of St Average and give them a huge box of chocolates when they go home with Jack 4 days after his birth.

Michelle is given the name of a child health clinic she can go to, to get Jack weighed and where she can access advice about breastfeeding. She is pleased about this because Jack still seems a bit confused about how to latch on and her nipples are very sore. Her mum, Jenny, is coming to stay for a couple of weeks, but Jenny is very unsure about how to support Michelle in breastfeeding Jack. Jenny's own experience left her thinking she was 'unable to make enough milk' and that formula was the only option in these circumstances.

Thus begins the new life of Michelle and Daniel as proud parents of little Jack Taylor . . .

REFLECTING ON MIDWIFERY PRACTICE SCENARIO ONE

Within the culture of maternity care in industrialised countries, where healthcare professionals who are strangers to the woman often provide fragmented care in busy, understaffed maternity units, the story in Midwifery Practice Scenario One is all too familiar. It describes well-meaning midwives and doctors struggling to provide a safe, kind service under conditions hampered by fragmented care, staff shortages, public expectations, medical dominance and all the other components of the stresses associated with maternity service provision in most large tertiary maternity units. At every stage of the story, these members of staff reinforce Michelle and Daniel's belief that Michelle will need some form of pain relief. In the spiralling cascade of intervention, Michelle is rendered passive and dependent on the expertise of strangers.

Re-constructing the birth of Jack Taylor

As this is not a 'real' story, there is the opportunity to wind back the clock and explore how the experience might have been different for Michelle, Daniel and their baby, Jack, had circumstances been otherwise. The re-telling of this story enables scrutiny of a range of changes to practice, some of which are within the grasp of the practitioner and others which would require significant changes to systems. The evidence for these strategies will be woven throughout the process of looking at how we might reconstruct the 'everyday story' of the birth of Jack Taylor.

Promoting physiology: place of birth

Given that the birth of Jack Taylor could be reconstructed in any way, it would be possible to tell a story where Michelle decides to give birth at home or in a midwifery-led birth centre. Studies comparing outcomes for women with uncomplicated pregnancies by intended **place of birth** consistently provide evidence that physiological birth is safely nurtured where women intend to give birth at home, in birth centres or small primary maternity units. A New Zealand study of outcomes for over 16,000 low-risk women booked with midwives providing care as lead maternity care providers in 2006 and 2007 identified that women planning to give birth in secondary and tertiary hospitals had a higher risk of caesarean section and forceps, ventouse and labour interventions than did those who planned to give birth at home or in a primary unit (Davis et al., 2011; Dixon et al., 2014).

In Australia, a large population-based study comparing outcomes for women with uncomplicated pregnancies during the years 2000 to 2012 demonstrated that, compared with planned hospital births, the odds of normal labour and birth were over twice as high in planned

birth centre births and nearly six times as high in planned home births, with no statistically significant differences in the proportion of intrapartum stillbirths, early or late neonatal deaths between the three planned places of birth (Homer, Cheah et al., 2019). An earlier population study using Australian national data showed that the overall rate of perinatal mortality was lower in alongside-hospital birth centres than in hospitals, irrespective of the mother's parity (Tracy et al., 2007).

Internationally, large studies have shown that home birth is a safe option for women with uncomplicated pregnancies, with protective features for promoting physiology (Birthplace in England Collaborative Group et al., 2011; de Jonge et al., 2015; Hutton et al., 2019; Janssen et al., 2009; Johnson & Davis, 2005; Reitsma et al., 2020). In New Zealand, women can choose to give birth at home within publicly funded maternity services. There are good reasons to suggest that publicly funded home birth should become more widely available for Australian women. The first national evaluation of a significant proportion of women choosing to give birth in publicly funded home birth found that 84% of the 1807 women who intended to give birth at home did so and 90% had a straightforward vaginal birth; the rate of stillbirth and early neonatal death was 1.7 per 1000 births when deaths because of expected fetal anomalies were excluded (Catling-Paul et al., 2013).

Given all the evidence that planned home birth is just as safe as birth in hospital for the majority of women, the promotion and support of home birth as a mainstream option for women with uncomplicated pregnancies, like Michelle, has to be a major tactic in promoting physiological birth. Resistance to such a proposal is enshrined in the discourse of contemporary maternity services.

Public awareness of the safety of home birth also needs to be addressed. As identified by the Albany Midwifery Practice, it is possible to convince people that home birth is a safe option, even where they would never have considered it before (Reed, 2015). Over 43% of women who booked with the Albany Midwifery Practice gave birth at home at a time when NHS home birth rates were below 3%. This community-based midwifery practice working in a caseload model was able to show that where known midwives engage with women and their supporters throughout pregnancy, in particular during a home visit in late pregnancy and where final decision making about the place of birth is reserved for labour, home birth can be seen as a safe option for the majority of women, with a significant decrease in operative birth and medical interventions (Homer et al., 2017).

REFLECTIVE THINKING EXERCISE

Internationally, home birth has been shown to be a safe option for a carefully selected group of women. Look up the recommended references on home birth and make a table of the outcomes achieved in three of the studies compared with those achieved in the hospital closest to where you work.

In order to make full use of reconstructing the birth of Jack Taylor, we will not simplify the story by turning it into one about home birth or birth centre care. However, we will enable Michelle to have continuity of carer with a midwife with whom she can build a trusting relationship (Homer et al., 2019a). We will imagine that Michelle has booked with a midwifery group practice that sees bringing women together in groups as a crucial strategy to develop a forum where they can learn from each other and develop friendships and support networks (Leap, 2010; Leap & Edwards, 2006; Schrader McMillan et al., 2009). The reconstructed story in Midwifery Practice Scenario Two speaks of the difference these factors make to how the story unfolds.

 Midwifery Practice Scenario Two

Midwifery continuity of carer for Michelle and Daniel

When Michelle suspects that she is pregnant, she goes to her local community centre, where she knows there are midwives who advertise a free pregnancy-testing service twice a week at set times. The midwives are in a group practice and have their own premises in the community centre where women can access advice and information and attend a variety of support groups. The midwifery group practice is linked to the publicly funded maternity service provided at St Average Hospital.

The midwife who confirms with Michelle that she is pregnant sets out the various options for maternity care and gives Michelle some written information so that she can go home and discuss these options with Daniel. It does not take Michelle and Daniel long to decide that they will book with the midwifery group practice. Fiona is the midwife assigned to be Michelle's primary midwife. She phones Michelle and arranges to come to her home to carry out the booking visit at a time when Daniel can be present.

By the end of this leisurely visit, Michelle and Daniel feel excited and very relieved. Fiona has made them feel that they are very special. She leaves the pregnancy record with Michelle and encourages her to fill in any parts that she wants to and to make a note of any questions she has for subsequent visits.

Fiona encourages Michelle and Daniel to attend the **antenatal groups** that the midwives run in their practice. Instead of classes where the midwives instruct the women, these antenatal groups are organised so that each week someone comes back to the group with

their new baby to tell their story. Michelle can go to the group as often as she likes, starting in early pregnancy, so she will hear many different stories. She will learn from other women and will make friends who will be her support network when she is at home with a new baby. Daniel decides he might go with Michelle to some of the evening groups now that he has met Fiona and likes her.

Michelle's confidence about giving birth starts to grow.

REFLECTING ON MIDWIFERY PRACTICE SCENARIO TWO

Promoting physiology: midwifery continuity of care

Some might question the importance of midwifery-led continuity of care given that, in Midwifery Practice Scenario One, Michelle and Daniel appear grateful and happy about the birth of their son. Although the members of staff at St Average were all strangers to Michelle and Daniel, they were friendly, kind and competent; it has long been argued by some that this is more important to women than continuity of care with a known midwife in labour (Green et al., 1998). Such an opinion can still be heard where there is resistance to the evidence promoting **midwifery continuity of care** models that include intrapartum care. In recent years, in some parts of Australia there is an increase in the development of models where midwives provide antenatal and postnatal midwifery continuity but do not attend the labours of the women in their caseload.

These challenges raise complex questions about how to evaluate women's experiences of birth in terms of their 'satisfaction' and how midwifery and the promotion of physiological birth might be implicated. It can be argued that women have a vested interest in evaluating their experience positively in the postnatal period and that, in many situations, it is impossible for women to know how their experience might have been otherwise (Sawyer et al., 2013; Wiegers, 2009). For example, research in South Australia has shown that women like Sophie (remember scenario one) choose private obstetric care because they have no knowledge of midwifery. However, once such women are exposed to midwife-led care, they identify that they would choose it in subsequent pregnancies (Zadoroznyj, 2000).

The anxiety of pregnant women who do not know which midwife will be there in labour for them, and whether this anxiety might make a difference to outcomes, has not been well captured by researchers on the whole. Confusion about the term 'midwifery continuity of care' and what it actually means in practice has added to the difficulty of making comparisons in research studies, particularly in exploring how women feel about their care (McLachlan et al., 2019). Furthermore, the notion of randomising women in studies does not lend itself to enquiry into choices, processes and relationships. A Cochrane review, however, has identified that midwifery-led care has the potential to make a significant difference to the promotion of physiological birth when comparisons are made with standard care from physicians and midwives, as identified in Box 19.1 (Sandall et al., 2016).

Increasingly there are efforts in Australia to change maternity care so that more women experience midwifery continuity of care. Had Michelle lived in New Zealand, however, she would have had considerably more chance of finding and getting to know a midwife who would be present during her labour. For over two decades, women in New Zealand have been able to access continuity of care from a lead maternity care provider as part of publicly funded maternity services; the majority continue to choose midwives for this role (Ministry of Health (MOH), 2021).

This is an important consideration because midwives can play a crucial role in promoting psychosocial wellbeing. This was first identified by Anne Oakley and colleagues (Oakley et al., 1990, 1996) in a randomised controlled trial (RCT) that studied the effect of midwives making themselves available, in a 'listening ear' capacity, throughout pregnancy to women who had previously given birth to low-birth-weight babies. The intervention had profound long-term consequences for the relationships and social lives of women, their children and their families. Midwives adopting a primary healthcare role as a public health strategy has been identified as an important consideration in planning the future of maternity services, particularly for women who do not sail through pregnancy on the wings of prosperity and good health: 'every women needs a midwife and some women need a doctor too' (Homer et al., 2019b; Sandall, 2012, p. 323).

Promoting physiology: midwifery caseload practice

In New Zealand, midwives who provide care in a caseload model transcend the divide between 'normal and abnormal' through a woman-centred approach; midwives follow women through their experience of pregnancy, labour and the early postnatal period, liaising with medical and other practitioners as and when this is deemed appropriate (Davis & Walker, 2011). A similar system of care provided in an Australian maternity service has been shown in an RCT to be safe and cost effective (Tracy et al., 2013). Another RCT in Australia identified that care provided in **midwifery caseload practice** models can reduce caesarean section rates for women deemed at low risk (McLachlan et al., 2012) and increase their satisfaction with antenatal, intrapartum and postnatal care (Forster et al., 2016). Non-randomised studies of midwifery caseload practice in Australia suggest that there are improved outcomes for women where they are able to establish relationships with midwives during pregnancy (Cornwell et al., 2008; Fereday et al., 2009; Turnbull et al., 2009).

The Albany Midwifery Group Practice in the United Kingdom has been held up as an example of a community-based midwifery group practice that operated a caseload practice model and made a difference to outcomes in a socially disadvantaged community (Homer et al., 2017; Huber & Sandall, 2006, 2008; Reed, 2002a, 2002b). An analysis of the practice outcomes of this community-based midwifery group practice identified that the midwives were very successful at facilitating normality in pregnancy and birth (Homer et al., 2017). Of the 2568 women included over the 12.5-year period, more than half were from Black, Asian and Minority Ethnic (BAME) communities. Almost all the women (95.5%) were cared for in labour by either their primary or secondary midwife and there were high rates of spontaneous vaginal birth (79.8%) and home birth (43.5%).

Promoting physiology: antenatal groups

In Midwifery Practice Scenario Two, Michelle and Daniel attend an antenatal group where information is shared in a non-didactic way. The evidence and rationale for this approach (Schrader McMillan et al., 2009) is outlined in a useful online resource pack for midwives and others setting up or facilitating antenatal groups (Department of Health UK, 2011)—see Online resources at the end of this chapter.

Antenatal groups offer a powerful tool for exploring the rationale and strategies for keeping birth normal

---

> **Box 19.1 Midwife-led continuity models versus other models of care for childbearing women**
>
> Women who had midwife-led continuity models of care were less likely to experience:
>
> - regional analgesia
> - instrumental vaginal birth
> - pre-term birth less than 37 weeks
> - fetal loss before and after 24 weeks plus neonatal death
> - amniotomy and episiotomy.
>
> Women who had midwife-led care were more likely to experience:
>
> - no intrapartum analgesia/anaesthesia
> - a longer mean length of labour
> - being attended by a known midwife in labour
> - higher rates of satisfaction.
>
> (Source: Sandall J et al., 2016)

413

(Leap, 2010; Leap et al., 2010a; Reed, 2002a, 2002b). A model of antenatal education and support in which women set the agenda (as opposed to being taught what the midwife has decided they should know about) can have far-reaching consequences for both women and midwives. Such groups are best situated in the community, but have also been run successfully in hospital antenatal clinics as an alternative to classes, and on antenatal and postnatal wards for women who are hospitalised (Leap, 2010).

Groups can also provide an ideal setting in which to provide antenatal care. The CenteringPregnancy® model was developed by midwife Sharon Schindler Rising in the USA (Schindler Rising, 1998). Combining antenatal care, education and support has been shown in RCTs to reduce social isolation and improve outcomes, particularly in disadvantaged groups (Ickovics et al., 2003, 2007, 2011, 2016; Powell Kennedy et al., 2009). CenteringPregnancy® is now provided in over 580 sites in North America and has been piloted in many other high and low income countries, including Australia (Teate et al., 2011), the Netherlands (Rijnders et al 2019) and the UK (Gaudion et al., 2011). Group antenatal care is recommended by the World Health Organization (2018) and you can access a plethora of videos on YouTube identifying examples of how it has been implemented.

In our reconstructed story, Michelle will also be able to attend a postnatal group that is run by child health nurses in the same community centre. She will carry on meeting the women she has met in the antenatal group there because she is very motivated to continue these friendships. This will provide her with a continuity of friendship and support.

Building confidence and support throughout pregnancy

We can return to the reconstruction of Michelle and Daniel's story and in Midwifery Practice Scenario Three we shall see how, at every stage of their interactions with Michelle and Daniel, their midwives engage in conversations that are likely to promote confidence. There are many good online resources that midwives can use as a guide when engaging in such discussions (see Online resources at the end of this chapter for some ideas).

 ## Midwifery Practice Scenario Three

Building confidence and support during pregnancy
Michelle has established a group of friends through attending the antenatal groups. She has heard many stories of women's births and looks forward to the day when it will be her turn to come to the group and tell her story. Daniel has met some new fathers too and heard some of their experiences of being at the labour, so he is feeling less anxious.

Michelle and Daniel were introduced to all the midwives in the group practice when they went to the community centre for their antenatal care. Sarah has been assigned to them as their second midwife and they have met her at the practice for alternate antenatal check-ups. As Fiona is their primary midwife, she is most likely to be there when their baby is born, but if she is having days off when Michelle goes into labour, Michelle and Daniel will be very happy to have Sarah be with them as they have come to know her too. Fiona has taken responsibility for keeping the overview of their pregnancy; she made sure that all Michelle's tests were completed and explained the results to her.

At 36 weeks, Fiona and Sarah go to Michelle and Daniel's home to talk about support in labour and in the early days following birth. At Fiona's instigation, all the relatives and friends who will be supporting Michelle come to that meeting. Fiona and Sarah talk about practical support in the first weeks following birth. They suggest rosters for bringing in food, taking away washing, shopping and walking the dog.

Fiona and Sarah also talk to the gathered people about how best to support Michelle in labour. They show photos of births and talk about pain. They explain that the midwives will not be rushing to try to take away Michelle's pain, that pain is purposeful, and that it would not be helpful to keep asking her if she wants something to take away the pain. They give Michelle's supporters ideas about how they can minimise disturbance to help Michelle withdraw into her body so that her own opiates and oxytocin can come into play. They talk about noise, moving around, transition and early breastfeeding—in effect, they explain why it is important to promote physiology and give plenty of suggestions about how best to facilitate this. Fiona and Sarah know that if they do not engage in these discussions then Michelle's labour supporters are likely to expect them to offer pain relief during Michelle's labour, and in their distress pester the midwives to 'do something' about the pain. They tell Daniel and the supporters that if at any stage they are worried they should look at their midwife: if she is looking calm, they can feel reassured that all is well. They will let them know if there are any concerns.

Fiona and Sarah also explain about 'prelabour' or early labour and the importance of not going into hospital too soon. They talk through what to do if the baby comes in a hurry before the midwife arrives, and make sure they know where this is written in Michelle's notes.

Fiona and Sarah tell the support people that, if Michelle's labour is going well, the midwives will offer her the opportunity to stay at home to have her baby, as they always carry all the equipment with them needed for a safe birth. They explain that if Michelle needs 'help' they can go to hospital, but otherwise the best place to enable physiology to flourish is in a woman's own home.

The midwives also explain that the majority of white women having first babies do not go into labour until they are at least a week to 10 days after the 'due date'. They talk about the possibility of 'prelabour' contractions and the importance of Michelle eating, drinking and getting lots of sleep while labour gets established. This advice includes when to call the midwives, with clear messages to avoid the hours between midnight and 7 a.m. unless they are worried or the contractions are coming every 2 to 3 minutes, lasting about a minute and Michelle can't talk through them.

Michelle is keen to use water in labour. She has heard stories in the group of how helpful women have found being in a deep tub. Fiona explains to everyone that if Michelle's labour is progressing well and she wants to stay in the tub to give birth, this is a safe option. The midwives offer to lend Michelle and Daniel one of the inflatable tubs that are available through their group practice.

By the end of this visit, everyone is clear about their possible roles in supporting Michelle. The photographs of a labour sequence have helped to promote discussion about the sorts of things to expect, and everyone is excited about approaching labour with an open mind. The midwives have imparted an important message that they trust in Michelle's ability to give birth to her baby and to cope well with whatever events unfold.

REFLECTING ON MIDWIFERY PRACTICE SCENARIO THREE

Promoting physiology: the 36-week home visit or 'birth talk'

The **36-week home visit** described in Midwifery Practice Scenario Three was studied by Joy Kemp (2003), who described the initiative as:

> . . . an alternative model of authoritative knowledge, one which acknowledged a role for intervention and technology but placed as central a philosophy of birth as a physiological, transformational and socio-cultural event.
>
> (Kemp, 2003, p. 4)

In her research, Kemp (2003) identified a range of productive activities involved in carrying out a 36-week home visit to make plans for labour and the early postnatal period, all of which have implications for promoting physiology:

- involving family members in support in labour and in the early days following birth, with practical suggestions for how this might take place
- discussions about approaches to being with women in **pain in labour** without rushing to take away pain and to ensure that physiology is promoted
- the use of photographs to encourage discussion about normal birth
- information to reduce premature admission to hospital and choice about place of birth in labour.

Kemp's (2003) study portrayed the 36-week birth talk as an integral part of the ongoing dialogue and relationship of mutual trust that occurs between a woman and her midwife throughout pregnancy, where the same midwife or midwives are going to be with the woman during labour (Kemp & Sandall, 2010). The concept is thus directly related to continuity of care that includes an intrapartum component. It is also one element of a midwifery model that aims to focus on birth as a social, rather than a medical, event (Kitzinger, 2006).

REFLECTIVE THINKING EXERCISE

Describe some of the activities and conversations involved in carrying out a 36-week home visit to make plans for labour and the early postnatal period, all of which have implications for promoting physiology.

Promoting and supporting physiology during labour

We return to Michelle's story when she is 41 weeks pregnant and will consider how Michelle's midwives continue to adopt an evidence-based approach to supporting Michelle in making decisions that promote physiological birth. A useful guide when considering this is a booklet developed by Canberra Hospital and Health Services (Division of Women, Youth and Children, ACT Health, 2014). This resource aims to provide maternity care givers with ready access to the best available evidence on clinical issues related to promoting physiological labour and birth. The 10 recommendations are reproduced in Box 19.2.

We shall now see how the evidence-based approaches to promoting physiological birth in Box 19.2 are reflected in the care Michelle receives in the reconstructed story of the birth of Jack in Midwifery Practice Scenario Four.

415

Box 19.2 Promotion, support and facilitation of normal birth: 10 evidence-based recommendations for midwives and medical officers

1. Women should be supported and encouraged to remain at home during the latent stage of labour until labour establishes.

2. Women should receive continuous physical and emotional support throughout labour, ideally from someone known to her and where possible from another woman.

3. Women should be supported and encouraged to remain mobile and adopt upright positions during the first stage of labour as well as rest as she desires.

4. Women should be encouraged to maintain oral fluid intake and eat a light, easily digested diet as desired during labour.

5. Women should be provided with access to warm water immersion during labour.

6. During second stage of labour women should be encouraged to adopt upright positions which she finds comfortable.

7. Women should be encouraged with physiological pushing rather than directed pushing in the second stage of labour.

8. Women should be offered a warm perineal compress during the second stage of labour and caregivers should adopt a 'hands poised' approach.

9. The benefits of active management of the third stage of labour compared with expectant management for low-risk women must be weighed against the benefits of delayed cord clamping.

10. All women should be informed of the benefits of breastfeeding, and breastfeeding should be initiated within the first hour after birth. Skin-to-skin contact between the mother and baby should be facilitated.

(Source: Division of Women, Youth & Children, ACT Health. Promotion, Support and Facilitation of Normal Birth, 10 Clinical Recommendations for Midwives and Medical Officers. Canberra: ACT Government; 2014)

 Midwifery Practice Scenario Four

Michelle gives birth to Jack

On a Sunday evening, a week past her due date, Michelle starts having some low, period-type pains. She thinks her waters may have broken. She phones Fiona and describes what has happened and tells her that the baby is wriggling around as usual. Fiona is very excited for Michelle and Daniel, and offers to call in and see them. She visits, carries out a reassuring check and confirms that Michelle is draining clear liquor. Fiona explains the evidence from studies comparing a waiting approach with accelerating labour, and together they make a plan to wait and see how events unfold. Michelle will keep in touch by telephone if she has any concerns, if her temperature rises or if labour gets underway. Otherwise Fiona will visit again the next day.

Michelle manages to get some sleep overnight, although by 6.30 in the morning the contractions are beginning to get stronger and closer together. She lets Daniel sleep, makes herself some breakfast and potters around the house. By the time Fiona visits again at midday, Michelle's contractions are coming every 3 minutes and are lasting about a minute. Michelle's mum Jenny is helping Daniel to rub Michelle's back during contractions and is making sure that she is sipping plenty of water. Michelle's friend Linda, who has had two babies and was also present at the 36-week home visit, is making sure that everyone has enough to eat and drink. After

performing some routine checks to ensure that Michelle and her baby are responding well to labour, Fiona watches quietly; she can tell that Michelle is in strong labour. She tells Michelle this and suggests that this would be a good time to think about going into hospital if this is still what she wants to do. She has with her all the equipment needed if Michelle decides she would like to give birth at home after all. Michelle is clear that she does want to have the baby in hospital, so they make plans for the journey.

Fiona goes ahead to the hospital and arranges to meet Michelle, Daniel, Jenny and Linda there in the next hour or so. She prepares a room in the birthing suite to make it as cosy as possible, takes the mattresses off the bed and places them in the corner, making a little nest of cushions and beanbags. She pushes the bed up against the wall; it is no longer the centre of attention in the room. The lights are dimmed, there is some ambient music playing very softly and the room smells of lavender (Fiona has previously checked that Michelle likes this smell). There is plenty of comfy seating around the edge of the room for Michelle, her supporters and midwives to rest on as labour unfolds. Fiona is wearing her own clothes—some loose track-pants and a T-shirt.

After Michelle settles in at St Average, her labour progresses well and she roams around the room, gets in and out of the deep bath and makes loud moaning noises. Fiona keeps a watchful eye, using an unobtrusive Doppler to monitor the baby's heartbeat. She offers Michelle a birthing ball, and heated wheat packs for comfort. As

Michelle's contractions get stronger and closer, she becomes withdrawn. Fiona quietly reassures her that she's doing well after each contraction and when Michelle pleads that she 'can't do it', Fiona keeps saying that she *can* do it, that this is normal and that she is doing really well.

Michelle starts to feel an urge to bear down and Fiona applies warm compresses to Michelle's perineum and encourages her to keep doing whatever her body is telling her to do. Michelle's contractions are strong and expulsive. Soon the baby's head can be seen. Fiona talks Michelle through breathing her baby's head out slowly—Michelle remembers the discussions they had about 'sighing the baby out' to slow down the birth of her baby and optimise the chance of her perineum stretching well.

When Michelle is giving birth, with her permission, Fiona invites Alexandria, the new resident, into the room to sit in the corner and watch as Michelle gives birth to Jack on all fours. Daniel puts his hands next to Fiona's as Jack emerges and helps to pass him through and place him in front of Michelle so that she can pick him up and take him to her when she is ready. Michelle confirms for everyone that her baby is a boy. She takes him to her and talks to him, exclaiming as she explores his little body, finding family likeness in features—'Look, he's got your ears, Daniel!' She is amazed at the cord, which is still pulsating.

Fiona gently reminds Michelle that soon she will feel a slight fullness in her vagina as the placenta separates. She reassures Michelle that pushing out the placenta will be easy, as it is soft, and that as soon as the placenta is out, they will cut the cord. Within a few minutes Michelle has delivered her placenta and, with Fiona's help, she cuts the cord herself, as Daniel is not keen to do this.

Jack is lying skin-to skin on Michelle's abdomen. After a while, he works his way up Michelle's torso in order to find her breast and have a first suckle. He is very alert and latches on enthusiastically. Everyone marvels at the placenta and membranes, as Fiona shows them its various wonders. There is much celebration all round.

REFLECTING ON MIDWIFERY PRACTICE SCENARIO FOUR

Promoting physiology: working with pain in labour

Michelle's midwives have made a conscious effort to address the crucial role that working with pain plays in keeping birth normal. It has been suggested that there is a need to change the culture in institutions around pain in labour through shifting the approach away from one of 'pain relief' to one of 'working with pain in labour' (Leap & Anderson, 2008; Leap et al., 2010b; Whitburn et al., 2014, 2017, 2019). A full exploration of this approach can be found in Chapters 25 and 26.

Over many years, qualitative research has highlighted the fact that the attitudes of midwives have a profound effect on women's experience of giving birth, in particular how they cope with pain in labour (Hodnett, 2002; Karlsdottir et al., 2014; Lundgren & Dahlberg, 1998). This influence can promote birth when the labouring woman and midwife have not met before, but where a trusting relationship has developed through midwifery continuity of care it is easier to promote women's confidence in their abilities (Leap et al., 2010a).

Promoting physiology: continuous support in labour

In Midwifery Practice Scenario Four, we see how Michelle's midwives provided her with continuous support in labour. The importance of this cannot be underestimated. A Cochrane systematic review of continuous support in labour concluded that women who receive continuous support have shorter labours and are more likely to have a spontaneous vaginal birth and report satisfaction with their experience of birth; they are less likely to use analgesia and epidurals, have a caesarean or instrumental birth or have a baby with a low Apgar score at 5 minutes (Bohren et al., 2017).

A literature review exploring women's views about what contributes to a positive birth experience and what behaviours women value most highly from the professional caring for them in labour identified that continuous support in labour is important to women (Ross-Davie & Cheyne, 2014a). Not only does high-quality support play a key role in promoting normal birth and reducing medical interventions, but it also improves women's perceptions of their birth experiences. This promotes a positive adaptation to motherhood, potentially reducing the risk of post-traumatic stress disorder and other perinatal mental health problems (Ross-Davie & Cheyne, 2014a).

It has been suggested that the culture and environment of hospital maternity units may inhibit the quality of support that hospital staff are able to provide; divided loyalties, additional duties besides labour support and the constraints of institutional policies and routine practices may play a role in continuous support in labour being the exception rather than routine practice (Bohren et al., 2017). Reality television shows reinforce anecdotal accounts of midwives being at the desk, leaving a woman's partner to provide her with continuous support. The importance of midwives being in the room in order to provide continuous support for women and their birth supporters was highlighted in an observational study in Scotland (Ross-Davie et al., 2014b). Midwives being out of the room was associated with:

- heightened anxiety, particularly if the midwife did not explain where she was going, why she was leaving or how long she would be away
- the pain of contractions being more difficult and women having tense interactions with their partner about what was happening
- a reduction in opportunities to build rapport leading to less supportive care when the midwife *was* in the room
- a reduction in the midwife's ability to monitor the progress of the woman's labour accurately.

Encouragement and the promotion of neurohormonal physiology

Undoubtedly, words of encouragement and reassurance during labour play a vital role in giving women confidence in their ability to cope with pain and this, in turn, increases women's ability to avoid the side effects of pharmacological analgesia and their disturbing effect on physiological processes. The role of the midwife in giving quiet encouragement—'midwifery muttering' (Leap, 2010)—is one of watchfulness and anticipation and her presence is important in reassurance for the woman and her supporters (Powell Kennedy et al., 2010).

This approach recognises the need for women to have privacy in order to avoid disturbance of the complex neurohormonal cascades of labour. Michel Odent (1992) first suggested that it is important to enable women to find a private, quiet, dark, comfortable space in which to labour and give birth. He explained this in terms of promoting labour-enhancing hormones that can be inhibited when there is stimulation to the busy thinking part of the brain, the neocortex, or when fear and anxiety lead to excessive catecholamine production. This makes sense to midwives, who often see women 'disappear into their bodies' and enter a state of altered consciousness as labour intensifies.

It may also be that the reassurance of midwives and reduction in anxiety contributes to the building of women's confidence and the biobehavioural state of 'calm and connection' associated with neurohormonal physiology, increased oxytocin, wellbeing and uncomplicated birth (Foureur, 2008; Hammond et al., 2013, 2014). Sarah Buckley (2015) provides a comprehensive overview of the hormonal science of labour and birth, identifying the far-reaching implications for lactation, attachment and parenting (see Online resources).

The role of midwives in facilitating situations and environments where neurohormonal processes can prevail has been explored by various authors in *Birth Territory and Midwifery Guardianship: theory for practice, education and research* (Fahy et al., 2008). A wide range of measures that promote physiology during labour are also outlined in *The Labor Progress Handbook: early*

Box 19.3 Promoting physiology in labour

Measures that can promote physiology during labour include:

- encouraging an atmosphere of privacy, calm and safety and the guaranteed presence of the midwife/birth supporters
- offering comfort devices such as heat/ice packs, warm blankets, birth ball, beanbag, bath, shower, tea, music, massage, wiping the woman's face and neck with a cool cloth
- encouraging immersion in water during labour and for birth in a deep tub that allows movement and different positions, including all fours
- the continued presence of a female companion, partner or 'doula', who is committed to promoting normal birth
- encouraging the woman to move around, adopt different positions, rest, make noises and eat and drink as she sees fit
- avoiding continuous electronic fetal monitoring (EFM) in uncomplicated labour and using intermittent auscultation instead
- where continuous EFM is necessary, still encouraging different positions, swaying
- staying at home as long as possible when hospital birth is planned
- understanding the anatomy, physiology and psychology of labour, and the techniques that can enhance these.

(Source: Based on Simkin P & Anchetta R, 2011)

---

interventions to prevent and treat dystocia (Simkin & Ancheta, 2011). Some of these strategies are outlined in Box 19.3.

CRITICAL THINKING EXERCISE

Using Boxes 19.2 and 19.3 as a guide, how many of the measures listed there are in place in your place of work? For those that are not in place, what evidence would you invoke in order to convince others of the importance of introducing them?

All the strategies to promote physiological birth that have been addressed so far in this chapter will flourish in an environment where there is collegiality and good support for practitioners. In reconstructing the story of the birth of Jack Taylor, there is an opportunity to fantasise about an ideal culture that supports practitioners in promoting physiological birth, as outlined in Midwifery Practice Scenario Five.

Midwifery Practice Scenario Five

Promoting physiological birth in an ideal culture . . .
Fiona knows that if she is worried or tired she can ask for help—this may be from another midwife in her practice. It may also be from one of the core midwives who staff the birthing service and support the midwives in the group practices when they bring women to St Average. If Fiona is concerned about Michelle's labour she will discuss the situation with one of the doctors, either in person or by phone. Such a supportive culture has been engendered at St Average by a concerted interdisciplinary approach in the last few years. There is also a 'zero-tolerance' approach to dominating behaviour and horizontal violence.

Every day at 2 p.m. at St Average, there is some form of interdisciplinary get-together or 'in-service' in the meeting room around the corner. This is organised by the Midwifery Consultant, is open to all staff, including midwives in community-based practices, and may involve any of the following activities:

- a monthly perinatal mortality meeting where midwives as well as doctors present cases for review; this includes reviewing admissions to the neonatal unit

- interesting case reviews, led by midwives, doctors or students on a rotational basis

- the reviewing of consensus guidelines for practice development—these have replaced protocols; they are evidence based and incorporate woman-centred approaches to practice

- student project presentations—students are encouraged to present their projects to all staff

- topic-based reviews of putting evidence into practice; these are guided discussion sessions or lively debates, and recent topics included:

- an interdisciplinary approach to reducing the rate of caesarean sections at St Average by encouraging women to entertain vaginal birth after caesarean section (VBAC) and external cephalic version (ECV), selective use of continuous EFM and informing all staff of the evidence about all of these

- changing the culture of 'pain relief' to one of 'being with women in pain in labour'

- regular practice sessions using the mannequins for emergency drills—staff are encouraged to attend the ALSO (Advanced Life Support in Obstetrics) course—or a similar obstetric emergency course—and continue to practise the 'hands on' simulations and mnemonics.

REFLECTING ON MIDWIFERY PRACTICE SCENARIO FIVE

Promoting a culture that cherishes physiology

In Midwifery Practice Scenario Five, we see an ideal supportive culture for the promotion of physiological birth. This involves breaking down hierarchical barriers, enabling safe situations for all practitioners to share their uncertainty as well as their expertise, and recognising different expertise and complementary roles. Such an approach also depends on the most powerful groups—doctors—relinquishing some of their power. Power cannot be given; it can only be taken, and this process involves mutual sensitivity to the dynamics and potential pitfalls surrounding collaboration on the part of all parties.

In units where interdisciplinary efforts are activated to reduce caesarean sections, success may well depend on raising consciousness and awareness of issues and philosophical approaches, plus a concerted effort from all disciplines. It seems that pulling together, a commitment to evidence-based practice, one-to-one support from midwives during labour, managing change and fostering goodwill are important strategies in reducing interference in labour and improving outcomes for women (Leap & Hunter 2022).

Changing the wider culture, both within and outside of institutions, to one that privileges normal birth is a daunting task in an era when caesarean and epidural rates are rising and these methods of childbirth are increasingly being identified in the media as the obvious choice for women in order for them to make full use of the benefits of modern technology. Promoting normal birth in the media is obviously important, but a more fundamental approach may be necessary. The promotion of normal birth may have to start in primary schools through visits by pregnant and breastfeeding women and midwives, in order to plant the seeds of thought that will grow into an adult ability to conceptualise birth as a social event with profound meaning for all involved.

Conclusion

This chapter has explored how promoting physiology involves far more than a series of techniques used in labour. It involves the raising of consciousness at every level in our institutions, healthcare services and governments in order to build systems and services that nurture the potential of birth to transform lives and strengthen women, their families and societies.

Review questions

1. In the context of your own practice, how can you enhance a culture that promotes physiological birth?

2. Imagine that you have been asked to visit a primary school to talk about 'having a baby'. What will you say?

3. You have been asked to prepare a 20-minute talk for the interdisciplinary lunchtime meeting. The topic is 'promoting physiological birth'. How will you defend your argument when the anaesthetists suggest that all women should be offered an epidural during labour?

4. Name some of the underlying power dynamics in your workplace that possibly subvert the efforts of midwives to promote physiological birth.

5. How have the dynamics you described in Question 4 evolved over recent centuries? (1000 words)

6. Describe what you understand by the terms 'technocratic' and 'medicalised' in terms of promoting physiological birth.

7. You have been asked to prepare a talk on home birth for the local Country Women's Association. What are the questions you might expect from a group of women who gave birth in the 1960s and 1970s?

Online resources

Buckley SJ. Hormonal Physiology of Childbearing: evidence and implications for women, babies, and maternity care. 2015. Online: https://www.nationalpartnership.org/our-work/resources/health-care/maternity/hormonal-physiology-of-childbearing.pdf.

Department of Health (Producer). Preparation for Birth and Beyond: a resource pack for leaders of community groups and activities. 2011. Online: https://www.gov.uk/government/uploads/system/uploads/attachment_data/file/215386/dh_134728.pdf.

Simkin P. Comfort in Labour: how you can help yourself to a normal satisfying childbirth. 2015. Online: https://www.nationalpartnership.org/our-work/resources/health-care/maternity/comfort-in-labor-simkin.pdf

References

Birthplace in England Collaborative Group. Perinatal and maternal outcomes by planned place of birth for healthy women with low risk pregnancies: the Birthplace in England national prospective cohort study. *BMJ Open Access.* 2011;343: doi:10.1136/bmj.d7400.

Bohren MA, Hofmeyr GJ, Sakala C, et al. Continuous support for women during childbirth. *Cochrane Database Syst Rev.* 2017;(7):CD003766. doi:10.1002/14651858.CD003766.pub6.

Carolan-Olah M, Kruger G, Garvey-Graham A. Midwives' experiences of the factors that facilitate normal birth among low risk women at a public hospital in Australia. *Midwifery.* 2015;31:112–121.

Catling-Paul C, Coddington R, Foureur M, et al. Publicly funded homebirth in Australia: a review of maternal and neonatal outcomes over 6 years. *Med J Aust.* 2013;198:616–620.

Cornwell C, Donnellan-Fernandez R, Nixon A. Planning and implementing mainstream midwifery group practices in a tertiary setting. In: Homer C, Brodie P, Leap N, eds. *Midwifery Continuity of Care: A Practical Guide.* Sydney: Elsevier; 2008: 107–126.

Darra S. 'Normal', 'natural', 'good' or 'good-enough' birth: examining the concepts. *Nurs Inquiry.* 2009;16(4):297–305.

Davis D. The decline in normal birth: our maternity system's failure to progress. *Aust Midwifery News.* 2013;12(3):9–10.

Davis D, Baddock S, Pairman S, et al. Planned place of birth in New Zealand: does it affect mode of birth and intervention rates among low-risk women? *Birth.* 2011;38(2):111–119.

Davis D, Walker K. Case-loading midwifery in New Zealand: bridging the normal/abnormal divide 'with woman'. *Midwifery.* 2011;27(1):46–52.

Davis-Floyd R. The technocratic, humanistic and holistic paradigms of childbirth. *Int J Gynecol Obstet.* 2001;75:S5–S23.

de Graaff LF, Honig A, van Pampus MG, et al. Preventing post-traumatic stress disorder following child-birth and traumatic birth experiences: a systematic review. *Acta Obstet Gynecol Scand.* 2018;97(6). doi:10.1111/aogs.13291.

de Jonge A, Geerts CC, van der Goes BY, et al. Perinatal mortality and morbidity up to 28 days after birth among 743 070 low-risk planned home and hospital births: a cohort study based on three merged national perinatal databases. *BJOG.* 2015;122(5):720–728.

Delbaere I, Cammu H, Martens E, et al. Limiting the caesarean section rate in low risk pregnancies is key to lowering the trend of increased abdominal deliveries: an observational study. *BMC Pregnancy Childbirth.* 2012;12:3. Online: http://www.biomedcentral.com/1471-2393/12/3.

Division of Women, Youth and Children, ACT Health. *Promotion, Support and Facilitation of Normal Birth, 10 Clinical Recommendations for Midwives and Medical Officers.* Canberra: ACT Government; 2014.

Dixon L, Prileszky G, Guilliland K, et al. Place of birth and outcomes for a cohort of low risk women in New Zealand: A comparison with Birthplace England. *NZCOM.* 2014;50:11–18. doi:10.12784/nzcomjnl50.2014.2.11-18.

Donnison J. *Midwives and Medical Men*. London: Heinemann; 1977.

Downe S, Finlayson K, Olodapo OT, et al., What matters to women during childbirth: A systematic review. *PLoS ONE*. 2018;13(4): e0194906.

Downe S, McCourt C. From being to becoming: reconstructing childbirth knowledge. In: Downe S, Byrom S, eds. *Squaring the Circle. Normal birth research, theory and practice in a technological age*. London: Pinter and Martin; 2019:69–100.

Fahy K, Foureur M, Hastie C. *Birth Territory and Midwifery Guardianship: Theory for Practice, Education and Research*. Edinburgh: Heinemann/Elsevier; 2008.

Fereday J, Collins C, Turnbull D, et al. An evaluation of Midwifery Group Practice. Part II: women's satisfaction. *Women Birth*. 2009;22(1):11–16.

Forster DA, McLachlan HL, Davey M-A, et al. Continuity of care by a primary midwife (caseload midwifery) increases women's satisfaction with antenatal, intrapartum and postpartum care: results from the COSMOS randomised controlled trial. *BMC Pregnancy Childbirth*. 2016;16:28. doi:10.1186/s12884-016-0798-y.

Foureur M. Creating birth space to enable undisturbed birth. In: Fahy K, Foureur M, Hastie C, eds. *Birth Territory and Midwifery Guardianship: Theory for Practice, Education and Research*. Edinburgh: Heinemann/Elsevier; 2008:57–78.

Gaudion A, Menka Y, Demilew J, et al. Findings from a UK feasibility study of the CenteringPregnancy® model. *Br J Midwifery*. 2011;19(12):796–802.

Green JM, Curtis P, Price H, et al. *Continuing to Care. The Organisation of Midwifery Services in the UK: A Structured Review of the Evidence*. Hale: Books for Midwives; 1998.

International Confederation of Midwives (ICM). *International Definition of a Midwife*. Revised and adopted at Toronto Council Meeting 2017. Online: https://www.internationalmidwives.org/assets/files/definitions-files/2018/06/eng-definition_of_the_midwife-2017.pdf

Gould D. Normal labour: a concept analysis. *J Adv Nurs*. 2000; 31(2):418–427.

Hammond A, Foureur M, Homer CSE, et al. Space, place and the midwife: exploring the relationship between the birth environment, neurobiology and midwifery practice. *Women Birth*. 2013;26:277–281.

Hammond A, Foureur M, Homer CSE. The hardware and software implications of hospital birth room design: a midwifery perspective. *Midwifery*. 2014;30:825–830.

Hodnett ED. Pain and women's satisfaction with the experience of childbirth: a systematic review. *Am J Obstet Gynecol*. 2002;186(5):S160–S172.

Homer CSE, Cheah S, Rossiter C, Dahlen H, Ellwood D, Foureur M, . . . Scarf V. Maternal and perinatal outcomes by planned place of birth in Australia 2000 – 2012: a linked population data study. *BMJ Open Access*. 2019;9:e029192. doi:0.1136/bmjopen-2019-029192.

Homer C, Leap, N, Brodie, P, et al. *Midwifery Continuity of Care*. 2nd ed. Sydney: Elsevier Australia; 2019a.

Homer C, Leap, N, Brodie, P, et al. Prologue: Why midwifery continuity of care matters for all women in all situations. In: *Midwifery Continuity of Care*. 2nd ed. Sydney: Elsevier Australia; 2019b: xxi–xxiv.

Homer CSE, Leap N, Edwards N, et al. Midwifery continuity of carer in an area of high socio-economic disadvantage in London: a retrospective analysis of Albany Midwifery Practice outcomes using routine data (1997–2009). *Midwifery*. 2017; 48:1–10.

Huber U, Sandall J. Continuity of care, trust and breastfeeding. *MIDIRS Midwifery Digest*. 2006;16(4):445–449.

Huber U, Sandall J. A qualitative exploration of the creation of calm in a continuity model of maternity care in London. *Midwifery*. 2008;25(6):613–621.

Hutton E, Reitsma A, Simioni J, et al. Perinatal or neonatal mortality among women who intend at the onset of labour to give birth at home compared to women of low obstetrical risk who intend to give birth in hospital: A systematic review and meta-analyses. *EClinicalMedicine*, 2019;14:59–70.

Ickovics JR, Kershaw TS, Westdahl C, et al. Group prenatal care and preterm birthweight: results from a two-site matched cohort study. *Obstet Gynecol*. 2003;102:1051–1057.

Ickovics J, Kershaw T, Westdahl C, et al. Group prenatal care and perinatal outcomes: a randomized controlled trial. *Obstet Gynecol*. 2007;110(2):330–339.

Ickovics JR, Reed E, Magriples U, et al. Effects of group prenatal care on psychosocial risk in pregnancy: results from a randomized controlled trial. *Psychol Health*. 2011;26(2):235–250.

Ickovics JR, Earnshaw V, Lewis JB, et al. Cluster randomized controlled trial of group prenatal care: perinatal outcomes among adolescents in New York City health centers. *Am J Public Health*. 2016;106:359–365.

Janssen PA, Saxell L, Page LA, et al. Outcomes of planned home birth with registered midwife versus hospital birth with midwife or physician. *CMAJ*. 2009;181(6–7):377–383.

Johnson KC, Davis B. Outcomes of planned home births with certified professional midwives: large prospective study in North America. *BMJ*. 2005;330(7505):1416–1422.

Karlsdottir SI, Halldorsdottir S, Lundgren I. The third paradigm in labour pain preparation and management: the childbearing woman's paradigm. *Scand J Caring Sci*. 2014;28:315–327.

Katz Rothman B. Women, providers and control. *J Obstet Gynecol Neonatal Nurs*. 1996;25(3):253–256.

Kemp J. *Midwives', Women's and Their Birth Partners' Experiences of the 36-Week Birth Talk: a Qualitative Study*. London: Florence Nightingale School of Nursing and Midwifery, King's College; 2003. (unpublished thesis).

Kemp J, Sandall J. Normal birth, magical birth: the role of the 36-week birth talk in caseload midwifery practice. *Midwifery*. 2010;26(2):211–221.

Kennedy HP. 'Orchestrating normal': the conduct of midwifery in the United States. In: Davis-Floyd R, Barclay L, Tritten J, eds. *Birth Models That Work*. Berkeley, CA: University of California Press; 2009:415–440.

Kitzinger S. *Birth Crisis*. Abingdon, Oxon: Routledge; 2006.

Kurz E, Davis D, Browne J. 'I felt like I could do anything!' Writing the phenomenon of 'transcendent birth' through autoethnography. *Midwifery*. 2019;68:23–29. doi:10.1016/j.midw.2018.10.003.

Kurz E, Davis D, Browne J. Parturescence: A theorisation of women's transformation through childbirth. *Women Birth*. 2021. doi:10.1016/j.wombi.2021.1003.1009.

Kurz E, Davis D, Browne J. The relationality of maternity care: A diffractive analysis of maternity care experiences. *Women Birth*. 2022;96–103. doi:110.1016/j.wombi.2021.1002.1004.

Leap N. Journey to midwifery through feminism: a personal account. In: Stewart M, eds. *Pregnancy, Birth and Maternity Care: Feminist Perspectives*. London: Books for Midwives; 2004:185–200.

Leap N. The less we do, the more we give. In: Kirkham M, ed. *The Midwife–Mother Relationship*. 2nd ed. Basingstoke: Palgrave Macmillan; 2010:37–54.

Leap N, Anderson T. The role of pain and the empowerment of women. In: Downe S, ed. *Normal Childbirth: Evidence and Debate*. 2nd ed. Edinburgh: Churchill Livingstone; 2008: 29–46.

Leap N, Edwards N. The politics of involving women in decision making. In: Page LA, Campbell R, eds. *The New Midwifery: Science and Sensitivity in Practice*. 2nd ed. London: Churchill Livingstone/Elsevier; 2006:97–123.

Leap N, Hunter B. *The Midwife's Tale: An Oral History From Handywoman to Professional Midwife*. 2nd ed. Barnsley, South Yorks, UK: Pen and Sword History; 2013.

Leap N, Hunter B. *Supporting Women for Labour and Birth: A Thoughtful Guide*. 2nd ed. London: Routledge; 2022.

Leap N, Sandall J, Buckland S, et al. Journey to confidence: women's experiences of pain in labour and midwifery continuity of carer. *J Midwifery Womens Health*. 2010a;55(3):234–242.

Leap N, Dodwell M, Newburn M. *Working with Pain in Labour: An Overview of Evidence. Evidence-based briefing paper*. 2010b. Online: https://www.nct.org.uk/sites/default/files/related_documents/Research%20overview-%20Working%20with%20pain%20in%20labour_6.pdf

Lundgren I, Dahlberg K. Women's experience of pain during childbirth. *Midwifery*. 1998;14(2):105–110.

Lyerly AD. Ethics and 'normal birth'. *Birth*. 2013;39(4):315–317.

McLachlan H, McCourt C, Coxon K, et al. Is midwifery care better for women and babies? What is the evidence? In: Homer C, Leap N, Brodie P et al., eds. *Midwifery Continuity of Care*. 2nd ed. Chatswood, NSW: Elsevier Australia; 2019.

Mander R, Murphy-Lawless J. *The Politics of Maternity*. Abingdon, Oxon: Routledge; 2013.

Marland H, ed. *'Mother and Child were Saved': the Memoirs (1693–1740) of the Frisian Midwife Catharina Schrader*. Amsterdam: Rodopi; 1987.

McLachlan H, Forster D, Davey M, et al. Effects of continuity of care by a primary midwife (caseload midwifery) on caesarean section rates in women of low obstetric risk: the COSMOS randomised controlled trial. *BJOG*. 2012;119(12):1483–1492.

Ministry of Health (MOH). *Maternity Care*. 2021. Online: https://www.health.govt.nz/your-health/pregnancy-and-kids/services-and-support-during-pregnancy/maternity-care

NCT/RCM/RCOG. Maternity Care Working Party. *'Making Normal Birth a Reality' Consensus Statement from the Maternity Care Working Party—our Shared Views About the Need to Recognise, Facilitate and Audit Normal Birth*. 2007. Online: http://bhpelopartonormal.pbh.gov.br/estudos_cientificos/arquivos/normal_birth_consensus.pdf.

Newnham E, McKellar L, Pincombe J. A critical literature review of epidural analgesia. *Evid Based Midwifery*. 2016;14(1):22–28.

Oakley A, Rajan L, Grant A. Social support and pregnancy outcome. *BJOG*. 1990;97:155–162.

Oakley A, Hickey D, Rajan L, et al. Social support in pregnancy: does it have long term effects? *J Reprod Infant Psychol*. 1996; 14:7–22.

Odent M. *The Nature of Birth and Breastfeeding*. Westport CT: Bergin & Garvey; 1992.

Page M, Mander R. Intrapartum uncertainty: a feature of normal birth, as experienced by midwives in Scotland. *Midwifery*. 2014;30:28–35.

Powell Kennedy H, Farrell T, Paden R, et al. I wasn't alone. A study of group prenatal care in the military. *J Midwifery Womens Health*. 2009;54(3):176–183.

Powell Kennedy H, Leap N, Anderson T. Midwifery presence: philosophy, science, and art. In: Walsh D, Downe S, eds. *Essential Midwifery Practice: Intrapartum Care*. Edinburgh: Elsevier; 2010:105–124.

Prosser SJ, Barnett AG, Miller YD. Factors promoting or inhibiting normal birth. *BMC Pregnancy Childbirth*. 2018;18:241. doi:210.1186/s12884-12018-11871-12885.

Reed B. The Albany Midwifery Practice (1). *MIDIRS Midwifery Digest*. 2002a;12(1):118–121.

Reed B. The Albany Midwifery Practice (2). *MIDIRS Midwifery Digest*. 2002b;12(3):261–264.

Reed B. Changing a birthing culture: Becky Reed explores why so many women with the Albany Midwifery Practice had home births. *AIMS J*. 2015;27(4):6–7.

Reitsma A, Simioni J, Brunton G, et al. Maternal outcomes and birth interventions among women who begin labour intending to give birth at home compared to women of low obstetrical risk who intend to give birth in hospital: A systematic review and meta-analyses. *E Clinical Medicine*, 2020;100039.

Rijnders M, Jans S, Aalhuizen I, et al. Women-centered care: Implementation of CenteringPregnancy® in The Netherlands. *Birth*. 2019;46:450–460.

Ross-Davie M, Cheyne H. Intrapartum support: what do women want? A literature review. *Evid Based Midwifery*. 2014a;12(2):52–58.

Ross-Davie MC, McElligott M, Little M, et al. Midwifery support in labour: how important is it to stay in the room? *Pract Midwife*. 2014b;17(6):19–22.

Sandall J. Every woman needs a midwife and some women need a doctor too. *Birth*. 2012;39(4):323–326.

Sandall J, Soltani H, Gates S, et al. Midwife-led continuity models versus other models of care for childbearing women. *Cochrane Database Syst Rev*. 2016;(4):CD004667. doi:10.1002/14651858. CD004667.pub5.

Sawyer A, Ayers S, Abbott J, et al. Measures of satisfaction with care during labour and birth: a comparative review. *BMC Pregnancy Childbirth*. 2013;13(1).

Schindler Rising S. Centering pregnancy: an interdisciplinary model of empowerment. *J Nurse Midwifery*. 1998;43(1):46–54.

Schrader McMillan A, Barlow J, Redshaw M. *Birth and Beyond: A Review of the Evidence About Antenatal Education*. UK: University of Warwick; 2009. Online: https://webarchive.nationalarchives. gov.uk/ukgwa/20130107105354/http://www.dh.gov.uk/prod_consum_dh/groups/dh_digitalassets/@dh/@en/documents/digitalasset/dh_110371.pdf.

Simkin P, Ancheta R. *The Labour Progress Handbook: Early Interventions to Prevent and Treat Dystocia*. 3rd ed. Chichester, West Sussex: Wiley-Blackwell; 2011.

Teate A, Leap N, Rising SS, et al. Women's experiences of group antenatal care in Australia—the Centering Pregnancy Pilot Study. *Midwifery*. 2011;27(2):138–145.

Thompson F. *Mothers and Midwives: The Ethical Journey*. Edinburgh: Books for Midwives; 2004.

Tracy SK, Dahlen H, Caplice S, et al. Birth centers in Australia: a national population-based study of perinatal mortality associated with giving birth in a birth center. *Birth*. 2007; 34(3):194–201.

Tracy SK, Hartz D, Tracy MB, et al. Caseload midwifery care versus standard maternity care for women of any risk: M@NGO, a randomised controlled trial. *Lancet*. 2013;382(9906): 1723–1732.

Turnbull D, Baghurst P, Collins C, et al. An evaluation of midwifery group practice. Part I: clinical effectiveness. *Women Birth*. 2009; 22(1):3–9.

Whitburn LY, Jones LE, Davy M-A, Small R. Women's experiences of labour pain and the role of the mind: An exploratory study. *Midwifery*. 2014;30:1029–1035.

Whitburn LY, Jones LE, Davey M-A, Small R. The meaning of labour pain: how the social environment and other contextual factors shape women's experiences. *BMC Pregnancy Childbirth*. 2017;17:157.

Whitburn LY, Jones LE, Davey M-A, et al. The nature of labour pain: An updated review of the literature. *Women Birth*. 2019; 32:28–38.

Wiegers TA. The quality of maternity care services as experienced by women in the Netherlands. *BMC Pregnancy Childbirth*. 2009;9:18.

Wilson A. *The Making of Man-Midwifery*. Cambridge, MA: Harvard University Press; 1995.

Witz A. *Professions and Patriarchy*. London: Routledge; 1992.

World Health Organization. *WHO recommendation on group antenatal care*. The WHO Reproductive Health Library: Geneva: World Health Organization; 2018.

Zadoroznyj M. Midwife-led maternity services and consumer 'choice' in an Australian metropolitan region. *Midwifery*. 2000;17:177–185.

Further reading

Downe S, ed. *Normal Childbirth: Evidence and Debate.* 2nd ed. Edinburgh: Churchill Livingstone; 2008.

Fahy K, Foureur M, Hastie C. *Birth Territory and Midwifery Guardianship: Creating Birth Space.* Oxford: Elsevier; 2008.

Leap N, Hunter B. *Supporting Women for Labour and Birth: A Thoughtful Guide.* London: Routledge; 2016.

Simkin P, Ancheta R. *The Labour Progress Handbook: Early Interventions to Prevent and Treat Dystocia.* 3rd ed. Chichester, West Sussex, UK: Wiley-Blackwell; 2011.

Index

Page numbers followed by "*f*" indicate figures, "*t*" indicate tables, and "*b*" indicate boxes.